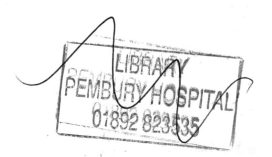

Nursing DOCUMENTATION

A NURSING PROCESS APPROACH

PATRICIA W. IYER, RN, MSN, CNA

President
Patricia Iyer Associates
Med League Support Services, Inc.
Flemington, NJ

NANCY H. CAMP, RN, MSN, C

Partner
Comprehensive Legal Nursing Consulting
Dowington, PA;
Nurse Educator
Valley Forge Military Academy and College
Wayne, PA

THIRD EDITION

with 145 illustrations

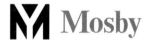

St. Louis   Baltimore   Boston   Carlsbad   Chicago   Minneapolis   New York   Philadelphia   Portland
London   Milan   Sydney   Tokyo   Toronto

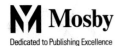

Mosby

Dedicated to Publishing Excellence

Publisher: Sally Schrefer
Editor: Lisa Potts
Developmental Editor: Aimee E. Loewe
Project Manager: Deborah L. Vogel
Production Editor: Sarah E. Fike
Manufacturing Supervisor: Debbie LaRocca
Book Designer: Bill Drone
Cover Designer: Teresa Breckwoldt

*NURSING RECORDS
" PROCESS
WY 102*

THIRD EDITION

Composition by: Graphic World Inc.
Printing/binding by: R. R. Donnelley & Sons Company

Mosby, Inc.
11830 Westline Industrial Drive
St. Louis, Missouri 63146

Library of Congress Cataloging-in-Publication Data

Iyer, Patricia W.
    Nursing documentation: a nursing process approach / Patricia W.
Iyer, Nancy H. Camp. — 3rd ed.
      p.   cm.
    Includes bibliographical references and index.
    ISBN 0-323-00223-4
    1. Nursing records.   2. Nursing records—Standards—United States.
I. Camp, Nancy Hand. II. Title.
    [DNLM: 1. Nursing Records. 2. Patient Care Planning. WY 100.5
I97n 1999]
RT50.I9 1999
610.73—dc21
DNLM/DLC
for Library of Congress   98-47696
                                 CIP

98 99 00 01 02 / 9 8 7 6 5 4 3 2 1

Contributors

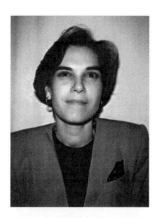

Barbara Ashley, RN, BSN, MSN, is the author of the Neonatal Documentation section of Chapter 10, Maternal-Child Documentation. She has more than 10 years of experience as a neonatal nurse clinician and has been a director of nursing for home healthcare agencies. She has worked as a legal nurse consultant for both defense and plaintiff law firms in the fields of medical malpractice, risk management, and personal injury. Ashley owns Texas Legal Nurse Consultants, Inc., in Houston, Texas. In addition to her consulting practice, she has been active in developing policies, procedures, and standards of care. She received her diploma in Nursing from St. Mary's School of Nursing, her BS in Nursing from Brigham Young University, and her MS from the University of Houston–Clear Lake. She is a member of the American Association of Legal Nurse Consultants.

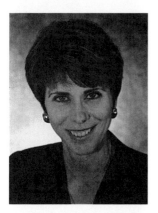

Donna Cairone, RN, BS, BSN, CNOR, RNFA, is the author of the section on Documentation in the Operating Room in Chapter 12, Perioperative Documentation. She is currently a perioperative staff nurse and Director of Infection Control/Employee Health at Mercy Community Hospital in Havertown, Pennsylvania. Her perioperative career began at the Hospital of the University of Pennsylvania. As a registered nurse first assistant (RNFA), she is the first assistant for various surgical specialists in addition to performing the traditional perioperative nurse's roles in the inpatient operating room and surgery center settings. Cairone is a graduate of Villanova University and received her BS in Nursing from the University of Pennsylvania. She is certified in operating room nursing, and she is a member of the American Association of Legal Nurse Consultants.

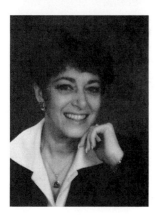

Rita Cavallaro, RN, C, LNHA, MS, is the co-author of Chapter 14, Documentation in the Long-Term Care Setting. Cavallaro's nursing career spans 32 years, and she has held various positions in medical-surgical, critical care, and long-term care nursing; education; and training. She has extensive experience in the diverse settings of long-term care management, program development, education, quality improvement, and OBRA compliance, in addition to extensive lecturing in her home state of New Jersey and across the country. She is currently a licensed nursing home administrator, interdisciplinary consultant, and Vice President of Accreditation of a long-term care consulting firm. Cavallaro serves on the Board of Directors of *The Director,* the official publication of the National Association of Directors of Nursing Administration in Long-Term Care and is a member of the faculty of the TOWNCO 100-hour Administrator's Course. She obtained her degree in Nursing from Holy Name Hospital School of Nursing, her BS from Saint Joseph's College in Windham, Maine, and her MS in Human Services: Gerontology from the College of New Rochelle in New Rochelle, New York.

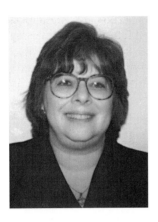

Gail Coplein, BA, JD, is the co-author of the section on Issues in Pediatric Documentation in Chapter 10, Maternal-Child Documentation. Coplein has a solo law practice in Princeton, New Jersey, which includes defense of professional liability matters and other healthcare and family law issues. She is a senior nursing student at the Helene Fuld School of Nursing, Capital Health System in Trenton, New Jersey. Coplein holds a BA from the University of Pennsylvania, where she was inducted into Phi Beta Kappa honor society, and a JD from the University of Miami Law School.

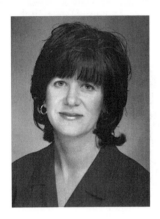

Joyce Hamlin, MSN, RNC, CS, is the co-author of the section on Issues in Pediatric Documentation in Chapter 10, Maternal-Child Documentation. She currently holds the position of Learning Resources Nurse Educator at the Helene Fuld School of Nursing, Capital Health System in Trenton, New Jersey. Hamlin, who is a certified clinical specialist in Pediatrics, has clinical experience covering all types of pediatric settings, including acute-care, community, and school health settings. She has been a faculty member at several colleges and universities in the Philadelphia area. She has co-authored several pediatric-related publications and has contributed to many nursing textbooks. Hamlin is a member of the Xi chapter of Sigma Theta Tau. She obtained a BS in Nursing from Carlow College in Pittsburgh and an MS in Nursing from the University of Pennsylvania.

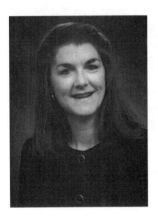

Ann Marie Santarelli-Kretovics, RN, BSN, MS, is the author of the section on Documentation in Intensive Care in Chapter 11, Critical Care Documentation. She has more than 25 years of experience in critical care nursing practice, including staff, education, and nursing administration positions. She is President of Santarelli and Associates, an independent nurse consulting practice that specializes in consultation to small businesses, including law firms. Santarelli-Kretovics earned her BS in Nursing from the Ohio State University College of Nursing and her MS in Organizational Development and Analysis from the Weatherhead School at Case Western Reserve University.

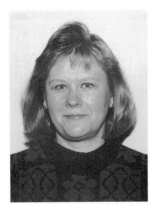

Jo Anne Kuc, RN, BSN, is the author of the section on Documentation in the Postanesthesia Care Unit of Chapter 12, Perioperative Documentation. Kuc is a published author and speaker who currently works part time in the Acute Pain Service Department at Ingalls Memorial Hospital in Harvey, Illinois. Her prior experience includes critical care and postanesthesia care unit nursing in both staff nurse and managerial capacities. She is the owner of Midwest Medical Legal Resources, Inc. Kuc received a BS in Nursing from Purdue University and is the secretary of the American Association of Legal Nurse Consultants. She is based in St. John, Indiana.

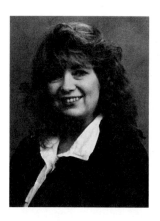

Joanne McDermott, RN, BSN, MA, is the author of the section on Obstetrical Documentation in Chapter 10, Maternal-Child Documentation. McDermott is currently clinically active in a busy labor and delivery unit in a medical center in the Kansas City area. Since 1975, McDermott has worked as a staff nurse, assistant head nurse, clinical coordinator, and assistant director of nursing in maternal-child health care. She received her MS in Nursing Education from New York University. McDermott provides consultation on maternal-child health nursing and legal issues in health care, and she performs risk management reviews of medical records. She is a member of the American Association of Legal Nurse Consultants and the Association of Women's Health, Obstetrical and Neonatal Nursing (AWHONN).

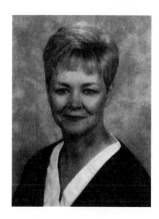

Patricia Meadows, RN, BSN, CEN, is the co-author of the section on Documentation in the Emergency Department in Chapter 11, Critical Care Documentation. She currently manages a three-campus emergency department that includes a level 1 trauma center, a national cardiac center and chest pain observation unit, and a women and children's emergency department with a pediatric observation center. She has been elected President of the West Virginia Emergency Nurses' Association. She earned her BS in Nursing from West Virginia University.

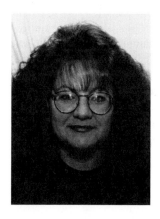

Pamela Meyer-Tulledge, RN, BSN, MA, is the co-author of the section on Psychiatric Documentation in Chapter 13, Psychiatric and Home Care Documentation. Meyer-Tulledge has more than 18 years of nursing experience with all age groups in the field of psychiatry. She has held several positions including psychiatric adult program administrator, psychiatric nurse manager, psychiatric nurse consultant, psychotherapist, and risk management and quality assurance program manager. Meyer-Tulledge is the founder and President of Meyer Medical Consultants in Tempe, Arizona. She has extensive experience in medical malpractice, psychiatric malpractice, toxic tort, product liability, wrongful death, personal injury, worker's compensation, and bad faith cases. In addition, she has reviewed cases as a psychiatric nurse expert witness. She earned her BS in Nursing from the College of St. Teresa in Winoma, Minnesota, and she obtained her MS in Human Resources from Ottawa University in Phoenix, Arizona. She is a member of the American Association of Legal Nurse Consultants.

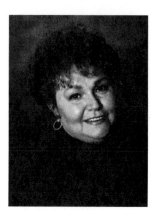

Joyce R. Newman, RN, C, CLNC, C-GN, is the co-author of Chapter 14, Long-Term Care Documentation. Since 1975, her experience has included psychiatric nursing, adult and juvenile corrections, drug and alcohol counseling, and in the past 14 years, long-term care. She is currently employed full time as the nurse manager of a 25-bed behavior management unit in a long-term care skilled nursing facility in southern New Jersey. She received her AAS and RN from Gloucester County College in New Jersey. Newman is ANA certified in gerontology and is a certified legal nurse consultant, owner of "jrn" associates, and a member of the American Association of Legal Nurse Consultants.

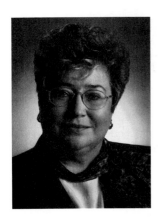

Rosie Oldham, RN, BS, is the co-author of the section on Psychiatric Documentation in Chapter 13, Psychiatric and Home Care Documentation. She has held several positions in nursing, including Director of Nursing of the Westbridge Center for Children, quality assurance coordinator, and risk management, and she also has developed criteria for physician and nursing peer review. Oldham is President of R & G Medical Consultants, Inc., and R & G Press in Peoria, Arizona. She has extensive experience providing litigation support internationally to law firms and insurance companies. Oldham is the author and publisher of the *Medical Legal Internet Directory.* Her firm provides trial exhibits, participates in settlement conferences, and assists with discovery, depositions, and trial preparation. Her firm specializes in large case volume. Oldham earned her Associates' Degree in Nursing at Glendale College in Glendale, Arizona, and her BS in Health Arts at the College of St. Francis in Joliet, Illinois. She is the Director at Large of the American Association of Legal Nurse Consultants and is a past President of the Phoenix Chapter of the American Association of Legal Nurse Consultants. She is listed in the International Who's Who of Entrepreneurs.

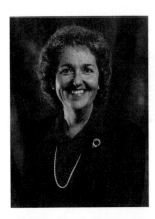

Donna Ambler Peters, RN, PhD, FAAN, is the author of the section on Home Care Documentation in Chapter 13, Psychiatric and Home Care Documentation. Peters, a nationally recognized author and public speaker, is currently the Senior Product Consultant for Delta Health Systems. Among her many accomplishments, she has served as Project Director at the National League for Nursing for a $1.2 million project funded by the Kellogg Foundation to develop outcomes for home health care. Peters has served as Program Officer for the Robert Wood Johnson Foundation and as Director of Nursing Research and Quality Assurance at the Johns Hopkins Hospital in Baltimore, Maryland. Outcomes, quality, and cost are her primary areas of expertise. Peters received her BS and Doctorate from the University of Pennsylvania and her MS from the University of Iowa. She is currently based in New Jersey.

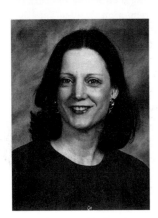

Mary Kathryn Sadler, RN, BSN, MBA, CEN, is the co-author of the section on Documentation in the Emergency Department in Chapter 11, Critical Care Documentation. She has 20 years of clinical practice and is currently working as a staff nurse in a busy level 1 trauma center emergency department. She is CEO and President of Medical-Legal Consulting in Charleston, West Virginia, and she is active in the West Virginia Emergency Nurses' Association as the newsletter editor and membership chair. Sadler earned her BS in Nursing from the University of Kentucky and her MBA from the University of South Carolina. She is a member of the American Association of Legal Nurse Consultants.

About the Authors

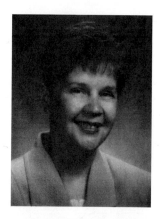

Patricia W. Iyer received her diploma from Muhlenberg Hospital School of Nursing in Plainfield, New Jersey, and her BS and MS in Nursing from the University of Pennsylvania in Philadelphia. She is President of Med League Support Services Inc., which provides legal nursing consulting services to personal injury, malpractice, and product liability attorneys. Ms. Iyer reviews nursing malpractice cases as an expert witness. She is a prolific author with numerous books published on a wide variety of nursing topics. Correspondence may be directed to the author at 260 Route 202-31, Suite 200, Liberty Court, Flemington, NJ 08822.

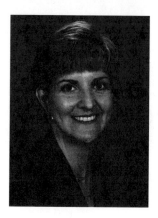

Nancy H. Camp received her diploma in Nursing from Presbyterian School of Nursing in Philadelphia and her BS from North Carolina Central University in Durham, North Carolina. She earned her MS in Nursing from Villanova University College of Nursing in Villanova, Pennsylvania, where her major area of study was nursing administration. During the past 20 years, Ms. Camp has held positions as a staff nurse, preceptor, clinical instructor, standards coordinator, and director of education. She has extensive consulting experience and has provided seminars and consultation services on a variety of topics, including nursing documentation, nursing standards development, and patient outcomes. Currently, Ms. Camp is a partner in Comprehensive Legal Nurse Consulting, which offers medical-legal services to malpractice attorneys. In addition, she maintains her clinical practice as a student health nurse and educator at Valley Forge Military Academy and College in Wayne, Pennsylvania. Ms. Camp has written another textbook on medical surgical nursing, and she contributed to *Expert Physical Examinations,* published by Mosby in 1997. Correspondence may be directed to the author at 14 Paul Nelms Drive, Dowingtown, PA 19335.

To Raj, Raj Jr, and Nathan Iyer, whose pride
in my accomplishments leads them to tell anyone who
will listen about my books.

To Dona Ramsey, a friend for 38 years, who has been
a constant source of encouragement.

To Sam Davis, Esq., whose lively interest in life, the law,
and medicine has stimulated my growth.

—Patricia Iyer

To my husband, John Camp, for his love and
encouragement, and the many father-son outings he took
so that I could write.

To my son, Matthew, for his laughter and love. Yes, Matt,
Mommy is *finally* finished!

To Donna Cairone, whose friendship is the greatest gift.

—Nancy Camp

Foreword

Documentation is one of the most important aspects of a healthcare provider's role in the healthcare arena. It serves multiple purposes in the intricate web of patients, facilities, services, providers, and payers. Documentation is evidence that the nurse's legal and ethical responsibilities to the patient were met and that the patient received quality care.

Of utmost importance, there is written proof of communication between the healthcare fields, doctors, nurses, and allied health professionals. Evidence that patient's rights are being protected is also critical with potential allegations of fraud, mistreatment, or abuse. Documentation serves as evidence that laws, rules, regulations, guidelines, statutes, policies, and procedures were followed regarding nursing practice. Such an issue can be a deciding factor in medical-legal claims, ethical dilemmas, and disciplinary actions before the State Boards of Nursing.

In today's world of healthcare economics, the focus of documentation is emphasized. Data from documentation are compiled for such activities as reimbursement, planning future health care, quality of care review, continuing education, research, and billing. Documentation is also scrutinized by major accrediting bodies such as Joint Commission on Accreditation of Healthcare Organizations (JCAHO), other federal and state regulatory bodies, and third party payers.

Documentation plays a role, and many times a pivotal point, in several areas of the law, including medical malpractice claims, personal injury suits, worker's compensation claims, Social Security hearings, custody matters, psychiatric proceedings, and criminal cases, to name a few.

Nurses practicing in today's litigious environment must remain aware and educated on the documentation process so as to avoid involvement in litigation and disciplinary proceedings. To accomplish this task, *Nursing Documentation: A Nursing Process Approach,* third edition, provides nurses with a comprehensive text filled with case examples, useful forms, and recommended formats to streamline and refine or redesign charting systems. With acuity levels of patients increasing, it only decreases the actual time nurses have to chart. Numerous mergers add to the anxiety of nurses because systems will be changed or integrated.

This book provides something for all levels of nursing—from the student to the very experienced. Its easy-to-read format and "user-friendly" style presents valuable day-to-day information that can be put into practice immediately. Best of all, this practical resource can be used over and over again by nurses who want to increase their charting skills, competency level, and accuracy, as well as allow more quality time for the most important person, the patient.

Tonia Dandry Aiken, RN, JD
Past President
American Association of Nurse Attorneys
** and Foundation;**
President
RN Development, Inc.
New Orleans, LA

Preface

The third edition of *Nursing Documentation: A Nursing Process Approach* was written to provide readers with current information about documentation. Several factors influence contemporary nursing charting practices. In addition, the increased acuity of patients and the nursing shortage have decreased the amount of time available for documentation. Nurses are seeking information on how to refine charting practices or redesign charting systems to streamline charting. As organizations merge, charting practices in the new corporate structure must be integrated. Furthermore, nurses should be aware that patients are now more likely to sue nurses and other healthcare personnel than in the past; therefore legal issues related to charting are increasingly important as nurses become more concerned about protecting themselves from liability. Finally, nurses should recognize that a wide variety of regulatory agencies are scrutinizing their charting, including the Joint Commission for the Accreditation of Healthcare Organizations (JCAHO), peer review organizations, insurance companies, utilization managers, and quality management/quality improvement personnel.

This text is intended for student nurses and practicing nurses who wish to increase and update their knowledge of documentation. Nurse managers, case managers, and administrators who are looking for methods to improve the efficiency and effectiveness of their charting systems will also find this book helpful.

This third edition provides a systematic overview of the essentials of documentation and has been thoroughly revised and updated. It includes approximately 50 new or updated forms that illustrate multidisciplinary assessment formats to provide the most current forms needed for proper and complete documentation.

Several new chapters have been added, including Chapter 10, Maternal-Child Documentation; Chapter 11, Critical Care Documentation; Chapter 12, Perioperative Documentation; and the Psychiatric Documentation section in Chapter 13, Psychiatric and Home Care Documentation. Chapter 10 covers special documentation concerns for children and pregnant women, such as proper documentation of electronic fetal monitoring, newborn care, child abuse, and neglect. Chapter 11 includes specific documentation needs in the emergency departments and intensive care units, such as proper documentation of triage, evaluation, and communication, and passive observation. In addition, Chapter 12 provides valuable information for postanesthesia care and operating room documentation, including documentation of recovery from spinal anesthesia, common postanesthesia problems, and preoperative emergencies. Furthermore, the psychiatric documentation section in Chapter 13 presents specific information for documentation of psychiatric care, such as documentation of suicidal or violent behavior, refusal of treatment, and medical management.

Throughout this edition, timely topics have been included, such as common litigation issues in home care, maternal and child care, critical care, perioperative care, psychiatric care, and long-term care. This information will help readers better understand the need for proper documentation and will ensure that nurses understand the pitfalls of incomplete or inaccurate documentation. In addition, updated information on the trends in charting, along with legal issues, reimbursement issues, and issues surrounding changing an existing documentation system, have been included.

Furthermore, new information has been added on the development and use of clinical pathways. Information on outcome-oriented charting and clinical path charting is also new to this edition.

Chapter 1 describes the factors that influence documentation practices and decisions about changing a documentation system. Chapter 2 discusses the documentation of assessment findings on the initial data base. Chapter 3 covers the documentation of nursing diagnosis and planning and also updates the new forms of care planning, including critical pathways. Chapter 4 describes the documentation of implementation and the design and use of flowsheets. Chapter 5 covers the documentation of the evaluation of patient responses—the aspect of charting that some nurses have found to be the most difficult.

Chapter 6 presents the legal aspects of charting, which are illustrated by nursing case law, in addition to highlighting defensive charting through the use of examples. Chapter 7 describes and compares the major charting systems currently in use and lists the factors that must be considered when selecting a documentation system. Chapter 8 presents current information about computerized medical records. Chapter 9 provides tips on implementing changes in a documentation system, which should be particularly helpful to staff development departments, members of documentation committees, and nurse managers.

While planning this third edition, it was realized the focus needed to be broadened to cover documentation in specialty areas of nursing. The chapters in the latter part of this book describe the clinical issues pertinent to a particular specialty and include examples of case law. Chapter 10 focuses on documentation issues specific to maternal-child nursing, including obstetrical, neonatal, and pediatric nursing. Chapter 11 describes critical care documentation in intensive care units and emergency departments. Chapter 12 covers perioperative documentation, including operating room suites and postanesthesia care units. Chapter 13 addresses documentation in psychiatric and home care nursing. Chapter 14 describes long-term care documentation.

ACKNOWLEDGMENTS

We are indebted to our contributors, who dedicated their time to share their knowledge of documentation in specialty areas. Examples of documentation forms are integrated throughout the text. As we gathered forms from a variety of sources, we learned that no one "perfect" form that every agency can use exists. We included the best examples from the forms available to us. We welcome any documentation forms sent by readers for possible inclusion in the fourth edition of this book. Much of the content of this edition is based on our experiences as educators, consultants, and agents for change. We have taught documentation programs throughout the United States and Canada and have learned a great deal from our participants.

We thank all of the nurses who have shared their forms and experiences. Finally, we are grateful to Jaime Schultz for her work on the manuscript and her ability to keep track of the multiple versions of each chapter as changes were made to the manuscript.

—Patricia W. Iyer and Nancy H. Camp

Contents

Figures

Forms

Home Care

Incident Reporting

Long-Term Care

Miscellaneous

Obstetrics

Pediatric

Perioperative Records

Psychiatric

Transfers

1

Overview of Documentation

Since the time of Florence Nightingale, nurses have viewed documentation as a vital part of professional practice. In her early writings Nightingale described the need for nurses to record "the proper use of fresh air, light, warmth, cleanliness, and the proper selection and administration of diet," with the goal of collecting, storing, and retrieving data to manage patient care intelligently (Seymour, 1954, p. 32). In Nightingale's time, documentation was used primarily to communicate implementation of medical orders, not to observe, assess, or evaluate the patient's status (as it is today).

During the 1930s Virginia Henderson promoted the idea of using written care plans to communicate patient care information. With the establishment of the Joint Commission for Accreditation of Healthcare Organizations (JCAHO)—formerly JCAH—in 1951 and with the trend toward formalization of nursing standards, documentation became a way to evaluate nursing care. Although we now view nursing documentation as essential to nursing, medical records personnel did not always view it as such. Consequently, nursing documentation was discarded after a patient's discharge.

Since the early 1970s nursing documentation has become more important, reflecting changes in nursing practice, regulatory agency requirements, and legal guidelines. In addition, with the advent of diagnostic related groupings (DRGs), nursing documentation has moved forward as a mechanism for determining monetary reimbursement for care. With the development of the nursing process as a framework for practice, documentation has evolved to become an essential link between the provision and evaluation of care. Most aspects of nursing documentation now remain a permanent part of the medical record; worksheets such as those used to record intake and output are one exception.

WHY DOCUMENT?

Professional Responsibility

Professional responsibility and accountability are among the most important reasons for accurate documentation. Documentation is part of the nurse's overall responsibility for patient care. The clinical record facilitates care, enhances continuity of care, and helps coordinate the treatment and evaluation of the patient. The American Nurses Association (1985) emphasized the role of documentation by stating:

The nurse is responsible for data collection and assessment of health status of the client; determination of the nursing care plan directed toward designated goals; evaluation of the effectiveness of nursing care in achieving the goals of care; and subsequent reassessment and revision of the nursing care plan (p. 10).

One of the most significant professional functions of the registered nurse is the evaluation of the patient's responses to nursing care. Professional nurses are responsible for managing increasingly complex patient issues and coordinating patient care among many levels of healthcare workers. Documentation must clearly communicate a nurse's judgment and evaluation of the patient's status. The nurse's ability to make a difference in patient outcomes must be demonstrated in practice and in charting. Hays (1989, p. 203) points out, "If we can achieve excellence in increasingly complex patient care, we can learn to describe it in words."

Legal Protection

Another reason for charting is that nursing documentation may be used in malpractice cases. The information charted by the nurse may deter a plaintiff from filing a suit against a healthcare provider. If the suit proceeds, nursing documentation may provide valuable evidence about a patient's condition and treatments. Documentation may be critical in determining whether a standard of care was met. (Standards of care are defined by nursing organizations and regulatory agencies.) Some nursing organizations have developed frameworks for providing and documenting nursing care.

Jurors and attorneys usually view the patient's chart as the best evidence of what really happened to a patient. Timely, accurate, and complete charting helps the patient secure better care and protects the nurse, physicians, and hospital from litigation. Documentation should be done deliberately and carefully, with the understanding that the chart is a legal document. One goal of this text is to help nurses streamline charting to avoid unnecessary duplication while still including all essential information to reduce liability. Specific information on the legal aspects of documentation can be found in Chapter 6.

Regulatory Standards

The Joint Commission is probably the most notable health care regulatory agency. Discussing documentation without addressing the Joint Commission requirements is impossible. Hospitals not accredited by the Joint Commission are not eligible for any government reimbursement funds such as Medicare. Part of the Joint Commission standards address nursing documentation; therefore one must know the current requirements to maintain compliance with the standards. In recent years the Joint Commission has embraced the concept of performance improvement, emphasizing the importance of outcomes and a multidisciplinary approach to care. This approach has changed the way many organizations structure patient care and, as a result, has changed documentation methods. References to Joint Commission requirements are included throughout this text.

A healthcare facility must comply with the documentation regulations issued by the department of health of that state. These standards vary from state to state and can be obtained by contacting the state department involved with surveying healthcare facilities.

Federal regulations may also affect documentation standards; for example, the U.S. Department of Health and Human Services issues requirements that affect the delivery of care to Medicare patients. Depending on the type of facility, accreditation standards of other regulatory agencies may apply.

Reimbursement

The evolution of managed care has changed the environment in which nurses work. In the past nurses did not have

a strong focus on cost containment. At one time, only a few items on a supply cart were chargeable. Today, some facilities require an accounting of every wound dressing and every incontinence pad. This emphasis on cost is increasing the awareness of not only *what* care is necessary but also *how* that care can be most efficiently provided.

Third-party payers such as Medicare, Blue Cross/Blue Shield, and other private insurance companies are increasingly interested in documentation. They scrutinize the clinical record to determine whether the billed services were necessary and to verify that they were delivered appropriately. With the advent of prospective payment systems (PPS) and DRGs, documentation has become critical. Accurate, thorough documentation facilitates appropriate DRG assignment and reimbursement.

Peer review organizations (PROs) and utilization management committees monitor length of stay, services rendered, and appropriateness of care. Unless there is thorough documentation by the healthcare provider to justify treatment and services, the healthcare agency could lose substantial revenue through denied reimbursement. For example, documentation helps to justify the need for services when the patient charges exceed the allotted cost or the length of stay is increased for a particular DRG. Progress notes play an important role in this review process. The PRO must substantiate every item on the hospital bill; therefore medication entries and documentation of other similar items has become essential.

Complete and thorough documentation is critical to accurate DRG assignment and reimbursement. The complexity of patient problems and the intensity of patient needs must be documented to ensure complete reimbursement. Regardless of the clinical setting, the nurse must be aware of documentation issues as they relate to reimbursement.

SOCIETAL FACTORS AFFECTING NURSING DOCUMENTATION

Many recent societal changes have affected the healthcare industry. Among these changes are increased consumer awareness, increased acuity of the hospitalized patient, and increased emphasis on healthcare outcomes.

Increased Consumer Awareness

The general population is being provided with a great deal of information on health care. Popular magazines and television shows educate patients about medical and nursing issues and treatment options. Healthcare consumers demand high-quality care at a reasonable cost. In addition, patients have become increasingly litigious, placing considerable pressure on healthcare facilities, physicians, and nurses to provide nearly flawless care. Consumers expect nurses to be knowledgeable, competent, and caring in approach while providing high-quality care in the most efficient and effective manner possible. The evidence of this care must be recorded in the medical record.

Increased Acuity of Hospitalized Patients

Changes in the reimbursement system have resulted in growth of outpatient services and increased acuity among patients receiving nursing care in hospital, long-term care, and home care settings. Most people using healthcare resources are older than 65 years. Elderly patients present more complex issues in care and management. As chronic illness increases, so does the demand for nursing services.

Compounding the situation is the decreasing length of stay associated with the managed care. Decreased length of stay increases nursing intensity, resulting in the need to set care priorities. Because patients are hospitalized for shorter periods, nurses must be able to gather pertinent data quickly, make accurate assessments, plan and implement appropriate care, and provide a written record.

Increasing patient acuity requires that we examine and change the tools we use for data collection. Accurate assessment and identification of patient needs are essential if high-quality care is to be provided. Documentation tools must be designed to gather data regarding potential problems and risk factors for an increasingly ill population. Discharge preparation and patient education must be emphasized to facilitate management of the patient at home. Documentation must confirm that the patient and family are prepared to assume home care responsibilities. Nursing documentation systems generally have not kept up with the rapid changes in health care; however, with the advent of clinical paths and mapping of patient care, documentation methods must change to keep pace.

Increased Emphasis on Outcomes

Documentation has assumed new importance with the current emphasis on monitoring the quality of health care as evidenced by patient outcomes. When financial resources were abundant and good care was assumed to be inherent, the evaluation of care was left to healthcare professionals or no evaluation was done at all. Prospective payment systems, medical malpractice lawsuits, and limited healthcare resources have made the quality of health care a major issue. Consumers, insurers, and government agencies are seeking more information on clinical performance and related dimensions of good care.

In the late 1980s the Joint Commission moved away from the traditional reliance on structural measures and embraced the concept of accrediting hospitals based on their overall performance outcomes. Proponents of this new emphasis on measuring the outcomes of clinical practice predict social benefits will increase. These benefits include better infor-

mation for healthcare practitioners and patients, improved guidelines for practice, and wiser decisions by purchasers of health care. The research of outcomes may help determine more about the effectiveness of different interventions and may help increase the efficiency of existing systems for monitoring the quality of care.

The following three important factors have led to the current emphasis on the assessment of effectiveness and outcomes:

- *Cost containment.* The emphasis on outcomes is seen as an index of the relative effectiveness of different interventions, allowing the elimination of unnecessary expenditure.
- *Renewed sense of competition.* A variety of healthcare agencies are becoming increasingly competitive. For example, health maintenance organizations (HMOs) have grown nearly twentyfold since 1970. These insurers are now competing vigorously for the healthcare buyers' dollar. Furthermore, purchasers of health care are trying to compare outcomes and quality as well as price.
- *Recognition of geographically variant standards.* Researchers have documented substantial geographic differences in the use of various medical procedures. As a result, major efforts are under way to define nationwide standards of care. Practice guidelines based on research are being issued by professional and governmental organizations.

Documentation is one mechanism used to evaluate care. Until recently, documentation was process oriented, emphasizing tasks performed by the caregiver. This approach does not adequately represent the patient's status. The development of standards and outcome criteria make it possible to evaluate the patient's status and generate documentation of progress or the lack of progress, which focuses the documentation on patient outcome.

The transition to *outcome charting* is a difficult one. In outcome charting, the nurse is expected to interpret data and evaluate the patient's response to care based on established outcome criteria. In the past, nurses were expected to document tasks, not make judgments; this is a difficult habit to break. In reality, many nurses still chart assessment data and nursing care but leave the analysis and evaluation to the person reading the notes. The need to evaluate and document outcomes is discussed at greater length in Chapter 5.

TRENDS IN CHARTING

Although documentation practices and healthcare procedures are rapidly changing, some conclusions can be drawn about trends in charting.

Reduction in Duplicate Charting

It is increasingly difficult to justify recording the same information in many places in the medical record. Forms are being designed to reduce and eliminate duplicate charting.

Bedside Charting

The immediate recording of pertinent data reduces duplicate charting and improves the accessibility and accuracy of information. Resistance to keeping records at the bedside is fading as healthcare professionals change their practices and perceptions about bedside records.

Multidisciplinary Charting

As the distinctions between departments begin to blur, a renewed team approach can affect documentation systems. Patient-focused care, which involves placing multiskilled workers at the patient's bedside, has stimulated a rethinking of documentation systems. Multidisciplinary forms and shared progress notes are emerging.

Clinical Paths

Case management/managed care has led to the development of a new documentation tool: the clinical path. One-page or two-page clinical paths act as road maps to direct care and reflect the multidisciplinary team approach. Documentation reflects the outcomes on the path and leads to more consistent evaluation of the patient's attainment of goals. Clinical paths are discussed in Chapter 3.

More Uniformity in Documentation

Joint Commission standards require that the same standard of care be used for patients with similar or identical needs, regardless of their location in a hospital. For example, a woman recovering from anesthesia after a cesarean birth should receive the same monitoring in the postanesthesia recovery room as she would in the labor and delivery suite. Nursing department staff members are scrutinizing forms to ensure that a uniform standard of care is reflected in the design of the forms.

Computerized Documentation

The computer has gained acceptance as a vital tool in the healthcare environment. Nurses in administration have recognized the advantages of using computers for documentation and are now purchasing software and hardware. This is discussed in detail in Chapter 8.

Fax Machines

Fax machines function as low-cost—but limited—alternatives to computerized documentation and permit the

---

Box 1-1
Reasons for Changing a Charting System

- Improve the quality of documentation.
- Reduce the amount of time nurses spend charting.
- Contain costs (for example, reduce overtime, improve reimbursement).
- Reduce duplication of information in the medical record.
- Institute multidisciplinary charting methods.
- Increase emphasis on patient outcomes.

---

faxing of orders, histories and physicals, laboratory results, and a variety of healthcare documents.

CHANGING AN EXISTING DOCUMENTATION SYSTEM

Reasons for Changing a System

The healthcare delivery landscape continues to evolve. Many factors may stimulate a nursing department to examine existing documentation forms, systems, and practices. Throughout this text, new ideas and strategies for documentation are introduced; however, change requires thoughtful and deliberate planning. Therefore the following points should be considered when determining whether or not a change in documentation is needed (Box 1-1):

1. The need to *improve the quality* of nursing documentation may require not only new or revised tools, but also new ways of thinking. Nurses must recognize that the written word conveys the judgment of the writer. Nurses must move beyond their comfort zone in charting tasks and learn to chart analysis and evaluation.
2. The need to *reduce the amount of time spent charting* is critical. Estimates suggest that nurses spend up to 40% of their time on paperwork (McDaniel, 1997). Excess time spent on documentation is better spent on other patient-care activities. By "downsizing" the need for labor-intensive charting requirements, the nurse is better able to manage patient care. A charting approach that reduces the amount of time spent on charting becomes essential in the high-pressure healthcare environment and facilitates documentation by ancillary staff.
3. The need to *contain costs* may require nurses to reexamine routine practices, such as documentation, to develop more efficient methods. Cost-containment efforts have resulted in new ways to decrease time spent charting and to improve documentation for reimbursement purposes.
4. The need to *reduce duplication* is essential. Think of the number of times a nurse must chart vital signs, intake and output, medications, and intravenous fluids. Charting duplicate information is very time consuming and is not cost effective. Many innovative flowsheets have been

designed in an effort to decrease duplication of information. Streamlined charting systems, such as charting by exception (described in Chapter 7), are becoming more widespread as nurses recognize the need to eliminate redundancy in the medical record.

5. The current emphasis on *multidisciplinary care* has resulted in changes in the traditional forms and systems used for documentation. New admission forms are being designed to incorporate assessment data from several disciplines and eliminate the need for the patient to be asked the same questions by different healthcare providers. See Chapter 2 for more detailed information on assessment tools.

6. The increasing *emphasis on patient outcomes* has necessitated a change in the content of nursing documentation. Nurses are expected to chart the patient's response to care, in addition to the care rendered. Plans of care have taken on new identities to facilitate this transition to outcome-focused charting. Critical paths, Care Maps, and clinical pathways abound as nurses work to incorporate documentation of patient outcomes into the daily routine.

Changes in a system must not be based on "knee-jerk" reactions to criticism. The authors have seen hospitals change adequate charting systems based on a casual comment from a Joint Commission surveyor. Be sure to distinguish Joint Commission requirements from a Joint Commission surveyor's personal preferences to avoid unnecessary changes. Further information regarding implementation of documentation changes can be found in Chapter 9.

Documentation Outcomes

Before making changes in a documentation system, the nurse should first determine the desired outcome. Deciding on the desired outcome of the change directs the planning and implementation process. Following are several outcomes to consider in conjunction with the reasons to change a documentation system listed previously.

The Chart Is Legally Sound

Nursing documentation must provide evidence of care and the patient's response to that care. In addition, the clinical record should include documentation that the nurse provided for the patient's safety. Documentation should indicate that the nurse did the following:

- Assessed the patient for risk factors for injury
- Planned strategies to protect the patient from harm
- Implemented strategies to protect the patient from complications such as falls or skin breakdown
- Notified the physician of critical changes in the patient's status
- Clearly documented the circumstances of an incident or unusual event

Furthermore, the type and frequency of documentation must comply with the institutional policies. Regardless of the method chosen (for example, Focus, SOAP [subjective data, objective data, assessment, plan], or PIE [problems, interventions, evaluation]), the documentation system should be easy to defend in court if the institutional policies are adhered to consistently. Specific information on a variety of charting systems is presented in Chapter 7.

The Chart Reflects the Nursing Process

The American Nurses Association and specialty nursing organizations emphasize the need to incorporate the nursing process into documentation. Charting systems and forms are being revised and new ones developed to achieve this outcome. Making decisions about care, evaluating the results, and revising nursing strategies to facilitate patient progress are all elements of the nursing process that must be documented in the record.

The Chart Describes the Patient's Ongoing Status from Shift to Shift

The chart is used as a communication tool among health professionals. The more accurate and complete the documentation, the greater the chance for continuity of care, which is vital in light of the increasing number of part time, agency, and per diem nurses providing care.

The Plan of Care and Chart Complement Each Other

Standards of care are used as the basis for care and documentation. Nurses are responsible and accountable for identifying problems and making nursing diagnoses at the time of admission and for following through with interventions and evaluation. However, sometimes no documentation is recorded to support those activities, giving the impression that problems were identified but not handled appropriately.

The Documentation System is Designed to Facilitate Retrieval of Information for Quality Improvement Activities and Research

The documentation system should allow the efficient collection of data to facilitate quality improvement activities. Flowsheets often are used for this purpose.

The Documentation System Supports the Staffing Mix and Acuity Levels in the Current Healthcare Environment

Many charting methods exist, although they do not all meet the same needs. In researching which method is best for your institution, consider the staffing mix, the nurse-to-patient ratios, the acuity levels of the patient population, and the nursing care delivery system. For example, charting by exception was developed in a hospital in which the staff were all registered nurses (RNs). In the current healthcare environment, many hospitals are using unlicensed assistive personnel (UAP) to handle a variety of patient care tasks. (The number of licensed personnel may be reduced to contain costs.) As a result, fewer licensed nurses are responsible for charting on more patients. This must be a consideration when planning a change in documentation methods.

These documentation outcomes can be used to evaluate an individual's documentation efforts or to evaluate a system of documentation, and they can also be used to evaluate strengths and limitations within documentation systems. (Most systems have strengths, although they may not be readily apparent.) Evaluating documentation practices based on these outcomes and the reasons for changing a documentation system makes it possible to maximize strengths and correct weaknesses.

SUMMARY

The healthcare environment and the nursing profession are changing rapidly. Documentation techniques must keep up with the trend toward high-quality care in an environment where cost containment is essential. Nursing documentation systems must reflect the many factors that influence nursing practice. Documentation outcomes and policies should reflect reality, including available resources. Nurses should analyze current nursing strategies with documentation in mind and seize the opportunity to participate fully in restructuring documentation forms, systems, and practices. This text provides the opportunity for nurses to do the following:

- Examine documentation within the framework of the nursing process.
- Learn about different charting systems, concepts, and requirements.
- View many sample forms.
- Discover implementation strategies to improve nursing documentation on an individual or systemic level.
- Understand the legal implications of documentation.

The authors hope that this information will stimulate thought and encourage nurses to look at documentation as the way in which nursing process comes to life.

REFERENCES

American Nurses Association: *Code for nurses with interpretive statements,* Washington, DC, 1985, The Association.

Hays J: Voices in the record, *Image* p 200, 1989.

McDaniel A: Developing and testing a prototype patient care database, *Computers in Nursing* 15(3):129, 1997.

Seymour L: *Selected writings of Florence Nightingale,* New York, 1954, Macmillan.

2

Documenting Assessment

The primary focus of this chapter is documentation of data on the initial acute care admission assessment forms. In this chapter, as well as in the rest of this text, a number of documentation forms are presented. These forms are examples that illustrate some of the approaches to documentation. Remember that the samples represent only a few of the ways these forms can be designed. The examples given here may be modified to meet a facility's needs. A complete index of forms follows the Contents page at the beginning of this text.

Careful assessment and documentation of the patient's needs can enhance the effectiveness of nursing care by the following:

- Describing the patient's needs to make accurate nursing diagnoses and set priorities, thereby using nursing time effectively
- Facilitating the planning of interventions
- Describing the family's needs and pinpointing factors that will enhance the patient's recovery and promote discharge planning
- Fulfilling professional obligations by documenting important assessment information

INITIAL DATA BASE: ADMISSION ASSESSMENT

The first step in the nursing process is assessment. The standards of care for assessment are defined by a number of regulatory agencies and professional nursing associations, including the American Nurses Association (ANA) and the Joint Commission for Accreditation of Healthcare Organizations (JCAHO). The ANA's standard for assessment includes measurement criteria that focus on the following (ANA, 1991):

1. Using the client's immediate condition or healthcare needs to define the priorities for data collection

2. Using appropriate assessment techniques to collect pertinent data
3. Involving the client, significant others, and other healthcare providers, as appropriate, to collect data
4. Using a systematic, ongoing data collection process
5. Documenting the relevant data in a manner that permits easy retrieval

The Comprehensive Accreditation Manual for Hospitals, which published the 1997 JCAHO standards in 1996, contains an entire chapter about the assessment process. The applicable standards are mentioned in this chapter.

A facility may use a variety of data bases to identify each patient's physical, psychologic, and social needs. One established practice in an acute-care facility serving a number of different patient populations is the use of several types of admission assessments. Some of these may include data bases for the patient seen in the following units or departments; same day or outpatient surgery, renal dialysis, pediatrics, short-stay admission, medical-surgical, critical care, emergency department, labor and delivery areas, and ambulatory care.

The initial data base should be designed for the most common population cared for in the clinical area. For example, if most patients admitted to a medical-surgical unit are elderly, the data base should focus on common problems seen in this population, such as high risk for impaired skin integrity, falls, and sensory impairments. If the usual patient population is not readily identified, the admitting office or finance office may be able to provide data on the typical age, sex, length of stay, and medical diagnoses of patients cared for by the facility or a specific nursing unit. The development of a typical patient profile is addressed in more detail in Chapter 3. As nursing computer information systems become more sophisticated, it will be possible to identify the most common nursing diagnoses for particular patient populations as well.

Multidisciplinary Data Bases

Another growing trend is to use the same admission data base, which has a multidisciplinary focus. This format consolidates the assessments of several disciplines. For example, Figure 2-1 presents an example of an admission assessment form that permits documentation by a variety of disciplines, including Audiology, Food and Nutrition, Occupational Therapy, Pastoral Care, Physical Therapy, Respiratory Services, Social Services, and Speech and Hearing. Development of multidisciplinary admission assessment forms must overcome some organizational challenges to create a form that meets the needs of the departments and satisfies regulatory standards. Care must be taken not to create an overwhelmingly long and cumbersome tool.

Time Frame for Completion of Data Base

The time frame for completing the initial data base is defined by policy and varies according to the clinical area. The time frame will depend on a variety of factors, including the types of patients treated by the hospital, the complexity and duration of their care, and the dynamics of the conditions surrounding their care (JCAHO, 1996). For example, the needs of a woman in active labor or a patient admitted to a critical-care unit should be assessed as soon as possible after arrival. An individual being admitted for long-term therapy may be assessed over a period of hours or days. According to the Joint Commission, the patient's history, physical examination, nursing assessment (done by a registered nurse), and other screening assessments are to be completed within 24 hours of admission as an inpatient. This time frame applies even on weekends and holidays. The nursing assessment may be performed before admission, as commonly occurs before planned surgery, provided that any significant changes in the patient's condition are documented at the time of the patient's actual admission. The original or a copy of the assessment form completed before admission should be included in the medical record (JCAHO, 1996). Figure 2-2 on p. 14 is an example of an admission assessment form that is completed before a planned same-day procedure.

Priority Assessment Issues

The increasingly complex healthcare needs of patients and shortened lengths of stay have highlighted the need for efficient collection of data. The initial encounter with the patient should focus on the following four priority "Ps" of assessment:

- Problems
- Patient's risk for injury
- Potential for self-care following discharge
- Patient and family education needs

Problems

An important purpose of collecting data at the time of initial assessment is to identify the patient's priority nursing diagnoses or problems. When developing initial assessment forms, keep in mind the length of time the facility expects to provide care for the patient. For example, when it is anticipated that a patient will be receiving long-term care, it is appropriate to obtain a complete data base. On the other hand, in acute-care facilities with short lengths of stay, spending a long time collecting volumes of data on admission is no longer practical. The initial data base should be carefully analyzed. Some of the questions may require collection of information about problems that cannot possibly be addressed in a short time.

Patient's Risk for Injury

A second purpose of the initial assessment is to detect and document factors that may contribute to patient injury. This commonly includes identifying the patient's risk for falls, pressure ulcers, suicidal or violent behavior, physical or emotional abuse, or substance abuse.

Falls. Patient falls account for a large percentage of all incidents reported by acute and long-term care facilities. Consequences of falls include prolonged hospitalization, increased healthcare costs, and liability problems. The elderly are at particular risk for injuries resulting from falls. Accidents are the fifth leading cause of death in those older than 65 years. "Approximately two thirds of accidents are falls. Of those hospitalized for a fall, only half will be alive 1 year later" (Rubenstein et al, 1988, p. 267). Recently more attention has been directed toward the identification of those at risk for falls. Box 2-1 on p. 16 lists characteristics that should be considered when identifying the patient at risk for falls.

The patient's risk for a fall must be assessed and documented on admission to an acute or long-term care facility and during the initial visit of a home care nurse. Falls have been found to be more common during the first few days of admission. Factors that can contribute to the increased incidence of falls after the patient's arrival may include an unfamiliarity with the environment, acute illness with accompanying weakness and disorientation, sensory deprivation caused by the absence of hearing aids and glasses, feelings of helplessness in a fast-paced environment, and the disruption of normal patterns of elimination (Iyer, 1988).

A number of documentation tools have been developed to identify the patient at high risk for falls. Commonly, points are assigned to certain risk factors. This type of form should be used on admission or whenever a significant change in the patient's health status increases the risk for falls. There are advantages and disadvantages to developing a separate form for assessing fall risk factors. If the facility is not ready to revise the data base simply to add the risk assessment, a separate form works well. On the other hand, nurses sometimes forget to initiate the risk assessment form.

Text continued on p. 16

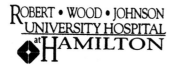

MULTIDISCIPLINARY HEALTH ASSESSMENT FORM

Date_____ Time of Arrival_____ A.M. / P.M.

TPR_____ B/P _____ Height _____ Weight _____ Clothing Sheet Completed _____

Mode of Admission: Amb. _____ Wch. _____ Stretcher _____ Admitting Source: ER _____ Home _____ Nursing Home _____ Other _____

ROOM ORIENTATION: Use of Call Bell _____   Use of Telephone _____   Hi-low Bed _____   Smoking Policy _____

Use of Intercom _____   Location of Bathroom _____   T.V. Rental _____   Visiting Policy _____

SIGNIFICANT OTHER_____

PATIENT HISTORY Obtained From_____ Relationship_____

SECTION I

1. Physician's Admitting Dx._____

2. Patient's Description of Illness/Injury: (Tell me why you are here?)_____

_____

3. Past Medical History: Hospitalization_____

_____

a. Medical (include recent infection)_____

b. Surgical_____

c. Current Medications

MEDICATION	DOSE	ROUTE	FREQUENCY	TIME & DATE LAST TAKEN
1.				
2.				
3.				
4.				
5.				
6.				
7.				

d. **Allergies:** Asthma _____   Hay Fever _____   Eczema _____   Soap _____   Latex _____

Food _____   Drugs _____   X-Ray Dye _____   Other _____

Explain Reaction_____

e. Blood Transfusion ☐ Yes ☐ No   If yes, ever had an adverse reaction?   ☐ Yes ☐ No

If yes, explain_____

f. Do You Smoke?   ☐ No ☐ Yes Cigarettes/Pipe/Cigar Amount/day _____ # of years _____ (Quit–date)_____

Do You Drink Alcohol? ☐ No Ⓢ Yes Type_____ Amount/day _____ # of years _____ (Quit–date)_____

Recreational Drugs? ☐ No Ⓢ Yes Type_____ Amount/day _____ # of years _____ (Quit–date)_____
(Other than prescription drugs)

Figure 2-1 Multidisciplinary assessment form. (Courtesy Robert Wood Johnson University Hospital at Hamilton, Hamilton Square, NJ.)
Continued

Robert Wood Johnson University Hospital at Hamilton

SECTION I PATIENT HISTORY (continued)

g. Occupation/Former Occupation_____

   Exposure to Occupational Hazards? ☐ No ☐ Yes – Explain_____

h. Family History: (Circle) Diabetes   Cancer   Hypertension

   Heart   Tuberculosis   Anemia

   Other_____

4. Advance Directive ☐ None ☐ No restrictions on life-sustaining treatment

☐ Restrictions on life-sustaining treatment

5. Fall Prevention Program: ☐ No risk factors

The patient will be placed in the fall program if:

☐ Age > 65 or < 3 years ☐ Poor nutritional status ☐ Incontinent ☐ Neuro/ortho dx ☐ Cardiovascular

☐ Analgesics/hypnotics ☐ Weakness ☐ Confusion ☐ Impaired vision ☐ Decreased mobility ☐ Hx of syncope/falls

Other_____

SECTION II REVIEW OF SYSTEMS
(Check at least one under each category)

COMFORT

Pain/Discomfort: ☐ Yes ☐ No

Where?_____

Type: ☐ Burning ☐ Dull ☐ Pressure ☐ Heavy ☐ Sharp ☐ Cramping ☐ Other_____

Intensity (circle) 1 2 3 4 5 6 7 8 9 10
                    L   H

Duration: ☐ Constant ☐ Intermittent

What relieves the pain? ☐ Rest ☐ Heat ☐ Cold ☐ Medication Specific:_____

Comments:_____

ACTIVITY

Walking: ☐ No Difficulty ☐ Stiffness ☐ Weakness ☐ Paralysis – **P/S** Acute ☐ Frequent Falls ☐ Loss of Balance

☐ Contractures ☐ Deformities **S** History of Fractures_____

Upper Extremity: ☐ No Difficulty ☐ Weakness **O** Paralysis ☐ Deformities Functional Grasp ☐ Yes **O** No

☐ Splints

Activity: ☐ Bedrest ☐ BRP ☐ Chair ☐ Ambulatory_____ **Support Devices:** ☐ No ☐ Yes_____

Ambulatory Devices: ☐ Walker ☐ Crutches ☐ Wheelchair ☐ Other_____

Levels in Home: ☐ 1 Story ☐ 2 Story Bath First Floor ☐ No ☐ Yes Steps to Entry ☐ No ☐ Yes

Comments:_____

OXYGENATION

Respiratory: ☐ No Difficulty ☐ Pain ☐ Cough ☐ Dyspnea ☐ Sputum **R** Tracheostomy

☐ Respiratory Equipment at Home ☐ No ☐ Yes If yes, what?_____

Circulatory: ☐ No Difficulty ☐ Edema ☐ Numbness ☐ Syncope ☐ Palpitations ☐ Murmur ☐ Pacemaker

Comments:_____

Figure 2-1, cont'd Multidisciplinary assessment form. (Courtesy Robert Wood Johnson University Hospital at Hamilton, Hamilton Square, NJ.)

Robert Wood Johnson University Hospital at Hamilton

SECTION II   REVIEW OF SYSTEMS (continued)
(Check at least one under each category)

NUTRITION

☐ No Nutrition Related Problems

Eating: [F] Poor Intake [F/H] Difficulty Swallowing [F] N/V/D > 3 Days

Alternate Nutrition: [F/S] Tube Feeding [F/S] TPN [F] Vent Support

[F] Braden Scale < 15

Weight: [F] Involuntary Weight Loss (> 10 lbs./6 mo.)

Medical: [F] Uncontrolled Diabetes [F] GI Disorder

Current Diet:_____

Comments:_____

ELIMINATION

Bowel: ☐ No difficulty ☐ Constipation ☐ Diarrhea Frequency of stool_____

☐ Incontinence ☐ Ileostomy ☐ Colostomy Comments:_____

Bladder: ☐ No difficulty ☐ Incontinence ☐ Hematuria ☐ Frequency

☐ Nocturia ☐ UTI ☐ Dribbling ☐ Catheter Type:_____ Size:_____

Comments:_____

SEXUAL/REPRODUCTIVE

Date of LMP_____

Date of Last Cervical Cancer Screen (Pap Smear)_____

Self Breast Exam: ☐ No ☐ Yes Date of Last Mammogram_____

Use of Contraceptives: ☐ No ☐ Yes – Type:_____

Prostate Problems: ☐ No ☐ Yes Testicular Self-Exam: ☐ No ☐ Yes

Pregnant: ☐ No ☐ Yes

Sexual/Reproductive Concerns/Comments:_____

PROTECTION

Mental Status: ☐ Oriented ☐ Agitated ☐ Combative ☐ Unresponsive ☐ Other:_____

☐ Cooperative ☐ Disoriented To *(circle)* person place and/or time ☐ Lethargic ☐ Unresponsive

☐ Seizures – Type and Frequency:_____

Safety: ☐ Side Rails Up ☐ Call Bell in Reach

Comments:_____

Vision: ☐ No difficulty ☐ Glasses ☐ Contact Lens ☐ Blurring ☐ Cataracts ☐ Glaucoma ☐ Diplopia ☐ Artificial Eye

Comments:_____

Hearing: ☐ No difficulty ☐ Deaf ☐ Limited ☐ Aid ☐ Pain ☐ Tinnitus ☐ Discharge

Comments:_____

Mouth/Teeth: ☐ No difficulty ☐ Caps ☐ Loose teeth ☐ Gum disease ☐ Dentures: ☐ Upper ☐ Lower ☐ Partial

Comments:_____

Integument: ☐ No Problems ☐ Rash ☐ Lesion ☐ Scars [S] Bruises ☐ Diaphoresis

[F] **Pressure Ulcer:** Location_____ Stage_____ Size_____

Color_____ Exudate_____ Odor_____ Dressing_____

Comments:_____

Figure 2-1, cont'd   Multidisciplinary assessment form.   *Continued*

Robert Wood Johnson University Hospital at Hamilton

SECTION II **REVIEW OF SYSTEMS** (continued)
(Check at least one under each category)

BRADEN SCALE

					Score
→ **Sensory Perception**	1 Completely Limited	2 Very Limited	3 Slightly Limited	4 No Impairment	
→ **Moisture**	1 Constantly Moist	2 Very Moist	3 Occasionally Moist	4 Rarely Moist	
→ **Activity**	1 Bedfast	2 Chairfast	3 Walks Occasionally	4 Walks Frequently	
→ **Mobility**	1 Completely Immobile	2 Very Limited	3 Slightly Impaired	4 No Limitations	
→ **Nutrition**	1 Very Poor	2 Probably Inadequate	3 Adequate	4 Excellent	
→ **Friction & Shear**	1 Problem	2 Potential Problem	3 No Apparent Problem		
				Total Score	

RESULTS: 15–16 Low Risk
12–14 Moderate Risk
< 11 High Risk ☐

If Score < 15, refer to Skin Care Prevention Procedure.

COMMUNICATION

Speech: ☐ Normal ☐ Problems _____

Language(s) Spoken: ☐ English ☐ Other(s)_____ Read English ☐ No ☐ Yes

S.O. Interpreter:_____

Memory Problems: ☐ No ☐ Yes_____

Recent: ☐ No ☐ Yes_____ Remote: ☐ No ☐ Yes

Barriers to Learning: ☐ No ☐ Yes_____ Motivated to Learn: ☐ No ☐ Yes

Learning Preferences: ☐ Written ☐ Audio-visual ☐ Discussion

Education Level (check the highest level): ☐ Grade School ☐ College
☐ High School ☐ Post Graduate

Are there any questions that you have at this time? ☐ No ☐ Yes_____

COPING

State problems or fears that are of concern to you:_____

Do you plan to return to your home when you leave the hospital? ☐ Yes [S] No – Where?_____

Cultural/Spiritual:

Are there any religious, traditional, ethnic, or cultural practices that need to be part of your care? ☐ No [C] Yes

Is there any way the hospital can assist you with your religious practices? ☐ No [C] Yes – How?_____

MANAGEMENT OF HEALTH

Do you live alone? ☐ No [S] Yes **Significant other able to help?** [S] No ☐ Yes Who?_____

Do you require any assistance in the following areas:

Bathing ☐ No [S] Yes Eating ☐ No [S] Yes Walking ☐ No [S] Yes Stairs ☐ No [S] Yes

Dressing ☐ No [O/S] Yes Toileting ☐ No [S] Yes Medications ☐ No ☐ Yes

What community services are you using now?

☐ None ☐ Community Support Group_____

[S] Meals on Wheels [S] Transportation [S] Rehab

[S] Home Care [S] Adult Day Care [S] Other_____

Do you feel you will need any of these services on discharge? ☐ No [S] Yes Which ones?_____

Nurse Signature_____ Date _____

Figure 2-1, cont'd Multidisciplinary assessment form. (Courtesy Robert Wood Johnson University Hospital at Hamilton, Hamilton Square, NJ.)

Robert Wood Johnson University Hospital at Hamilton

SECTION III   **PHYSICAL ASSESSMENT**
(completed by RN)

Cardiovascular: Heart Sounds: ☐ Regular   ☐ Irregular

☐ Edema:_____

Peripheral Pulses: ☐ Present L _____   R _____

☐ Absent (location):_____

Respiratory: Lung Sounds: ☐ Clear   ☐ Crackles   ☐ Wheezes

☐ Rhonchi   ☐ Diminished:_____

Gastrointestinal: Bowel Sounds: ☐ Present   ☐ Absent

Abdomen: ☐ Soft   ☐ Rigid   ☐ Tender   ☐ Distended

Neurological: Pupils: ☐ Equal   ☐ Unequal   Hand Grasps: ☐ Equal   ☐ Unequal   ☐ Strong   ☐ Weak

PATIENT PROBLEMS LIST

	SIGNATURE
1.	
2.	
3.	
4.	

PLAN OF CARE

Identify Nursing Care Plan:_____

EDUCATION/TEACHING NEEDS

_____

_____

RN Signature_____ Date _____ Time _____

	Notified	DATE/TIME/INITIAL	SCREENING SIGNATURE	DATE
Audiology **(A)** 6827	☐	/ /		
Food and Nutrition **(F)** 6557, 6444	☐	/ /		
Occupational Therapy **(O)** 6828	☐	/ /		
Pastoral Care **(C)** DIAL "0"	☐	/ /		
Physical Therapy **(P)** 6640	☐	/ /		
Respiratory Services **(R)** 6490	☐	/ /		
Social Services **(S)** 6590	☐	/ /		
Speech and Hearing **(H)** S-6643, A-6827	☐	/ /		

Figure 2-1, cont'd   Multidisciplinary assessment form.

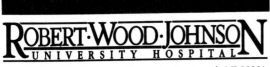

One Robert Wood Johnson Place, New Brunswick, NJ 08901

SAME DAY HEALTH ASSESSMENT FORM
ADMISSION / PROCEDURE RECORD

PREADMISSION PHONE CALL DATE TIME ☐ AM ☐ PM	PERSON CONTACTED (*RELATIONSHIP IF OTHER THAN PATIENT*)	PROCEDURE

ARRIVAL TIME
☐ AM
☐ PM   ☐ LEAVE VALUABLE AT HOME   ☐ RESPONSIBLE ADULT TO ACCOMPANY / DRIVE PT HOME   ☐ BRING ADVANCED DIRECTIVE (*IF APPLICABLE*)

☐ CHECK WITH DOCTOR REGARDING MEDICATIONS   ☐ PAT_____   ☐ DIET INSTRUCTIONS_____

RN SIGNATURE PRINT NAME	☐ UNABLE TO CONTACT PATIENT (*LIST REASON*) RN SIGNATURE PRINT NAME

DO YOU HAVE ANY ALLERGIES?   ☐ NO   ☐ YES (*IF YES, LIST & EXPLAIN TYPE OF REACTION BELOW*)

☐ FOOD_____

☐ MEDICATIONS_____

☐ LATEX _____

☐ DYE / CONTRAST MEDIA _____

	HEIGHT	WEIGHT	LMP

☐ OTHER

HISTORY OF CHICKEN POX? ☐ NO ☐ YES   IF NO, HISTORY OF EXPOSURE IN THE PAST 3 WEEKS ☐ NO ☐ YES   RECENT COLD, FEVER, I.D. EXPOSURE ☐ NO ☐ YES

MEDICATIONS IN USE: ☐ NONE

DRUG NAME	DOSE	FREQUENCY	DRUG NAME	DOSE	FREQUENCY

PATIENT / FAMILY HISTORY   √ = YES   O = NO   — = N/A   P = Patient   F = Family

☐ P ☐ F DIABETES MELLITUS   ☐ P ☐ F KIDNEY DISEASE   ☐ P ☐ F HYPERTENSION   ☐ P ☐ F SEIZURE DISORDER

☐ P ☐ F CARDIAC DISEASE   ☐ P ☐ F ASTHMA   ☐ P ☐ F CANCER

☐ P ☐ F ANESTHESIA Hx   ☐ P ☐ F GLAUCOMA   ☐ P ☐ F GI

SMOKING ☐ NO ☐ YES IF YES, HOW MUCH & HOW LONG?	QUIT DATE
ALCOHOL ☐ NO ☐ YES IF YES, HOW MUCH & HOW LONG?	QUIT DATE
DRUGS ☐ NO ☐ YES IF YES, HOW MUCH, HOW LONG, WHAT TYPE? (*NOTE: RECREATIONAL DRUGS OTHER THAN PRESCRIPTION DRUGS*)	QUIT DATE

PREVIOUS SURGERIES / ILLNESSES / HOSPITALIZATIONS: ☐ NONE

DATE / YEAR TYPE	DATE / YEAR TYPE

RN SIGNATURE (*IF OTHER THAN ABOVE*)	PRINT NAME

Figure 2-2   Same day procedure assessment form. (Courtesy Robert Wood Johnson University Hospital, New Brunswick, NJ.)

ADMISSION			SOURCE OF INFORMATION *(STATE NAME AND RELATIONSHIP IF OTHER)*
DATE	TIME	☐ AM ☐ PM	☐ PATIENT ☐ OTHER

ARRIVED BY	ACCOMPANIED BY: NAME	RELATIONSHIP
☐ AMBULATORY ☐ WHEELCHAIR ☐ STRETCHER		

ADVANCED DIRECTIVE
☐ NONE ☐ ON CHART ☐ OTHER LOCATION

*   *SEE NURSE'S NOTES FOR ADDITIONAL COMMENTS*

DISCHARGE PLANNING / ENVIRONMENTAL FACTORS

PROSTHESIS	☐ NO ☐ YES	_____	
GLASSES	☐ NO ☐ YES	CONTACT LENSES ☐ NO ☐ YES	
HEARING AIDS	☐ NO ☐ YES	☐ R ☐ L	
DENTURES	☐ NO ☐ YES	PARTIAL / FULL	
LOOSE TEETH	☐ NO ☐ YES	CAPS ☐ NO ☐ YES	
ASSISTIVE DEVICES	☐ NO ☐ YES	_____	
PACEMAKER	☐ NO ☐ YES	DATE IMPLANTED_____	

HIGHEST LEVEL OF EDUCATION _____

OCCUPATION _____

EXPOSURE TO OCCUPATIONAL HAZARDS? ☐ NO ☐ YES

PRIMARY LANGUAGE ☐ English ☐ Other

VITAL SIGNS

T   P   R   BP

WHEN INDICATED, STATUS OF PERIPHERAL PULSES

NUTRITION

NPO SINCE _____ *(DATE / TIME)* ☐ N/A   IF PO INTAKE, INDICATE TYPE / TIME _____

SPECIAL DIET AT HOME   ☐ NO ☐ YES / TYPE _____

PROTECTION

HAVE YOU EVER HAD A BLOOD TRANSFUSION? ☐ NO ☐ YES IF YES, HAVE YOU EVER HAD AN ADVERSE REACTION? ☐ NO ☐ YES (IF YES, DESCRIBE)

MENTAL STATUS: ☐ ALERT & ORIENTED   ☐ CONFUSED   ☐ APPREHENSIVE   ABILITY TO COMPREHEND: ☐ NO ☐ YES

☐ Hx OF VIOLENCE   ☐ SUICIDAL IDEATION   ☐ HALLUCINATION   ☐ OTHER_____

☐ CALL BELL WITHIN REACH   ☐ SIDE RAILS UP

PERTINENT OBSERVATIONS ABOUT PHYSICAL OR PSYCHOSOCIAL STATUS _____

CULTURAL / SPIRITUAL

ARE THERE ANY RELIGIOUS, TRADITIONAL, ETHNIC, OR CULTURAL PRACTICES THAT NEED TO BE PART OF YOUR CARE? ☐ NO ☐ YES_____

IS THERE ANY WAY THE HOSPITAL CAN ASSIST YOU WITH YOUR RELIGIOUS PRACTICES? ☐ NO ☐ YES_____

MEDICATIONS

MEDICATIONS TAKEN TODAY _____

prep RESULTS _____

IV STARTED SOLUTION / AMOUNT / RATE	NEEDLE TYPE / GAUGE	LOCATION
TIME ☐ AM ☐ PM	BY	

SELF CARE ABILITIES

PATIENT AND OR SIGNIFICANT OTHER VERBALIZE KNOWLEDGE OF CURRENT MEDICATION REGIME AS PRESCRIBED BY PHYSICIAN

☐ YES   ☐ NO REFER TO NURSE'S NOTES FOR ACTION TAKEN

PATIENT AND OR SIGNIFICANT OTHER VERBALIZE UNDERSTANDING OF PROCEDURE AND EXPECTED OUTCOMES?   ☐ YES ☐ NO

PROCEDURE VERIFIED AS _____

VERIFICATION

I VERIFY THE INFORMATION I HAVE GIVEN ABOUT MY LAST FOOD/ LIQUID INTAKE IS CORRECT. I VERIFY THAT I HAVE A RIDE HOME.

SIGNATURE OF PATIENT   *(INDICATE NAME & PHONE NUMBER OF DRIVER)*

X

PRE PROCEDURE CHECK LIST   √ = YES   O = NO   — = N/A

_____ H & P	_____ LYTES	_____ IDENTIFICATION BAND ON
_____ CONSENT	_____ BILIRUBIN	_____ ALLERGY BAND ON
_____ M.D. ORDERS	_____ BUN / CREAT	_____ GLASSES / CONTACT LENSES REMOVED
_____ CONSULTS / ANESTHESIA	_____ TYPE & Rh	_____ VOIDED
_____ CBC	_____ CHEST X-RAY	_____ DENTURES REMOVED
_____ Pro time / PTT	_____ EKG	_____ OLD CHART WITH PATIENT
_____ URINALYSIS	_____ CLOTHING REMOVED & SECURED	_____ MEDS GIVEN / CHARTED
_____ URINE PREGNANCY	_____ VALUABLES TO_____	_____ INTERIM SUMMARY
		_____ MEDS SENT WITH PATIENT

ADMITTED BY RN SIGNATURE	PRINT NAME	TIME	TO PROCEDURE ROOM ☐ AM ☐ PM	RN SIGNATURE	PRINT NAME

Figure 2-2, cont'd   Same day procedure assessment form.

Admission assessment forms that include a method to assess the patient's risk for falls remind nurses not to overlook this important risk factor.

Pressure Ulcers.   One of the recurring concerns in nursing practice is the prevention of pressure ulcers. Like falls, pressure ulcers lengthen hospitalization time and increase healthcare costs and the risk of death from sepsis. Family members may equate the development of pressure ulcers with poor nursing care and initiate a lawsuit, alleging that neglect led to the skin breakdown. The following case illustrates this type of situation:

> The plaintiff, a 92-year-old woman, entered the defendant hospital in January and spent most of the next 9 months in the hospital. Within the first few weeks, her skin began to break down. Ultimately the patient developed stage IV ulcers on both hips and her sacrum, ankles, and heels. She succumbed from sepsis. The plaintiff contended that there were multiple deviations from the standard of care. Photographs of her bedsores were enlarged and shown to the jury. The jury returned a $1,130,000 verdict, with $1,000,000 awarded for pain and suffering and $130,000 as compensatory damages (Unpublished verdict, *Eason v. Interfaith Hospital,* 1998).

A number of risk factors are associated with the development of a pressure ulcer, including immobility, hypoalbuminemia, obesity, decreased hemoglobin, nutritional factors (such as inadequate dietary intake and impaired nutritional status), infection, incontinence, altered level of consciousness, and fracture. Two commonly used scales—the Norton scale and the Braden scale—which are incorporated into Figure 2-3—have been extensively tested. Their use provides a consistent format for systematically assessing risk factors for pressure ulcers. Either tool may be incorporated into the admission assessment or used on skin integrity assessment forms. Some facilities have developed a separate form for ongoing documentation of the pressure ulcer stages that can be used on admission or whenever the patient's condition deteriorates.

Documenting the condition of the patient's skin on admission and periodically thereafter is vital. The frequency with which such reassessment should be done varies with the health status of the individual. If the patient becomes less mobile or other risk factors appear, the risk of developing a pressure ulcer should be reviewed. "Accurate and complete documentation of all risk assessments ensures continuity of care and may be used as a foundation for the skin care plan" (*Pressure Ulcers in Adults,* 1992). The size (in inches or centimeters), depth, location, and appearance of any existing pressure ulcers should be described. The ulcer should be staged using the commonly accepted system presented in Box 2-2.

Some facilities are using the additional precaution of photographing all pressure ulcers found at the time of admission. Such photographs should be dated. These data may be needed if there is a question about whether a pressure ulcer developed before or during the current hospitalization. The photographs and documentation also establish a baseline to evaluate changes in skin integrity.

Suicidal Tendencies and Violence.   A third aspect of identifying the patient at risk for injury involves patients with a potential for harming themselves or others. Nurses often detect symptoms of emotional or psychiatric problems. When concern arises about the patient's emotional stability, the nurse should document the following: any information provided by the patient concerning previous psychiatric problems, treatments, or hospitalizations; the patient's perception of the situation; and the nurse's assessment of the patient's interpersonal strengths and limitations. Consider the following example:

Patient admitted with chief complaint of rectal bleeding. States he was hospitalized at State Hospital in 1993 because he wanted to kill himself. Says he still has these thoughts and keeps a loaded gun at home. Patient has been receiving outpatient counseling at local mental health clinic. Lacks insight into his problems.

Given this assessment, the nurse would identify the patient's risk for injury and initiate appropriate interventions, including notifying the physician of the patient's comments. The nursing assessment should include data about risk factors for violence. A psychotic patient or patient with a history of violence, substance abuse, or suicide attempts may be more prone to violent outbursts. Questions about these risk factors should be included in the data base. Although these factors are commonly incorporated into the data base for a patient with a psychiatric diagnosis, any patient may have these risk factors. The nursing assessment must show that the presence of signs indicating a potential for violence have been noted. If warranted by the patient's condition, further documentation should indicate that action was taken to protect the patient and others from harm.

ADMISSION ASSESSMENT

INTEGUMENTARY: ❑ WNL
Skin color within patients norm. Skin intact. Mucus membranes moist and intact. No evidence of nail changes, ecchymosis, rashes or redness.
No pain. *Identify skin changes by placing appropriate letters on figure. Refer to Scale.*

SCALE
Ecchymosis	E	Rash	RH
Reddened	R	Scars	S
Laceration	L	Incision	I
Abrasion	A	Amputation	X
Blisters	B	Avulsion	V
Ulcers	U	Petecheiae	P

Skin color: ❑ Pale ❑ Cyanotic ❑ Jaundiced ❑ Mottled ❑ Ruddy
Turgor: ❑ Adequate ❑ Poor
Nails: ❑ Clubbing ❑ Thickened ❑ Discolored
Mouth/Lips: ❑ Lesions ❑ Bleeding gums
Describe Skin and mucus membrane abnormalities:
If pressure ulcer present, describe size (width, length, depth, color, drainage, skin intact or broken)
_____
_____
_____
_____

BRADEN SCALE FOR PREDICTING ULCER RISK

CATERGORY	CRITERIA
Sensory Perception: Ability to respond meaningfully to pressure-related discomfort	1. Completely Limited 2. Very Limited 3. Slightly Limited 4. No Impairment
Moisture: Degree to which skin is exposed to moisture	1. Constantly Moist 2. Moist 3. Occasionally Moist 4. Rarely Moist
Activity: Degree of physical activity	1. Bedfast 2. Chairfast 3. Walks Occasionally 4. Walks Frequently
Mobility: Ability to change and control body position	1. Completely Immobile 2. Very Limited 3. Slightly Limited 4. No Limitations
Nutrition: Usual food intake pattern	1. Very Poor 2. Probably Inadequate 3. Adequate 4. Excellent
Friction and Shear:	1. Problem 2. Potential Problem 3. No Apparent Problem

TOTAL SCORE: _____

CONSULT
If any of the following are checked, obtain an ET nurse consult:
❑ Braden Score ≤ 16
❑ New or established ostomy or urinary diversion
❑ Hx of urinary incontinence
❑ Pt. weight of > 350 lbs.

Important: For a new ostomy, place consult preoperatively for marking of ostomy site by ET nurse.
Consult placed by: _____
Date/Time: _____

Reassess prn as status changes and record score on flow sheet.

FUNCTIONAL ASSESSMENT
If patient is independent in all areas, check ❑ WNL

	Independent	Needs Assistance	Dependent
Bathing			
Dressing			
Toileting			
Gait / Mobility			
Balance			
Eating			
Communication of needs			
Swallowing			

If any of the above are new problems and/or improvement in the area is a goal by the patient or family, request a Rehab consult.

CONSULT
Occupational Therapy: Bathing, Dressing, Toileting
Physical Therapy: Gait/Mobility
Speech Therapy: Communication of needs, Swallowing

Consult requested by: _____
Date/Time: _____

CONSULT
If any of the following are checked, obtain Discharge Planning Consult:
❑ Unexplained bruises, injuries
❑ Unkempt, dirty, poor hygiene
❑ Behavior clues which may indicate suspected abuse/neglect/domestic violence.
See policy regarding reporting abuse/neglect.

Consult placed by: _____
Date/Time: _____

Risk for Fall Assessment
❑ No need identified
❑ History of recent fall
❑ Difficulty with mobility
❑ Confused, altered mental state
❑ Weakness, vertigo, fainting
❑ Sensory perception deterioration: (speech, hearing, sight)
❑ Noncompliant behavior, substance abuse

If any of the above are identified, implement Risk for Fall Precautions per "Safety Precaution for Patients at High Risk" policy.

Date implemented: _____
Initials: _____

Mission
A MEMBER OF THE MISSION + ST. JOSEPH'S HEALTH SYSTEM

Adult/Geriatric Patient History and General Information
Readmissions within 30 days: Update

Figure 2-3 Braden scale for identifying risk for skin breakdown and section to document cues for abuse. (Courtesy Mission and St. Joseph's Health System, Asheville, NC.)

Box 2-2

Stages of Pressure Sores

Stage I

Nonblanchable erythema of intact skin; the heralding lesion of skin ulceration. *Note:* Reactive hyperemia normally can be expected to be present for one half to three fourths as long as the pressure-occluded blood flow to the area (*Pressure ulcers in adults,* 1992). This should not be confused with a Stage I pressure ulcer.

Stage II

Partial-thickness skin loss involving epidermis and/or dermis. The ulcer is superficial and shows symptoms such as an abrasion, blister, or shallow crater.

Stage III

Full-thickness skin loss involving damage or necrosis of subcutaneous tissue that may extend down to, but not through, underlying fascia. The ulcer shows symptoms such as a deep crater with or without undermining of adjacent tissue.

Stage IV

Full-thickness skin loss with extensive, destructive tissue necrosis or damage to underlying muscle, bone, or supporting structures such as a tendon or joint capsule. *Note:* Undermining and sinus tracts may also be associated with Stage IV pressure ulcers.

Clinical Practice Guidelines: Pressure ulcers in adults, 1992, Rockville, Md, 1992, Department of Health and Human Services.

Tips for Charting

Documentation should include the following (Calfee, 1996):

- Direct quotations from the patient, family, or visitors related to suicidal thoughts, actions, and motives
- Data gathered about the patient's risk factors for suicide
- Actions taken to remove items that could harm the patient
- Individuals who were notified about the concerns, such as the attending physician or supervisor

In the following case the assessment of the healthcare workers was a significant factor in a patient's claim that he was unjustly committed to a psychiatric facility:

> The plaintiff was a 25-year-old man who worked as a medical records clerk. He was involuntarily committed to the defendant's psychiatric hospital. He was released 34 days later after a court hearing. The plaintiff claimed that the applicable laws required him to be mentally ill to be committed and that the defendants had no evidence of mental illness to justify his commitment. The defendant contended that the plaintiff refused to cooperate with testing and evaluations; therefore the hospital could only look at the plaintiff's actions in making a determination about his

mental state. The defendants claimed that the plaintiff exhibited signs of mental illness. A defense verdict was reached (Laska, 1998, p. 20).

It is likely that the observations of the nurses and doctors documented in the medical record were used to justify this patient's commitment.

Abuse. People of all ages may be the victims of abuse, from young children to the elderly. Abuse may fit into one of four categories: physical, psychological, financial, or neglect (Lynch, 1997). Nurses encounter victims of abuse in a variety of settings, including the office, the home, the workplace, the emergency department, and acute and long-term care settings. Over the course of the last several years, Joint Commission standards have highlighted the need to identify possible victims of abuse. The 1997 standards define the need to use criteria developed by the hospital in identifying possible victims of abuse and to recognize that these victims have special needs relative to the assessment process. The criteria should focus on observable evidence and not be based on allegation alone. The following situations should be addressed: physical assault, rape or other sexual molestation, domestic abuse, and abuse or neglect of children and elders (JCAHO, 1996).

In general, those who are most likely to be abused are dependent on the abuser. Risk factors for elder abuse include the following: both the victim and the abuser having a history of mental illness; shared living arrangements; family history of violence; dependency; and lack of financial resources. Poor health and cognitive impairment on the part of the victim can also contribute to the risks (Lynch, 1997). The abuser may be under unusual stress or have psychiatric or substance-abuse problems. Adult victims of abuse are typically isolated from contact with others who would intervene if they knew about the abuse. The nurse should suspect abuse whenever the patient refers to violence in the home or has injuries inconsistent with the explanation of the patient or family. Bruises in areas covered by clothing, cigarette burns, and unusual fractures may raise the suspicion of abuse. Abused young children may be more likely to be underweight and anemic from neglect. The patient's interactions with family members should be observed, because the victim may exhibit fear in the presence of the abuser. In these situations, trying to interview the patient privately is advisable. The nurse should look for evasion when the patient or family is questioned about how the injury occurred. The patient's explanations about the cause of the physical problems should be documented.

The description of the nature of the injuries and the patient's behavior should be precise. For example:

(Adult female) patient has a variety of yellow-green and black-blue bruises over her breasts and abdomen. Patient avoided eye contact and said she was injured when she walked into a door.

The integumentary section of the assessment form should be used to document the size, shape, and appearance of bruises, lacerations, or injuries in unusual areas such as the neck or genitals. Look for and document pattern injuries that are left when an object used to strike a person leaves an imprint, or parallel injuries, such as bruises on both arms in the same area. Burns should be described; for example, cigarette, iron, rope and immersion burns may be noted (Lynch, 1997). Many facilities include a specific section on the admission assessment form that provides an area to document any concerns about abuse or neglect (see Figure 2-3).

Photographs are sometimes taken with the patient's permission to preserve evidence of the appearance of the bruises. Be sure to fulfill legal obligations to report suspected cases of abuse. The medical record should include the following: consents from the patient, parent, or legal guardian for collection of information and evidence, as needed; data regarding notification of authorities; and referrals made to community agencies.

Frost and Willette (1994) studied medical records of home care patients in a search for documentation regarding patients who were at risk for abuse and neglect. They concluded that providing a specific area on the assessment form often elicited one or more factors that described increased vulnerability of the patient. The resources and abilities of the individual to deal with these problem areas were frequently not noted, however. The authors recommended providing a space on the assessment form that asks the nurse to address physiological, mental, psychological, caregiver, interpersonal, and other environmental factors that may contribute to the increased risk of a vulnerable adult. Furthermore, the authors recommended that the assessment of environmental factors, the analysis of resources, and the evaluation of the assistance that was provided to the patient and caregiver by those resources would provide more information. The healthcare provider could use this information to determine whether or not the level of risk warranted a nursing diagnosis in this area and whether or not intervention was needed.

Substance Abuse. The abuse of substances is an increasingly common problem in our society. Patients with substance-abuse problems may be encountered in all areas of nursing care. Substances that are commonly abused include narcotics, sedatives, alcohol, and street drugs. The desire to use narcotics may be based on positive reinforcement (the desire for a high) or negative reinforcement (the desire to alleviate pain or discomfort, including that of withdrawal). Nonmedical use of sedatives and tranquilizers has been reported in 3.5% and 5.1% of the population, respectively. Sedatives may be addictive. For example, use of a benzodiazepine (antianxiety drug), especially Xanax, even at the therapeutic dosage for a month or more can produce physical dependence (Trachtenberg, Fleming, 1994).

The dimensions of this issue are enormous. The 10% of the population who drink the most heavily accounts for 50% of the alcohol consumed in the United States. Many of the medications that elderly patients take, including antidepressants and tranquilizers, interact with alcohol, often synergistically. Such interactions can result in aspiration pneumonia, falls, hip fractures, and motor vehicle accidents. Substance abuse is often misdiagnosed in the elderly because symptoms such as changes in cognition, behavior, or physical functioning tend to be attributed inaccurately to an underlying medical condition or simply old age. The leading cause of death among people between 15 and 24 years old is violence, including accidents, homicides, and suicides. Many of these deaths can be attributed to the use of drugs and alcohol.

Part of the assessment process includes inquiring about drug and alcohol use. The patient is far more likely to respond to questions regarding drugs if the nurse remains empathic, respectful, and nonjudgmental. When using a direct approach the nurse should ask specifically about the amounts and frequency of alcohol use and other drug use in the past month, week, and day. Details should be documented, including how old the patient was when the substances were first used, the duration and intensity of use, and patterns and consequences of use. Patterns of use may include loss of control over the amount or frequency of use, inability to be abstinent, and relapses (JCAHO, 1996).

If the patient denies recent use, asking about previous history to determine whether the patient has ever abused alcohol or used other drugs is appropriate. Even currently substance-abusing clients in denial may be able to reveal excessive substance use in the distant past. Use of multiple prescriptions from several doctors and the use of illicit drugs should be specifically investigated. Key signs of substance abuse include consumption of five or more drinks at a time, or use of marijuana more than five times in the client's life. (Statistically, using marijuana more than five times seems to correlate with an increased likelihood of substance abuse.)

Four key questions to ask include the following:

1. Have you felt that you ought to cut down on your drinking or drug use?
2. Have people annoyed you by criticizing your drinking or drug use?
3. Have you felt bad or guilty about your drinking or drug use?
4. Have you ever had a drink or used drugs first thing in the morning (eye opener) to steady your nerves, get rid of a hangover, or get the day started?

Use interview techniques to build rapport and minimize the patient's defensiveness. Eventually the patient may reveal problems such as marital difficulties of health, legal, or financial trouble, which may signify a drug or alcohol problem. Medical consequences of alcohol and drug use should be documented. Determine and document the patient's level of insight about the correlation between the medical complications of substance abuse and the use of substances. Responding to this information with a sympathetic approach may encourage a considerable degree of openness in the patient.

The patient may be asked about the effects of drug or alcohol use on the patient's life. Problems may exist with his or her health, family, job, or financial status or with the legal system. The patient may admit to a history of blackouts or motor vehicle accidents. Document information regarding the treatment the patient has received for the abuse problem and the effectiveness of the treatment.

The medical records should be carefully evaluated when there is a suspicion of drug-seeking behavior. Characteristics that correlate with abuse or suspected abuse, according to the *Journal of Pain Symptom Management* (1996), include the following:

- Doctor shopping
- Prescription loss
- Visiting without an appointment
- Frequent calls to the physician's office
- Multiple drug intolerances or "allergies"
- Frequent requests for drug escalation

Clues in the Medical Records

Drug-seeking behavior may be suspected when a pattern of entries like these—based on actual medical records—are found in office or clinic records:

- Patient states he lost his bottle of Percodan (oxycodone) and needs a new prescription.
- Patient states she accidentally spilled her Percocet/Tylox on the floor and needs a new prescription.
- Patient wants a new prescription for MSContin (morphine) because her husband has been taking her supply.
- Pharmacy called: When patient brought script to drug store, it looked like the number "1" was changed to "4". They refused to fill prescription. Dr. Kipp was informed.
- Patient arrived without an appointment. He stated his back pain was severe and he wanted an injection for pain.
- Mr. Pille has called the office three times in the last three days seeking a new prescription for pain medication. He states the Tylenol #3 (acetaminophen with codeine, 15 mg) does not work with codeine and he would like to have a script for Percodan (oxycodone).
- Mr. King is allergic to Demerol (meperidine), morphine, Talwin (pentazocine) and Nubain (nalbuphine).
- Mrs. Swing says she would like to have a prescription for Percocet/Tylox, 100 tabs, with 6 refills.

Elements of a Psychosocial Assessment

When appropriate, a psychosocial assessment should be performed. This process would include information about the following (JCAHO, 1996):

- Motivation to change or accept treatment
- Obstacles or resources that would impact recovery, including substance abuse by other family members
- Religious and spiritual beliefs
- A history of physical or sexual abuse
- Sexual history and orientation
- Leisure and recreational activities and childhood history
- Military service and financial status
- The social, peer-group, and environmental setting from which the patient comes
- Family circumstances, including the composition of the family group
- Current living situation
- Other social, ethnic, cultural, health, and emotional factors

Potential for Self-Care Following Discharge

Assessment and documentation of discharge-planning needs begin at the initial encounter with the patient and continue throughout the provision of care. It is important to identify the patients who are most likely to need assistance with discharge planning. A high-risk group in one facility may not be so in another facility. The types of patients and the services they require vary with location, socioeconomic status, and support systems of the populations served by the facility. These factors should be taken into account when discharge-planning questions are designed and incorporated into assessment tools. Some agencies include this assessment as part of the initial data base, whereas others have separate discharge-planning assessment forms (Figure 2-4).

Answers to the questions in Box 2-3 are usually documented as part of the initial assessment. When the patient is oriented and articulate, eliciting this information is relatively easy. Assessment of confused, comatose, or chronically ill patients who have little awareness of how to care for themselves can pose a bigger challenge. Additional sources of information, such as family members or significant others, are usually needed to complete the data base and document discharge needs. When gathering information from sources other than the patient the nurse should clearly document the name of the person, the data provided by the person, and the person's relationship with the patient; for example:

Son, Sam Davis, states the patient is being given the following medications at home: Lasix, 40 mg qd; Digoxin, 0.25 mg qd; and Humulin NPH Insulin, 40 units at 0730 hours and 10 units at 1700 hours.

LAFAYETTE HOME HOSPITAL, INC.
LAFAYETTE, INDIANA

Stamp and Room

HEALTH CARE TEAM DISCHARGE SCREEN FOR NICU, NSY, L/D, POST PARTUM
(Circle Points, Date and Update if applicable)

CIRCLE POINTS	LIVING ARRANGEMENT	CIRCLE POINTS	SOCIAL STATUS
5	Single Parent	5	Non Compliant
5	Mother is 18 or under	5	Behavioral problems
10	Disabled or mentally retarded parent	5	Bonding problem
5	Unemployed parent/low economic situation	20	Adoption of newborn
5	Home Environment (Absence of heat, elect., etc)	5	Psycho-Social problems
5	Others	20	Suspected abuse/neglect
CIRCLE POINTS	**DIAGNOSTIC GROUP**	20	< 16 year old mother
	Birth Complication	5	Late or no prenatal care
5	a) Maternal	5	Admitted to NICU
5	b) Infant, including anomalies, < 33 wks GA	5	Others
5	Others	--10	Community Health Clinic Pt.

Instruction:		POINTS	REFERRAL SENT/DATE	NO REFERRAL INDICATE DATE	SIGNATURE
Add all circled points and determine Discharge Risk Factor High Risk Patient ≥ 20 points: Send referral to Social Work via SMS Low Risk Patients < 20 points: Nursing intervention Request Social Work from MD if indicated					

Figure 2-4 Discharge screen. (Courtesy Lafayette Home Hospital, Lafayette, Ind.)

Box 2-3

Discharge Planning Factors

- How well has the patient been coping with a chronic health problem?
- In what type of environment does the patient live?
- Where is the patient's bedroom located in relation to stairs?
- Is the patient homeless?
- Is running water available to the patient?
- Do stairs lead up to the house?
- Who is available to help the patient manage self-care?
- Is the patient responsible for the care of another person, such as an elderly parent or small child? If so, what arrangements may need to be made to assist this individual?
- Where will the patient go after discharge?
- Does the individual know how to use the community resources such as Meals on Wheels, visiting nurses, or community health centers?

Initial assessment forms usually include a section for documentation of previous admissions. If a patient states that he or she was recently hospitalized, it is important to gather additional information by reviewing old charts. Assessment of discharge needs is particularly important when a patient has been readmitted within a short time for the same condition. Reimbursement problems may result if a regulatory group, such as a peer review organization, determines that faulty discharge planning or premature discharge was a factor in the readmission. The results of the previous discharge plan, the stability of the patient's health, the patient's understanding of self-care, and the patient's knowledge of community resources should be evaluated. In addition, the patient who has no family or friends to depend on for support may need referral for discharge planning.

The documentation of self-care abilities provides information about the patient's needs to those involved in discharge planning. The initial assessment form provides a central source of information needed for discharge planning. A variety of healthcare professionals use these data, including nurses, physicians, dietitians, social workers, discharge planners, and therapists. With all information centrally located, health workers can easily retrieve data through the clinical record. The documentation of discharge planning, which follows the assessment of discharge needs, is discussed in Chapter 3.

Advance Directives

Definitions

When a patient is no longer competent, it may be possible to establish his or her wishes by consulting documents such as advance directives. There are two types of advance directives: *treatment directives,* which are also called

"living wills," and *appointment directives,* which are also called power of attorney or healthcare proxies. Living wills allow a competent adult to give directions for future care in the event that the person is incapacitated by terminal illness or impending death. The directions are limited to the instructions in the document. A *medical power of attorney* (also called a *healthcare proxy*) appoints a trusted person, usually a relative or close friend, to make medical decisions for the patient if the patient becomes incapacitated. This individual can clarify living wills or make decisions independent of the patient's wishes (Haynor, 1998).

Legal Requirements

Federal legislation called the *Patient's Self-Determination Act (PSDA),* which became effective in 1991, requires hospitals, long-term care facilities, home health, hospice, and other eligible programs such as HMOs to provide information regarding the patient's rights at the time of admission. These state laws provide the right to make decisions concerning acceptance or refusal of treatment and the patient with the right to give advance directives. The agency is required to provide information concerning its implementation of such patient's rights and to document any such declaration in the patient's medical records. The provision of care cannot be contingent upon whether or not the patient has executed an advance directive (*Risk management handbook for living wills,* 1992). In addition, federal law requires that the agency provide staff and community education on issues concerning advance directives.

Questioning a patient on admission as to the existence of any advance directives has become common practice for a healthcare facility. If the patient or family has a living will or a healthcare proxy, this information should be provided and kept on file. On subsequent admissions the patient maybe asked to verify that these records are still valid. "Documenting this process is a critical step in promoting compliance with the patient's wishes and it may be necessary for reimbursement as well" (Haynor, 1998, p. 27). A policy or procedure should be in place to alert healthcare professionals to the existence of advance directives. A computer alert or a manual system may contain this information. The living will or healthcare directive should be inspected for the following:

- The form should be dated and signed.
- The form should be witnessed or notarized.
- The patient should have specified directions for a terminal condition.
- The patient should confirm that the information is current (if the directive came from a previous medical record).
- Additional instructions should be included regarding specific treatment (for example, intubation, dialysis, surgery, antibiotics, mechanical ventilation, or do not resuscitate orders).

If the patient has a form specifying a power of attorney for health care decisions, it should be reviewed for the following:

- The form should be dated and signed.
- The form should be witnessed or notarized.
- The power of attorney should cover health care decisions (not just financial affairs).
- The patient should confirm that the information is current (if the form came from a previous medical record).
- The power of attorney should be durable (that is, the agent's authority will not end if the patient becomes incapacitated).
- Any specifics should be defined stating which powers are given or are limited (Stubbs, 1995).

Absence of Advance Directives

The more likely situation that a nurse will encounter is the absence of an advance directive. In a recent study of about 9000 patients, investigators found that only 10% of the patients had written advance directives. When patients did have an advance directive, 75% of the physicians were unaware that it existed—even though it was part of the patient's medical records. Only 3% of the advance directives were specific enough to affect care decisions. If the patient does not have an advance directive, the nurse should encourage the patient to state his or her wishes to the healthcare providers and family. In most states the documentation in the medical record of a competent patient's wishes is as valid as a written living will (Haynor, 1998); for example:

> Patient states that, if his heart stops suddenly, he wants to be "allowed to die without a resuscitation effort."

The liability issues surrounding advance directives relate to the failure to carry out the requirements of the law, including the following: failure to adequately supervise the use of informational materials and statements of the staff concerning advance directives; coercing the patient or resident to make an advance directive; and accepting advance directives made under undue influence by a third party or by someone who is mentally incompetent.

As with informed consent, an advance directive may be revoked at any time—in writing, orally, or by any action that indicates that the patient no longer wants the advance directive to be in effect. The advance directive goes into effect after it has been given to the agency and the attending physician has determined that the patient lacks decision-making ability.

Tips for Charting

1. If providing information about advance directives *is the responsibility of the nursing staff in the facility,* the nurse should document the following: that an inquiry was made about the existence of an advance directive; that the location of the advance directive is known; and that information was provided about advance directives if the patient requested it. Many facilities have incorporated information about advance directives into the admission data base (Figures 2-5 and 2-6).

2. If the patient or resident is mentally incompetent, the nurse should determine whether the patient has a healthcare proxy who might know of the existence of an advance directive and be able to supply a copy. In the absence of the family or healthcare proxy the nurse should document a decision not to provide information to the mentally incompetent patient/resident.

3. If the nurse notices evidence of undue influence on the patient's decisions regarding treatment, it should be documented.

4. If the patient becomes distraught by a discussion of advance directives, the nurse should provide the required information as outlined but offer an opportunity for further discussion or counseling at a later date. The patient's reaction should be recorded in the medical record.

5. The nurse should document his or her evaluation of the patient's comprehension of information relating to advance directives.

6. If the patient was referred to others for additional information about advance directives, document the referral.

7. If the competent patient has a change of heart about the provisions of the advance directive, this document can be changed at any time. The nurse should document any comments made by the patient, such as "I want to change my advance directive," and follow through as indicated.

8. The nurse should include written evidence of the patient's wishes, such as copies of advance directives, in the clinical record. Oral evidence can be included in the form of letters written by people who heard the patient make relevant statements.

9. The nurse should ensure that this evidence is described in detail, including the dates of the conversation, the participants, the circumstances, and the types of treatment and medical conditions discussed.

Patient and Family Education Needs

The assessment of learning needs provides the foundation for the individualized teaching plan. The data collected during the first interaction with the patient are supplemented and validated by subsequent encounters with the patient. To determine the appropriate approach for teaching, the patient's vocabulary and verbal content used when answering questions should be noted. The patient's body language and willingness to communicate may also help determine medical and nursing needs.

The following three factors are important in the documentation of assessed learning needs:

1. *Health beliefs, attitudes,* and *social factors* may help or hinder the patient's ability to follow the medical

ACTIVITY / SELF-CARE	ACTIVITY / SELF-CARE	**Mobility Status** ☐ Ambulatory ☐ Assist Needed _____ ☐ Wheelchair ☐ Bedrest **Assistive Devices** ☐ No ☐ Yes (describe)_____ **Comments** _____ _____ **Activities of Daily Living That Need Assistance** ☐ Feeding ☐ Grooming ☐ Toileting ☐ Other ☐ Bathing ☐ **NONE** ☐ Dressing

Mobility Status
☐ Ambulatory
☐ Assist Needed _____
☐ Wheelchair
☐ Bedrest

Activities of Daily Living That Need Assistance
☐ Feeding   ☐ Grooming
☐ Toileting   ☐ Other
☐ Bathing   ☐ **NONE**
☐ Dressing

Assistive Devices   ☐ No   ☐ Yes (describe)_____
Comments _____
_____

REST / SLEEP

Sleep
☐ Difficulty falling asleep
☐ Difficulty staying asleep
☐ Not rested after sleep

☐ Other _____
☐ **No Problem**
How long do you usually sleep? _____
What helps you sleep? _____

Comments _____

INFECTION

Recent exposure to communicable diseases   ☐ No   ☐ Yes (describe) _____
Comments _____

NURSING PSYCHOSOCIAL ASSESSMENT

EMOTIONAL NEEDS / ROLE / COPING

What concerns you most about your illness/hospitalization? _____
_____

How does your illness/hospitalization affect your family/significant others? _____
_____

Who are your resources for emotional support?   ☐ Spouse   ☐ Other _____
                                                 ☐ Family   ☐ NONE
Marital Status   ☐ Single   ☐ Married   ☐ Widowed   ☐ Divorced   ☐ Separated
Children   ☐ No   ☐ Yes   Number _____   Ages _____
Do you have any religious requests during this hospitalization?   ☐ No   ☐ Yes, describe _____

KNOWLEDGE DEFICIT / TEACHING / DISCHARGE

What do you know about your present illness? (describe)_____
_____

What further information would you like about your present illness?   ☐ NONE   ☐ Yes _____
_____

How long do you expect to be in the hospital? _____
When you leave the hospital, where will you stay?   ☐ Home Alone   ☐ Nursing Home   ☐ with Family/Others
☐ Hospice   ☐ Rehabilitation Facility   ☐ Unsure   ☐ Other _____
Potential referrals for discharge
☐ Social Service   ☐ Religion & Health   ☐ Support/Self-help Groups
☐ Physical Therapy   ☐ Home Health Service   ☐ Other _____
☐ Dietician   ☐ NONE
Potential self-care/equipment needs   ☐ No   ☐ Yes, describe _____
Comments _____

Advance Directives
Do you have a Durable Power of Attorney for Healthcare named?   ☐ No   ☐ Yes (name) _____
_____

Do you have a Living Will?   ☐ No   ☐ Yes   **Are you an Organ Donor?**   ☐ No   ☐ Yes
Referral Made to _____

Is your family aware of this hospital admission?   ☐ No   ☐ Yes_____

Initials of RN completing Nursing Admission Assessment _____ Date _____ Time _____

Figure 2-5 Portion of an admission assessment form that includes information on advance directives. (Courtesy EHS Trinity Hospital, Chicago.)

HOSPITALIZATION/SURGERY WHICH OCCURRED DURING LAST ADMISSION

Completed by:_____ Date/Time_____

Include dates _____
_____
_____
_____
_____

PSYCHOSOCIAL / SPIRITUAL / CULTURAL / SELF PERCEPTION Completed by:_____ Date/Time_____
❏ No Changes

The following changes are noted: _____
_____
_____
_____
_____

CONSULT ❏ Pt. request chaplain visit

Chaplain consult placed by: _____ Date/Time_____

HEALTH PERCEPTION / HEALTH PRACTICES   ❏ No Changes   Completed by:_____ Date/Time_____

The following changes are noted: _____
_____
_____
_____
_____

CONSULT This is a smoke free hospital. Would you like assistance with this during your stay? ❏ Yes ❏ No

Consult placed with Smoking Cessation Program by: _____Date/Time_____

PATIENT SELF DETERMINATION ACT CHECKLIST   ❏ No Changes   Completed by:_____ Date/Time_____

The following changes in the Living Will and/or Health Care Power of Attorney are noted: _____
_____
_____

If patient has Living Will, is a copy on the chart?   ❏ Yes ❏ No   **Are you an organ donor? ❏ Yes ❏ No**
If patient has Health Care Power of Attorney, is a copy on the chart?   ❏ Yes ❏ No   **❏ Undecided**
                                                                                         ❏ Would like more information.
What else do we need to know about your wishes? _____
_____

RESPIRATORY ❏ No Changes   Completed by:_____ Date/Time_____

The following changes are noted: _____
_____
_____
_____

CONSULT **OBTAIN RESPIRATORY CONSULT for items checked below:**   (Not applicable to Critical Care)

Use at home: ❏ Chest PT ❏ BIPAP/CPAP: settings: _____ ❏ Home Ventilator ❏ Transtracheal O_2

Consult placed by:_____ Date/Time_____

Mission
A Member of the Mission + St. Joseph's Health System
Adult/Geriatric Patient History
and General Information
Readmissions within 30 days: Update

Figure 2-6 Portion of an admission assessment form that includes information on advance directives. (Courtesy Mission and St. Joseph's Health System, Asheville, NC.)

regimen. Examples of factors that may *help* the patient follow treatment recommendations include a willingness to follow the healthcare regimen, understanding from a supportive family, and the individual's belief that he or she is in control of his or her own destiny. Examples of factors that may *hinder* the ability to follow treatment recommendations include superstitions, poverty, language barriers, cultural practices, illiteracy, old wives' tales, and the belief that fate and luck control one's destiny instead of the individual. These could be documented in the following manner:

Health beliefs	Patient believes that copper bracelets reduce arthritis symptoms and refuses to take antiinflammatory agents.
Attitudes	Patient states that there is no point in learning how to do dialysis at home because he or she is going to die anyway.
Social factors	(Adult) patient has completed third grade and is unable to read.

2. *The ability to learn, follow directions, and recall information* may be hindered by several factors, including the effects of aging, sensory deficits, cognitive limitations, the effects of sedation and analgesics, sleep deprivation, pain, stress, memory loss, limited attention span, impaired judgment, and sensory overload. These could be documented in the following manner:

Ability to learn and follow directions	Patient is a college graduate who owns a dry cleaning business. Patient is hard of hearing and does not have a hearing aid with her.
Ability to recall information	Patient is unable to recall names or types of medications she is taking. Patient states that physician told her what she is taking, but that she can never remember these details.

3. *Readiness to learn about condition, self-care measures, and priority learning needs* may be hindered by several factors, including lack of motivation, denial of the need to learn, substance abuse, self-destructive patterns, depression, anxiety, stress, fear of change, and social isolation. These could be documented in the following manner:

Readiness to learn	Patient says she wants to learn how to manage diabetes.
Self-care measures	Patient states that he does not want to learn how to change colostomy bag, saying, "My daughter takes care of that."
Priority of learning needs	Patient says she is very interested in finding out how to do CPR for the sake of her infant.

Box 2-4

Elements to Document When Assessing Patient Education Needs

- *Chief complaint:* knowledge of disease process, reason for seeking health care; awareness of signs and symptoms as they relate to primary diagnosis
- *Diet:* knowledge of dietary restrictions, adherence to diet
- *Medications:* ability to describe medications, including purpose, schedule, and side effects; adherence to medication regimen; use of over-the-counter medications or illegal drugs
- *Physical activity:* awareness of the impact of activity on disease as well as how disease affects lifestyle
- *Treatments:* ability of the patient or significant other to manage continuing care needs after discharge

---

Documentation of patient education needs. The assessment of learning needs is documented on the initial assessment form. Documentation continues on the progress notes or patient education flowsheet as new information is gained. The key points that should be documented are listed in Box 2-4.

The description of patient-education needs may be documented in appropriate sections of the initial assessment form (decentralized documentation) or in one section labeled "Teaching Needs" (centralized documentation). With *decentralized* charting of teaching needs, pertinent comments can be placed in specific categories of data. However, in this approach the information that identifies learning needs is scattered throughout the form, and the information must be retrieved from several places to develop a teaching plan. *Centralized* charting of teaching needs is typically presented as a summary statement at the end of an assessment form. The section labeled "Teaching Needs" acts as a cue to remind the nurse to address patient education needs. Using this format the nurse can synthesize all the information provided by the patient and identify the high-priority teaching needs. If this format is used, sufficient space for documentation must be included on the form.

Patient education needs that are identified after admission to the hospital or after care is initiated may be documented in progress notes or on a centralized form. Cordell and Smith-Blair (1994) described a centralized patient education form that was divided into three sections: educational assessment, educational goals, and knowledge or skill criteria to be met by discharge. Preprinted forms were developed for teaching plans used most frequently at the hospital. The authors found that documentation of patient education increased dramatically after the implementation of the forms.

Chapter 3 provides more information on documentation of the teaching plan. Evaluation of patient education is discussed in Chapter 5.

FORMAT FOR ADMISSION ASSESSMENT FORMS

Admission assessment forms are traditionally designed to gather information according to body systems. Assessment based on body systems flows from the medical model of health care. This is a physician-oriented way of perceiving a patient as a biophysical being with an illness in one or more body systems. The body systems typically evaluated include the following:

- Ears, eyes, nose, and throat
- Respiratory
- Integumentary
- Reproductive
- Genitourinary
- Cardiovascular
- Musculoskeletal
- Neurologic
- Gastrointestinal

Formats

Admission assessment formats usually fit into one of three designs: open-ended assessment, closed-ended assessment, or physical assessment.

Open-Ended

A typical format is to list the system followed by a blank line in which the nurse enters information about the patient's specific complaints as well as the symptoms the patient denies having. Figure 2-7 shows a portion of an open-ended body systems form. This approach is based on the assumption that the nurse is knowledgeable about the types of questions to be asked for each category. A benefit of this type of format is that the nurse can record information specific to the patient with the most efficient use of space.

One of the drawbacks of the open-ended assessment approach is that the nurse's questions will vary according to his or her knowledge. The form provides no cues as to what type of information should be obtained for each body system. In addition, filling in a blank line is more time-consuming than checking off a series of boxes. North and Serkes (1996) reported that half of the 48 nursing admission assessment forms they studied were incompletely filled out. They commented that the nursing staff had difficulty preparing the forms because of a lack of clarity about what inquiries should be made and because of the many narrative entries that were required. They cited specific problems such as lack of focus in data collection, absent or incomplete problem lists, failure to identify priorities for care during the current hospitalization, and lack of linkage between the patient's initial care plan and the problems that were found on the admission assessment

form. In fairness, many of these issues can be associated with other formats as well.

Closed-Ended

Another approach to structuring the admission assessment is an assessment form containing specific cues or questions designed to assess each body system (Figure 2-8). The form usually contains a number of symptoms for each body system, each with an accompanying box to check if the symptoms are present. The form typically includes a box to be checked if the patient denies having problems with that particular body system. In addition, space should be provided for a detailed description if the patient confirms that specific symptoms are present in that system. Some assessment forms combine closed-ended and open-ended formats.

Physical Assessment

As nurses learned physical assessment skills the initial data bases began providing space to document their findings. Recent body systems assessment forms provide spaces for documenting physical assessment findings. A format that works well is to divide the page into two columns. The history associated with each body system is documented on one side of the page, and physical assessment findings are described on the other. A further refinement of this format with the normal or expected findings associated with each body system listed, is shown in Figure 2-9. In such a form the nurse documents only the deviations from normal. Charting by exception, which incorporates this type of assessment form, is described in more detail in Chapter 7.

Nursing Model

Nursing is directed toward assessing the patient's biophysical, psychosocial, psychological, environmental, learning, and discharge planning needs. One drawback of the medical model is that using it to assess areas of nursing responsibility and deriving nursing diagnoses is difficult. The nurse must manipulate the data, reorganize it, and use it to identify the most important nursing diagnoses. In the 1980s nurses began to recognize that assessment forms could be based on a nursing model using nursing diagnoses.

The term *nursing diagnosis* first appeared in the general nursing literature in the 1950s. During the 1960s few references to nursing diagnosis could be found in the literature. By the 1970s nurses recognized the need for a frame of reference for nursing diagnosis. The North American Nursing Diagnosis Association (NANDA) met for the first time in 1973 to create a nursing diagnosis language. At this time the literature began to support the concept of nursing diagnosis and encourage its application in clinical practice and education. The years since 1975 have been spent developing and refining nursing diagnoses,

Text continued on p. 31

GENITOURINARY   ❑ No Changes   Completed by:_____   Date/Time_____

The following changes are noted: _____
_____
_____
_____
_____

ENDOCRINE DISORDERS   ❑ No Changes   Completed by:_____   Date/Time_____

The following changes are noted: _____
_____
_____
_____
_____

CONSULT — **If any of the following are checked, obtain a diabetic nurse consult:**
❑ Newly diagnosed diabetic   ❑ History of not adhering to prescribed treatment   ❑ Changing from oral agent to insulin
❑ Lack of financial resources to manage diabetes
Consult placed by:_____Date/Time:_____

CANCER   ❑ No Changes   Completed by:_____   Date/Time_____

The following changes are noted: _____
_____
_____
_____
_____

HEMATOLOGIC DISORDERS/INFECTIOUS DISEASE   ❑ No Changes   Completed by:_____   Date/Time_____

The following changes are noted: _____
_____
_____
_____
_____

SPEECH   ❑ No Changes   Completed by:_____   Date/Time_____

The following changes are noted: _____
_____
_____

VISION   ❑ No Changes   Completed by:_____   Date/Time_____

The following changes are noted: _____
_____

HEARING   ❑ No Changes   Completed by:_____   Date/Time_____

The following changes are noted: _____
_____
_____

Mission
A Member of the Mission + St. Joseph's Health System
**Adult/Geriatric Patient History
and General Information
Readmissions within 30 days: Update**

Figure 2-7   Open-ended admission assessment. (Courtesy Mission and St. Joseph's Health System, Asheville, NC.)

GASTROINTESTINAL/GENITO URINARY

Diet at home: ☐Regular_____ ☐Fluid restriction_____/24 hours ☐Other_____

Supplement: ☐Yes ☐No

Appetite: ☐Good ☐Fair ☐Poor

Weight: ☐No Change ☐Gain ☐Loss ☐How much_____ Time frame_____

Oral mucosa: ☐Healthy color ☐Coated ☐Dry, cracked ☐Odorous ☐Lesion

Complains of: ☐None ☐Nausea ☐Vomiting ☐Indigestion

Difficulty with ☐No Problem ☐Chewing ☐Swallowing ☐Tasting ☐Following diet

Feeding tubes/devices_____

Bowel habits: ☐Stools/day ____ ☐Soft/formed_____ ☐Last BM____ ☐Constipation ☐Diarrhea
☐Incontinent ☐Hemorrhoids ☐Bloody stools ☐Color_____

Abdomen: ☐Soft ☐Firm ☐Tender ☐Distended ☐Girth_____

Bowel sounds: ☐Present ☐Absent ☐Comments _____

Ostomies/tubes: ☐Present, type_____

Bladder habits: ☐No problem ☐Self cath ☐Hemodialysis ☐Hematuria ☐Urgency
☐Nocturia ☐Dysuria ☐Polyuria ☐Anuria ☐Burning
☐Dribbling ☐Discharge ☐Peritoneal dialysis ☐Other_____

Urinary devices/treatments:_____

Comments:_____
_____

RESPIRATORY

Breath sounds:

☐No Problem ☐Crackles(R/L) ☐Wheezes (R/L) ☐Diminished(R/L) ☐Absent(R/L) ☐Use of Accessory Muscles

Cough: ☐No Problem ☐Productive ☐Nonproductive ☐Sputum color_____

Shortness of Breath:☐No Problem ☐With exercise ☐Without exercise ☐Sleeps on _____pillows

Tracheostomy: ☐None ☐Present

Comments_____

CARDIOVASCULAR

Chest pain - ☐No ☐Yes (Describe)_____
_____

☐Pacemaker, rate_____ ☐Apical rate/rhythm Regular_____ Irregular____ ☐Other _____
☐Radial rate/rhythm Regular_____ Irregular____

LIMB	No problem	Red	Mottled	Blanched	Warm	Cold	Varicosities
Right Arm							
Left Arm							
Right Leg							
Left Leg							
Right dorsalis pedal pulse ☐Strong		☐Weak			☐Absent		
Left dorsalis pedal pulse ☐Strong		☐Weak			☐Absent		

HGH
HAZLETON GENERAL HOSPITAL
700 East Broad Street, Hazleton, PA 18201
(717) 450-HELP

Figure 2-8 Closed-ended admission assessment. (Courtesy Hazleton General Hospital, Hazleton, Pa.)

ADMISSION ASSESSMENT

Normal Definitions WNL = Within Normal Limits	Abnormal Choices Use only if assessment is not normal according to definition.

PSYCHOSOCIAL: ❑ WNL
Calm, interactive, cooperative.

❑ Agitated   ❑ Withdrawn   ❑ Combative   ❑ Sad   ❑ Angry   ❑ Anxious
❑ Other: _____

RESPIRATORY: ❑ WNL
Respirations unlabored and symmetrical with regular rhythm and depth. Bilateral breath sounds clear and equal. No pain with respirations. Sputum minimal and clear. Nailbeds and mucus membranes pink.

Respiration: ❑ WNL ❑ SOB ❑ Labored ❑ Use of accessory muscles ❑ Ventilator Assisted
Cough: ❑ WNL ❑ Productive ❑ Nonproductive
Secretions: ❑ WNL Consistency:_____ Amount:_____ Color: _____
Mucus membranes: ❑ WNL   ❑ Pale   ❑ Dusky   ❑ Cyanotic
Nailbeds: ❑ WNL   ❑ Pale   ❑ Dusky   ❑ Cyanotic
Painful respirations: describe: _____
Airway/adjunct: _____
If abnormal breath sounds, describe: _____

CARDIOVASCULAR: ❑ WNL
Regular apical pulse, S1 & S2 audible. Without extra heart sounds. No chest pain. Capillary refill ≤ 2 seconds. No edema. No calf tenderness. Neck veins flat at 45°. Skin warm and dry.

Rhythm: ❑ WNL ❑ Irregular   ❑ Other rhythm: _____
Heart Sounds: ❑ WNL   ❑ Murmur   ❑ S3   ❑ Extra Sounds:_____
Edema: ❑ WNL ❑ Periorbital ❑ Generalized   ❑ Pitting: Amount: _____ Location: _____
Capillary refill: ❑ WNL   ❑ > 2 Seconds Location: _____
Calf tenderness: ❑ R ❑ L   +Homans: ❑ R ❑ L   Neck veins: ❑ JVD at 45°
Skin: ❑ WNL ❑ Dry ❑ Moist ❑ Clammy ❑ Hot ❑ Cool ❑ Cold
Pain: Describe: _____

GASTROINTESTINAL: ❑ WNL
Abdomen soft. Bowel sounds present in all 4 quadrants. No abdominal pain. Tolerates prescribed diet. BMs within own normal pattern, consistency and color.

Abdomen: ❑ WNL ❑ Tender ❑ Distended ❑ Soft ❑ Firm ❑ Rigid ❑ Nausea
         ❑ Emesis   Flatus: ❑ Yes ❑ No
Abdominal pain: Describe: _____

Bowel Sounds	RUQ	LUQ	RLQ	LLQ
Present				
Absent				
Hypoactive				
Hyperactive				

Ostomy/Stoma condition: _____
Bowel movement: Describe: _____

GENITOURINARY: ❑ WNL
Able to void. Continent. Urine clear, yellow to amber. Nondistended bladder. No pain. Vaginal discharge scant, clear and non-odorous or no penile discharge.

If Vas Cath/Tenckhoff: Without redness or swelling.

❑ Unable to void   ❑ Distention   ❑ Incontinent Uses: ❑ Diapers ❑ Pads
Urine: Odor: ❑ Foul ❑ Strong   Clarity: ❑ Cloudy ❑ Sediment Color: _____
❑ Foley: Size: _____ Date inserted: _____
❑ Dialysis Access: ❑ Gortex Graft ❑ AV Fistula   ❑ Palpable thrill, audible bruit
❑ Vas Cath   ❑ Tenckhoff   Vas Cath/Tenckhoff: ❑ WNL   ❑ Describe if outside normal limits:
_____
❑ Ostomy/Stoma condition: _____
Vaginal/Penile discharge: Describe if present/abnormal: _____
Genital lesions: Describe if present: _____

NEUROLOGICAL: ❑ WNL
Alert and oriented to person, place and time. Follows simple commands. Behavior appropriate to situation. Pupils equal and reactive to light. Active ROM of all extremities with symmetry of strength. No paresthesia. Verbalization clear, meaningful and understandable. Can track with eyes. Able to swallow own secretions. Normal cough and blink reflex. No pain.

MUSCULOSKELETAL: ❑ WNL
Normal ROM of all joints. No muscle weakness. Absence of inflammation in joints. Neurovascular status intact to all extremities. Ambulatory without assistance. Palpable pulses in all extremities.

Orientation: ❑ WNL   ❑ Disoriented to: ❑ Person   ❑ Place   ❑ Time
   Follows simple commands: ❑ Yes ❑ No ❑ At times   Can track with eyes: ❑ Yes ❑ No
LOC: ❑ WNL   ❑ Arouses to touch ❑ Arouses to pain ❑ Arouses to voice ❑ Does not arouse
Pupils: ❑ WNL   ❑ Unequal R: ❑ Reactive ❑ Nonreactive   L: ❑ Reactive ❑ Nonreactive
Speech: ❑ WNL ❑ Slurred ❑ Aphasic ❑ Dysphasia ❑ Inappropriate ❑ Artificial Airway
Swallow: ❑ WNL ❑ Chokes on liquids   ❑ Chokes on solids   ❑ Dysphagia
Reflexes: ❑ WNL ❑ Absent cough ❑ Absent blink ❑ Absent gag
❑ Non Ambulatory ❑ Ambulatory with assistive device: _____
Pain: Describe: _____
Additional findings/deficits: _____

	RUE	LUE	LLE	RLE
Weakness				
Flexion				
Extension				
Flaccid				
Inflammation				
Capillary refill > 2 seconds				
Pulse: Absent, Diminished, Bounding				
Paresthesia				
Extremity temp cool				
Color: Pale, Mottled, Cyanotic				

2 3 4 5 6 7 8 9
● ● ● ● ● ● ● ●
Size MM: R _____   L _____
Pupillary Reaction:
R= Reactive N= Nonreactive R _____ L _____
TYPE AND LOCATION
Traction: _____
Brace: _____
Cast: _____
Splint: _____

Mission
A Member of the Mission + St. Joseph's Health System
**Adult/Geriatric Patient History
and General Information
Readmissions within 30 days: Update**

Figure 2-9 Portion of admission assessment. (Courtesy Mission and St. Joseph's Health System, Asheville, NC.)

educating nurses in their use, and developing strategies for implementing them in nursing practice. The NANDA group, which meets every 2 years, has shaped the evolution of nursing diagnosis by serving as a mechanism for the development and acceptance of nursing diagnoses for clinical testing. Additional discussion of nursing diagnosis appears in Chapter 3.

Admission assessment forms based on nursing diagnoses follow a common pattern of placing nursing diagnoses next to each applicable section of the admission assessment form. As the nurse collects the assessment data, the appropriate nursing diagnoses are used to identify actual or potential problems. This design format encourages the identification of the problems that will be the focus of nursing care.

CHARTING TIPS FOR COMPLETING INITIAL ASSESSMENTS

The following are charting tips that can be used to complete the initial assessment:

1. Describe the physical assessment findings in sufficient detail. Avoid the use of words such as "a little" and "a lot," which are open to interpretation and must be clarified to be meaningful.
2. When there is not enough room on the form to describe findings, leave that section blank. Rather than crowding information into a small space in handwriting that may be impossible to read, write "See progress notes."
3. Describe what is seen, heard, felt, and smelled during assessment. Do not interpret the patient's behavior unless these conclusions can be validated; for example, writing "patient crying during interview" is better than "patient crying because she is depressed" unless this conclusion can be verified.
4. Use the PQRST system to gather data about the patient's pain and to document findings. The *PQRST* mnemonic can be used to remember the important aspects of assessment (data do not necessarily have to be documented in PQRST order):

   - *Provocative/Palliative.* What causes it? What brings it on? What relieves it?
   - *Quality/Quantity.* How does it feel, look, or sound? What amount is present?
   - *Region/Radiation.* Where is it located? Where does it spread to?
   - *Severity.* How intense is it on a scale from 1 to 10? How does it affect activities?
   - *Timing.* When did it begin? How long does it last? Is the onset sudden or gradual? How often does it occur? (*Assessment,* 1984).
5. When documenting the assessment of pain, use a pain scale (Figure 2-10). Kohr and others (1995) found that pain control was complicated by a lack of consistency

in describing the severity of the pain. Their solution was to use a scale from 0 to 5 with a precise description assigned to each number. They then developed a graphic pain management record in the form of a pain intensity flowsheet.

Document the patient's description of the pain based on the pain scale used. When interviewing pediatric patients, use the word "hurt" interchangeably with "pain." Explain the pain scale and ask the child to mark the line to indicate how much pain he or she has. An alternative method is to have the child point to faces that are smiling, neutral, or frowning, in increasing severity of pain, respectively.

6. When describing the patient's chief complaint, use his or her own words. This will provide others with insight into the patient's level of understanding and reaction to the illness. Allow at least 2 to 3 inches of space in an admission assessment form for recording the chief complaint. Describe the onset, treatment, and present nature of the problem.
7. Document symptoms that the patient denies and the negative findings from the physical examination. This may assist with the formulation of nursing diagnoses.
8. If the patient cannot provide information during the initial assessment, note the reason why; for example, note that the patient was confused and unable to provide a history. Leaving a section blank may imply that the form was not completed because the nurse was in a hurry or lacked the knowledge and skills to complete the assessment. Describing the factors that impeded the data collection protects the nurse. Try to obtain the information from available family members or close friends. Both the Joint Commission and the ANA standards of care mention the need to obtain (and document) data from significant others when indicated.
9. It is helpful to direct pediatric assessment forms to a specific age or developmental group. Forms are commonly developed for the following age groups: infant to 3 years, 4 to 12 years, and 13 to 18 years.
10. Consider eliminating the recording of clothing lists in an acute-care facility. Current trends are toward asking the patient to sign a statement indicating that clothing and valuables are his or her own responsibility. Facilities for long-term care, which often have more personal belongings to track, continue to use clothing lists. When a patient enters a facility with expensive jewelry or large amounts of money, the nurse should clearly document the disposition of the valuables. This is particularly important when the patient is physically or mentally unable to keep track of personal property. The problem can be partially solved by encouraging the patient's family to take personal belongings home with them. Patients undergoing planned hospitalizations can be informed in the preadmission process that they should leave their valuables at home.

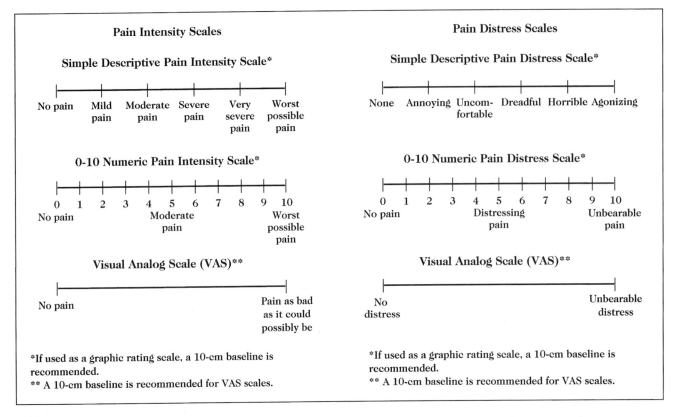

Figure 2-10 Pain scales for use in assessing pain. (From Clinical Practice Guideline: *Acute pain management,* Rockville, Md, 1992, U.S. Department of Health and Human Services.)

11. Ensure that the initial assessment contains a section for recording allergies. Document the patient's description of the allergic response and help the patient distinguish between an allergic reaction and side effects. Although duplication in charting is discouraged, the recording of allergies is an exception. Allergy information should be placed on the assessment form, the medication administration record, the treatment kardex, and the front of the chart.

12. The hospital pharmacy usually requires data on height, weight, current medications, and drug allergies when a patient is admitted. To avoid transcribing this information onto a separate piece of paper, consider creating an assessment form with a carbonized second sheet that can be sent to the pharmacy.

13. Registered nurses (RNs) may delegate aspects of the initial data collection to licensed practical nurses (LPNs). Typically, LPNs take vital signs, height, and weight, and provide instructions to orient the patient to the new environment. However, RNs are still responsible for completing the admission assessment. Design the admission assessment form in such a way that the LPN can sign the section of the form that he or she completes.

14. Provide a space to document whether the patient has an advance directive.

REASSESSMENTS

Once the admission assessment is completed, the process of ongoing reassessments begins. Hospital policy defines how frequently patients are reassessed. The intervals vary depending on the acuity of the patient and the type of care that is needed. Significant changes in the patient's condition, responses, and diagnostic testing trigger the reassessment process. Reassessments are documented in the progress notes and on a variety of flowsheets.

The documentation of reassessments frequently becomes a factor in malpractice cases. A discrepancy between the nurse's assessment and the physician's assessment was a factor in the following case:

The 45-year-old man died of undiagnosed internal injuries after he fell 10 feet from the deck of his house. Although chest x-rays were performed during his week-long hospitalization, no abdominal films were ever taken. The doctor contended that he saw the patient daily, but the records did not contain notes documenting the visits. The patient's treatment consisted of pain medication and bedrest.

On the evening before he was to be discharged, the patient complained of abdominal pain. His family testified that his abdomen was noticeably distended. The family contacted a nurse, who immediately contacted the doctor after examining the abdomen. The doctor assumed that the pain and swelling were due to the broken ribs and attributed the abdominal distention to constipation and internal inflammation from the pain medications. On the day of discharge a second nurse noted abdominal distention. This was contraindicated in the doctor's discharge note, wherein he alleged that he had examined the man and did not find either abdominal pain or distention. The patient was discharged to his home.

Within 3 days after he returned home, the patient went to the emergency room with complaints of abdominal pain and distention. This was recorded in the medical records as rib pain. His blood pressure was elevated, and he was pale and febrile. An abdominal x-ray showed swelling. He was diagnosed with fractured ribs and sent home. Within 18 hours he died at home. An autopsy confirmed the cause of death as internal injuries, suffered at the time of the fall, which were allowed to progress and become worse. A $1.44 million verdict was returned (Laska, 1997).

In this case, it is readily apparent that the jury had to weigh the credibility of the documented reassessments of the nurses with the testimony and documentation of the physicians. The identities of the patient and defendants were protected in the reporting of this case (*Anonymous* v. *Anonymous*) so it is unclear whether the nurses were named as defendants.

The lack of reassessment documentation was a significant factor in the result of the following case:

A 54-year-old schoolteacher was admitted to the hospital for nausea and vomiting. Her surgeon diagnosed a probable small bowel obstruction and performed laparoscopic surgery. Postoperatively, antiembolism stockings were applied to her legs. She began complaining of numbness and tingling in her legs. The doctor was allegedly notified but does not recall being given that information. The nurse on duty never checked the pulses or assessed the strength of the patient's legs during the nurse's eight hour shift, even though the patient became very agitated and could not move her legs. Later that morning the doctor arrived and noted absent pulses in the patient's legs up to the femoral arteries. Although the doctor made an immediate diagnosis of acute arterial occlusion, he did not order anticoagulation or perform an embolectomy because he was not confident in his diagnosis. Ultimately the patient's right leg had to be amputated. The jury returned a $2 million verdict for the plaintiffs. The hospital and the doctor were named in the suit (Laska, 1997b).

The absence of documentation of pulses and movement in the patient's legs was undoubtedly a factor in the conclusions of negligence on the part of the nurse in this case.

SUMMARY

Assessment involves gathering information about a patient's needs to identify nursing diagnoses and plan nursing care. The problems, potential for injury, potential for self care following discharge, and patient and family education needs of the patient should drive the setting of priorities for assessment. A variety of formats for admission assessments have been used to structure and document the assessment process. Reassessment of key information at appropriate intervals demonstrates the use of the nursing process.

REFERENCES

American Nurses Association: *Standards of clinical nursing practice,* Washington, DC, 1991.

Assessment: Springhouse, Pa, 1984, Springhouse.

Calfee B: Documenting suicide risk, *Nursing 96* p 12, July 1996.

Cordell B, Smith-Blair N: Streamlined charting for patient education, *Nursing 75,* 1994.

Eason v. Interfaith Hospital, 1998.

Frost M, Willette K: Risk for abuse/neglect: documentation of assessment data and diagnoses, *J Gerontol Nurs* p 37, August 1994.

Haynor P: Meeting the challenge of advance directives, *Am J Nurs* p 26, March 1998.

Iyer P: Preventing falls in the elderly, *S Calif Nurs News* p 15, October 1988.

Joint Commission on Accreditation of Hospitals: *Comprehensive accreditation manual for hospitals: the official handbook,* Oakbrook Terrace, Ill, 1996, The Association.

Kohr J: Measuring your patient's pain, *RN* p 39, April 1995.

Laska L, ed: Failure to diagnose abdominal injuries from fall which caused rib fractures, *Medical Malpractice Verdicts, Settlements and Experts* p 9, February 1997a.

Laska L, ed: Florida schoolteacher undergoes laparoscopic surgery for bowel obstruction, *Medical Malpractice Verdicts, Settlements and Experts* p 49, October 1997b.

Laska L, ed: Medical records clerk committed to psychiatric ward after threatening to kill five co-workers, *Medical Malpractice Verdicts, Settlements and Experts* p 20, January 1998.

Lynch S: Elder abuse: what to look for, how to intervene, *Am J Nurs* 97(1):27, 1997.

North S, Serkes P: Improving documentation of initial nursing assessment, *Nursing Management* 27(4):30, 1996.

US Department of Health and Human Services: *Pressure ulcers in adults: prediction and prevention,* Rockville, Md, 1992, Author.

Risk management handbook for living wills, Lafayette, La, 1992, Gachassen and Hunter.

Rubenstein L et al: Falls and instability in the elderly, *J Amer Geriatr Soc* p 267, 1988.

Trachtenberg A, Fleming M: Diagnosis and treatment of drug abuse in family practice, *American Family Physician,* 1994.

ADDITIONAL READINGS

Not documented, not done, *Nursing 96* p. 76, October 1996.

Stubbs Sr MF: Protecting your patient's wishes, *Nursing 95* p 75, February 1995.

3

Documenting Nursing Diagnosis and Planning

Although the formats and methods may change, planning care remains a key step in the nursing process. With accurate and thorough planning, the nurse is able to provide individualized care. Expressing the plan of care in writing promotes continuity and consistency of care. A plan of care based on the admission assessment and subsequent nursing diagnoses provides the nurse with information essential for the provision of high-quality care.

Information in this chapter includes the following:

- Suggestions for developing care plans
- Ideas for streamlining the care-planning process
- Discussions of multidisciplinary care planning and critical paths
- Descriptions of the essential features of documenting patient education and discharge planning

COMPONENTS OF THE PLANNING PROCESS

The planning phase of the nursing process involves the following: formulating nursing diagnoses, establishing desired patient outcomes, selecting appropriate interventions, and documenting the plan of care. Each of these components is discussed in the following text.

Nursing Diagnoses

Formulation

The nursing diagnosis usually consists of three components: human responses (or problems), related factors, and signs and symptoms (Figure 3-1).

Human Responses

The human response is a term used to define a problem that the nurse has identified through assessment. The vast majority of human responses identified by the North American Nursing Diagnosis Association (NANDA) define problems that nurses are licensed to treat because they are qualified by virtue of their education. A group within NANDA has directed its attention toward defining patients' strengths as well as problems. In response to these concerns, human responses oriented toward wellness have been added to the NANDA list.

After gathering and analyzing assessment data, the nurse formulates the nursing diagnosis by selecting the appropriate human response from the list of accepted nursing diagnoses. If the nurse is unable to locate a human response on the NANDA list (or other system in use at the facility), he or she should develop a statement that defines the patient's problem.

Related Factors

Related factors can be reflected in physiologic responses and influenced by psychosocial and spiritual elements. The identification of related factors is just as important as the correct identification of the human response. In the planning process of nursing diagnoses, whereas the human response guides the selection of the appropriate outcome, the related factors guide the choice of intervention (Figure 3-2). If the nurse cannot identify the related factors because of insufficient data, the term *unknown etiology* can be used to indicate that more data are needed; for example, "anxiety related to unknown etiology."

The term *related to* links the human response and the related factors. This relationship implies that if one part of the diagnosis changes, the other part may also change (Taptich, Iyer, Bernocchi-Losey, 1994). "Related to" does not express a direct cause-and-effect relationship.

The human response may be associated with a wide variety of related factors, such as *impaired mobility related to fatigue* or *impaired mobility related to decreased visual acuity.* In this example the human response is the same but the interventions reflect the difference between related factors.

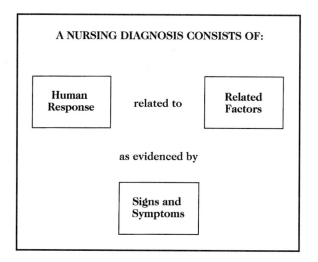

Figure 3-1   Three components of a nursing diagnosis.

Signs and Symptoms

Also referred to as *defining characteristics,* signs and symptoms comprise the third part of the nursing diagnosis. They are linked to the related factor with the words "as evidenced by" or the acronym AEB. Just as many possible related factors can exist, the list of signs and symptoms associated with a human response can be extensive. The nurse should document only the most significant signs and symptoms to avoid lengthy nursing diagnoses.

Outcomes

In the next part of the planning phase, the nurse establishes patient outcomes, which provide a mechanism for evaluating the patient's progress and changes in the patient's status. Outcomes are based on the nursing diagnoses and direct the nursing care. With an increased emphasis on evaluating outcomes of care, the nurse must obtain the knowledge and develop the skills to formulate effective outcomes.

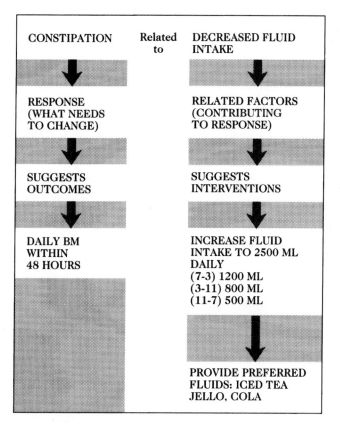

Figure 3-2   Diagram illustrating how the problem (human response) suggests outcomes and the related factor suggests intervention. (From Taptich B, Iyer P, Bernocchi-Losey D: *Nursing diagnosis and care planning,* ed 2, Philadelphia, 1994, WB Saunders.)

Tips for Writing Outcomes

Nurses should adhere to the following guidelines to construct meaningful patient outcomes (Box 3-1):

1. Outcomes should be *patient oriented.* Outcomes describe the expected behavior that should occur when the patient and family have resolved the nursing diagnosis. Most nurses no longer confuse nursing goals with patient outcomes, as seen in the following example:

Nursing goal	Patient outcome
Prevent skin breakdown.	No evidence of skin breakdown over bony prominences exists.

Outcomes are now clearly phrased to define patient behaviors, not nursing behaviors.

2. Outcomes should be *realistic.* The nurse must be realistic in writing patient outcomes because a partial change in behavior may be the only goal attainable. In addition, a short patient stay may limit what can be accomplished in the healthcare facility. Some outcomes may have to be completed after discharge, extending the continuum of care into the patient's home environment.

3. Outcomes should be *measurable* and *observable.* Without measurable patient outcomes the nursing process cannot be completed. The nurse should avoid using the terms *understands* and *appreciates* because these terms are difficult to measure. The following examples are inappropriate:

The patient understands diabetes.
The patient appreciates the importance of taking insulin.

Instead, write outcomes that are easy to validate, for example:

The patient can describe the signs and symptoms of hypoglycemia.
The patient demonstrates correct insulin injection technique.

Only when outcomes are measurable can the nurse determine whether they have been achieved (Taptich, Iyer, Bernocchi-Losey, 1994).

4. Outcomes should be *clear* and *concise,* written in a way that is easily understood by both staff and patients. The nurse should avoid lengthy, ambiguous wording, and use simple language to communicate what is expected of the patient.

5. Outcomes should be established *mutually* between the nurse and patient because mutual goals facilitate active participation and communication of expectations between the nurse and the patient. The probability of a patient achieving the goals is enhanced if he or she is included in the planning process. The patient's participation in outcome setting can be documented in a number of ways (as described in Box 3-2).

6. Outcomes should be *time bound.* The inclusion of a time frame directs the evaluation of outcome achievement at a predetermined interval. Time frames can be stated in a number of ways (for example, "within 2 hours," "within 3 days," "throughout hospitalization," "within 1 month," or "by the time of discharge"). The nature of the outcome and a realistic evaluation of the probability of achieving it should be considered when establishing the time frame.

Outcome Measurement Criteria

The desired patient outcome is formulated as a statement that expresses the positive outcome the patient and healthcare team will work together to achieve. However, determining whether a patient has actually achieved the stated outcome can be subjective in the absence of specific outcome measurement criteria, which are the benchmarks used to determine the degree of outcome achievement. For example, if an outcome states that "the patient will regain an effective breathing pattern," what criteria will be used to determine if that outcome has been achieved? Specific

---

Box 3-1

Guidelines for the Formulations of Outcomes

Outcomes should be . . .

- Patient oriented
- Realistic
- Measurable and observable
- Clear and concise
- Mutually established
- Time bound

Box 3-2

How to Document Patient Participation in Outcome Setting

- Establish a policy of asking the patient to sign the plan of care, signifying agreement with the outcomes. This practice is most common in psychiatric and long-term care facilities, but it is gaining acceptance in acute-care settings.
- Create a column on the plan of care titled "Patient agrees with outcomes." When the patient is unable to participate, the nurse may include the family or significant others in a discussion of the outcomes. The reasons why the patient or family were not involved in setting the outcomes should be described in the progress notes.
- Establish a policy that the discussion of outcomes should be documented in the progress notes. (This method is not as successful as the others. A line for a signature or a column to be marked on the care plan cues the nurse to document the patient's involvement in setting outcomes.)

criteria such as respiratory rate, laboratory values, and statements for the patient can be used to measure outcome achievement. Box 3-3 illustrates the use of outcome measurement criteria (Camp, Iyer, 1995).

Interventions

The final component of the planning phase is the selection of interventions. After the nursing diagnoses and outcomes are established, interventions that help the patient achieve the outcomes should be selected and documented. Box 3-4 outlines the characteristics of appropriate interventions.

Nursing interventions should be specific enough to direct anyone giving care to the patient. Each outcome should have a set of interventions designed to achieve it. The interventions should describe the type of care to be given, the frequency with which the intervention is to be done, and who is to be responsible for providing the care. The interventions should clearly state all actions to be taken to achieve the outcomes (Doenges, Moorhouse, 1988).

With an increasing number of part-time, per diem, and float pool nurses caring for patients, accuracy and completeness of the nursing interventions is essential.

Tips for Writing Interventions

1. As stated previously the interventions are generated from the related factors in the nursing diagnosis. For example, the nursing diagnosis "high risk for impaired skin integrity related to immobility" should prompt the nurse to develop interventions to treat the immobility, such as turning the patient or moving the patient out of bed. By treating immobility the nurse may be able to prevent skin integrity problems.
2. Nursing interventions should be specific. The interventions are meant to direct the care provided by the nursing

staff. Therefore action verbs should be used to communicate the expectations for care and the frequency of interventions. Nurses often write vague interventions such as "encourage fluids" and leave the specifics to the discretion of the caregiver. Specific interventions such as "give 200 ml of juice every 2 hours" are more meaningful.

3. Interventions should be individualized. The purpose of planning care is to assist nurses in addressing differences in the care of patients with similar problems. Interventions should be based on the patient's individual needs. For example, a child and an elderly person may both have the same nursing diagnosis; however, the interventions would differ, perhaps significantly, because of differences in the patients' ages and development.
4. Interventions should be realistic for the patient and nurse and should consider the patient's length of stay, the patient care resources available, and the expected outcomes. Implementing the interventions in the time allotted with the available staff should be possible. The interventions should be realistically phrased to reflect available resources. For example, "assess skin condition every 2 hours" means that a registered nurse (RN) should check the patient's skin every 2 hours. If the intervention states "observe skin condition every 2 hours," a licensed practical nurse (LPN) or nursing assistant could carry out that intervention. A difference does exist between assessment and observation.
5. All interventions should be dated and initialed, which enables the nurse to establish accountability for professional practice and provides other caregivers with an opportunity to obtain clarification from the person who initiated the interventions.

In summary, the planning phase of the nursing process has three components: the formulation of nursing diagnoses, the establishment of patient outcomes, and the selection of appropriate interventions. Expectations for care can be effectively documented using the recommendations addressed in this text to write the nursing diagnoses, outcomes, and interventions.

Box 3-3

Outcome Measurement Criteria

Desired Patient Outcome

The patient will regain an effective breathing pattern.

Outcome Measurement Criteria

- Respiratory rate of 12-20 breaths per minute
- Unobstructed breathing
- Decreased use or nonuse of accessory muscles
- Absence of dyspnea, shortness of breath, cyanosis, tachycardia, or chest tightness
- Oxygen saturation above 90%
- Arterial blood gases within normal range

Box 3-4

Guidelines for Formulation of Interventions

Interventions should be . . .

- Generated from the related factors
- Specific
- Individualized
- Realistic
- Dated and initialed

CARE PLANNING

Purpose

The purpose of the plan of care is to provide a core of information on the patient's nursing diagnoses, outcomes, and planned interventions. The plan of care is a communication tool for everyone involved in patient care. The interaction of nurses with one another is limited, so they rely heavily on the plan of care to ensure continuity of care for the patient. Because of increases in cross-training efforts designed to contain costs, nurses assigned to work in areas where they have little practical experience can benefit from written plans developed by expert clinicians (Greenwood, 1996). The plan of care should guide care and document the planning phase of the nursing process.

The plan of care should ideally be based on the admission assessment and should be initiated during the admission process (or shortly thereafter). The introduction of the diagnostic related grouping (DRG) designations has decreased length of stay, necessitating rapid assessment and interventions for patient problems. Once the plan of care has been established, it must be updated regularly to remain current and useful. A number of individuals review care plans, and the information obtained helps to validate admissions, services provided, length of stay, and DRG assignment and to ensure the delivery of high-quality care. For example, insurance companies, peer review organizations (PROs), regulatory agencies, malpractice attorneys, and utilization management personnel routinely read the plan of care and associated documentation (Taptich, Iyer, Bernocchi-Losey, 1994). The identified nursing diagnoses, outcomes, and interventions may be compared with the documentation in the progress notes. Such an evaluation may be used to determine whether the patient's significant problems were identified and whether nursing measures were effective in relieving them. Additional documentation, including flowsheets and progress notes, may be reviewed to verify that the nurse carried out the plan of care.

The Role of the RN and LPN

The American Nurses Association (ANA), the Joint Commission for the Accreditation of Healthcare Organizations (JCAHO) and many acts regulating nursing practice have addressed the issue of planning care. The consensus is that the RN is responsible for initiating the plan of care. Based on educational preparation, the RN is the most qualified person to plan care mutually with the patient. The role of the LPN in adding to an established plan of care is less clear and continues to be inconsistently handled in healthcare agencies across the United States.

EVOLUTION OF CARE PLANNING

Box 3-5 outlines the evolution of care planning.

Box 3-5

Evolution of Care Planning

- Individualized care plan: handwritten; contains basic nursing interventions and medical orders; often discarded when the patient is discharged.
- Standardized care plan: preprinted plan based on nursing diagnosis or disease process; no space for individualization; not consistently reviewed or revised.
- Modified standard care plan: preprinted plan consists of nursing diagnosis, outcomes, and interventions; space available for individualization; provides more flexibility.
- Multidisciplinary care plan: used initially in long-term care and psychiatric settings; provides a place for each discipline to document its plan; used during team conferences to discuss patient progress.
- Clinical paths: a predetermined, multidisciplinary plan of care written to address the medical diagnosis; predicts outcomes and interventions for specified time intervals; includes teaching and discharge planning; may be used as a documentation tool as well.

Individual Care Plans

Individual care plans are created for each patient based on individual needs. This approach was the only option when the concept of care planning first emerged. The nurse collected data at the time of admission, identified problems, and formulated the individual, handwritten plan of care. The format is usually a three-column design with the column headings *Patient Problems/Nursing Diagnosis, Patient Outcomes,* and *Nursing Interventions.* Many nurses struggled to transform these blank columns into a care plan. The care plan was attached to a kardex, which usually was not a permanent part of the medical record; thus both were discarded when the patient was discharged. As a result, no documentation of ongoing nursing care was kept other than the nurses' notes. In addition, the care plan was primarily a collection of basic nursing measures or record of the implementation of medical orders that did not reflect the care of the patient as a total person, and it was not routinely reviewed and revised as needed (Kobs, 1997). Motivating nurses to spend time developing a document that was thrown out at the end of the patient's stay was difficult. However, by the end of the 1980s the vast majority of healthcare facilities were keeping the care plan as a permanent part of the clinical record.

Standardized Care Plans

As nursing continued to change, the pendulum swung from using individual care plans to using standardized care plans in an effort to meet the needs of both nurses and patients. The term *standardized care plan* refers to a preprinted plan of care for a group of patients with the same medical or nursing diagnosis. Certain commonalities exist among patients with the same diagnosis, which allows nurses to establish standards of care for particular groups of patients. The first standardized care plans, which did not allow for individualization, were frequently "rubber-stamped" by the nurse and placed in the patient's record to meet the requirement for a care plan.

Modified Standard Care Plans

The standard care plan evolved into a more meaningful tool when it was modified to include spaces for individualization. The plan of care can be modified by the following actions:

- Adding the related factor and the signs and symptoms to the nursing diagnosis
- Adding frequency to clarify the time frames stated on the outcomes
- Adding frequency, amount, time, and patient preferences to the nursing interventions
- Documenting nursing diagnoses, outcomes, and interventions specific to the individual patient

Modified standard care plans reduce the amount of time needed for care planning (compared with individualized care plans), their quality is usually higher because they are written by clinical experts, and they can be used as a clinical teaching tool for nurses unfamiliar with the setting or patient population. While modified standard care plans are an improvement, they can be quite lengthy, and they must be designed to include only the essential information. Using the word-processing capabilities of computers, the nurse can edit standardized care plans to produce an individualized document.

Multidisciplinary Care Planning

Another phase in the evolution of care plans has been the emergence of multidisciplinary care plans, which have been used most commonly in long-term care and psychiatric settings. However, multidisciplinary care planning and documentation has become more widespread with the trend toward collaborative practice. In addition, the emphasis on quality improvement and the use of cross-departmental teams to address patient care issues (as recognized by the Joint Commission) lends itself well to a multidisciplinary approach. Figure 3-3 illustrates a multidisciplinary patient teaching record that facilitates documentation by several disciplines. This form could be used to document teaching.

Demise of the Care Plan

Care planning has become a controversial issue in nursing: Problem solving and planning are an integral part of nursing, but the traditional process of care planning is no longer efficient or effective. Sovie (1989) challenges nurses

to examine the rituals such as care planning that pose problems in nursing practice.

In 1991, prompted by decreasing length of stay, advancing computer technology, and increasing patient noncompliance with care plan requirements, the Joint Commission revised the accreditation criteria to help streamline hospital operations. Among criteria they changed was the requirement for the prototypical care plan. The nurse must still show that a plan of care is in place, but he or she has greater flexibility in how to accomplish this. The 1997 Joint Commission standards state that care planning may be performed using any of the following tools for care (JCAHO, 1996):

- Handwritten notes
- Electronic records
- Preprinted forms
- Standards of practice
- Algorithms
- Care paths or clinical pathways
- Individualized, preprinted plans of care

Kobs (1997) points out that, according to the Joint Commission, the use of standardized care plans is perfectly acceptable. The expectation is that the care is individualized to meet the patient's needs. If the patient needs only those interventions outlined in the plan, the documentation may read "Care rendered per asthma plan." If the patient needs additional interventions, they should be documented on the plan.

Greater emphasis is also being placed on patient and family education and discharge planning, which is addressed later in this chapter and in Chapter 5. With the changes occurring in health care, more efficient and effective methods of planning and communicating patient needs and outcomes of care with the entire healthcare team must be developed.

CURRENT TRENDS IN CARE PLANNING

New care-planning strategies are emerging as a result of the quality and cost-containment initiatives in the healthcare setting. The responsibility for developing a plan of care no longer rests solely upon the nursing department. A multidisciplinary team approach to care planning is being adopted throughout the country. Healthcare facilities are developing patient profiles, using practice guidelines, implementing case management models, and introducing critical pathways to enhance communication between healthcare team members and improve the quality of care.

Development of Patient Profiles

The relevance of care planning can be increased by defining the profile of the patients served by a facility. The team can develop the care plan, which accurately describes appropriate care for patients in a particular DRG category, based on

Clark Memorial
Hospital
Jewish Hospital Health Network Partner

INTER DISCIPLINARY PATIENT/FAMILY HEALTH EDUCATION RECORD

REFERRED TO SOCIAL SERVICES NO_____ YES_____	RE:
REFERRED TO CLINICAL EDUC. NO_____ YES_____	RE:

EDUCATION NEEDS		WHO	HOW		RESPONSE	
CODE MED	SAFE & EFFECTIVE USE OF MEDICATIONS	CODE PT PATIENT	CODE D	DEMONSTRATION	CODE Q	ASKED QUESTIONS
P/P	PRE/POST OP TEACHING	S SIGNIFICANT OTHER	P	PAMPHLET	VR	VERBALIZED RE CALL UNDER-STANDING
ACT	ACTIVITY LEVEL	B BOTH	TV	TV/VIDEO	R	RESTLESS DIFFICULTY LISTENING
DIET	KNOWLEDGE OF DIET		V	VERBAL INSTRUCTIONS	DI	SEEMS DISINTERESTED
SCT	KNOWLEDGE OF SELF-CARE TECHNIQUES	**READINESS BARRIERS**	W	WRITTEN INSTRUCTIONS	DR	DENIAL/RESISTANCE
ILL	KNOWLEDGE OF ILLNESS/CONDITION					
T/P	KNOWLEDGE OF TESTS/PROCEDURES	1 COGNITIVE 2 CULTURAL 3 EMOTIONAL			DA	DEMONSTRATED ABILITY
RX	WHEN & HOW TO OBTAIN FURTHER TREATMENT/COMMUNITY RESOURCES	4 FINANCIAL 5 MOTIVATIONAL 6 RELIGIOUS 7 AGE RELATE	MED	MEDICATION INSTRUC. SHEET	NR	NEEDS REINFORCEMENT
RES	RESPONSIBILITIES OF PATIENTS IN THEIR CARE	8 AUDITORY 9 LANGUAGE 10 PAIN	GR	GROUP WORK	A	ATTENTIVE VERBAL RESPONSE
D/C	PERTINENT DISCHARGE INSTRUCTIONS OF CONTINUING CARE NEEDS	11 READING 12 VISUAL 13 SEDATION	O	OTHER	NA	NOT APPLICABLE
O	OTHER					

DATE	ED. NEEDS	WHO	INFORMATION TAUGHT	HOW	BARRIER	RE-SPONSE	SIGNATURE/ TITLE
			– – – – – – – – – – – –		PT		
					S		
			– – – – – – – – – – – –		PT		
					S		
			– – – – – – – – – – – –		PT		
					S		
			– – – – – – – – – – – –		PT		
					S		

Figure 3-3 Multidisciplinary patient teaching record. (Courtesy Clark Memorial Hospital, Jeffersonville, Ind.)

DATE	ED. NEEDS	WHO	INFORMATION TAUGHT	HOW	BARRIER	RE-SPONSE	SIGNATURE/ TITLE
			– – – – – – – – – – – –		PT		
					S		
			– – – – – – – – – – – –		PT		
					S		
			– – – – – – – – – – – –		PT		
					S		
			– – – – – – – – – – – –		PT		
					S		
			– – – – – – – – – – – –		PT		
					S		
			– – – – – – – – – – – –		PT		
					S		
			– – – – – – – – – – – –		PT		
					S		
			– – – – – – – – – – – –		PT		
					S		
			– – – – – – – – – – – –		PT		
					S		
			– – – – – – – – – – – –		PT		
					S		
			– – – – – – – – – – – –		PT		
					S		
			– – – – – – – – – – – –		PT		
					S		
			– – – – – – – – – – – –		PT		
					S		
			– – – – – – – – – – – –		PT		
					S		
			– – – – – – – – – – – –		PT		
					S		
			– – – – – – – – – – – –		PT		
					S		

_____   _____
DATE   SIGNATURE OF PATIENT / PARENT / LEGAL GUARDIAN

Figure 3-3, cont'd   Multidisciplinary patient teaching record.

the patient profile. The result is a relevant and useful tool to guide care and documentation.

The patient profile provides information about typical DRGs, length of stay, patient characteristics, sources of admission, and course of hospitalization. These data permit the facility to develop care plans that are appropriate for patients with certain DRGs. The realities of managed care require that the healthcare team examine several variables before developing the plan of care.

DRG and Length of Stay

The DRG and associated length of stay (LOS) must be determined before a plan develops for a particular population. The team should determine the high-volume DRGs—that is, those patients most frequently treated—for the facility. For each DRG, the LOS should be determined. The admissions, finance, or medical records departments can provide information on the DRG and LOS.

Without knowing the DRG and LOS writing a realistic plan of care is impossible. For example, the healthcare team must address numerous problems, including psychosocial issues, for a patient admitted for radical mastectomy. However, if the patient will be hospitalized for a period of only 4 days, priorities and critical elements of the patient's care must be addressed within that time frame.

Characteristics

The next step is to examine the characteristics of a population that shares a particular DRG, including the average age, predominant sex, and any other common characteristics of the patients. This information can be obtained with a retrospective audit of admissions for patients having that DRG. As these data are collected, a profile will emerge that describes the average patient in that category. For example, a hospital in metropolitan New York discovered that its typical diabetic patient was a male amputee who was homeless.

Sources of Admission

Next, the source of admission for the majority of patients in a particular DRG must be determined (for example, emergency department, same day surgery, or the physician's office). This factor may affect initial planning and interventions. The healthcare team should also determine the percentage of patients processed through preadmission testing. All of these data are in the medical records.

Course of Hospitalization

Once the patient's admission status has been determined, that patient's course of hospitalization should be explored.

Factors that assist in the development of patient profiles are summarized in Box 3-6. Once all of this information has been collected, a clear profile of the average patient should emerge. The plan of care can be developed to truly reflect

---

Box 3-6

Elements of a Patient Profile

- DRG and length of stay
- Average age of population
- Gender
- Source of admission (e.g., emergency department, same day surgery, physician's office)
- Percentage of patients processed through preadmission testing department
- Percentage of patients who experienced complications
- Type of complications experienced by patients
- Particular physician group responsible for the majority of admissions in a particular DRG category

---

the type of patient within that DRG who is routinely treated in the facility.

Practice Guidelines

Practice guidelines (also referred to as *protocols*) describe the management of patient-care issues, such as skin integrity, safety, postoperative care, or administration of specific medications. The practice guidelines may address independent nursing care or collaborative practice issues; for example, the practice guidelines for patient safety outline independent nursing assessment and interventions intended to protect the patient from harm. Practice guidelines for the management of patients receiving chemotherapy, however, describe medical orders and associated care along with the independent nursing management of the patient. The interdependence of this type of practice guideline reflects the collaboration of the healthcare team in the management of a specific patient problem.

Practice guidelines are currently being developed by professional organizations and individual healthcare facilities. Once implemented, these guidelines may serve as an adjunct to the plan of care, an outline for patient management, and a valuable communication tool for the healthcare team.

Case Management

The profound changes in healthcare reimbursement practices have provided the impetus for nursing professionals to examine current nursing care delivery systems. The case management model has led to the shift from task-oriented nursing care to outcome-oriented care delivery.

Definition and Goals

Case management is the organization of care in a way that ensures a specific patient outcome may be achieved within the prescribed time frame utilizing the appropriate resources (Zander, 1988). In case management systems the care is coordinated by a nurse case manager who follows the course of the patient through the entire illness, through all units in which the patient receives care (Hampton, 1993). The nurse case manager is responsible for coordinating care while maintaining a balance between quality and the cost.

Before implementation the facility must decide what will be accomplished by developing a case management model. Giuliano and Poirier (1991), Cesta et al (1998), and Birdsall and Sperry (1997) identify the following goals for case management:

1. Achievement of positive patient outcomes using a case management plan
2. Well-coordinated continuity of care using collaborative practice
3. Continuity across the continuum of care in various settings
4. Appropriate use of resources to reduce wasted time, energy, and materials
5. Timely discharge within the prescribed length of stay or earlier (if possible)
6. Enhancement of professional development and satisfaction

Framework

The framework for case management involves the following: a multidisciplinary team approach to care; the development of a comprehensive case management plan; the implementation of a clinical path to guide care; and the concurrent analysis, evaluation, and adjustment of the care being rendered.

Multidisciplinary Team. Representatives from areas such as nursing, medicine, dietary, pharmacy, respiratory and physical therapy, social services, utilization review, and quality management collaborate to develop a plan for managing patient care. These interdisciplinary clinical experts determine the sequence and timing of interventions and outcomes for particular medical diagnoses or DRGs and promote the appropriate and effective use of resources (Flynn and Kilgallen, 1993). Once the plans are implemented the multidisciplinary group meets regularly to review the plans and the outcomes of care to determine if the plans are effective.

Clinical Path. The comprehensive case management plan is a standardized plan of care that includes the following: predictions for patient needs and nursing diagnoses outcomes for patients, definitions of time frames, and nursing and medical interventions. This plan is then summarized into a one-page or two-page clinical path. The clinical path is a proactive, multidisciplinary set of daily prescriptions for the care of a specified patient population from the time of preadmission to postdischarge. The clinical path identifies key nursing interventions, treatments, consultations, diagnostic tests, teaching, and discharge planning activities and indicates when these must occur to achieve the desired outcomes within the expected LOS. This form of care plan works best when the LOS and clinical outcomes can be predicted and defined.

As stated, the clinical path is the communication tool used to guide the care of the patient from the time of admission to discharge. Clinical paths help to determine a predictable sequence of interventions to avoid oversights that might compromise effective discharge planning (Giuliano and Poirier, 1991). The clinical path is used on every shift on each consecutive unit to plan and monitor the flow of care. Figure 3-4 is an example of a clinical path developed for a patient undergoing a total hip replacement.

Format. The most common clinical path format is set up in a grid. Across the top of the page is the time frame (for example, preadmission, day 1, day 2, day 3). Down the left side of the paper are events, treatments, outcomes. If an event spans more than one day, a solid or dotted line with an arrow on the right end is used in the grid to indicate this. The expected LOS for the DRG often is defined at the top of the page.

The following two trends are currently affecting the format of clinical paths:

1. Many facilities are defining outcomes and interventions for each day of the clinical path. These daily outcomes are added to the bottom of each page of the clinical path or are written on a separate page.
2. Software companies are marketing programs that allow computer analysis of clinical paths.

Variances. Nurses can evaluate the patient's daily progress based on the established standards in the case management plan and clinical path. The nurse identifies a variance in care when an activity or outcome is not achieved within the time frame noted on the clinical path. The variance is justified or actions are taken to rectify it (Zander, 1988). Variances and corrective actions (or justifications) are documented and analyzed by the multidisciplinary team to improve care.

Legality. The use of clinical paths as a permanent part of the record continues to cause controversy. Clinical paths may or may not be retained as a permanent part of the record unless they are included in the healthcare team's documentation. "A documentation system showing that the clinical path was actually followed could be a substantial ally to the defense" in the event of a malpractice suit (Forkner, 1996, p. 36). A charting system to ensure that variances in the patient's recovery are clearly explained may prevent the patient or family from attributing adverse patient outcomes to a nurse's negligence. Forkner (1996) stresses that patients and families need to understand that care is unpredictable and clinical paths may have to be modified. Some facilities place a disclaimer on the clinical path, stating that the clinical path is a general guideline only and that care is individualized and revised based on a patient's specific needs.

The Medical Center at Princeton   Pt. Label   Case Type: __TOTAL HIP REPLACEMENT__   Page 1 of 5   LOS: __12 Days__

Multidisciplinary Plan   MD Review _____   Pt./S.O. Review _____   Date: _____

CAREGIVER INTERVENTIONS

	Day 1 (Pre-Op)				Day 1 (Post-Op)				Day 2		
	Date:	M	U	N/A	Date:	M	U	N/A	Date:	M	U	N/A
Assessments/ Consults	Anesthesia. Medical Clearance.								Social Service to see patient.			
Tests	Admitting Bloods, CXR, EKG, Hip films in OR.				CBC lytes, PACU (if indicated), HIP films in PACU.				PT, PTT and CBC.			
Treatments	Antiembolic stockings.				Foley, Drains, O2 (if indicated), Incentive Spirometer, DSD, TED's and Trapeze.				Foley, Drains, Incentive Spirometer, DSD and TED's, and DIC O2.			
Medications	Pre-Op. Optional DVT prophylaxis.				DVT prophylaxis, IV antibiotics, IM analgesics or PCA, IV Fluids, IV antibiotics and stool softeners.				DVT prophylaxis, IM analgesics or PCA, IV antibiotics, and stool softeners.			
Nutrition	NPO.				Clear fluids and advance as tolerated.				As tolerated.			
Safety/Activity	Ad lib.				Bedrest with abductor pillow and trapeze.				Bedrest with abductor pillow and trapeze. Order physical therapy evaluation.			
Teaching	Incentive Spirometer, Cough and deep breathing, and Isometric Exercises.				Reinforce leg strengthening exercises, Coughing and deep breathing, and Incentive Spirometer.				Reinforce leg strengthening exercises and total hip precautions.			
Discharge Coordination	Assess home environment.				Intervention and planning with RN and MD as well as patient and family. Social Service consult.							

OUTCOME STATEMENTS

PROBLEM/FOCUS	Day 1 (Pre-Op) Date:				Day 1 (Post-Op) Date:				Day 2 Date:			
		M	U	N/A		M	U	N/A		M	U	N/A
Knowledge Deficit	Patient verbalizes understanding of Pre-Op teaching and Post-Op routine.				Patient demonstrates use of: A) Abduction Pillow/Trapeze B) Incentive Spirometry and C) Leg Strengthening Exercises.				Patient continues to utilize: A) Abductor Pillow/Trapeze B) Incentive Spirometer and C) Leg Exercises.			
Immobility	Patient verbalizes proper body mechanics while in bed.				Patient demonstrates proper use of abductor pillow. Patient repositioned every two hours.				Patient demonstrates proper use of abductor pillow. Patient repositioned every two hours. P/T independent with lower extremity isometrics.			
Nutrition	Patient verbalizes understanding of being NPO after midnight. Patient tolerating PO food and fluids.				Patient maintained NPO prior to surgery.				Patient tolerates diet as ordered. Remains free of N and V.			
Neuro-Vascular Assessment	Patient has positive CMS of affected limb.				Patient utilizing TED stockings, positive CMS.				Patient utilizing TED stockings, positive CMS.			
Pain	Patient will verbalize an understanding of pain medication and PCA usage.				Patient utilizes PCA machine or IM pain medication. Patient reports satisfaction with comfort measure.				Patient utilizes PCA machine or IM pain medication. Patient reports satisfaction with comfort measures.			
Infection	Maintains temperature and WBC WNL.				Maintains temperature WNL. Urine is clear, yellow, odorless and without sediment. Maintains clear lung sounds.				Maintains temperature WNL. Dressing dry and intact. Urine is clear, yellow, odorless and without sediment. Maintains clear lung sounds.			

Figure 3-4 Clinical path for a patient undergoing a total hip replacement. (Courtesy The Medical Center at Princeton, Princeton, NJ.)

Equally controversial is the debate over whether clinical paths should be treated as guidelines, which implies that they are desirable options, or used as standards that must be followed. If a clinical path is used as a standard and the healthcare provider deviates from the clinical path without adequate justification, the deviation can be used to prove negligence of duty by the nurse and may be seen as the cause of the adverse outcome. However, if the patient's condition changes, deviation from the path may become necessary. The nurse must clearly document the assessment findings and substantiate the reason for deviating from the path *at the time of the deviation.* Conforming to a clinical path does not automatically result in immunity from liability: Nurses are still bound by duty to make judgments in providing care based on the individual patient's unique needs (Forkner, 1996; Noonan, 1997). The nurse's best defense against litigation is still factual, timely, and accurate documentation.

Benefits. The use of the clinical path approach to care has benefits for the facility, the healthcare team, and the patient. The obvious benefit to the healthcare facility is adequate reimbursement for care rendered. Clinical paths provide a mechanism for monitoring care and identifying problems that could interfere with the achievement of outcomes and timely discharge. The early identification of variances and the appropriate intervention result in the responsible use of resources and the maximum reimbursement for services. The benefits to the healthcare team from the use of clinical paths are shown in Box 3-7.

The central figure in the development of clinical paths is always the patient. An integral part of the success of clinical paths is patient and family involvement. Forkner (1996) stresses the importance of clinical paths as a way to strengthen the relationship between the patient and the healthcare team. Nothing is more effective in preventing malpractice allegations than effective communication with the patient and family. The clinical path should be shared with the patient and family at the time of admission to clarify expectations and establish mutually acceptable goals for care. An ongoing discussion should be maintained throughout the hospitalization. Patient control and participation are enhanced if the patient and family understand the activities and goals to be accomplished (Hampton, 1993).

Benefits to the patient include the following:

- Patients who are involved in and educated about their care tend to progress toward positive outcomes more effectively than those who are not.
- Improved patient satisfaction results when patients have a better understanding of their care and one person consistently oversees their care.
- Discharge planning and patient education begin earlier.

Overall, case management and clinical paths foster the achievement of quality patient care while addressing the economic concerns facing healthcare facilities.

Box 3-7

Benefits of Case Management and Clinical Paths to the Healthcare Team

- Communication and collaboration among health professionals is promoted.
- Continuity across the continuum of care is promoted because all caregivers are working from the same plan to achieve the same goals with the patient, regardless of the clinical setting (Raiwet et al, 1997).
- Documentation of care becomes consolidated, streamlined, and consistent if it is based on the clinical path. Some facilities use the clinical path as a documentation tool, whereas others use flowsheets to document interventions and a charting-by-exception model to document variances.
- The traditional nursing care plan can be replaced because clinical paths with outcomes and interventions *are* the plan of care.
- Professionalism in nursing is enhanced when nurses assume the role of case manager.
- Clinical paths serve as readily available, up-to-date, multidisciplinary teaching tools.
- Clinical research and quality improvement concerns can be identified and studied by the multidisciplinary team (Redick et al, 1994).

Development of Clinical Paths. Several approaches to the development of clinical paths have been developed, including the following:

1. Multidisciplinary committees who meet frequently to discuss and plot care elements
2. Nursing committees who draft clinical paths and involve other disciplines in their review and refinement

The principles used in making changes to a documentation system (as defined in Chapter 9) directly apply to the development of clinical paths. The authors have determined that the process of developing clinical paths is painful in the beginning. The first few clinical paths are difficult to define as the group identifies system issues, creates a format, uncovers territorial concerns, and deals with the defensiveness and fears brought about by the implementation of "cookbook medicine." Healthcare facilities that have gone through this process have determined that starting with a limited number of paths (until the process becomes more familiar to the staff) is often better.

The origin of clinical or critical paths, deeply rooted in nursing, is the result of a blend of the traditional nursing care plan, the need to provide care within a structured framework, and a means for establishing a standard of care for all patients (Birdsall, Sperry, 1997). No single "right" way to develop clinical paths exists. The steps defined in Box 3-8 present a sequence of steps that some healthcare facilities

---

Box 3-8

Steps in Developing Critical Paths

1. Identify the specific multidisciplinary caregivers for a particular patient population, then appoint one or more physician liaisons or ask for volunteers.
2. Analyze the practice pattern of each discipline for the current process and outcome and compare it with the optimal process and outcome. Use the utilization management staff to determine the LOS.
3. Determine when key interventions occur during the patient's stay.
4. Identify the barriers to providing these interventions, including those of the system, practitioner, and patient.
5. Define the measurable clinical outcomes that the patient is expected to achieve each day.
6. Compare current patterns with optimal patterns.
7. Sequence the key interventions needed to achieve the outcomes by discharge. Involve computer information systems personnel when establishing the format for the clinical path to determine how the path can be automated.
8. Identify the contributions of each discipline to the achievement of the outcomes. Develop a path, then ask the risk manager to review it.
9. Teach nurses about the use of the clinical path, the principles of case management DRGs, and reimbursement mechanisms.
10. Test the clinical path using a pilot program.
11. Document and analyze any variances for issues that can be resolved through changing the system or practitioner behavior.
12. Report variance detail as part of the quality improvement program.

---

have found to be successful in developing clinical paths. References and additional readings at the end of this chapter provide more information on this topic.

DOCUMENTATION OF DISCHARGE PLANNING

This section addresses discharge planning in terms of why, when, and how it should be documented.

Why Document?

The prospective payment system has increased the importance of early discharge planning. If discharge needs are not identified in a timely fashion and discharge arrangements are delayed, the patient will remain in the facility and receive services longer than necessary or will be prematurely discharged without receiving adequate preparation. Documentation of discharge planning may be scrutinized by the peer review organization (PRO) if the patient is readmitted with the same diagnosis shortly after discharge.

When to Document

Discharge planning should be done as early in the process as possible. Discharge needs should ideally be considered before a patient is admitted. Smeltzer and Flores (1986) describe a preadmission discharge planning program that incorporates discharge assessment and planning before admission for surgery. In this program, nurses in the preadmission testing department are accountable for initiating and documenting discharge planning.

When initiating discharge planning before admission is impossible, such as in the case of an unexpected illness, discharge planning should begin at the time of admission. The identification of patients who need discharge planning is discussed in Chapter 2.

How

A form with cues that remind healthcare providers to implement and document discharge planning may be helpful. Discharge planning is often included on a separate form in the medical record. This form usually describes the following:

- Initial assessment of the need for discharge planning
- Attempts to place the patient in the appropriate facility for continuing care or to arrange for home care as needed
- Data provided by family members during interviews

Communication between care providers and discharge planning personnel is essential for successful discharge planning. Most hospitals incorporate multidisciplinary discharge conferences as part of their routine, which provides team members with an opportunity to share current information about the patient's status and particular discharge needs. Most of this information is communicated verbally during the conference. Staff members for each discipline are responsible for documenting discharge information specific to that discipline. However, duplication of information is a problem with this method. Incorporating discharge information from all disciplines into one form ensures communication between personnel and enhances the continuity of care.

DOCUMENTATION OF PLANNING FOR PATIENT EDUCATION

This section focuses on documentation of teaching plans. The identification of patient education needs is discussed in Chapter 2. After assessing the learning needs of the patient and family, the nurse identifies the high-priority learning needs and documents those priorities that will be addressed by the healthcare team. Lower-priority needs may be referred to other agencies or resources for follow-up. The nurse then develops a written teaching plan with clearly defined outcomes, which enables the nurse to evaluate the patient's achievement of the outcomes or need for further

---

education. Additional reasons for documenting patient education plans are listed in Box 3-9.

Learning Outcomes

Any number of outcomes can describe the end result of the teaching plan. Learning outcomes are written in accordance with the guidelines for outcomes discussed earlier in this chapter (see Box 3-1). They must be measurable, observable, and clearly communicate the expected behavior. Learning outcomes address the three domains of behavior: cognitive, psychomotor, and affective.

The cognitive domain of behavior includes the concepts that increase the patient's knowledge of his or her self and disease. Facts, principles, and other types of knowledge comprise the cognitive area of teaching. The psychomotor domain of behavior consists of the manual skills used by the patient to maintain his or her health or provide for his or her physical needs. These include activities such as changing dressings, giving injections, and effective treatments. The affective domain of behavior consists of emotions, attitudes, and self-acceptance. The teaching process may involve altering a patient's self-perceptions and helping the patient to accept limitations, particularly those associated with a chronic disease.

The following are examples of outcomes for each domain:

Domain	Outcome
Cognitive	Identifies three risk factors for heart disease and selects low cholesterol foods from menu.
Psychomotor	Demonstrates acceptable technique for suctioning a tracheostomy, accurately follows steps for performing blood glucose monitoring.
Affective	Discusses feelings about having epilepsy and demonstrates positive coping mechanisms for interacting with family.

After the outcomes have been identified in measurable and observable terms, the next step is development of a content outline. This process may consist of listing the topics that will be taught along with the resources that will be used.

Patient Education Forms

Patient education forms have been developed to do the following:

- Gather data about patient education into one central document for easy retrieval
- Create consistency in charted information
- Promote interdisciplinary collaboration and communication
- Provide efficient documentation of patient education

Components

Patient education forms usually consist of the following components:

- A summary of patient factors with a positive or negative effect on the patient's capabilities to learn the content
- Strategies used to teach the patient
- Learning outcomes
- Evaluation of the patient's progress toward achieving the outcomes
- Dates and signatures

Types

Figure 3-5 illustrates one approach to the documentation of patient education plans. Standardized teaching forms are useful when the nurse is providing education about a complex issue (for example, ostomy care or a chronic illness, such as diabetes or heart disease). A teaching plan is often developed to provide more in-depth information for the nurse to use as a reference when teaching the patient. The patient education record provides the nurse with a standard form to document the outcomes of the teaching.

Teaching forms may be designed to address the different domains and outcomes of learning. Using phrases such as "patient demonstrates" defines the psychomotor outcomes. Phrases such as "patient verbalizes" defines the cognitive objectives. A section labeled "Progress, Lack of Progress, Patient Teaching, and Evidence of Learning," provides space to document achievement of outcomes. (This is discussed in Chapter 5.) These are just a few examples of the ways nurses are documenting their patient education responsibilities, which are an essential part of comprehensive

MERCY Community Hospital
Ostomy/Self-Management
Patient/Family Teaching Record

Patient/Family Expected Outcomes By the end of Instruction, the Patient/Family will be able to:	Date	Responsible Discipline and Signature	Teaching Methods	Evaluation Follow-Up	Content Outline and Resources
DIAGNOSIS/PROBLEM					
Define Ostomy **Define Stoma**		Nursing E.T. Nurse			**Ostomy** — surgically created opening into intestinal tract through abdominal wall; may be temporary or permanent. **Stoma** — visible portion of ostomy.
Describe Patient specific type of ostomy		Nursing E.T. Nurse			**Colostomy**: opening into colon for fecal elimination. **Ileostomy**: opening into lower portion of small intestine for fecal elimination.
MEDICATION					
Verbalize comprehension of at least 4 recommendations to follow with medication use.		Pharmacy Nursing E.T. Nurse			• Notify medical person re: presence of ostomy. • Time released medications not recommended. • Use liquid medications when possible. • **MOM** is the strongest laxative to use **(TRY dietary measures first).** • If rectum is removed: — no enemas — no rectal temperatures — no rectal suppositories.

ADDRESSOGRAPH	**Code: Teaching Methods** **D: Discussion** **AV: Audiovisual** **H: Handout**	**Evaluation/Follow-up** **1. Outcome achieved** **2. Outcome unachieved** **3. Reteach/Reinforce materials** **4. Non-applicable**

Figure 3-5 Patient/family teaching record. (Courtesy Mercy Community Hospital, Havertown, Penn.)

Continued

Patient/Family Expected Outcomes By the end of Instruction, the Patient/Family will be able to:	Date	Responsible Discipline and Signature	Teaching Methods	Evaluation Follow-Up	Content Outline and Resources
Explain at least 3 dietary modifications to be made		Dietitian E.T. Nurse			• Some foods are gas and/or odor forming. They include eggs, onions, garlic, beans, raw fruits, beer. Monitor use and eat in moderation. • Maintain fluid intake of 6-8 glasses per day. • Adjust eating preferences to coincide with activities. • Chew all foods well.
TREATMENTS					
Demonstrate care of ostomy		Nursing E.T. Nurse			• **Emptying** • **Clamping** • **Changing setup**
DISCHARGE PLANS					
Describe adaptations for activities of daily living		Nursing E.T. Nurse			Provide Ostomy Care Management Packet (video available) Always carry extra supplies Protect stoma from injury of direct blow. Prior to sexual activity, empty pouch, roll-up and secure with tape. Add extra tape to pouch margins during bath time.
Identify supplies needed and where to obtain supplies		Nursing			List of supplies (will be individualized per patient needs). Physician should write prescription for supplies prior to discharge. Will need to contact local pharmacy or medical supply service.
State how to get help after discharge		Nursing E.T. Nurse Social Work			E.T. Nurse - Mercy Community Hospital (610) 645-3931 Social Work will assist with arrangements for nurse visits if indicated.

ADDRESSOGRAPH	**Code: Teaching Methods** **D: Discussion** **AV: Audiovisual** **H: Handout**	**Evaluation/Follow-up** 1. **Outcome achieved** 2. **Outcome unachieved** 3. **Reteach/Reinforce materials** 4. **Non-applicable**

Figure 3-5, cont'd   Patient/family teaching record.

patient care. Additional examples may be found in Chapters 5 and 11.

SUMMARY

This chapter provides information on the planning phase of the nursing process. Planning must be deliberate and thoughtful to be effective. To facilitate the documentation of planning, various methods are discussed, including traditional approaches, such as care planning, and current trends, such as using case management and clinical paths to manage patient care. Documentation of planning should include both discharge and education needs to manage patients effectively in the hospital and at home. Planning patient care provides an opportunity for nurses to define nursing practice and set the standards for excellence.

REFERENCES

Birdsall C, Sperry S: *Clinical paths in medical-surgical practice,* St Louis, 1997, Mosby.

Camp N, Iyer P: *Patient outcomes in medical-surgical nursing,* Springhouse, Pa, 1995, Springhouse.

Cesta T et al: *The case manager's survival guide,* St Louis, 1998, Mosby.

Doenges M, Moorhouse M: *Nurse's pocket guide: nursing diagnoses with interventions,* Philadelphia, 1988, FA Davis.

Flynn AM, Kilgallen ME: Case management: a multidisciplinary approach to the evaluation of cost and quality standards, *J Nurs Care Qual* 8(1):58, 1993.

Forkner DJ: Clinical pathways: benefits and liabilities, *Nurs Manage* 27(11): 35, 1996.

Giuliano K, Poirier C: Nursing case management: critical pathways to desirable patient outcomes, *Nurs Manage* 22(3):52, 1991.

Gordon M: *Manual of nursing diagnosis, 1993-1994,* St Louis, 1993, Mosby.

Greenwood D: Nursing care plans: issues and solutions, *Nurs Manage* 27(3):33, 1996.

Hampton D: Implementing a managed-care framework through care maps, *J Nurs Adm* 23(5):21, 1993.

Joint Commission for Accreditation of Healthcare Organizations: *1997 Comprehensive accreditation manual for hospitals,* Oakbrook Terrace, Ill, 1996, Author.

Kobs A: Nursing care plans: are they required? *Nurs Manage* 28(5):30, 1997.

Noonan R: Liability issues associated with care pathways and practice protocols, *J Legal Nurse Consult* 8(2):2, 1997.

Raiwet C et al: Care maps across the continuum, *Can Nurse* p 26, January 1997.

Redick E et al: Expanding the use of critical pathways in critical care, *DCCN* 13(6):316, 1994.

Smeltzer C, Flores S: Preadmission discharge planning, *J Nurs Adm* 16(1): 18, 1986.

Sovie M: Clinical nursing practices and patient outcomes: evaluation, evolution, and revolution, *Nurs Econ* 7(2):79, 1989.

Taptich B, Iyer P, Bernocchi-Losey D: *Nursing diagnosis and care planning,* ed 2, Philadelphia, 1994, WB Saunders.

Zander K: Nursing case management: strategic management of cost and quality outcomes, *J Nurs Adm* 18(5), 1988.

ADDITIONAL READINGS

Coluciello M, Mangles L: Clinical pathways in subacute settings, *Nurs Manage* 28(6):52, 1997.

Crummer M, Carter V: Critical pathways, the pivotal tool, *J Cardiovasc Nurs* 7(4):30, 1993.

Driscoll D, Caico C: Critical pathways and mother-baby coupling, *Nurs Manage* 27(12):22, 1996.

Eggland E: Charting smarter: using new mechanisms to organize your paperwork, *Nursing* p 35, September 1995.

Gage M: The patient-driven interdisciplinary care plan, *J Nurs Adm* 24(4):26, 1994.

Iyer P, Taptich B, Bernocchi-Losey D: *Nursing process and nursing diagnosis,* ed 3, Philadelphia, 1995, WB Saunders.

Kinney M: Clinical practice guidelines: a vehicle for improving patient care, *Nurs Dynamics* 2(3):11, 1993.

Lumpkins R, Veal J: Interdisciplinary collaboration: strengthening documentation, *Nurs Manage* 26(10):48L, 1995.

Lumsdon K, Hagland M: Mapping care, *Hospitals and Health Networks* p 34, October 20, 1993.

Woodyard LW, Sheetz J: Critical pathway patient outcomes: the missing standard, *J Nurs Care Qual* 8(1):51, 1993.

Worthy M, Siegrist-Muller L: Integrating a "plan of care" into documentation systems, *Nurs Manage* 23(10):68, 1992.

Documenting Implementation

Documenting implementation involves charting the interventions selected to meet the patient's needs. The interventions may be included in the written plan of care, standards of care, protocols, or clinical paths. Charting interventions, using either a flowsheet or progress notes, provides information used to monitor the care that the patient received. Documenting implementation provides evidence of the care rendered, facilitates appropriate reimbursement, and promotes continuity of care.

The documentation of implementation is a broad subject. The chapters covering specialty area documentation, 10 through 14, which comprise the second half of this book, address the charting of interventions. This chapter focuses on the following: the nursing intervention classification (NIC) system, critical documentation issues related to falls and the use of restraints, documentation of psychosocial care, and the development of forms to enhance documentation of nursing interventions.

NURSING INTERVENTION CLASSIFICATION

Purpose

With the development of computerized nursing information systems, creating a standardized method for classifying nursing interventions has become increasingly important. Before nursing documentation can become fully computerized, a common language must be established to clarify and communicate the role of the nurse in healthcare settings. While a common language for nursing diagnoses and patient outcomes has already been established, continuation of the development of a system for classifying interventions is essential to capturing the essence of nursing. Incorporating standard interventions or a minimum data set into computerized patient records will provide data that can be used to describe nursing practice and determine the contribution of nursing to patient outcomes and quality of care (Moorehead,

Delaney, 1997; Daly et al, 1997). Chapter 8 provides additional information on computerized documentation.

Description

The NIC project, developed in 1992 by researchers at the University of Iowa, is a standardized language for nurse-initiated and physician-initiated nursing treatments. The classification system represents both general and specialized nursing practice, and defines interventions all nurses use regardless of the setting (Iowa Intervention Project, 1993).

The interventions are arranged into groups using a three-level taxonomy. The first level consists of six domains that include basic physiological needs to health system issues. The second level contains 26 classes that are grouped according to their relationship with each of the six domains. Figure 4-1 provides an example of a domain and its related classes. The third level is made up of individual interventions, each having a label, a definition, and a set of activities indicating that the intervention was carried out. Figure 4-2 is an example of an intervention and the associated activities.

More than 300 interventions were mapped, labeled, and placed into appropriate categories to facilitate their incorporation into computerized nursing information systems. An intervention may have any of the 26 separate activities, and the specific activities are selected and implemented based on the nurse's clinical judgment and the patient's needs (Daly et al, 1997).

Advantages of Nursing Intervention Classification

The following list details advantages of NIC:

1. Establishing a common language for communicating and clarifying nursing activities enhances efforts

	DOMAIN 1	DOMAIN 2	DOMAIN 3	DOMAIN 4	DOMAIN 5	DOMAIN 6
Level 1 Domains	**1. PHYSIOLOGICAL: BASIC** Care that supports physical functioning	**2. PHYSIOLOGICAL: COMPLEX** Care that supports homeostatic regulation	**3. BEHAVIORAL** Care that supports psychosocial functioning and facilitates life-style changes	**4. SAFETY** Care that supports protection against harm	**5. FAMILY** Care that supports the family unit	**6. HEALTH SYSTEM** Care that supports effective use of the health care delivery system
Level 2 Classes	A *Activity and Exercise Management:* Interventions to organize or assist with physical activity and energy conservation and expenditure B *Elimination Management:* Interventions to establish and maintain regular bowel and urinary elimination patterns and manage complications due to altered patterns C *Immobility Management:* Interventions to manage restricted body movement and the sequelae D *Nutrition Support:* Interventions to modify or maintain nutritional status *Physical Comfort Promotion:* E Interventions to promote comfort using physical techniques F *Self-Care Facilitation:* Interventions to provide or assist with routine activities of daily living	G *Electrolyte and Acid-Base Management:* Interventions to regulate electrolyte/acid base balance and prevent complications H *Drug Management:* Interventions to facilitate desired effects of pharmacological agents I *Neurologic Management:* Interventions to optimize neurologic functions J *Perioperative Care:* Interventions to provide care before, during, and immediately after surgery K *Respiratory Management:* Interventions to promote airway patency and gas exchange L *Skin/Wound Management:* Interventions to maintain or restore tissue integrity M *Thermoregulation:* Interventions to maintain body temperature within a normal range N *Tissue Perfusion Management:* Interventions to optimize circulation of blood and fluids to the tissue	O *Behavior Therapy:* Interventions to reinforce or promote desirable behaviors or alter undesirable behaviors P *Cognitive Therapy:* Interventions to reinforce or promote desirable cognitive functioning or alter undesirable cognitive functioning Q *Communication Enhancement:* Interventions to facilitate delivering and receiving verbal and nonverbal messages R *Coping Assistance:* Interventions to assist another to build on own strengths, to adapt to a change in function, or to achieve a higher level of function S *Patient Education:* Interventions to facilitate learning T *Psychological Comfort Promotion:* Interventions to promote comfort using psychological techniques	U *Crisis Management:* Interventions to provide immediate short-term help in both psychological and physiological crises V *Risk Management:* Interventions to initiate risk-reduction activities and continue monitoring risks over time	W *Childbearing Care:* Interventions to assist in understanding and coping with the psychological and physiological changes during the childbearing period X *Lifespan Care:* Interventions to facilitate family unit functioning and promote the health and welfare of family members throughout the lifespan	Y *Health System Mediation:* Interventions to facilitate the interface between patient/family and the health care system a *Health System Management:* Interventions to provide and enhance support services for the delivery of care b *Information Management:* Interventions to facilitate communication among health care providers

Figure 4-1 NIC taxonomy: domains and classes. (From Iowa Intervention Project—McCloskey JC, Bulechek GM, eds: *Nursing intervention classification [NIC]*, ed 2, St Louis, 1996, Mosby.)

Incision Site Care

DEFINITION: Cleansing, monitoring and promotion of healing in a wound that is closed with sutures, clips, or staples

ACTIVITIES:

Explain the procedure to the patient using sensory preparation

Inspect the incision site for redness, swelling, or signs of dehiscence or evisceration

Note characteristics of any drainage

Monitor the healing process in the incision site

Cleanse the area around the incision with an appropriate cleansing solution

Swab from the clean area toward the less clean area

Monitor incision for signs and symptoms of infection

Use sterile, cotton-tipped applicators for efficient cleansing of tight-fitting wire sutures, deep and narrow wounds, or wounds with pockets

Cleanse the area around any drain site or drainage tube last

Maintain the position of any drainage tube

Apply closure strips, as appropriate

Apply antiseptic ointment, as ordered

Remove sutures, staples, or clips, as indicated

Change the dressing at appropriate intervals

Apply an appropriate dressing to protect the incision

Facilitate the patient's viewing of the incision

Instruct the patient on how to care for the incision during bathing or showering

Teach the patient how to minimize stress on the incision site

Teach the patient and/or the family how to care for the incision, including signs and symptoms of infection

---

BACKGROUND READINGS:
Perry, A.G., & Potter, P.A. (1990). **Clinical nursing skills and techniques.** St. Louis: Mosby.
Sorensen, K., & Luckmann, J. (1986). **Basic nursing: A psychophysiologic approach** (2nd ed.) (932-964). Philadelphia: W.B. Saunders.

Figure 4-2   Example of one intervention from NIC. (From Iowa Intervention Project, McCloskey JC, Bulechek GM, eds: *Nursing intervention classification [NIC],* ed 2, St Louis, 1996, Mosby.)

to implement computerized nursing information systems.

2. A common language for interventions promotes the comparison and evaluation of nursing care among various settings.

3. The taxonomy provides a structure that can be easily coded to facilitate data collection.

4. The NIC structure includes a class called *Health System Management,* which identifies interventions related to the delivery of care, such as multidisciplinary care conferences, order transcription, quality improvement activities, and preceptor responsibilities (to name just a few). Although these activities take place away from the patient's bedside, they are done on behalf of the patient and consume considerable nursing time. Identifying these indirect care activities will help to make a more accurate determination of costs and to provide a more complete picture of nursing responsibilities (Iowa Intervention Project, 1993).

With the movement toward more fully integrated computerized nursing information systems, nurses must be able to describe the problems, interventions, and patient outcomes that result from nursing care. Using a common language to describe nursing interventions is one step toward accomplishing that goal. The reader is encouraged to refer to the references and additional readings at the end of this chapter to obtain more information about the NIC project.

PSYCHOSOCIAL CARE

Documenting

An area of nursing care routinely overlooked in documentation is psychosocial care. Perhaps because of the combination of patient reassurance and emotional support with other "more important" interventions, nurses often discount the significance of the interaction and fail to chart it.

Nurses provide needed psychosocial care and rarely take credit for the investment of time and energy they make in this regard. Psychosocial interventions are no less a part of nursing practice than assessing findings, providing physical care, administering medications, and teaching patients.

Charting Tips

Documenting psychosocial care need not be overwhelming or labor-intensive. Jost (1995) offers the following suggestions for recognizing and documenting psychosocial interventions:

1. Include a brief statement about the main theme of the conversation. For example, "Patient discussed feelings of frustration related to the long hospital stay." Include a direct quote from the patient if it helps to clarify the patient's concerns. Charting the entire conversation is not necessary.

2. Chart pertinent nonverbal cues and behaviors of the patient, such as wringing of the hands, clenched fists, worried facial expression, frequent sighs, pacing, and fidgeting.

Box 4-1

Common Phrases Used to Document Psychosocial Interventions

- Listened supportively
- Helped patient identify or express feelings
- Helped patient identify alternative choices
- Encouraged patient not to become overwhelmed by long-term possibilities
- Clarified, confirmed, or reviewed information for the patient
- Reinforced positive coping skills of the patient
- Helped patient identify support systems
- Reassured patient that his or her responses are a normal reaction
- Diffused the patient's anger by allowing him or her to verbalize

---

3. Use objective statements to describe the patient's behavior. Avoid drawing conclusions or labeling the behavior based on personal feelings. For example, instead of charting that the patient is "depressed," record specific behaviors, such as crying or withdrawal from touch.
4. Briefly state the method of intervention using descriptive words, such as "listened supportively," or "reinforced appropriate coping skills" (Box 4-1).
5. Document the patient's immediate response to the interventions, keeping in mind that the response may not be a change in the emotion or behavior, but rather that the patient was able to verbalize his or her feelings.

Charting psychosocial interventions provides an opportunity for nurses to communicate valuable information about the patient and to account for the time and effort expended in meeting the patient's various healthcare needs.

CRITICAL DOCUMENTATION ISSUES

Falls

Patient falls are one of the main causes of litigation against nurses. Although falls can occur in any patient population, they are most common in the elderly. Identification of patients at high risk for falls is addressed in Chapter 2. Once a patient has fallen, nursing documentation should indicate additional measures taken to prevent further falls. Once a fall has occurred, nurses are held to a higher standard of care because they should now be aware that the patient is at a higher risk for a fall. A variety of helpful strategies are used to prevent falls, including the use of siderails, restraints, and mechanical devices that provide a warning signal when a patient attempts to climb out of bed.

Documenting Preventive Measures

Ongoing documentation of preventive measures is essential and should include the following information: the bed position, the number of siderails used, the placement of the call bell, the use of restraints, and the use of any other safety devices, such as bed alarms. This documentation provides evidence that the nurse was aware of the patient's risk for falls and attempted to provide for his or her safety. Most facilities now include a section on the daily flowsheet to facilitate documentation of patient safety interventions. Instructions given to the patient or family regarding the patient's risk for falls and the need to call for assistance should be recorded in the progress notes. When the nurse implements and documents the preventive measures taken, defense attorneys can argue that a diligent effort was made to protect the patient.

The following case illustrates the benefit of documenting preventive measures and the patient's progress:

A woman in her early seventies was admitted to a New York hospital with complaints of abdominal pain. She underwent abdominal surgery and was recovering without difficulty. Two days before discharge, she got out of bed, fell in her room, and suffered a fractured hip. She later died of unrelated causes. Her family alleged that she should not have been allowed to get out of bed without supervision until she was fully recovered. The defendant argued that the patient had been out of bed, in accordance with doctor's orders, 5 days before the incident. The defendant further contended that no supervision was necessary because she was ambulating well on her own at the time. A defense verdict was reached (Laska, 1998a).

The following case illustrates the need for appropriate assessment and intervention when a patient is at high risk for falls:

A 74-year-old woman with Alzheimer's disease was admitted to the hospital after she fell at home. While unattended on a gurney, she tried to get up and fell again, fracturing her wrist. The plaintiff's attorney argued that the hospital failed to take precautions to protect the patient in spite of her history of falls and statements from the family. The jury awarded the plaintiff more than $100,000 in damages (Eskreis, 1998).

Documenting a Fall

If a patient falls despite all precautions, physical assessment findings and the treatment rendered should be documented in the medical record and in an incident report. The critical observations to be made after a fall are listed in Box 4-2.

In addition, the nurse should evaluate the circumstances surrounding the fall and review the patient's medications for possible adverse effects and interactions. Box 4-3 provides questions to ask the patient and points to be included in the documentation of a fall.

The following example illustrates the need for timely and accurate intervention after a fall:

Box 4-2

What to Assess After a Fall

Integumentary System

Observe the patient for bruises, lacerations, or abrasions.

Musculoskeletal System

Note any pain or deformity in the patient's extremities, particularly the hip, arm, leg, or lumbosacral spine. Particularly note if one of the patient's legs is externally rotated, abducted, and shortened compared with the other leg.

Cardiovascular System

Assess the patient's blood pressure while the patient is lying down and sitting (or standing, if permitted). Look for a drop of 20-30 mm Hg in the patient's systolic blood pressure, which might indicate orthostatic hypotension. Check the patient's pulse for irregularities.

Neurologic System

Assess the patient for any obvious neurologic changes, such as slurred speech, decreased strength in the extremities, or changes in mental status.

A 67-year-old woman was admitted to the hospital for removal of a brain tumor. She was recovering from the surgery without difficulty when, after numerous attempts to ring for the nurse, she fell trying to get to the bathroom unassisted. The nurse assisted her back to bed and notified the doctor on call. The nurse's note indicated that the patient's vital signs were stable and the patient had no cuts or bruises. The physician's note was sketchy at best, with no reference to physical assessment findings. The patient was complaining of pain in her right leg. She was given an ice bag and Motrin (ibuprofen) for the pain. Over the next two days the patient complained of excruciating pain but was assisted in and out of bed as ordered. On the third day the woman's primary physician consulted an orthopedic surgeon, who determined immediately that the woman had broken her hip. His note indicated that the leg was externally rotated and foreshortened, which are classic signs of a fractured hip. Finally, 96 hours after the fall, the patient had surgery to repair the fracture. The case was settled out of court and the patient was awarded damages in excess of $70,000 (Unpublished verdict, Picone v. Presbyterian Hospital of New York, 1995).

Documenting Refusal of Safety Devices

Because falls are associated with a large number of lawsuits, the charting of information related to safety devices should be clear and specific. In a number of situations a patient, family, or physician may request that siderails, restraints, or mechanical devices not be used. The nurse is expected to exercise clinical judgment in evaluating such requests, including evaluation of the patient's safety and mental status. When the nurse believes that requests for restraints are reasonable, it is appropriate that the nurse comply with

---

Box 4-3

Documentation After a Fall

The following important information should be gathered and documented after a fall.

- Evaluate the circumstances surrounding the fall. Determine whether the patient had any symptoms before the fall. Ask the patient if any of the following symptoms were present:
  Dizziness
  Generalized weakness or one-sided weakness
  Slurred speech
  Impaired vision
  Loss of consciousness
  Lightheadedness
  Palpitations
  Aura/warning
  Shortness of breath
  Chest pain
- Determine what the patient was doing just before the fall, such as the following:
  Sitting up suddenly to get out of bed
  Climbing over the side rails or the end of the bed
  Hyperventilating
  Flexing the head backward
  Climbing or descending stairs
- Ask the patient what happened after the fall, including the following:
  Were there environmental factors that contributed to the fall?
  Did the patient lose control of his or her bladder or bowels?
  If alone, did the patient get up without assistance?
  What part of the patient's body was injured?
  Were there any witnesses to the fall who could supply additional details?
- The answers to these questions should be included on the incident report and charted in the progress notes.
- Document the time that the physician was notified of the fall. The physician is responsible for documenting a description of the patient's injuries on the progress notes and incident report. Document the time and name of the supervisor who was notified of the incident and the time that the family was notified.

---

them. Some facilities require a siderail release form to be filled out as well; for example:

| 2300 hours | Pt. alert, oriented × 3, steady on feet, no c/o dizziness. Pt. requests that siderails be lowered at all times. Siderail release signed.—C. Evesham RN |

However, assessment of the patient may lead the nurse to believe that not to use side rails, restraints, or other devices would jeopardize the patient. In such a situation the nurse should discuss concerns with the appropriate people such as clinical nurse specialists or managers and explore alternative strategies. Such a situation requires careful documentation, including the following:

- Justification for the use of restraints
- Explanation of the risks of not using restraints
- Name of the person who refused to allow use of restraints
- Name of the person(s) whom the nurse informed of this problem

For example:

1400 hours	Pt.'s daughter objects to pt. being "tied down."
	I explained risks of not restraining pt. (i.e., chance of falls).
	Daughter agreed that when she is visiting patient the restraint will be removed. She will inform nursing staff when she leaves at the end of her visit so restraint may be reapplied.—P. Adams, RN

Restraints

Physical or chemical restraints are used to prevent falls, removal of tubes by the patient, wandering, or violent episodes, or to maintain body alignment. Known hazards of physical restraints include loss of mobility and muscle mass, skin breakdown, impaired circulation, impaired respiratory status, decline in functioning, incontinence, and strangulation.

Chemical restraints, such as antipsychotic drugs and sedatives, may increase the risk of falls by causing sleepiness, poor judgment, or confusion. The effectiveness of restraints is in question because of concerns that restraints may do more harm than good. The psychological consequences of restraints may include feelings of humiliation and fear, which may lead to combativeness. As a result of their examination of the use of restraints, many acute care and long-term care facilities are experimenting with new methods of providing safety without the use of restraints. Lower beds, removable lap trays, special seating devices, alarms on doors and beds, different bed rails, and "sitters" are being used to avoid tying patients down. A study of 12,000 residents of 276 nursing homes shows that, when differences in impairment and care needs are taken into account, residents who are restrained need more nursing care than those who are not restrained. The research concludes that implementing approaches to care that avoid the use of restraints does not produce higher costs, but that removing restraints actually reduces costs (*Reducing the use of physical restrains in nursing homes,* 1993). The use of restraints is discussed in more detail in Chapter 14.

Standards Governing the Use of Restraints

The federal government passed regulations governing the use of restraints as part of the Omnibus Budget Reconciliation Act. The Food and Drug Administration (FDA) also issued warnings and recommendations in November 1991 for the use of restraints. Many state departments of health have taken up this issue and have mandated policies that affect the ordering and use of restraints. Standards relating to restraints are included in the Joint Commission for the Accreditation of Healthcare Organizations (JCAHO) manual for hospitals. The goal is to limit the use of restraints and use the least-restrictive method of restraint whenever possible. The following list is a partial compilation of the standards of the Joint Commission (1997) addressing the use of restraints:

TX 7.1   Restraint or seclusion use within an organization is limited to those situations with adequate, appropriate clinical justification.

TX 7.1.3.2   Individual orders for restraint and seclusion use are consistent with organization policy.

TX 7.1.3.2.1   Patient rights, dignity, and well-being are protected during restraint or seclusion use.

TX 7.1.3.2.2   Restraint or seclusion is based on the assessed needs of the patient.

TX 7.1.3.2.3   The least-restrictive safe and effective restraint or seclusion method is employed.

TX 7.1.3.2.4   Restraint or seclusion is used correctly by competent, trained staff.

TX 7.1.3.2.5   Patients in seclusion or restraints are monitored and reassessed appropriately.

TX 7.1.3.2.6   Patient needs are met during the time of restraint or seclusion use.

TX 7.1.3.2.7   Restraint or seclusion use is ordered by a licensed independent practitioner.

TX 7.1.3.2.8   Orders for seclusion and restraint use define specific time limits.

TX 7.1.3.3   Documentation in the medical record reflects organization policy.

The decision to apply restraints must be made based on an assessment of the patient. In a life-threatening emergency, or when the patient is attempting to hurt others, nurses are legally justified in applying restraints immediately and later contacting the physician for an order. The nurse should continue to monitor the patient closely, recognizing that the patient may be capable of removing the restraints or getting out of the bed while still restrained.

The following case illustrates the need for adequate assessment and intervention regarding the need for restraints:

A 78-year-old Michigan man was hospitalized for bronchitis. During his lengthy hospitalization, he fell at least twice. He sustained bilateral intracerebral hematomas and bilateral subdural hygromas, which were determined to be the cause of his death. The plaintiff alleged that the hospital fell below the standard of care by failing to restrain the patient. The verdict in favor of the plaintiff was for $466,000 (Laska, 1998b).

Nursing documentation must specify why restraints were used. Proper entries into the record can justify the use of restraints and therefore minimize the liability risks associated with their use. Claims of false imprisonment can be countered by clear documentation.

Tips for Charting the Use of Restraints

The following list includes tips for charting the use of restraints:

1. Document attempts made to calm the patient in an effort to avoid the use of restraints. Describe the outcome of these attempts.
2. Inform the family of the need for restraints if the patient is mentally incompetent. Document this conversation; for example:

| 1700 hours | Janice Wright, daughter of resident, informed of need to use belt restraint while resident is in wheelchair. Daughter agreed with use of restraint. —P. Zanetti, RN |

3. Include the following points in documentation when the restraint is first applied:

   Reasons for the use of the restraints (with a specific description of the patient's behavior)
   Alternative interventions that were used first and why these were ineffective
   Type of restraint used
   Time of application of the restraint
   Patient's response to the restraint

   For example:

1900 hours	Pt. observed to be climbing out of bed. Instructed to remain in bed. Given bedpan. Said she would stay in bed. Call bell within reach.
1915 hours	Again seen trying to get out of bed. Confused as to time and place. Says she needs to go downstairs for breakfast. Chest restraint applied. Resting at present.
2000 hours	Asleep with chest restraint intact. —J. Zee, RN

4. Adhere to the agency's policies relating to the obtaining of a physician's order for restraints. Many agencies require such an order to specify the type of restraint used, the reason for the use of the restraint, and the duration of use. When the order for restraint needs to be renewed, follow through by notifying the physician of the need for a new restraint order. One acute-care facility developed a stamp to be placed on the chart to notify the physician of the need to reorder restraints (Figure 4-3).
5. Whenever a patient requires forcible restraint, such as the use of leather restraints on all four extremities, ensure that the chart contains a clear, vivid description of the behavior leading to the use of such restraint. The chart should indicate the following:

   Why the restraints were needed
   The number and names of persons who came to assist in the application of the restraints
   Injuries (if any) incurred in the effort to restrain the patient

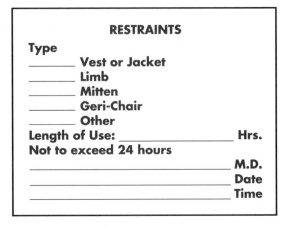

Figure 4-3 Stamp used to remind physician to reorder restraints. (Courtesy Robert Wood Johnson University Hospital at Hamilton Hospital, Trenton, NJ.)

6. Follow agency policy regarding ongoing documentation of observations of a restrained patient. Be sure that the clinical record reflects the frequency with which the patient was evaluated. The chart should state that the nurse:

   Assessed the skin under the restraint
   Noted that respiratory and circulatory status were not impeded by the restraint
   Noted symptoms that justified the need for continued use of the restraint
   Released and reapplied the restraints every 2 hours and performed range-of-motion exercises before replacing the restraints
   Repositioned the patient at frequent intervals
   Provided opportunities for the patient to use the urinal or bedpan

This type of documentation may be needed to help justify the use of restraints. The more abusive and combative the patient's behavior toward the staff, the more likely that the plaintiff may assert that the staff was punishing the patient. If the patient is injured in the process of being restrained, the staff may be held liable if a jury determines that excessive and unnecessary force was used to restrain the patient, as the following case illustrates:

A 32-year-old woman with a long history of mental illness and drug abuse recently had had a tracheostomy. One evening in the hospital, she became agitated and knocked down the charge nurse. Seven staff members responded, and she [the patient] was restrained and medicated.

Two hours later the patient was partially released from restraints to eat, but she tore at her tracheostomy site. She was allowed to walk about while wearing a straitjacket, but she harassed the staff. Later, the straitjacket was removed and the patient was allowed to wander about the ward. She continued to bother staff and other patients and, at one point, disrobed and walked about nude until the staff intervened. At 5:30 AM the patient urinated on the floor of the nursing station. An LPN put her back in her room. To place her in restraints, the nurse knelt on the patient and then gave her an injection.

About one-half hour later, the nurse checked the seclusion room and ran out looking pale. "Code blue," the nurse yelled, and help was summoned. CPR was unsuccessful, and the patient expired. An autopsy was performed. The autopsy report indicated that the patient had bruising on the neck and ligature marks on her wrists and ankles. An [sic] hepatic tear with bleeding was also discovered, but the medical examiner signed the case out as "asphyxiation by mechanical compression." The nurse was charged with manslaughter and criminally negligent homicide and was found guilty (Hill, 1991).

Patient Rounds

Even when a patient has not been placed in restraints or secluded, hospital policy dictates that the nurse must make frequent observations, or rounds, to monitor the patient's well-being. The mandated length of time between observations varies from one facility to another. This period may be as short as 30 minutes or as long as 2 hours. The nurse is responsible for following hospital policy in checking on the patients and for documenting that rounds were made. The nurse may sometimes make the appointed rounds but fail to document them; this can be a problem for the nurse if something untoward happens to the patient because the documentation would not support the nurse's claim that rounds were actually made.

Some facilities have incorporated a section on the daily flowsheet entitled "hourly rounds" or "patient observations," in which the nurse enters the time and initials to indicate that rounds were actually made. Avoid signing off in advance for rounds that have not actually taken place. A nurse working 11 PM to 7 AM documented that the rounds were made and the patient was fine, only to go in at the end of the shift to find the patient had died sometime much earlier in the shift.

DOCUMENTING IMPLEMENTATION USING FLOWSHEETS

Providing and documenting interventions is an integral part of nursing practice. A considerable amount of time is required to chart pertinent findings, patient safety interventions, and psychosocial care, not to mention the routine, repetitive aspects of daily care. To ease the burden and reduce the length of narrative charting, flowsheets were created.

Purpose

Flowsheets are used to collect assessment data, document nursing interventions, or both. Box 4-4 outlines several uses for flowsheets.

If used correctly, flowsheets can save the nurse considerable time when charting. Documentation of routine and repetitive aspects of patient care and assessment occupies much of the nurse's time. This routine data lends itself well to flowsheets. Avoid repeating flowsheet

---

Box 4-4
Purpose of Flowsheets

- To provide quick, efficient documentation of data or interventions
- To consolidate data that would otherwise be scattered throughout the medical record
- To facilitate continuity of care
- To reduce duplication in charting
- To protect the legal interests of the patient and the nurse
- To provide an immediate assessment of the patient's status
- To provide for easy comparison of baseline assessment data with subsequent assessment findings
- To document information that will lead to an evaluation of the patient's progress in achieving outcomes

---

data in the progress notes, because this practice defeats the purpose of using flowsheets and creates unnecessary work.

Nursing care records should provide a complete data base of patient status and nursing care interventions for a specified time period (usually 24 hours). If the form is designed to permit easy comparison of patient status from one shift to the next, the nurse will be able to quickly identify significant changes in patient status. Include key terms on a flowsheet to provide cues for care. For example, nursing care records in medical-surgical units often include a section for documenting whether the siderails were up or down and whether the call bell was within reach of the patient. Restraint flowsheets are often used as well. These serve as reminders to the nurse to address important safety issues.

Figure 4-4 illustrates a flowsheet that combines a variety of information in a format that is easy to use. The first page of the form uses a charting-by-exception approach (as discussed in Chapter 7) by defining normal assessment patterns and providing checklists to document patient assessments. The second page outlines ongoing care needs, such as activities of daily living (ADLs) and safety management. Page three includes a section for documenting frequent monitoring and patient rounds in addition to the documentation of treatments and equipment. The last page provides a space for progress notes and a list of suggested information to be included in the progress notes. Additional examples of flowsheets and related documentation tools are found throughout this text.

FLOWSHEET DEVELOPMENT

Initial Considerations

The first step in developing or revising a flowsheet is to determine the purpose of the form (Box 4-5, p. 64). Determine what is to be accomplished by creating the form, then

Text continued on p. 64

5189

Iredell Memorial Hospital
NURSING CARE RECORD
Daily Patient Assessment

EDEMA SCALE
1—No Indentation
2—Slight Indent/quickly disappears
3—Moderate Indent/remains 10-15 sec.
4—Deep Indent/remains 1-2 min.
5—Deep Indent/remains 7 min. or more

PULSE SCALE
+4=Bounding
+3=Strong, Palpable
+2=Weak, Palpable
+1=Intermittent, Palpable
0=Absent
D=Doppler

PAIN SCALE:
S=Sleeping
0=No Pain
1=Mild
2=Discomfort
3=Moderate
4=Severe
5=Excruciating

Date:

Time of Assessment: _____   **Time** of Assessment: _____   **Time** of Assessment: _____
BP/Time: _____ | _____   **BP**/Time: _____ | _____   **BP**/Time: _____ | _____

DAY	EVENING	NIGHT

Normal Integumentary Pattern
Skin: color within normal limits, warm, dry, intact, skin turgor elastic.

DAY: ☐ Within normal limits · ☐ Hot ☐ Flushed ☐ Diaphoretic · ☐ Jaundiced ☐ Cool ☐ Clammy · ☐ Dusky ☐ Pale ☐ Cyanotic · ☐ Inelastic Skin Turgor · ☐ Other_____ · ☐ Braden Scale _____ · ☐ Incision _____ · ☐ Dressing _____ · ☐ Tubes/Drains _____ · ☐ Cast _____

EVENING: ☐ Within normal limits ☐ NA · ☐ Hot ☐ Flushed ☐ Diaphoretic · ☐ Jaundiced ☐ Cool ☐ Clammy · ☐ Dusky ☐ Pale ☐ Cyanotic · ☐ Inelastic Skin Turgor · ☐ Other_____ · ☐ Braden Scale _____ · ☐ Incision _____ · ☐ Dressing _____ · ☐ Tubes/Drains _____ · ☐ Cast _____

NIGHT: ☐ Within normal limits ☐ NA · ☐ Hot ☐ Flushed ☐ Diaphoretic · ☐ Jaundiced ☐ Cool ☐ Clammy · ☐ Dusky ☐ Pale ☐ Cyanotic · ☐ Inelastic Skin Turgor · ☐ Other_____ · ☐ Braden Scale _____ · ☐ Incision _____ · ☐ Dressing _____ · ☐ Tubes/Drains _____ · ☐ Cast _____

Normal Respiratory Pattern
Resp. unlabored & symmetrical; reg. rhythm & depth. Secretions clear, thin, no cough. No abnormal breath sounds

DAY: ☐ Within normal limits · ☐ Dyspneic ☐ Tachypneic · ☐ Orthopneic ☐ Irregular · ☐ Other_____ · ☐ Abn. breath sounds, describe location: · ☐ Use accessory muscles · ☐ Non-Productive cough · ☐ Productive cough: Sputum: ☐ Frothy ☐ Thick ☐ Green ☐ Yellow ☐ Bloody ☐ Other_____ · 02 _____ LPM Via_____

EVENING: ☐ Within normal limits ☐ NA · ☐ Dyspneic ☐ Tachypneic · ☐ Orthopneic ☐ Irregular · ☐ Other_____ · ☐ Abn. breath sounds, describe location: · ☐ Use accessory muscles · ☐ Non-Productive cough · ☐ Productive cough: Sputum: ☐ Frothy ☐ Thick ☐ Green ☐ Yellow ☐ Bloody ☐ Other_____ · 02 _____ LPM Via_____

NIGHT: ☐ Within normal limits ☐ NA · ☐ Dyspneic ☐ Tachypneic · ☐ Orthopneic ☐ Irregular · ☐ Other_____ · ☐ Abn. breath sounds, describe location: · ☐ Use accessory muscles · ☐ Non-Productive cough · ☐ Productive cough: Sputum: ☐ Frothy ☐ Thick ☐ Green ☐ Yellow ☐ Bloody ☐ Other_____ · 02 _____ LPM Via_____

Normal Cardiovascular Pattern
Heart rhythm reg., peripheral pulses positive bilaterally, no edema.

DAY: ☐ Within normal limits · ☐ Abn. peripheral pulses Scale _____ · Location: _____ · ☐ Edema (location/scale) _____ · ☐ Calf tenderness ☐ R ☐ L · ☐ Other_____ · ☐ Telemetry rhythm _____ · Apical Rate _____

EVENING: ☐ Within normal limits ☐ NA · ☐ Abn. peripheral pulses Scale _____ · Location: _____ · ☐ Edema (location/scale) _____ · ☐ Calf tenderness ☐ R ☐ L · ☐ Other_____ · ☐ Telemetry rhythm _____ · Apical Rate _____

NIGHT: ☐ Within normal limits ☐ NA · ☐ Abn. peripheral pulses Scale _____ · Location: _____ · ☐ Edema (location/scale) _____ · ☐ Calf tenderness ☐ R ☐ L · ☐ Other_____ · ☐ Telemetry rhythm _____ · Apical Rate _____

Normal ROM Pattern
Full ROM all joints. No muscle weakness, absence joint edema.

DAY: ☐ Within normal limits · ☐ Abn. ROM/joints _____
EVENING: ☐ Within normal limits ☐ NA · ☐ Abn. ROM/joints _____
NIGHT: ☐ Within normal limits ☐ NA · ☐ Abn. ROM/joints _____

Normal Elimination Pattern
GI: Abd. soft, BS positive, all four quadrants. NO N/V diarrhea or constipation.

DAY: ☐ Within normal limits · ☐ Nausea ☐ Vomiting ☐ Diarrhea · ☐ Constipation · Abd. ☐ Distended ☐ Tender ☐ Pain · ☐ Abn. bowel sounds _____ Describe location:_____ · ☐ Other_____ · ☐ Bladder distended ☐ Burning · ☐ Frequency ☐ Dysuria ☐ Foley · ☐ Vaginal Drng. _____ · ☐ Other_____

EVENING: ☐ Within normal limits ☐ NA · ☐ Nausea ☐ Vomiting ☐ Diarrhea · ☐ Constipation · Abd. ☐ Distended ☐ Tender ☐ Pain · ☐ Abn. bowel sounds _____ Describe location:_____ · ☐ Other_____ · ☐ Bladder distended ☐ Burning · ☐ Frequency ☐ Dysuria ☐ Foley · ☐ Vaginal Drng. _____ · ☐ Other_____

NIGHT: ☐ Within normal limits ☐ NA · ☐ Nausea ☐ Vomiting ☐ Diarrhea · ☐ Constipation · Abd. ☐ Distended ☐ Tender ☐ Pain · ☐ Abn. bowel sounds _____ Describe location:_____ · ☐ Other_____ · ☐ Bladder distended ☐ Burning · ☐ Frequency ☐ Dysuria ☐ Foley · ☐ Vaginal Drng. _____ · ☐ Other_____

GU: Voiding without difficulty or Foley patent & draining. No bladder distention.

Normal Cognitive/Perceptual Pattern
Alert, active, calm, oriented to person, place, time, follows commands, speech clear, no pain.

DAY: ☐ Within normal limits · Disoriented to: ☐ Person ☐ Time ☐ Place · ☐ Does not follow commands · ☐ Pain (location/scale) _____ · LOC: ☐ Lethargic ☐ Unresponsive · ☐ Anxious · Speech _____ · Other _____

EVENING: ☐ Within normal limits ☐ NA · Disoriented to: ☐ Person ☐ Time ☐ Place · ☐ Does not follow commands · ☐ Pain (location/scale) _____ · LOC: ☐ Lethargic ☐ Unresponsive · ☐ Anxious · Speech _____ · Other _____

NIGHT: ☐ Within normal limits ☐ NA · Disoriented to: ☐ Person ☐ Time ☐ Place · ☐ Does not follow commands · ☐ Pain (location/scale) _____ · LOC: ☐ Lethargic ☐ Unresponsive · ☐ Anxious · Speech _____ · Other _____

Signature/Initial _____   Signature/Initial _____   Signature/Initial _____
Signature/Initial _____   Signature/Initial _____   Signature/Initial _____

Figure 4-4 Nursing care record organized according to functional health patterns. (Courtesy Iredell Memorial Hospital, Statesville, NC.)

ONGOING NURSING CARE

DAY	EVENING	NIGHT

SAFETY MANAGEMENT PATTERN

DAY

- ☐ **No Needs**
- ☐ **Needs being met with alternatives. Describe:**

_____

- ☐ **Protective Device**   ☐ **Pt. Refuses** (Summarize in Narrative)
  - ☐ To prevent pt. rolling out of bed
  - ☐ As a reminder to call for help
  - ☐ Medical immobilization that is part of specific policy and procedure for all patients
  - ☐ Postural/Adaptive Support
- ☐ **Restraint Device**
  - ☐ To control physical activity to prevent injury to self/others
  - ☐ Medical immobilization that is medically necessary for this individual patient
  - ☐ Meets intent through use of protocol, OR
  - ☐ Ordered by physician
- ☐ **Assessed and continues to meet intent for use**
- ☐ **Alternatives ineffective. Least restrictive device chosen. List device(s) in use:** _____

EVENING

- ☐ **No Needs**
- ☐ **Needs being met with alternatives. Describe:**

_____

- ☐ **Protective Device**   ☐ **Pt. Refuses** (Summarize in Narrative)
  - ☐ To prevent pt. rolling out of bed
  - ☐ As a reminder to call for help
  - ☐ Medical immobilization that is part of specific policy and procedure for all patients
  - ☐ Postural/Adaptive Support
- ☐ **Restraint Device**
  - ☐ To control physical activity to prevent injury to self/others
  - ☐ Medical immobilization that is medically necessary for this individual patient
  - ☐ Meets intent through use of protocol, OR
  - ☐ Ordered by physician
- ☐ **Assessed and continues to meet intent for use**
- ☐ **Alternatives ineffective. Least restrictive device chosen. List device(s) in use:** _____

NIGHT

- ☐ **No Needs**
- ☐ **Needs being met with alternatives. Describe:**

_____

- ☐ **Protective Device**   ☐ **Pt. Refuses** (Summarize in Narrative)
  - ☐ To prevent pt. rolling out of bed
  - ☐ As a reminder to call for help
  - ☐ Medical immobilization that is part of specific policy and procedure for all patients
  - ☐ Postural/Adaptive Support
- ☐ **Restraint Device**
  - ☐ To control physical activity to prevent injury to self/others
  - ☐ Medical immobilization that is medically necessary for this individual patient
  - ☐ Meets intent through use of protocol, OR
  - ☐ Ordered by physician
- ☐ **Assessed and continues to meet intent for use**
- ☐ **Alternatives ineffective. Least restrictive device chosen. List device(s) in use:** _____

NUTRITION / METABOLIC PATTERN

DAY

BREAKFAST Diet _____
Supplemental Feeding: ☐ Yes ☐ No
☐ NPO for _____
Food taken per ☐ Self ☐ Assist ☐ Fed
☐ All ☐ ¾ ☐ ½ ☐ ¼ ☐ None ☐ Refused
Tolerated diet s̄ difficulty ☐ Yes ☐ No
Swallows s̄ difficulty ☐ Yes ☐ No
Explain if no _____
☐ Calorie count
LUNCH Diet _____
Supplemental Feeding: ☐ Yes ☐ No
☐ NPO for _____
Food taken per ☐ Self ☐ Assist ☐ Fed
☐ All ☐ ¾ ☐ ½ ☐ ¼ ☐ None ☐ Refused
Tolerated diet s̄ difficulty ☐ Yes ☐ No
Swallows s̄ difficulty ☐ Yes ☐ No
Explain if no _____ ☐ Calorie count

EVENING

SUPPER Diet _____
Supplemental Feeding: ☐ Yes ☐ No
☐ NPO for _____
Food taken per ☐ Self ☐ Assist ☐ Fed
☐ All ☐ ¾ ☐ ½ ☐ ¼ ☐ None ☐ Refused
Tolerated diet s̄ difficulty ☐ Yes ☐ No
Swallows s̄ difficulty ☐ Yes ☐ No
Explain if no _____
☐ Calorie count
☐ HS Snack

NIGHT

☐ **NA** Diet _____
Supplemental Feeding: ☐ Yes ☐ No
☐ NPO for _____
Food taken per ☐ Self ☐ Assist ☐ Fed
☐ All ☐ ¾ ☐ ½ ☐ ¼ ☐ None ☐ Refused
Tolerated diet s̄ difficulty ☐ Yes ☐ No
Swallows s̄ difficulty ☐ Yes ☐ No
Explain if no _____
☐ Calorie count

ELIMINATION PATTERN

DAY

Voids: ☐ Yes ☐ No ☐ Cath ☐ Other _____
Urine: ☐ Straw ☐ Amber ☐ Bloody ☐ Clear ☐ Cloudy
Incontinent/Urine: ☐ Yes x _____ ☐ Urine strained
Stool: ☐ Yes x _____ ☐ No
Describe _____
Incontinent/Stool: ☐ Yes x_____ ☐ No
Enema: Time _____ Type _____
Results: _____
Tolerated enema s̄ difficulty ☐ Yes ☐ No
Explain if no _____

EVENING

Voids: ☐ Yes ☐ No ☐ Cath ☐ Other _____
Urine: ☐ Straw ☐ Amber ☐ Bloody ☐ Clear ☐ Cloudy
Incontinent/Urine: ☐ Yes x _____ ☐ Urine strained
Stool: ☐ Yes x _____ ☐ No
Describe _____
Incontinent/Stool: ☐ Yes x_____ ☐ No
Enema: Time _____ Type _____
Results: _____
Tolerated enema s̄ difficulty ☐ Yes ☐ No
Explain if no _____

NIGHT

Voids: ☐ Yes ☐ No ☐ Cath ☐ Other _____
Urine: ☐ Straw ☐ Amber ☐ Bloody ☐ Clear ☐ Cloudy
Incontinent/Urine: ☐ Yes x _____ ☐ Urine strained
Stool: ☐ Yes x _____ ☐ No
Describe _____
Incontinent/Stool: ☐ Yes x_____ ☐ No
Enema: Time _____ Type _____
Results: _____
Tolerated enema s̄ difficulty ☐ Yes ☐ No
Explain if no _____

ACTIVITY / EXERCISE PATTERN

DAY

Bath: Time_____ ☐ Refused ☐ Deferred
Type: ☐ Sponge ☐ Shower ☐ Tub ☐ Betadine Bath/Shower
Capabilities: ☐ Self ☐ Assist ☐ Complete by staff
☐ Oral Care ☐ Foley Care ☐ Peri Care
Denture Care: ☐ Upper ☐ Lower
AE Hose: ☐ Yes ☐ No ☐ Removed & reapplied
Skin Breakdown Prevention Protocol: ☐ Yes ☐ No
Tolerated hygiene s̄ difficulty: ☐ Yes ☐ No
Explain if no _____
Ambulate: ☐ Self ☐ Assist **Time:**_____
Up Chair: ☐ Self ☐ Assist **Time:**_____
☐ Bedrest Repositioned: ☐ Self ☐ Assist
Tolerated activity: ☐ Yes ☐ No
Explain if no _____

EVENING

Bath: Time_____ ☐ Refused ☐ Deferred
Type: ☐ Sponge ☐ Shower ☐ Tub ☐ Betadine Bath/Shower
Capabilities: ☐ Self ☐ Assist ☐ Complete by staff
☐ Oral Care ☐ Foley Care ☐ Peri Care
Denture Care: ☐ Upper ☐ Lower
AE Hose: ☐ Yes ☐ No ☐ Removed & reapplied
Skin Breakdown Prevention Protocol: ☐ Yes ☐ No
Tolerated hygiene s̄ difficulty: ☐ Yes ☐ No
Explain if no _____
Ambulate: ☐ Self ☐ Assist **Time:**_____
Up Chair: ☐ Self ☐ Assist **Time:**_____
☐ Bedrest Repositioned: ☐ Self ☐ Assist
Tolerated activity: ☐ Yes ☐ No
Explain if no _____

NIGHT

Bath: Time_____ ☐ Refused ☐ Deferred
Type: ☐ Sponge ☐ Shower ☐ Tub ☐ Betadine Bath/Shower
Capabilities: ☐ Self ☐ Assist ☐ Complete by staff
☐ Oral Care ☐ Foley Care ☐ Peri Care
Denture Care: ☐ Upper ☐ Lower
AE Hose: ☐ Yes ☐ No ☐ Removed & reapplied
Skin Breakdown Prevention Protocol: ☐ Yes ☐ No
Tolerated hygiene s̄ difficulty: ☐ Yes ☐ No
Explain if no _____
Ambulate: ☐ Self ☐ Assist **Time:**_____
Up Chair: ☐ Self ☐ Assist **Time:**_____
☐ Bedrest Repositioned: ☐ Self ☐ Assist
Tolerated activity: ☐ Yes ☐ No
Explain if no _____

ROLE / RELATIONSHIP PATTERN

DAY

Visitors / Family: ☐ Yes ☐ No
Communication pattern: ☐ Effective ☐ Ineffective
Explain _____

☐ **Standards of care given**

Signature/Initials _____
Signature/Initials _____
Signature/Initials _____

EVENING

Visitors / Family: ☐ Yes ☐ No
Communication pattern: ☐ Effective ☐ Ineffective
Explain _____

☐ **Standards of care given**

Signature/Initials _____
Signature/Initials _____
Signature/Initials _____

NIGHT

Visitors / Family: ☐ Yes ☐ No
Communication pattern: ☐ Effective ☐ Ineffective
Explain _____

☐ **Standards of care given**

Signature/Initials _____
Signature/Initials _____
Signature/Initials _____

Figure 4-4, cont'd Nursing care record organized according to functional health patterns.

Continued

NURSING PROCEDURES / TREATMENTS																			DATE						
Initial Appropriate Blocks **TREATMENTS / INTERVENTIONS / PROTOCOLS**	7:00 AM	8:00	9:00	10:00	11:00	12:00 NOON	1:00 PM	2:00	3:00	4:00	5:00	6:00	7:00	8:00	9:00	10:00	11:00	12:00 MN	1:00 AM	2:00	3:00	4:00	5:00	6:00 AM
INITIAL IF COMPLETED, EFFECTIVE OR WNL *If ineffective or abnormal (requires narrative note)																								
Patient rounds																								
Sleep / Rest Pattern (S-sleeping Q-quiet R-restless)																								
Repositioned / Turned																								
Protective(q2h) or **Restraint** (q1h) Rounds (Check Circulation / Skin Status / Hydration / Toileting)																								
Device Removed / Skin Care Given (Protective x 1 q8h; Restraint x 2 q8h)																								
Pathway / Care Plan evaluated and appropriate																								
Pain medication effective																								
Fingerstick reading ☐ N/A																								
Scheduled Insulin ☐ N/A																								
Sliding Scale Insulin ☐ N/A																								
Telemetry Alarms Reviewed/Checked ☐ N/A																								
Neuro-Vascular Check ☐ N/A																								
IV Site WNL ☐ N/A																								
IV Rate																								
IVAC Pump Venous Pressure																								
IVAC Pump Maximum Pressure Limit																								
Dr. Visited																								
Dr. Visited																								

SPECIMENS TO LAB / DIAGNOSTIC TESTS

Time	7-3	Time	3-11	Time	11-7

(*) **Asterisk** each time patient is charged for equipment/supplies   **EQUIPMENT/SUPPLIES**   (✔) **Check** if not applied or changed on your shift, but in use

7-3		3-11		11-7	
☐ IV pump	☐ K-Pad ☐ Overhead Trapeze	☐ IV pump	☐ K-Pad ☐ Overhead Trapeze	☐ IV pump	☐ K-Pad ☐ Overhead Trapeze
☐ Feeding pump	☐ Humidifier ☐ Electrodes	☐ Feeding pump	☐ Humidifier ☐ Electrodes	☐ Feeding pump	☐ Humidifier ☐ Electrodes
☐ Tubing changed	☐ Heel/elbow protectors	☐ Tubing changed	☐ Heel/elbow protectors	☐ Tubing changed	☐ Heel/elbow protectors
Suction:	☐ Bed Cradle	Suction:	☐ Bed Cradle	Suction:	☐ Bed Cradle
☐ Gauge	☐ Special Care Bed	☐ Gauge	☐ Special Care Bed	☐ Gauge	☐ Special Care Bed
☐ Canister		☐ Canister		☐ Canister	
☐ Tubing changed	☐ Other _____	☐ Tubing changed	☐ Other _____	☐ Tubing changed	☐ Other _____

SIGNATURE	TITLE	INITIALS	SIGNATURE	TITLE	INITIALS

Figure 4-4, cont'd Nursing care record organized according to functional health patterns. (Courtesy Iredell Memorial Hospital, Statesville, NC.)

NURSING PROGRESS RECORD

ADDRESSOGRAPH

Documentation to include:
—Continued use of restraint
—Time of application of restraint, type of restraint, reason for the restraint if initiated on that shift
—Psychosocial problems
—Changes from initial assessment, interventions, evaluations
—Calls to physician
—Evaluative statement on treatments, interventions
—Initial application of equipment/devices
—PRN/One time meds and evaluating effectiveness
—Patient status to and from surgery, endoscopy dept., treadmill & pts. transferred on same floor
—Signing consent, evaluation level of understanding
—All other data pertinent to patient's care not documented elsewhere
—Patient status summary note at end of shift

TIME	MEDS	

Figure 4-4, cont'd Nursing care record organized according to functional health patterns.

consider the content of the form. Decide what information should be included in the form to achieve the desired result.

Next consider the primary users of the form. Determine whether the form will be used only by nursing personnel or expanded to meet the needs of a multidisciplinary group. Consider organizing the information on the form in the most logical way so that the primary users will find it helpful. For example, if the nurses are performing head-to-toe assessments, the information should be organized accordingly to facilitate documentation.

One of the benefits of using flowsheets is that the duplication of documentation is reduced. When a form is being developed or revised, consider whether information from two forms could be consolidated into one flowsheet. Many facilities combine assessment data, fluid balance information, routine care and treatments, and progress notes into one flowsheet to eliminate the need for several different forms.

Finally, when developing or revising a flowsheet, always create a set of guidelines that explain how to use the form correctly. This step is essential to the successful implementation of new forms.

Developmental Steps

The creation or revision of a form requires time for planning and implementation. Rosenthal (1992) identifies the following key steps in the development of a form (Box 4-6):

1. Collect and critique forms from other organizations and review the literature to find examples of documentation tools.
2. Compose and revise rough drafts of the flowsheet until the staff reaches a consensus on the final draft version.
3. Ask the medical records department to review the selected draft. Revise the draft, if necessary, based on input from medical records personnel.
4. Present the flowsheet to major physician groups to verify that the form is user-friendly. (Failing to include in the discussions when creating a nursing flowsheet can be a mistake.) Revise the draft if necessary, based on the input received from the physician groups.
5. Present the form to the appropriate committees (for example, critical care, medical, or records staff) for approval. Find out when each committee regularly schedules its meetings. Because some committees meet

only quarterly or bimonthly, missing a meeting can delay the implementation of a new flowsheet.

6. Provide staff education programs to aid in the introduction of the new flowsheet and review the guidelines for using the form. If possible, create a case study so that the staff has an opportunity to use the form in a classroom setting and have their questions answered.
7. Test the flowsheet in a pilot program for a set time in designated units. Obtain permission from the medical records department to use the pilot form as part of the medical record until the final revisions have been made; this will eliminate the need for duplicate documentation. Pilot programs are discussed in more detail in Chapter 9.
8. Collect data to make needed revisions and refine the use of the flowsheet. Suggestions for revision by the staff are common and desirable after they have had a chance to use the form. With this in mind, print only enough copies of the form for the pilot program to avoid waste.
9. Revise the flowsheet as needed and repeat the education program to update the staff on the results of the pilot program and to explain the revisions.
10. Evaluate the staff's acceptance of the flowsheet and provide ongoing support and education as needed.

FLOWSHEET DESIGN

The process of creating the right design for a particular flowsheet or form has many variables. This section contains some general suggestions for the design of flowsheets.

1. Determine how much space the content of the form will require. Consider whether the format will be mostly check-off, fill-in-the-blank, or open-ended questions, or a combination of one or more of these styles.
2. Design a form that is simple to use and easy to read. Avoid overcrowding the page or using small type, which may be difficult to read. Ensure that the size of

the print is sufficiently large. Avoid using words in all capital letters when designing forms because words printed in this manner are much harder to read.

3. Decide whether the form will be used vertically or horizontally. Vertical forms usually provide more length to list information, whereas horizontal forms usually provide more space for narrative entries. The selection of the vertical or horizontal format will depend in part on the type of chart holder used and the way in which the medical records are stored after discharge. If possible, select either the vertical or horizontal format for all forms to create a uniform presentation. (Allow for exceptions as necessary.)

4. Use boldface and italic type to emphasize section headings or other important information. Consider using a heavy line (rule) to separate main sections of the form. However, be selective when using boldface type, underlining, and italic type for emphasis because of the tendency to ignore this type of print when it is overused.

5. Consider the spacing of information. Maintain ¼ inch between lines the nurse will be writing in to allow enough space for a variety of handwriting styles. Allow at least ½ inch for the left margin if the form is to be kept in a loose-leaf binder.

6. Determine whether the form will be more than one page long. When designing the form, consider the orientation of the top and bottom of a two-page form and whether the form will be turned over or turned up during use. (If this is not determined in advance, it will create frustration when the form is implemented.) Number the pages of a multipage form to eliminate questions about order in which the charting should occur. This is particularly important for those trying to photocopy the chart, retrieve information, or investigate chronologic events.

7. Consider whether the information on the form will be communicated between departments. If so, forms with multiple carbon copies may be used to eliminate duplication or unnecessary photocopying.

8. Include blank spaces to permit individualization in the recording of data and documentation of patient findings.

9. If multidisciplinary progress notes are not used, consider providing space for such notes on the reverse side of a flowsheet. This format works particularly well for multipage critical-care flowsheets, postanesthesia records, and labor and delivery forms. Combining flowsheets and progress notes keeps all documentation in one place and allows correlation of data with the documentation on the progress notes. This will not work, however, if all disciplines involved in the care, record information in the same progress notes section.

10. Consider keeping the basic structure of the form the same throughout the nursing areas and modifying the format for use in specialty areas. This helps to verify that the same standard of care was given by personnel throughout the organization, and it also provides some consistency in documentation.

11. Think globally when creating or revising forms. Avoid designing forms without consulting others because the creation of a new form will have an impact on other services and departments. Furthermore, collaboration with other departments may generate new ideas for multidisciplinary forms.

12. Involve the computer information systems personnel in the review of drafts of the flowsheet if the facility has computerized its medical records or is planning to do so.

13. Obtain input from the staff members who will be using the form.

14. Proofread the finished product carefully. Once the form has been printed in volume, encountering misspelled words will be annoying.

15. Understand that developing and implementing a new flowsheet will take longer than initially anticipated. Therefore ensure that enough time has been allocated in your initial plan.

SUMMARY

Documenting implementation of the nursing process is essential to providing a clear, chronologic description of events during the patient's hospitalization. Thorough nursing assessments and complete documentation of nursing interventions and the patient's response to treatments provides the best defense in the event of malpractice litigation. Designing efficient, user-friendly forms to record the data further enhances the nursing process.

REFERENCES

Daly J et al: Nursing intervention classification implementation issues at five test sites, *Comput Nurs* 15(1):23, 1997.

Eskreis TR: Seven common legal pitfalls in nursing, *Am J Nurs* 98(4):34, 1998.

Hill H: Use of restraints. In Henry G, ed: *Emergency medicine risk management,* Dallas, 1991, American College of Emergency Physicians.

Iowa Intervention Project: The NIC taxonomy structure, *Image* 25(3):187, 1993, Author.

Joint Commission for the Accreditation of Healthcare Organizations: *1997 comprehensive accreditation manual for hospitals,* Oakbrook, Ill, 1996, Author.

Jost K: Psychosocial care: document it, *Am J Nurs* p 46, July 1995.

Laska L: Failure to supervise convalescing patient allegedly leads to fall from bed, *Medical Malpractice Verdicts, Settlements, and Experts* p 21, January 1998a.

Laska L: Patient repeatedly falls in hospital: head injuries cause death, *Medical Malpractice Verdicts, Settlements, and Experts* p 23, January 1998b.

Moorehead S, Delaney C: Mapping nursing intervention data into the nursing interventions classification (NIC): process and rules, *Nurs Diagn* 8(4):137, 1997.

Reducing the use of physical restraints in nursing homes: will it increase costs? *Am J Public Health* 83(3):342, 1993.

Rosenthal K: ICU-CCU flowsheet, *Crit Care Nurse* p 58, December 1992.

ADDITIONAL READINGS

Addy-Keller J, McElwaney E: A new documentation tool, *Nurs Manage* 24(11):46, 1993.

Coenen A et al: Mapping nursing interventions from a hospital information system to the nursing interventions classification (NIC), *Nurs Diagn* 8(4):145, 1997.

Grobe S: The nursing intervention lexicon and taxonomy: implications for representing nursing care data in automated patient records, *Holistic Nurs Pract* 11(1):48, 1996.

McDaniel A: Developing and testing a prototype patient care database, *Comput Nurs* 15(3):129, 1997.

Morris A, Thomas S: A med/surg nursing record: convenient, adequate—and accepted, *Nurs Manage* 23(5):68, 1992.

5

Documenting Evaluation

Patients are assessed to gather pertinent data needed to identify and document the patient's high-priority nursing diagnoses. Development and documentation of the plan of care follows. The plan can be written in a variety of formats, as discussed in Chapter 3, including the following:

- A handwritten, individually developed nursing-care plan
- A standard care plan tailored to the patient's needs
- A critical path, which details a multidisciplinary plan of care and may include outcomes
- A practice guideline, which guides care of the patient

The plan of care provides a written framework for the delivery of care. Progress notes and flowsheets are used to document the delivery of care. Evaluation is the final step of the nursing process, and it flows from the outcomes defined in the plan of care. This chapter discusses five aspects of evaluation documentation: why what when where and how outcomes are documented.

WHY OUTCOMES ARE DOCUMENTED

Clinical records contain documentation of the evaluation of a patient's status for several number of reasons. The American Nurses Association standards (ANA, 1991) include an expectation that nurses will evaluate the patient's progress with respect to the achievement of outcomes. The ANA standard for evaluation contains the requirement that the nurse document both the patient's response to the interventions and revisions in the diagnoses, outcomes, and plan of care.

The Joint Commission for the Accreditation of Healthcare Organizations (JCAHO) standards include the requirement that a patient's medical record contain documentation of the patient's response to the care provided (JCAHO, 1996).

Societal factors have placed new emphasis on the achievement of outcomes, which has increased the scrutiny of evaluation documentation. The definition and evaluation of outcomes or results is a fundamental activity in any type of organization, including healthcare agencies. Traditionally, outcomes have not received as strong an emphasis in health care because of the difficulty associated with defining and measuring both the process of care and the results. Healthcare organizations find it easy to hide behind the rationalizations that the existing care processes are too complex to measure and that the human variables that influence outcomes, such as preexisting disease, cannot be controlled.

The current healthcare environment forces us to examine more closely the effectiveness of treatment at both the societal and individual levels. As the cost of health care continues to rise, the attention being directed to the evaluation of patient care outcomes as a way to define the quality of health care is increasing. Efforts to downsize nursing staffs have increased the emphasis on justifying the staffing mix (ratio of licensed to unlicensed personnel) and educating of the staff.

The most common reason for evaluating and documenting the achievement of outcomes is to determine the results of specific care and treatment of individual patients and families. Another purpose is to test or improve the effectiveness of services provided by a healthcare organization to a specific patient population. This area is addressed by utilization management and quality assurance/improvement programs, allowing a facility to determine if the length of stay (LOS) can be reduced while maintaining the quality of the outcomes. Comparison of an organization's outcomes with those of other organizations allows an organization to better understand and improve its own systems. The more closely outcomes are studied, the more apparent it becomes that they are affected by many complex variables.

WHAT OUTCOMES ARE DOCUMENTED

Outcomes fall into one or more of the domains defined in Box 5-1. Outcomes can be measured on different levels and

---

Box 5-1

Domains of Outcomes

Physiological Status

Documentation of assessment parameters, including blood pressure, breath sounds, blood glucose levels, skin integrity, healing of pressure ulcers, and response to treatment

Psychosocial Status

Behavior of the patient and family, including observations about anxiety level, interactions with others, attitudes, and coping mechanisms

Functional Abilities

The ability to perform activities of daily living, including toileting, grooming, cooking, bathing, and walking

Patient Satisfaction

Reactions and perceptions of the patient and family to the quality of nursing care

Knowledge of Self Care

Understanding of the patient and family regarding treatments, symptoms to be reported to the healthcare provider, self-care measures to maintain good health, and diet

Symptom Control

The ability of the patient, family, or nurse to control symptoms such as pain, fatigue, nausea, constipation, diarrhea, and itching

Satisfaction

Perceptions of the patient and family concerning the quality of care being provided

Home Maintenance

Daily functioning of the patient and family in the home, including cooking, cleaning, shopping, and paying bills

Goal Attainment

Comparison of the expected outcomes of care with the actual outcomes, measured at designated intervals or at discharge

Safety Maintenance

Prevention of falls, skin breakdown, medication errors, accidents or injuries, infections, unplanned readmissions, sentinel events (described in Chapter 6), and other complications

Length of Stay (LOS)

Patient's actual LOS compared with the expected LOS

---

for different purposes. Several difficulties currently complicate the measurement of outcomes, including the lack of the following:

- Agreement concerning a common set of elements to use to create a data base for measuring outcomes
- Agreement on precise definitions of outcomes
- Systematic documentation regarding the achievement of outcomes
- Communication between agencies (for example, between home care and acute-care facilities), which prevents measurement of long-term outcomes

These difficulties are being addressed in a number of ways. Attempts are being made to define a uniform set of data elements for medical records. Researchers at Wright State University College of Nursing and Health have developed the Core Data Set, which is composed of data elements collected from all patients receiving health care. This framework provides a uniform data set that has been recommended for use in a variety of healthcare settings to provide a longitudinal data record of an individual's health care. Use of this core data set permits comparisons between inpatient and outpatient care and between various treatment approaches and ensures that a consistent definition is used for data elements (Uddin, Martin, 1997).

The Joint Commission has encouraged the establishment of a system to measure the performance of healthcare facilities and services. Known as the Indicator Measurement System (IMSystem), the indicators of this system are focused on the quality of care; are recognized as clinically important; are relevant to a variety of healthcare organizations; and have been extensively tested for feasibility, reliability, and validity. The measures that are being tracked by healthcare organizations fall into one of seven domains: perioperative, obstetric, cardiovascular, oncology, trauma, medication use, and infection control. Examples of some of the measures that may be influenced by nursing care include the following:

- Perioperative (complications within 2 postoperative days)
  Central nervous system deficits
  Peripheral neurologic deficits
  Acute myocardial infarction (MI)
  Cardiac arrest
  Death
- Obstetric
  Cesarean section delivery
  Vaginal birth after previous cesarean section
- Cardiovascular
  Acute MI in the emergency department (ED): timing of prophylactic therapy
  Postoperative LOS for a coronary artery bypass (CABG) patient or a percutaneous transluminal coronary artery bypass (PTCA) patient
  Death after CABG, PTCA, or MI
- Oncology
  Female breast cancer: estrogen receptor analysis (ERA) results recorded in the medical record
- Trauma
  Vital signs in the ED

Glasgow Coma Scale score in the ED
Timing of computerized tomography (CT) of the head, neurosurgical procedures, orthopaedic procedures, and abdominal procedures
- Medication use
Timing of prophylactic antibiotic administration for selected surgical procedure groups
Demonstration of self-monitoring of blood glucose levels and self-administration of insulin
Measured drug blood levels of digoxin, theophylline, phenytoin, and lithium
- Infection control
Surgical site infection in selected surgical procedures
Pneumonia in patients on ventilators
Primary blood stream infections in patients with central or umbilical lines (McGreevey, Nadzam, Corbin, 1997)

Evaluation and documentation of the outcomes defined above tend to be more concrete than documentation relating to psychosocial outcomes. Outcomes that fit into the psychosocial domain include the following (Eggland, 1997):

- Relief of symptoms, such as anxiety or agitation, through the use of medications and therapy
- Improved ability to cope with stressful situations
- Improved ability to function and prevent further disability
- A sense of physical, mental, and emotional well-being
- Appropriate expression of feelings
- Improved interactions and communication with family, staff, and friends

WHEN TO EVALUATE OUTCOMES

Evaluation is categorized as either formative or summative. Formative evaluation occurs on a periodic basis during the provision of care, whereas summative evaluation occurs at the end of an activity, such as an admission, discharge, or transfer to another area, or at the end of a specific time frame, such as the end of a teaching session.

Formative Evaluation

The frequency with which a nurse evaluates progress depends on the following factors: policies, regulatory standards, healthcare setting, charting system, standards of care/practice guidelines, nursing diagnosis or problem, time frame specified by the outcome, and nursing interventions.

Policies

Policies of a healthcare agency may dictate the frequency with which the nurse should document an evaluation of the patient's progress. This policy may be defined in a number of ways. The agency may have general documentation policies that dictate the frequency of evaluation (for example, a requirement that the plan of care be evaluated hourly, daily, and weekly).

Regulatory Standards

Standards of regulatory agencies may also be used to dictate the time frame for evaluation. For example, the Joint Commission requires agencies to define a time frame for reassessing the patient and evaluating the abilities of the patient or significant other to perform self-care activities. Examples of Joint Commission standards (1996) that comment on evaluation include the following:

TX 1.3 The patients' progress is periodically evaluated against care goals and the plan of care, and when indicated, the plan or goals are revised.

TX 2.4 The patient's postprocedure status is assessed on admission to and before discharge from the postanesthesia recovery area.

TX 3.9 Medication effects on patients are continually monitored.

TX 4.5 Each patient's response to nutrition care is monitored.

TX 5.4 The patient is monitored during the postprocedure period.

TX 6.4 The patient's readiness to end rehabilitation services is determined based on written discharge criteria.

TX 7.4.1 Qualified staff review, evaluate, and approve all behavior management procedures.

Charting System and Forms

The charting system used by the facility may define how often the nurse should document an evaluation. For example, as discussed in Chapter 7, problems, interventions, and evaluation (PIE) charting recommends that outcomes be evaluated every 8 hours and summarized once every 24 hours.

The format of the medical record forms may also dictate the frequency of charting outcomes. For example, Lavin and Enright (1996) describe a flowsheet used in an inpatient chemical-dependency unit. The double-sided page consists of three columns and one page is used per shift. The left column lists the typical symptoms experienced by patients undergoing detoxification from drugs or alcohol. The middle column provides spaces for recording nursing interventions used to treat the symptoms. Standard interventions are preprinted on the form. The far right column is used to record the patient's responses or outcomes. Ongoing problems or additional information is documented in the progress notes.

Standards of Care and Practice Guidelines

Standards of care and practice guidelines may specify how frequently outcomes are to be evaluated. For example, a practice guideline for treatment of impaired skin integrity may suggest that the nurse evaluate and document the condition of the patient's skin every 8 hours.

Nursing Diagnosis or Problem

The type of nursing diagnosis or problem may influence the frequency of evaluation. When defining the patient's nursing diagnosis, as discussed in Chapter 3, the nurse identifies the most important (high-priority) problems. The human responses with the greatest effect on the patient's well-being are given the highest priority. The patient's basic physiological needs, including the need for food, air, elimination, and circulation, are usually the most urgent. These needs generally should be addressed before concentrating on psychosocial needs. The frequency of evaluation will vary as the patient's condition changes and as new diagnoses are made.

In the following case the development of a new problem did not trigger the expected evaluation of the patient's condition:

A woman in her late fifties fell at home. Doctor A performed surgery at an acute-care hospital, then admitted her to a rehabilitation facility in another county. Shortly after her admission there, she complained of severe neck pain, which never abated. Despite this, she was discharged. About 10 days after discharge, Dr. A readmitted her to the acute-care hospital and ordered an MRI of the neck. The MRI was never done, however. She gradually became paralyzed, but Dr. A told her family it was "in her head" and he would make a walker available, because she needed to walk. Nursing personnel noted in the records that she "refused" to use her legs. On the fifth day she experienced cardiopulmonary arrest caused by central nervous system paralysis. After she had been resuscitated, she was ultimately diagnosed with a massive cervical infection. She survived for 1½ years. The final settlement was for $1.2 million, with the acute-care hospital paying $350,000, the rehabilitation facility paying $250,000, and the rest being paid by the doctors (Laska, 1997a, p. 6).

Time Frame

As discussed in Chapter 3 the time frame tells the nurse when to evaluate the outcome. The inclusion of time frames, such as "within 24 hours," "by the time of discharge," or "by the third teaching session," provides a great deal of guidance for the nurse who will be evaluating the outcomes. Time frames are also defined in critical paths.

Nursing Interventions

Nursing interventions may specify how frequently the patient's status should be monitored or other nursing actions should be taken. For example, the nursing intervention of auscultating breath sounds every shift indicates that the clinical records should contain a description of breath sounds. Specific, clear interventions facilitate documentation by outlining the expected nursing actions.

Summative Evaluation

Summative evaluation is typically performed at the time of transfer or discharge of the patient. Critical thinking and clinical judgment must be used when the patient's status is incompatible with the planned discharge. The following case in California illustrates this point:

A 68-year-old diabetic woman stepped on a nail at her home. The patient developed an infection in her foot and was admitted to the hospital. During the hospitalization she developed nausea and vomiting with a resulting drop in her potassium level to 2.7 (the normal range is 3.5-5.0). On the sixth day of her admission, she was discharged. Although her doctor claimed that her temperature was normal at the time of her discharge, subsequent review of her medical record showed that her temperature was 100.9° F at the time of her discharge. After complaining of continued pain, swelling, and fever, she was readmitted to the hospital the next day. She developed nausea and fatigue, and her blood pressure dropped to 85/52 at 4 PM on the fourth day of her admission. The nurses did not notify a doctor of this change in her condition. At 8:50 PM she went into cardiopulmonary arrest. Although she was resuscitated, she did not regain consciousness before she died 4 days later. Her potassium level was found to be 2.4 at the time of the arrest. The jury returned a verdict of $250,000 against the doctor and hospital (Laska, 1997b).

In this case, errors in the formative and summative evaluations contributed to the outcome (inadequate evaluation of the patient's condition).

Allegations that a cast was too tight at the time of discharge were factors in the following case in Philadelphia:

The plaintiff underwent reconstructive surgery for a sprained ankle that would not heal properly. The plaintiff was discharged from the hospital the day after surgery, but she returned that night complaining of severe pain. It was determined that she was suffering from compartment syndrome in her right leg resulting from the cast being too tight. The plaintiff claimed that superficial peroneal nerve damage resulted in permanent foot drop. When the plaintiff alleged that she had complained of her cast being too tight while she was in the hospital, the defendants contended that the syndrome had developed after her release. The hospital records indicated that she had very little pain at the time of her discharge. The hospital staff were found ninety-nine percent liable and the surgeon was found one percent liable. The award was $1.2 million (Laska, 1997c).

Transfer Forms

The Joint Commission standards (1996) state that the hospital is to ensure that appropriate patient care and clinical information is exchanged when patients are admitted, referred, transferred, or discharged. One common method of ensuring that this exchange of information occurs is the use of transfer forms (Figure 5-1) and discharge forms. Transfer forms are used to communicate important information about the patient's status when the patient is moved within the facility, between two facilities, or between the patient's home and an institution. Transfer of a patient from one ED to another is discussed in Chapter 11.

Discharge Forms

The needs of the patient should be evaluated at the time of discharge from a healthcare facility. These needs will direct

Saint John's Health System
Anderson, IN 46016

History of Injury or Illness:	Unresolved Nursing Diagnosis:
_____	_____
_____	_____
_____	_____
_____	_____
_____	_____

Allergies: _____

Current Medications/IV's & Last Dose Given:	Other Current Orders (Treatments, O_2, Therapy, etc.):

Vitals: BP_____   T_____   P_____   R_____   Code Status _____

Studies/Reports Attached ❑

CBC ❑   Urinalysis ❑   ECG ❑   Other ❑ _____Mantoux ❑ Date Given:_____

ABG'S❑   Electrolytes ❑   Discharge Summary ❑   Chest X-Ray ❑ Date: _____

Assessment: (Circle If Normal Or Complete As Indicated By Patient's Condition)

Diet/Feed:_____   Sight:_____

Speech:_____   Activity: _____

Hearing:_____   Bowel/Bladder Control:_____ Date Last BM_____

Mental Status:_____   Prosthesis Or Appliance:_____

Nurses' Signature: _____

Date:_____

WHITE - Chart copy   **YELLOW -** Send with patient

★ A copy of the Face Sheet must accompany this form.

768-36-496   Patient Information Transfer Form

B-C Note	C-Lab	D-X-Ray	E-Diag	F-Surgery	G-Therapy	H-Orders	I-Nurses	J-Misc.

Figure 5-1   Sample of transfer form. (Courtesy St. John's Health Care Corporation, Anderson, Ind.)

the provision of continuing care. The different types of discharge forms are discharge summaries and discharge instruction sheets.

Discharge Summaries. Discharge summaries are used in some facilities and are intended to document the completion of the discharge process to ensure that all appropriate steps have been completed. They are *not* meant to summarize the course of the illness. They can be designed as a quick checklist with space provided for commenting on significant items. Patient education flowsheets are often combined with discharge status summaries to create efficient forms (Figure 5-2).

Discharge Instruction Sheets. Discharge instruction sheets list discharge instructions for diet, treatments, medications, activities, and follow-up appointments (Figure 5-3). The follow-up appointment information should specify who the healthcare provider will be and when the patient is to be seen, for example, "patient is to see Dr. Fellos in 2 weeks." Usually these forms have two copies: one for the patient and one for the medical record. The record should include a notation that these instructions were provided to the patient or a place for the patient to sign to confirm that the instructions were received and understood. Joint Commission requirements (1996) stress that discharge instructions should be given to the patient, to the family (when appropriate), and to the organization or individual responsible for the patient's continuing care, including extended-care facilities, home care agencies, and home companions.

Discharge instruction sheets are used in a variety of healthcare settings. These sheets are important in that they document the fulfillment of the nurse's professional responsibility to provide instructions and they shift the responsibility for following these instructions to the patient. Malpractice suits initiated because of poor outcomes provide evidence that arranging for follow-up after the patient is discharged clearly is more prudent than leaving aftercare to the patient or family's discretion. Specific instructions given in a language that the patient can understand are better than general advice. A written record of the conversation with the patient at the time of the patient's discharge can be vital in defending the actions of healthcare professionals. Tips on the development of discharge instruction sheets are shown in Box 5-2 on p. 75.

The use of discharge instruction sheets has raised issues in some settings about the degree of communication and collaboration between nurses and physicians. Sometimes confusion exists as to which discipline is responsible for discharge teaching and instructions. These issues must be resolved in order to promote cooperation and to facilitate documentation of discharge teaching.

In the following case, careful discharge instructions provided ED staff with a valid defense when the patient did not follow the instructions given to him, resulting in extensive surgery after his appendix ruptured:

A 26-year-old California man went to the defendant hospital's ED with complaints of abdominal pain and vomiting. After a thorough evaluation, he was diagnosed with possible gastritis. He was given oral and written instructions to seek follow-up care with his own doctor within 2 days. The patient failed to seek follow-up care as directed, but instead, returned to the ED 6 days later, where he was diagnosed with a perforated appendix. After an emergency appendectomy and partial colon resection, he filed suit against his doctors and the hospital. He claimed that the printed instructions were inadequate and outdated and that he did not understand or recall the verbal instructions because he was under the influence of Demerol (meperidine) at the time. The defendants contended that the printed instructions that the plaintiff signed clearly advised him to seek follow-up care within 2 days and that he was alert and oriented at the time of discharge. The verdict was for the defense (Laska, 1998).

Postdischarge Evaluation

In some healthcare settings documenting calls to patients following discharge to evaluate their status is common. This may be done in the ED, the outpatient surgery department (Figure 5-4, p. 76), the medical procedures unit, or any other unit. These forms usually consist of a series of questions about the patient's status and a space to fill in any instructions that were given to the patient. Often an area for the nurse to document information about the patient's satisfaction with his or her experience in the unit is also included. Policy should dictate how many attempts should be made to reach the patient before abandoning the effort. Each attempt to reach the patient should be documented to indicate that the effort was made. The absence of a report of follow-up phone calls in the medical record could be interpreted as a failure to make such calls.

WHERE OUTCOMES ARE DOCUMENTED

The evaluation of outcomes is documented in flowsheets and in progress notes. Chapter 4 presents content on the design of flowsheets, and Chapter 7 discusses the various charting systems and how evaluation is documented in each type of system.

HOW OUTCOMES ARE DOCUMENTED

Progress notes document the patient's status in relation to the desired outcomes. The patient's responses are compared with the outcomes defined by the plan of care. The following are some concepts typically addressed in the progress notes, including some examples of evaluative comments:

- Progress toward achieving outcomes (for example, "incision shows no sign of infection")
- Response to prn medications (for example, "verbalized relief of pain 45 minutes after injection of morphine"

Saint John's Health System
Anderson, IN 46016

PATIENT HEALTH CARE EDUCATION/DISCHARGE SUMMARY

Patient Diagnosis: _____

Other Learning Needs: _____

Instructed: patient _____ other_____

PATIENT OUTCOME CODES: P-Progressing (instruction given), **NPA**-Needs Periodic Assistance, **NC**-Non-compliant,
NCA-Needs Constant Assistance, **A**-Achieved, **RD**-Return Demonstration, **N/A**-Non-Applicable, *****-See Nurse's Note

	Adm.	Progress Updated	Disch.

Disease Process: _____

_____

Treatments/Procedures: _____

_____

Wound/Skin Care: _____

_____

Diet: _____

_____

Elimination: _____

_____

Activity: _____

_____

Other: _____

_____

Discharge Medications (Name, Dosage, Schedule, Purpose)

Initial Identification

Follow-up/Outpatient Appt. _____

Social Service Referral ☐ Yes ☐ No _____

Patient Signature: _____ Date: _____ Time: _____

601-75-294   Patient Health Care Education/Discharge Summary

B-C Note	C-Lab	D-X-Ray	E-Diag	F-Surgery	G-Therapy	H-Orders	I-Nurses	J-Misc.

Figure 5-2   Sample of discharge summary. (Courtesy St. John's Health Care Corporation, Anderson, Ind.)

NORTHWEST COVENANT MEDICAL CENTER
MULTIDISCIPLINARY PATIENT DISCHARGE INSTRUCTIONS

Discharge Date:_____

DIET:
- ❏ No restrictions   ❏ Special Diet_____
- ❏ Increase Fluids

ACTIVITY:
- ❏ No Restrictions
- ❏ Other:_____

WOUND CARE/TREATMENTS:
_____
_____

MEDICATIONS	STRENGTH	INSTRUCTIONS

FOLLOW-UP

Dr. _____ would like to see you in
_____ days. Call _____ for an appointment.

Other Doctor(s):_____

Diagnostic Tests After

Discharge:_____

Other Instructions:_____
_____

Doctor Signature:_____

NURSING INSTRUCTIONS

Patient has Prescriptions   ❏ YES   ❏ NO

Patient's own medications obtained from Pharmacy   ❏ YES ❏ NO

Patient verbalizes understanding of Physician Instructions   ❏ YES   ❏ NO
_____
_____

Patient Signature_____

R.N. Signature_____

WHITE - PATIENT   CANARY - CHART   PINK - DOCTOR

Figure 5-3 Multidisciplinary patient discharge instructions. (Courtesy Northwest Covenant Medical Center, Denville, NJ.)

Box 5-2
Tips on the Development of Discharge Instruction Sheets

- Ensure that the instructions are clear. Ask someone who is not a healthcare provider to read them to confirm that they are understandable. Remember that the average reading level of the individuals in the general public is about that of a fifth-grader. Include what the patient should not do and the risks of noncompliance with the instructions.
- Clearly state that the patient must seek help if the condition becomes worse, concerns develop about symptoms, or the recovery does not proceed as expected.
- Provide a place on the instruction sheet for the patient or family to sign. After providing the instructions, ask the patient to sign the form and explain that the patient's signature indicates that he or she understands the instructions. This statement should also appear on the form above or below the signature line.
- Document if the patient refuses to listen to the instructions or sign the instruction form. Attempt to determine who will be responsible for caring for the person, if applicable, and provide that person with instructions. Notify the physician of the actions taken and document the events in the patient's clinical record.
- Store the medical record copy of the instruction form with the rest of the chart.

or "vomiting subsided 1 hour after received Compazine [prochlorperazine]")
- Responses to change in activity (for example, "able to walk from bed to bathroom without becoming dyspneic")
- Tolerance for treatments or position change (for example, "unable to tolerate having head of bed lowered from 90 degrees to 45 degrees, became short of breath," or "complained of pain when Foley catheter was inserted")
- Ability to perform activities of daily living, particularly those that may influence discharge planning (for example, "unable to wash self independently because of left-side weakness" or "requires a walker to ambulate to bathroom")
- Response to diet or advancement of diet (for example, "consumed all of full-liquid lunch; stated she was hungry and wanted more solid food")

DOCUMENTATION OF PATIENT EDUCATION

Patient education is an important function of the delivery of nursing care. The goals of teaching are focused on improving health by promoting healthy behavior and involvement in healthcare decisions (JCAHO, 1996). Documentation of patient education is necessary to communicate

important information to other healthcare professionals and avoid duplication of effort. Factors that have been reported to be effective in increasing patient education documentation include the following (Casey, 1995):

- Make patient education a part of a nurse's job description.
- Include patient education as a factor in merit raises and promotions.
- Reinforce patient education through quality improvement activities.
- Include patient education as part of the standards of practice.
- Reinforce patient education through administrative attention to documentation.
- Revise documentation forms to place an emphasis on teaching.
- Provide staff development and education focused on patient education.

The process of teaching, whether informally, as care is provided, or in a structured teaching session, consists of presenting content and evaluating the responses of the patient, significant other, or both. At the conclusion of teaching, depending on the information presented, the nurse should be able to document the following:

- An increase in the patient's knowledge of medication administration, use of medical equipment, food-drug interactions, nutrition, community resources, and symptoms that should be reported to the healthcare provider
- An increase in the ability of the patient, family, or both to perform self-care skills and use rehabilitation techniques to increase the patient's level of functioning
- The patient's response to the information provided

The act of providing information does not guarantee learning in and of itself, which is why evaluating the patient's response to teaching is necessary. The nurse must evaluate whether learning has occurred and document the results of his or her judgment. However, it should be noted that compliance may not necessarily follow even though the patient has learned the content.

Methods of Evaluation

The methods of evaluation described in Box 5-3 will assist the nurse in deciding whether learning has resulted from the teaching.

How to Document Patient Education

The nurse should be specific in describing what the patient has been taught and should include the evaluation of learning. The following illustrates both poorly worded and well-written examples (Cirone, 1997):

ROBERT WOOD JOHNSON
UNIVERSITY HOSPITAL
New Brunswick, New Jersey 08903-2601

POST DISCHARGE PHONE CALL
SAME DAY UNIT

PROCEDURE	DATE OF PROCEDURE

POST-DISCHARGE PHONE CALL

DATE	TIME	☐ NO CALL REQUIRED

PERSON CONTACTED (NAME AND RELATIONSHIP)	TELEPHONE ( )

YES	NO	N/A	
☐	☐	☐	NAUSEA, VOMITING _____
☐	☐	☐	INCREASED TEMPERATURE _____
☐	☐	☐	PAIN _____
☐	☐	☐	PROCEDURE SITE DRAINAGE _____
☐	☐	☐	HEMATOMA _____
☐	☐	☐	BLEEDING _____
☐	☐	☐	NUMBNESS OF EXTREMITY _____
☐	☐	☐	DIFFICULTY IN VOIDING _____
☐	☐	☐	RETURN APPOINTMENT MADE _____

Description of any problems since discharge and how handled _____
_____
_____
_____
_____

Instructions given to patient by caller

☐ Call your physician for any problems, questions or concerns

☐ Other _____

Evaluation of response to instructions _____
_____
_____
_____

RN Signature   Print Name

_____

UNSUCCESSFUL CALL ATTEMPTS			
DATE	TIME	SIGNATURE/PRINT NAME	REASON

Figure 5-4 Postdischarge evaluation form following same day surgery. (Courtesy Robert Wood Johnson University Hospital, New Brunswick, NJ.)

Box 5-3 **Methods of Evaluating the Success of Patient Education** • *Return demonstrations* are most useful in evaluating psycho-motor skills (for example, injection techniques and dressing changes). They provide feedback to the nurse and allow for the correction of the patient's mistakes. • *Written tests* are objective tools used to measure knowledge. They may be threatening to some patients and are not useful for patients with limited reading and vocabulary skills (unless the tests are written in simple terms). • *Diaries* are maintained by the patient to record data (for example, blood pressure, blood sugar, eating patterns, and weight). Diaries are helpful in evaluating the patient's ability and willingness to follow self-care regimens to manage an illness or maintain health. • *Discussions* involve asking the patient to recall what he or she has been taught, which enables the nurse to correct the patient's misconceptions and evaluate the patient's memory. • *Observations* of verbal and nonverbal behavior, role-playing, and attitudes expressed through behavior give clues to learning. • *Questionnaires* are used to evaluate in the patient's attitude changes (for example, increased self-confidence) and to provide feedback for the instructor of a patient education class. • *Problem-solving* and *simulations* involve providing the patient with theoretical situations and asking him or her to describe how the situation should be handled.	*what* the nurse is planning to do or did do about it. For example: After instruction, patient was unable to demonstrate the correct injection technique. Patient said he was unable to read the syringe without his reading glasses. Patient's daughter will bring in glasses tonight. Teaching will resume tomorrow.—S. Wiley, RN

SUMMARY

Evaluation of the patient's status is an important ongoing part of the nursing process. Clearly defined outcomes direct how and when to evaluate the achievement of expected outcomes, provide a framework for documentation, and are increasingly being used as a tool to evaluate the performance of the nursing staff and as a basis for comparison with other healthcare agencies. The scope of patient education documentation has broadened to include documenting that the patient, family, or both comprehended the teaching that was provided to them. (Patient education forms now include this concept.) Nurses must continue to focus on refining documentation to demonstrate their role in assisting the patient toward recovery, stabilization of health, or a peaceful death.

REFERENCES

American Nurses Association: Standards of Clinical Nursing Practice, ANA, Kansas City, Mo, 1991.

Casey F: Documenting patient education: a literature review, *J Contin Educ Nurs* 26(6):257, 1995.

Cirone N: Documenting return demonstrations, *Nursing 97* p 17, December 1997.

Eggland E: Documenting psychiatric and behavioral outcomes, *Nursing 97* p 25, April 1997.

Joint Commission for the Accreditation of Healthcare Organizations: *1997 Comprehensive accreditation manual for hospitals,* Oak Brook Terrace, Ill, 1996, Author.

Laska L: Failure to diagnose inflammation and infection in cervical spine, *Medical Malpractice Verdicts, Settlements, and Experts* p 6, May 1997a.

Laska L: Failure to properly manage complications from foot injury blamed for cardiac arrest, *Medical Malpractice Verdicts, Settlements, and Experts* p 22, June 1997b.

Laska L: Patient's leg cast too tight, *Medical Malpractice, Settlements, and Experts* p 36, October 1997c.

Laska L: California man diagnosed with perforated appendix after discharge from emergency room, *Medical Malpractice Verdicts, Settlements, and Experts* p 14, January 1998.

Lavin J, Enright B: Charting with managed care in mind, *RN* p 47, August 1996.

McGreevey C, Nadzam D, Corbin L: The Joint Commission for the Accreditation of Healthcare Organizations' indicator measurement system, *Comput Nurs* p 87, March/April 1997.

Uddin D, Martin P: Core data set: importance to health services research, outcomes research, and policy research, *Comput Nurs* 15(2):S38, 1997.

ADDITIONAL READINGS

Dennison R: A nurse's guide to common postoperative complications, *Nursing 97* p 56, November 1997.

Jennings B: Patient outcomes research: seizing the opportunity, *Nurs Manage* 24(5):96, 1993.

Vague	Clear
Preoperative teaching	Use of incentive spirometer demonstrated by patient with acceptable return demonstration.
COPD education done	Abdominal breathing exercises demonstrated. Patient is able to perform exercises satisfactorily upon request.
Medications taught	Instructed patient about purposes and side effects of digoxin. Patient was able to repeat this information at the end of discussion.
Taught to perform finger stick	Following demonstration, patient performed self blood glucose monitoring with adequate blood sample 2 out of 3 times.

Attempts to teach a patient may fail for a number of reasons. When evaluation reveals that teaching was ineffective, three elements should be included in the documentation on the progress notes or patient education record: *how* the nurse determined that the teaching was unsuccessful, *why* the nurse thinks the teaching failed, and

Jost K: Psychosocial care: document it, *Am J Nurs* p 47, July 1995.

Katz J: Back to basics: providing effective patient teaching, *Am J Nurs* p 33, May 1997.

Lowe A, Baker J: Measuring outcomes: a nursing report card, *Nurs Manage* p 38, November 1997.

Miller B, Capps E: Meeting JCAHO patient education standards, *Nurs Manage* p 55, May 1997.

Phillips C: Post-discharge follow-up care on patient outcomes, *J Nurs Care Qual* 7(4):64, 1993.

Pobojewski B et al: Documenting nursing process in the perioperative process: continuity of care, patient evaluation, *AORN J* 56(1):98, 1992.

Scharf L: Revising nursing documentation to meet patient outcomes, *Nurs Manage* 28(4):38, 1997.

6

Legal Aspects of Charting Techniques

A legible, accurate medical record is a crucial healthcare document, communicating important information about the patient to a variety of professionals. In the event of a lawsuit the medical record may form the basis of the plaintiff's case or defense of the nurse, physician, or facility. The medical record is used as an important piece of evidence in the evaluation of a nursing or medical malpractice claim. Total, sole reliance on the medical record to evaluate the quality of nursing care is not without risks. Nurses may not only provide care that is not documented, but also document care that was not provided. Excellent documentation is not a substitute for providing nursing care, but excellent clinical care must be accompanied by appropriate documentation.

This chapter presents charting techniques and strategies to improve documentation. Specific "do's" and "don'ts" of charting are discussed and illustrated with reports of malpractice suits. These techniques should be considered when charting information on a variety of documentation tools.

DOCUMENT THE CLINICALLY SIGNIFICANT DETAILS

The main purpose of nursing documentation is to convey significant information about the patient. The medical record is used to document the nursing process and fulfill the nurse's professional obligations to communicate vital information. Entries in the notes should contain specific information that provides a description of the patient and the nursing care rendered. The evaluation of the patient's status should be incorporated into the entries.

SIGN EVERY ENTRY

The nurse's name should appear at the end of each entry. A line should be drawn from the end of the entry to the nurse's name so that no information can be inserted into the entry.

The approved method is for the nurse to write the initial of his or her first name, the full last name, and the status, such as RN (registered nurse), SN (student nurse), LPN (licensed practical nurse), or SPN (student practical nurse). Students should write the initials or abbreviated name of their nursing program; for example, "U Conn" for University of Connecticut. When charting continues from one page to the next, the bottom of the first page should be signed with the nurse's name. At the top of the next page, the date, the time, and the words "continued from previous page" should be written; for example:

7/29 1300 hours   (Continued from previous page.) Returned to bed with siderails up and call light within reach.—B. Waltham, RN

WRITE NEATLY AND LEGIBLY

An important purpose of documentation is to communicate with the healthcare team. Sloppy, illegible handwriting creates confusion and wastes time. More seriously, patient injuries may result if crucial information is misunderstood or miscommunicated because of illegible handwriting. Unclear handwriting can form the basis for a lawsuit. Illegible handwriting can come back to haunt the nurse at several points during a lawsuit. Even if a nurse provides the appropriate care, illegible nurse's notes could result in the following:

If an incident proceeds to a lawsuit, the plaintiff's attorney may take the illegible notes to a photocopying service to create a large poster. At the trial the plaintiff's attorney could present the poster in court and ask the nurse to read his or her writing on the medical record. The nurse could become distressed when it becomes clear that the writing is impossible to read—even for him or her. The plaintiff's attorney might show the jury the poster and say,

"See . . . the nurse can't read the handwriting. How do we know what is written here? If the nurse didn't take time to write clearly, it is evident that my client did not receive the needed care." The poster could be positioned in front of the jury during the entire trial, presenting a constant message of sloppy writing. The jury might doubt the credibility of the nurse, believing that sloppy charting equals sloppy care, and return a verdict for the plaintiff.

Healthcare facilities are addressing illegible handwriting in a number of ways. Some facilities send staff with bad handwriting to handwriting school. Computerized medical records, which incorporate printing of orders and progress notes, can reduce difficulties associated with handwriting. Simple, effective solutions to the handwriting problem include emphasizing the use of printing instead of writing and asking healthcare professionals to scan notes and orders habitually before closing the medical record. Physicians who are known to be poor writers should be encouraged to read their orders to a nurse before leaving the unit.

USE PROPER SPELLING, GRAMMAR, AND APPROPRIATE MEDICAL PHRASES

Progress notes that are filled with misspelled words and incorrect grammar also create negative impressions. Readers may infer that the nurse has a limited education or intellect or that he or she is careless and distracted when charting. Plaintiff attorneys may capitalize on spelling and grammatical errors the same way they exploit illegible handwriting.

Many mistakes are simple spelling errors, such as those found in Box 6-1. Other errors, such as those in Box 6-2, are senseless and avoidable. Spelling and grammatical errors can be combated in a number of ways, including the following:

1. Keep both a standard and medical dictionary in charting areas.
2. Post a list of frequently misspelled words. Individualize the list by selecting terms and medications used frequently on the unit (Kerr, 1987).
3. Write clear, concise sentences. Avoid useless, unnecessarily long words.
4. Clearly identify the subject of the sentence. Do not be afraid to include the word "I," as in "I contacted the family. . . ." Determining what actions were performed by the nurse, as opposed to the patient, physician, or other healthcare professionals, is sometimes very difficult.

DOCUMENT IN BLUE OR BLACK INK AND USE MILITARY TIME

The use of blue ink or black ink has become trendy in many healthcare settings. Red ink and green ink, traditionally used to document on shifts other than the 7:00 AM to 3:00 PM shift,

---

Box 6-1
Avoid These Spelling Errors

"Foley draining *fowl* smelling urine."
"I had a "barbaric" enema."
"I have a *linguine* hernia."
"Patient taking regular *foot* by mouth."
"Patient ate half of the food on the tray while lying in *skeletal* traction."
"Patient lying on *eggshell* mattress."
"Abdominal *mess* palpated in lower left quadrant."
"Patient suffered from *hyperamnesia* of pregnancy."
MD order: "Walk patient in *hell*."
"No *brewery* heard in right arm."
"*Fecal* heart tones heard."
"Patient observed to be *seeping* quietly."
"Patient suffered from pelvic *inflationary* disease."

---

are used less commonly because of the difficulty encountered in making legible photocopies of clinical records.

To further define the exact time of day, the use of military time, or the 24-hour clock (1300 hours instead of 1:00 PM), has become more widespread. This eliminates the use of AM and PM and the potential for confusion if the AM or PM is inadvertently omitted.

USE AUTHORIZED ABBREVIATIONS

Most healthcare facilities have a list of approved abbreviations. This list should be available to all healthcare workers who document in the medical record, from unit secretaries and student nurses to physicians. "A major purpose of the chart—communication—cannot be accomplished when abbreviations cannot be deciphered by anyone other than the author" (Solberg, 1986, p. 9). The nurse should review the list of abbreviations periodically to ensure that it reflects current practice. Because many medical abbreviations have more than one meaning, when in doubt, spell it out.

USE GRAPHIC RECORD TO RECORD VITAL SIGNS

The graphic (or vital sign) record should be used to record *all* vital signs instead of placing some vital signs in the progress notes and some in the vital signs record. The exception to this guideline occurs when flowsheets are used in specialty areas, such as critical care or labor and delivery units, instead of graphic records that span several days. The consistent use of flowsheets and forms promotes communication by keeping all related information in one predictable place. If the graphic record used has times printed at the top of each column (e.g., "8-12-4-8-12-4"), the nurse should work with the documentation committee to delete these times from the form. By eliminating the times, the nurse can use this one form for recording frequent vital signs, a

---

Box 6-2

Examples of Errors in Grammar or Incorrect Use of Words

Valuables disposition: "Pleasant."

"She had a cabbage done."

Description of hemorrhoids: "Big Time."

MD order: "Dulcolax suppository po prn."

MD order: "May shower with nurse."

"Respirations deep and regular—no breath sounds."

"Patient resting in bed with visitors."

"Patient discharged with prescription on foot."

"Patient having resp difficulty using ass. muscles."

"Patient's ring cut off finger and finger handed to Mom."

"Large brown BM up walking in halls."

"Vaginal packing out. Doctor in."

"She was probably identified and taken to the operating room."

"The patient states there is a burning pain in his penis, which goes to his feet." (L. Gibs)

"The patient has been depressed since she began seeing me in 1993." (L. Gibs)

"She has no rigors or chills, however, her husband states she was very hot in bed last night." (L. Gibs)

"The patient was able to remove his neck but it does cause some discomfort." (M. Shea)

"TheRapist in to see patient." (M. Shea)

"Resuscitation attempts failed. Patient pronounced. Patient requests an autopsy." (M. Shea)

The following examples come from Black, 1997:

"While in the emergency department, she was examined, X-rated, and sent home."

"The pelvic exam was done on the floor."

"By the time he was admitted, his rapid heart had stopped, and he was feeling better."

"After consultation, Dr. Doe felt we should sit tight on the abdomen, and I agree."

"Patient has chest pain when she lies on her side for over a year."

"On the second day, the painful knee was better and in the third day it had completely disappeared."

"Patient was alert and unresponsive."

"Healthy appearing, decrepit 69-year-old female."

"When she fainted, her eyes rolled around the room."

"Rectal examination revealed a normal-sized thyroid."

"The patient had waffles for breakfast and anorexia for lunch."

"Indwelling urinary catheter draining clear yellow roses."

"Both breasts are equal and reactive to light and accommodation."

"The baby was delivered, the cord clamped and cut and handed to the pediatrician, who breathed and cried immediately."

Skin: "Somewhat pale, but present."

"She stated that she had been constipated for most of her life until 1989, when she got a divorce."

"Patient complains of indigestion since last night when he ate a stake."

"Examination of genitalia reveals he is circus-sized."

"The patient lives at home with his mother, father, and pet turtle, who is presently enrolled in day care three times a week."

"The skin was moist and dry."

"Examination of genitalia was completely negative except for the right foot."

"Bleeding started in the rectal area and continued all the way to Los Angeles."

"Patient was in his usual state of good health until his airplane ran out of gas and crashed."

If he squeezes the back of his neck for 4 or 5 years, it comes and goes."

Discharge status: "Alive but without permission."

Data from Black J: *Nursing 97* p 53, December 1997.

---

temperature taken 1 hour after an elevated one, and vital signs taken when blood is administered.

An Illinois case revolved around the documentation of vital signs, as described in the following:

A 71-year-old Illinois woman with a history of hypertension and congestive heart failure was admitted to the hospital for surgery to remove a bowel obstruction. She was found unresponsive in her room after the surgery and was transferred to the intensive care unit (ICU), apparently the victim of a pulmonary embolism. The monitor strip from a Holter monitor that had been used to track her mild cardiac arrhythmia revealed a tachycardia that continued for 1 hour before her heart stopped, and a 1-hour interval between the time her heart stopped and her condition was discovered.

The decedent's four adult daughters claimed that she would not have died if the nursing staff had taken and recorded her vital signs in accordance with doctor's orders. The defendant argued that even if the woman's tachycardia had been discovered at the outset and treatment had been started, her death could not have been prevented. The jury returned a $650,000 verdict against the hospital (Laska, 1997b).

RECORD THE PATIENT'S NAME ON EVERY PAGE

The nurse can avoid inserting the wrong pages into the patient's records by stamping or labeling both sides of every page with the patient's identifying information. Use of a page with another patient's addressograph can result in disastrous consequences including inappropriate treatment orders and inaccurate documentation.

TAKE CARE WHEN NOTING HIV STATUS

The confidentiality of HIV-testing results is protected by state statutes in various parts of the country. Many facilities avoid placing information about a positive HIV status in the medical record. This policy may prohibit such entries anywhere on the medical record, including on the kardex, medication administration record, or front of the chart. The use of a code, such as colored dots, to signify a positive HIV status may similarly be prohibited.

AVOID TAKING VERBAL OR PHONE ORDERS

Misunderstandings or documentation of incorrect orders are prevalent when orders are received verbally or by phone. Another risk with phone orders is that the physician may misdiagnose the problem and provide inappropriate orders. Taking orders this way is an even greater problem when the physician has signed out to a covering physician who does not know the patient. Most agencies attempt to discourage verbal orders in circumstances other than emergencies. Every facility should have well-known and enforced policies that specify the criteria for dictating and accepting verbal and phone orders.

Occasionally a nurse may take a verbal order that the physician denies having given. Nurse managers may be able to enforce policies regarding verbal orders. If the nurse does not know the physician or if the physician is not reliable, the order should be written. Another nurse can listen in or witness the order, then cosign the documentation of the verbal or phone order. Repeating the order back to the physician along with the patient's name is always a good idea (Paxman, 1993). The guidelines for documenting a phone or verbal order are shown in Box 6-3.

The absence of a telephone order was a significant factor in the following Louisiana obstetrics case:

When Karen Dent arrived, the labor and delivery nurse notified the woman's obstetrician that the woman was in labor. There was no available room for Mrs. Dent in the obstetrical unit, so she was sent to a nonobstetrical unit. The doctor claimed that he gave phone orders to the nurse to notify his partner of the admission because the partner was scheduled to attend to patients within the next 15 minutes after Mrs. Dent arrived. The doctor also claimed that he left an order that the patient was to stay on the nonobstetrical unit for 15 minutes only.

Approximately 1 hour after her arrival on the nonobstetrical unit, Karen Dent delivered a baby girl with the help of an obstetrical nurse. No physician was present at the delivery. The infant died 2 days later. Mrs. Dent filed a suit for wrongful death of her infant and received $250,000 in an out-of-court settlement and $400,000 in a court verdict. The court found that the attending physician was negligent for failing to inform the nurses that another obstetrician would be taking charge of the patient.

The obstetrical nurse testified that she could not recall the events of that day other than by reading the information she

---

> ### Box 6-3
>
> #### Guidelines for Documenting a Phone or Verbal Order
>
> 1. Write the date and time of the order.
> 2. Document the order as it is being given to you.
> 3. Read the order back to the physician to verify accuracy.
> 4. Document "V.O." for a verbal order or "T.O." for a telephone order, followed by the name of the physician, your name, and your status (T.O. Dr. Waitley/R. Mooney, RN)
> 5. Transcribe the order according to your agency's policy. This order should be confirmed on the phone as follows: "Dr. Waitley, you have ordered Halcion zero-point-five milligrams P.O. for Bertha McGuire. Is that correct?"

---

recorded on the patient's chart. If the doctor had given an order for a specific length of time the patient was to be kept on the nonobstetrical unit, she would have charted it. The court held that the absence of the order was adequate evidence for the jury to conclude that the doctor never provided the order (Tammelleo, 1992b).

In this case the nurse was able to provide an effective defense: She would have documented a phone order if it had been given.

TRANSCRIBE ORDERS CAREFULLY

Accurate transcription of orders is essential. Although unit secretaries may transcribe orders, the RN has the ultimate responsibility for the accuracy of transcription. Care must be taken to read each order and carry out the necessary steps to implement the order. Checking off each order as it is processed or documenting a number next to the order as assigned by the computer is a common practice.

Much room exists for error in the transcription of medication orders, which can have serious consequences; for example:

A newborn in Ohio suffering from respiratory distress syndrome was placed on a ventilator and given theophylline. The infant was inadvertently given a tenfold overdose of theophylline. He showed noticeable development delays at birth and was still unable to walk or speak at age 4. The child's parents claimed he suffered brain damage as a result of the theophylline overdose. The case was settled for $100,000 (Laska, 1997c).

QUESTION INAPPROPRIATE ORDERS

The RN is expected to have the knowledge to question the appropriateness of orders and spot errors; the role of the nurse as the patient's advocate requires this. The American Nurses Association's Code for Nurses (1985) states that the nurse assumes responsibility and accountability for nursing judgments and actions. The nurse is to exercise informed judgment and use individual competence and qualifications as criteria for seeking consultation, accepting responsibilities, and delegating nursing activities to others. The Code further states that the nurse is obligated to "safeguard the patient and public when health and safety are affected by incompetent, unethical, or illegal practice of any person."

The following Massachusetts case commented on the responsibility of the nurse to spot conflicting orders:

The patient was a man who underwent a midlumbar osteotomy, which involved the insertion of fixation hooks and rods in his spine. His orthopedic surgeon intended and so ordered that he stay in bed for 4 or 5 days after surgery. On the third postoperative day an orthopedic resident wrote an order that the patient be put in a soft orthopedic support and moved into a chair that day. The orthopedic surgeon acknowledged the order of the resident for the soft support but did not see the order to move the patient from the bed to the chair. The charge nurse transcribed both orders. When the staff nurse assigned to the patient helped him out of bed, the hooks and rods slipped out of position. Surgery to correct the damage was not successful. The plaintiff sued both doctors and the charge nurse. When the defense won the case, the plaintiff appealed.

In the second trial the plaintiff's expert witness testified that the charge nurse's duty of care to the patient included recognizing the inconsistent orders and reporting them to the doctors. The trial was returned to the lower court for further proceedings (*A failure to communicate,* 1997).

This case makes it clear that the transcription of medical records cannot be a mechanical act. Thoughtful nursing judgment must be applied to the analysis of medical orders, and appropriate clarification of orders must occur.

Guidelines for transcription of orders are shown in Box 6-4.

Inaccuracies in medication errors can have potentially fatal results. Acting as a patient advocate to question medication orders if they look inappropriate is the responsibility of the nurse. If a physician orders an incorrect dose of medication, the nurse should follow these steps:

1. Contact the physician and discuss the reasons why the dose is being questioned.
2. If needed, contact the nursing supervisor.
3. Document in the progress notes that the physician was notified and record any new orders received; for example:

Jay Miller, age 40, is admitted to a neurological unit with a seizure disorder. His physician orders a loading dose of phenytoin (Dilantin) 1000 mg at 75 mg/minute to be mixed with 100 ml of normal saline. The nurse who is caring for the patient recognizes that the rate of administration should not exceed 50 mg/minute. The nurse contacts the physician and documents the following information on the progress notes:

1100 hours	Call placed to Dr. Allen concerning Dilantin dosage. Dilantin order changed to 50 mg/min.—C. Lilly, RN

> ### Box 6-4
>
> #### Guidelines for the Transcription of Orders
>
> 1. Think through the implications of the orders and question inappropriate orders.
> 2. Be careful to select the correct nameplate when stamping forms.
> 3. Have another person, such as a unit secretary or a nurse, double-check the orders you transcribe to ensure that it was done accurately.
> 4. If a physician's order is unclear, ask for clarification. Do not waste time asking others for their interpretations.
> 5. Be certain to include the date medication is to be discontinued. Additional days of unwarranted medication may create or worsen adverse medication effects.
> 6. Follow a policy of checking physicians' orders once every 24 hours to ensure that all the orders are transcribed correctly. This is commonly done by hospital night shifts. A line is drawn across the order sheet to indicate that all orders above the line have been checked for accuracy.

4. If the physician cannot be reached and the nurse has decided to withhold the medication, write in the progress notes that an attempt to reach the physician was made, and then the rationale for withholding the medication should be entered; for example:

Sam Parks is receiving Digoxin, 0.25 mg. This morning his apical pulse was noted to be 48 beats/minute. After unsuccessful attempts to contact his physician, the nurse charts the following information:

0930 hours	Digoxin withheld because of low pulse rate. Call placed to Dr. Boone's office regarding low pulse rate. Message left with office nurse to contact nursing unit.—F. Wong, RN

Following this episode the progress notes would contain evidence of the continued monitoring of the patient until the respiratory rate showed sustained improvement. Document the details of the episode, including the attempts to resolve the problem, in a memo to the nursing supervisor.

The following Massachusetts case raises the issue of whether orders for excessive dosage of Haldol were recognized and questioned by the nurses who transcribed the orders:

A 49-year-old man entered a major teaching hospital for debridement of an infection of his little finger. Upon awakening from anesthesia, the man became combative. The resident psychiatrist began administering intravenous Haldol (haloperidol) for the agitation. During the next 16 hours, 1270 mg of Haldol were administered, which is a far greater dose than any ever reported in the medical literature. The patient was not being monitored by a cardiac monitor during this time. The next morning he experienced an arrhythmia, which led to a cardiac arrest and left him in a semivegetative state. He later died. A settlement for $1,050,000 was reached (Laska, 1997m).

When inappropriate orders are at issue, details concerning the patient's clinical status should be documented in the medical record; however, stopping there is insufficient, as the following case illustrates:

The patient came to the hospital with symptoms of tuberculosis. The doctor believed that tuberculosis had been eliminated in the United States so never ordered a chest x-ray study. The nurse, who had 30 years of experience, strongly suspected that the patient had tuberculosis. She carefully documented the deteriorating status of the patient, and she told the charge nurse that she suspected the patient had pneumonia and documented this fact in the chart. Neither the charge nurse or staff nurse questioned the physician. The patient's condition worsened until he was put on a ventilator. Although he survived, he was left debilitated.

The patient filed suit against the physician, nurse, and hospital. After the physician reached an out-of-court settlement, the suit proceeded against the nurse and the hospital. The jury found that the nurse had a duty not only to record her observations, but also to follow up on her concerns directly with the doctor. The jury awarded $180,000 as well as $750,000 in punitive damages. (Horsley, 1997, p. 59).

Punitive damages are designed to punish and deter the defendant from tampering with records, and they are not covered by insurance policies. This leaves the defendant with a large out-of-pocket bill and serious financial consequences.

As this case illustrates, acting as a patient advocate and going up the chain of command to protect the patient is important.

DOCUMENT OMITTED CARE OR MEDICATIONS

If tests or procedures are not performed or medications are not given, the nurse should document the omission and the reasons for the omission. Any action that followed should be described, if applicable. The documentation of reasons for omission of medications is frequently overlooked. Figure 6-1 shows a medication administration record that provides a convenient space for recording the reasons for omission of medications. Documenting the reasoning that led up to the decision to withhold a medication based on the nurse's judgment is particularly important; for example:

1000 hours   Librium withheld. Patient extremely le-
               thargic. Dr. Leonard notified of lethargy
               at 1100. Librium was discontinued.
               —J. Ellis, RN

Ask questions if the administration of a medication has not been recorded; do not assume the medication was omitted and give it without checking. Options include asking the patient if the medication was received and calling the pharmacy to find out if they have already furnished the dose.

DOCUMENT COMPLETE INFORMATION ABOUT MEDICATIONS

The nurse should document the dose, date, time, and initials for each medication administered. Failure to document a dose of medication may result in administration of the same dose twice or the administration of medications which potentiate each other, as the following case illustrates:

Following neurosurgery, the patient developed syncope while being assisted in standing up to get into a wheelchair for transfer from the SICU to the hospital floor. The nurse thought the patient was experiencing symptoms of narcotic overdose and gave her Narcan (naloxone). She called the doctor, who concluded that the woman had experienced orthostatic hypotension. The doctor changed the pain medications from morphine to Vicodin (hydrocodone) and Demerol (meperidine). The patient was given both medications after being transfered to the new unit. She was later found in full respiratory arrest and could not be resuscitated. The family argued that she had been overdosed with morphine while in the SICU and should not have been given the Demerol, which caused her death. Conflicting records existed in the nursing notes, including 13 mg of morphine that were unaccounted for in the SICU. The family was billed for two administrations of Vicodin instead of just one, as was noted in the medical record. The hospital settled during the trial for $200,000, and the physician was found to be not negligent by the jury (Laska, 1997g).

Following hospital policies regarding documentation of medications is vitally important in preventing double doses or missed doses of medications.

DOCUMENT ALLERGIES TO MEDICATIONS AND FOODS

Facility policy usually defines how allergy information is documented. Commonly used areas for documenting allergies are the admission assessment, the medication administration record, the front of the patient's chart, and sometimes the top or bottom of every physician order sheet. Facilities with computerized medical records may have a warning system to flag an order that is contrary to a known allergy of the patient.

DOCUMENT SITES OF INJECTIONS

The sites of all intramuscular and subcutaneous injections should be documented. The attorney for a plaintiff who sustains injury from injections will comb the medical record for the name of the nurse who used a particular site. Several nurses may be needlessly involved in a suit because they gave injections without recording the site. All nurses who gave injections to the plaintiff may be named as potential defendants in a lawsuit. Figure 6-2 provides a medication record designed to allow documentation of the site of injections, vital signs, and blood sugar readings.

Text continued on p. 89

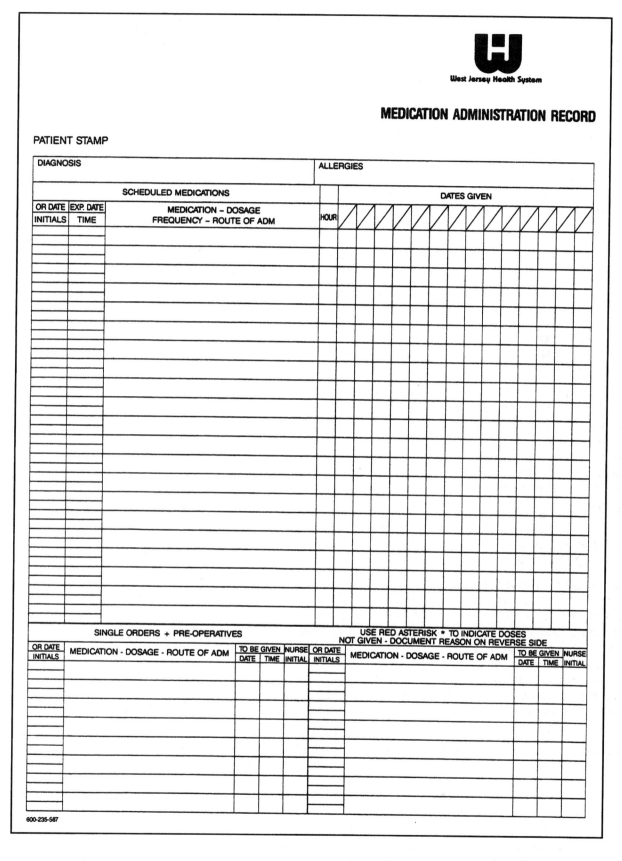

Figure 6-1 Medication administration record. (Courtesy West Jersey Health System, Voorhees Division, Voorhees, NJ.)

Continued

INITIALS	FULL SIGNATURE	TITLE	INITIALS	FULL SIGNATURE	TITLE

INJECTION SITES
ABBREVIATIONS SUBCUTANEOUS
LUA - LEFT UPPER ARM
LUT - LEFT UPPER THIGH
LUQ - LEFT UPPER QUADRANT
LUM - LEFT UMBILICUS
RUA - RIGHT UPPER ARM
RUT - RIGHT UPPER THIGH
RUQ - RIGHT UPPER QUADRANT
RLQ - RIGHT LOWER QUADRANT
RUM - RIGHT UMBILICUS

INTRAMUSCULAR
RD - RIGHT DELTOID
RGM - RIGHT GLUTEUS MAXIMUS
RVL - RIGHT VASTUS LATERALIS
RVG - RIGHT VENTRAL GLUTEUS
LD - LEFT DELTOID
LGM - LEFT GLUTEUS MAXIMUS
LVL - LEFT VASTUS LATERALIS
LVG - LEFT VENTRAL GLUTEUS

PRN MEDICATIONS   *PRN'S ARE CHARTED IN NURSE'S NOTES

OR DATE INITIALS	EXP DATE TIME	MEDICATION– DOSAGE – FREQUENCY ROUTE OF ADM		DOSES GIVEN
			DATE	
			TIME	
			SITE	
			INIT	
			DATE	
			TIME	
			SITE	
			INIT	
			DATE	
			TIME	
			SITE	
			INIT	
			DATE	
			TIME	
			SITE	
			INIT	
			DATE	
			TIME	
			SITE	
			INIT	
			DATE	
			TIME	
			SITE	
			INIT	
			DATE	
			TIME	
			SITE	
			INIT	

OMITTED MEDICATIONS

DATE	TIME	MEDICATION OMITTED	INITIALS	REASON FOR OMISSION

Figure 6-1, cont'd   Medication administration record. (Courtesy West Jersey Health System, Voorhees Division, Voorhees, NJ.)

(ADDRESSOGRAPH)

Page _____ of _____

HACKETTSTOWN COMMUNITY HOSPITAL

MEDICATION RECORD

Form 8597 3/92

Allergies _____

Vital signs and/or injection site <u>MUST</u> be recorded.

T	=	Time	Accu	=	Accuchek
I	=	Initials	Sched	=	Schedule
VS	=	Vital Signs			

Date Ordered	Date Exp.	Medication Dose Route Frequency	Sched	Date:		Date:		Date:		Date:		Date:	
				T/I	Site VS Accu/ Dose	T/I	Site VS Accu/ Dose	T/I	Site VS Accu/ Dose	T/I	Site VS Accu/ Dose	T/I	Site VS Accu/ Dose

Initial Codes:

_____ _____ _____ _____

_____ _____ _____ _____

_____ _____ _____ _____

Figure 6-2 Medication administration record. (Courtesy Hackettstown Community Hospital, Hackettstown, NJ.)

Continued

(ADDRESSOGRAPH)		**INJECTION CHART**

Injection Site Code:

1 - Right Gluteus	6 - Left Thigh
2 - Left Gluteus	7 - Abdomen
3 - Right Deltoid	8 - Left Hip
4 - Left Deltoid	9 - Right Hip
5 - Right Thigh	

PRN MEDICATION

Date	Medication Route - Dose	Freq	Date: T/I/Site	Date: T/I/Site	Date: T/I/Site	Date: T/I/Site	Date: T/I/Site
Ordered		12-8					
		8-4					
Expired		4-12					
Ordered		12-8					
		8-4					
Expired		4-12					
Ordered		12-8					
		8-4					
Expired		4-12					
Ordered		12-8					
		8-4					
Expired		4-12					
Ordered		12-8					
		8-4					
Expired		4-12					
Ordered		12-8					
		8-4					
Expired		4-12					
Ordered		12-8					
		8-4					
Expired		4-12					
Ordered		12-8					
		8-4					
Expired		4-12					
Ordered		12-8					
		8-4					
Expired		4-12					

SINGLE ORDER STAT PRE-OP MED - ETC

Order Date	Medication Dose & Route	Given Date	Given Time	Given Site	Given Init	Order Date	Medication Dose & Route	Given Date	Given Time	Given Site	Given Init

Figure 6-2, cont'd   Medication administration record. (Courtesy Hackettstown Community Hospital, Hackettstown, NJ.)

RECORD ALL DETAILS OF INTRAVENOUS THERAPY AND BLOOD ADMINISTRATION

Failure to carefully monitor IV therapy and blood administration are common sources of nursing liability. Patients at high risk for injury from IV fluids or medications include neonates, infants, the elderly, and those receiving medications that can be caustic to the tissues. Follow the agency's standards regarding the frequency with which the IV site should be described. Thorough documentation permitted a successful defense of the nurses involved in the following Ohio case:

The plaintiff, age 50, was treated for pyelonephritis by intravenous therapy. One week after treatment, following discharge from the hospital, her left hand began to discolor at the site of the intravenous therapy. The hand continued to worsen, ultimately requiring multiple debridement procedures and skin graft surgery. The plaintiff developed permanent scarring and limited function and movement of the hand. She alleged that she had complained of pain in the area of the therapy from the time the IV was placed until after it was removed and that the IV infiltrated, resulting in the injury to her hand. The defendant contended the following: the plaintiff did not complain of pain during the hospitalization; the complaints of pain were not noted on the plaintiff's hospital charts; and IV infiltration is an inherent risk of IV therapy and does not necessarily result from negligence. The verdict was for the defense (Laska, 1997l, p. 21).

A recent study (Roach, Larson, Bartlett, 1996) reported the results of observing nurses performing and documenting IV site care. These nurses knew they were being observed. Compliance with all of the steps of the IV site care itself was only 23.3%. The results also revealed that nurses in these five critical care units demonstrated compliance with documentation requirements ranging from 53.3% to 85.7%. The data were based on observation of a total of 116 site-care episodes. The documentation elements which were evaluated included the following:

- Was the date and time written on the initial dressing?
- Was the dressing change and site appearance recorded in the chart?
- Did the chart and dressing agree?

These nurses in this study knew they were being watched and still these results were obtained, which raises concerns about the compliance with hospital policies regarding documentation of IV site care.

Tips for charting IV therapy are found in Box 6-5, and tips for charting peripherally inserted central catheter (PICC) lines are found in Box 6-6.

Periodic observations about the IV site should be documented on flowsheets or progress notes to indicate that the nurse assessed the site according to policy. Flowsheets should be designed to permit documentation of the specifics of IV therapy. If unit or agency policy requires observation of the IV site at certain intervals, room should be provided to document this on the flowsheet; for example, a flowsheet that provides space for hourly IV site checks reminds nurses to observe and document their findings. When an IV infiltrates or phlebitis develops, the nurse should describe the nursing interventions that were initiated. Documenting actions taken when tissue necrosis could result from infiltration is particularly important; for example:

A Texas woman was admitted to the hospital for abdominal pain. An IV line was started in her right hand so she could receive medications. She developed an IV infiltration over several hours, and although she tried to alert the nursing staff of her steadily increasing pain, swelling, numbness, and discoloration to her right hand and arm, the infiltration was allowed to worsen and deteriorate, resulting in compartment syndrome. An emergency

---

Box 6-5

Documenting IV Therapy

The following should be documented concerning IV therapy:

- Site location
- Site condition (e.g., evidence of tenderness, redness, edema, or drainage)
- Tubing and dressing changes
- Rate changes
- Time, size of the needle, and name of the person who inserted the IV device
- Amount, type of IV solution, and the name of the nurse who hung the solution

---

Box 6-6

Documentation for PICC Lines

Insertion

- Time, size of the needle, and name of the person who inserted the PICC line
- Site location
- Length of the PICC
- Location of the PICC tip (usually the superior vena cava or subclavian vein)
- Length of the external segment of the PICC
- Patient teaching

Ongoing Documentation

- Condition of the site
- Length of the external segment of the PICC
- Type of dressing and cap, and dates of changes
- Presence and quality of blood return or blood sampling
- Type and amount of flushing solution and frequency
- Infusion problems and interventions

Data from Sansivero G: Taking care of PICCs, *Nursing 97* p 28, 1997.

Box 6-7

Documenting Blood Transfusions

- The identity of the two nurses who verified that the blood bag matched the patient identification and blood type
- The time the transfusion was started and completed
- Vital signs before, during, and after the transfusion
- Any difficulties identified during the administration of the blood and any actions taken to correct the problem (e.g., slow transfusion, infiltration)
- Instructions given to the patient to report signs of a blood transfusion reaction
- Any signs of a blood transfusion reaction and actions taken

---

fasciotomy, skin grafts (and other related surgery), and permanent nerve damage in her hand and arm were the consequences. The case was settled for $650,000, which involved the hospital writing off $100,000 in medical expenses (Laska, 1997d).

If a problem such as infiltration, phlebitis, or extravasation of irritating medication occurs, the nurse should clearly document that the appropriate steps were taken. If a patient is injured by an IV incident, the medical record will be scrutinized to determine if the appropriate standards of care were followed.

Blood administration creates a high potential for liability suits if the appropriate procedures are not followed. The two most serious concerns are (1) administration of blood to the wrong patient and (2) failure to detect a transfusion reaction or another complication associated with blood administration. The administration of blood to the correct patient can be ensured by careful adherence to the agency's policies relating to the identification of the person receiving blood. When shortcuts are taken, including checking the blood and blood slip at the nurses' station instead of in the patient's room or not checking the identification number on the bag with the hospital chart, the potential for mistakes is high.

Potential sources of errors include the following: mix-ups in identity between two people in the hospital with the same name; failure to adhere to type and crossmatch procedures; and delay in recognizing transfusion reactions. Tips for documentation concerning blood transfusions are shown in Box 6-7.

REPORT ABNORMAL LABORATORY RESULTS

Critically abnormal or "panic" laboratory results should be reported to the physician. When a patient is injured because an abnormality is untreated, the medical record may be evaluated. A common practice is for laboratory personnel to ask for and document the name of the nursing staff member who is notified of an important value. This person is then responsible for notifying the appropriate person of the

abnormality and for documenting this follow-through; for example:

1130 hours	Call placed to Dr. Hwang to inform her of 109 sodium value. Orders received. See IV flowsheet.—C. Borden, RN

In the following case, critically abnormal blood values were not acted upon by both the doctors and nurses caring for the patient:

A 70-year-old California man was evaluated in the emergency department (ED) for acute epigastric pain. His medical history included coronary artery bypass, aortic valve replacement, and chronic use of Coumadin (warfarin). After a diagnosis of gallstones was made, a laparoscopic cholecystectomy was performed. Significant bleeding occurred during the procedure, and the condition of the patient was followed after surgery by three doctors: the surgeon, gastroenterologist, and cardiologist. During the 3 days after surgery, the patient's hemoglobin dropped from 15.4 to 9.3. His hematocrit dropped from 45 to 27. Despite the precipitous drop in these levels, no one discontinued the heparin he had been placed on after surgery, and no one ordered a blood transfusion. Each of the defendants assumed that one of the others would handle those problems. The patient died 6 days after surgery. On autopsy, 2200 ml of blood was found in his abdomen. The doctors all argued that it would have been risky to discontinue heparin in view of the danger of clot formation in the decedent's replaced aortic valve, but each of them claimed that another should have been responsible for management of the patient. The settlement totaled $300,000. The hospital provided $65,000, the surgeon contributed $175,000, and the cardiologist and gastroenterologist each paid $30,000 (Laska, 1997j).

It could be argued that the nurses caring for this man should have contacted the doctors regarding the drop in hemoglobin and hematocrit and asked for interventions to address the abnormal test results. Clear documentation of calls placed to physicians is important, as outlined previously. Going up the chain of command when the doctor does not respond is also an essential step in obtaining help for a patient.

CHART PROMPTLY

The nurse should perform charting as close as possible to the time of an observation or provision of care. When charting is postponed until the end of the shift, important details are often forgotten. Information that is charted immediately is more likely to be accurate and complete than information charted in the rush at the end of a shift. In acute care, flowsheets at the bedside facilitate charting throughout the shift. Some hospitals also place progress notes at the bedside to assist with prompt charting. Others question this practice because of concerns about maintaining confidentiality. Some facilities have installed fold-down desks outside patient rooms to provide both a writing surface and a secure place for charting materials. Bedside terminals facilitate timely, ongoing documentation. In the absence of terminals or flowsheets at the bedside, notations on worksheets can be useful as reminders of key phrases and times. This information should be later transcribed onto the progress notes.

AVOID BLOCK CHARTING

Block charting is defined as entering progress notes under a broad time frame, such as 7 AM to 9 AM or 7 AM to 7 PM. Specific times next to entries establish when the nurse saw the patient. Times are particularly important when significant events or changes in the patient's condition occur. In the event of a lawsuit, attorneys and expert witnesses will scrutinize each entry associated with a specific time frame. For example, if a fetal monitor shows late decelerations (ominous signs of fetal distress), the attorneys will examine each entry on the strip and flowsheet to determine how much time transpired before action was taken. Block charting makes it very difficult to establish when specific events occurred.

In the following case the time of a nurse's entry was crucial to establishing when the physician was in the ED:

An 18-year-old male was brought to the ED after receiving multiple gunshot wounds. Around 5:20 PM, the ED doctor called the on-call thoracic surgeon, Dr. Paniker, who later claimed he was in surgery with another patient in another hospital at the time. Dr. Paniker told the ED doctor to stabilize the victim and transfer him to a trauma center. Dr. Paniker arrived at the hospital shortly after 7:00 PM to treat another gunshot victim and did not recall ever seeing the 18-year-old patient, although nurses' notes indicated that he was in the ED with him. The young man was transferred to another hospital around 7:20 PM and died 2 hours later. The plaintiff claimed that Dr. Paniker failed to timely come to the ED, and when he did arrive, he failed to take the man to surgery immediately. The plaintiff pointed to a note that stated "Paniker 5:20 PM. Here in ED" to argue that Dr. Paniker was in the ED at 5:20 PM. Dr. Paniker was unable to produce records concerning the identity of the patient upon whom he was operating on at the other hospital. A $525,000 settlement was reached with the hospital and ED doctor. The jury awarded a $4.621 million verdict against Dr. Paniker (Laska, 1997o).

CHART AFTER DELIVERY OF CARE

Documenting the performance of a procedure before it is performed should be avoided. The information in the record may be inaccurate once the procedure has been performed and will not reflect the patient's responses to the intervention. Charting in advance will also affect the credibility of the medical record.

FILL IN BLANKS ON CHART FORMS

If the chart form has a blank to be filled in, the nurse should enter data in that space. Chart forms that include sections traditionally left blank by the staff should be changed. A blank space raises questions. Was the data obtained? Was that aspect assessed? If the information does not apply to the patient, facility policy should be followed; however, drawing a line through the space or writing the abbreviation "NA" (not applicable) should be appropriate.

DOCUMENT EXACT QUOTES

When documenting in the progress notes the nurse should directly quote what a patient or family member says, which is important for the following reasons:

1. The quotes provide an indication of the patient's or family's mental status and degree of orientation. This can be a significant indication of the patient's ability to comprehend instructions or understand patient education.
2. The subjective information that the patient provides about symptoms may aid in diagnosis of the patient's problems. For example,

A Louisiana patient's use of the term *burning* (versus the term *pain*) was a pivotal issue in a lawsuit against nurses and a doctor. A cast was applied to the leg of a school bus driver. Approximately 24 hours later her husband found blisters near the top of her leg underneath the cast. When the cast was removed 1 hour later, third-degree burns from the plaster-of-paris cast were found on her leg. The suit against the doctor was dismissed. A jury trial against the hospital resulted in a verdict in favor of the hospital. When the plaintiff appealed the verdict, the Court of Appeals affirmed (supported) the verdict, finding the nurses to be not negligent. The plaintiff stated she told the nurses that her leg was burning. The nurses documented that the plaintiff made complaints of pain. Each nurse testified that she would have documented a complaint of burning if the plaintiff had used this word. Both the plaintiff's 12-year-old daughter and her husband did not remember the plaintiff using the word *burning*. The Court found that the jury obviously believed the nurses' testimony, which was corroborated by their notes (Tammelleo, 1992c).

ELIMINATE BIAS FROM WRITTEN DESCRIPTIONS OF PATIENTS

Documentation should be based on fact, not opinion and assumptions. Words that reveal a negative attitude toward the patient should be avoided, including complainer, abusive, drunk, lazy, spoiled, problem patient, difficult, hostile, rude, demanding, aggressive, crazy, obnoxious, nasty, and disagreeable. If a jury reads progress notes with these types of words, they may infer that the patient received substandard care because the nurses disliked the patient. Instead of using negative words that can be interpreted as uncaring, objectively describe the patient's behavior. For example, instead of charting that the patient was drunk, describe the specific symptoms, such as staggering, slurred speech, and alcohol on the breath.

DOCUMENT CHANGES IN THE PATIENT'S CONDITION

Nursing documentation should reflect all phases of the nursing process. The assessment phase consists of data collection, whereas the evaluation component includes making a determination of whether the patient's condition has changed. Recognition that the patient's condition has worsened should be described in the nursing documentation, and appropriate actions should then be taken. The nurse's evaluation of the condition of the patient may be contrasted with the physician's evaluation. The actions of the health-care team in reacting to the changes (or alleged changes) in condition are often factors in a malpractice suit; for example:

A 5-year-old girl died after being treated at a local ED. The cause of death was claimed to be a bite from a brown recluse spider that was not recognized or treated. The medical examiner concluded that the death resulted from cardiac dysrhythmia caused by myocarditis. The physicians acknowledged that this might have been related to the spider bite, but they denied that it was clearly the cause and claimed their treatment of the girl was proper.

When the girl came to the hospital that morning, she was treated with Tylenol (acetaminophen) and discharged when her fever went down. She returned to the ED in the afternoon when her fever again spiked. She began to vomit again. Additionally, a blemish on her upper right arm was visible. (This site is thought to have been the location of the spider bite.) The doctors transferred her from the ED to a nursing unit, but she died after a sudden cardiac arrest in the early evening. The plaintiffs contended that the doctors should have aggressively treated the girl for a brown recluse spider bite, including administering IV fluids and steroids. They also claimed that the hospital's nurses failed to aggressively observe the girl for changes in symptoms, and they failed to chart changes in the girl's condition and inform the doctors of the changes. The doctors claimed that, although they included a spider bite in their differential diagnosis, this was not a definite diagnosis and their treatment was proper. They contended that she did not show the usual signs of toxic shock. No spider was ever found, and the bite mark did not show the necrosis usually associated with a brown recluse spider bite. The jury returned a defense verdict for all of the defendants (doctors and nurses) (Laska, 1998a).

BE PRECISE IN DOCUMENTING INFORMATION REPORTED TO PHYSICIANS

A nurse is obligated to report serious symptoms to the physician. Reporting significant findings and changes to the appropriate physician is essential. The documentate concerning this contact is essential to demonstrate that the nurse fulfilled his or her professional obligations to communicate with the healthcare team. The entries (or lack thereof) are often crucial in a malpractice suit. A nurse's documentation of the steps taken to secure the attention of a physician were pivotal in the following suit:

A hospitalized 26-year-old Maryland woman with a history of hydrocephalus needed a ventricular shunt to drain cerebral spinal fluid from her ventricles. Several revisions of the shunt had occurred over the years. When the patient's headache worsened, the neurologist was called by the staff nurse. The doctor prescribed medication, but he did not examine the patient despite the nurse's urging. The nurse called a house physician, who examined the patient and found her to be normal. He did not consider the shunt to be the source of the problem. When the nurse called the neurologist back, the doctor stated that he believed the headache was due to the lumbar puncture that had been performed in the ED. The doctor did not come in to examine the patient. The patient went into a coma and died. The parties settled for $1,000,000. Neither the nurse nor the hospital were named as defendants in the suit (Laska, 1997h).

The time of a phone call informing a physician of a change in the patient's condition should always be documented on the clinical record to demonstrate the sequence of events. Included in the note should be the specific symptoms that were reported to the physician.

1700 hours	At 1650 hours, Dr. Michels was notified of patient's symptoms: BP 90/40, pulse 120, pale, clammy skin. Dressing saturated with blood.—P. Tie, RN

Note that the nurse in this example wrote the name of the physician and time the physician was notified. The wording makes it clear that the nurse initiated the call to the physician and is preferable to the phrase, "Doctor called," which makes it unclear as to whether the nurse or the physician initiated the phone call. In addition, when several doctors are involved in the care of a patient, "Doctor called" gives no information about which doctor was contacted. This phrase should not be used in nurses notes because of the confusion that this term causes.

The physician may not always give the expected response. In such a situation, it is important not to use the chart to criticize the physician's judgment or not to include damning quotations. For example, instead of charting the response "I know about that, don't bother me again," the nurse should write "No new orders received." If the situation warrants further action, the nurse is obligated to pursue the matter up the chain of command.

When the chain of command is used, the names of the individuals notified must be documented. Instead of documenting "Nurse manager informed" or "Supervisor notified," the name of the individual should be documented. This information will help later if the events of the shift must be reconstructed and the names of people who can corroborate the facts must be provided.

Conversations in which the physician is informed of the patient's lack of improvement or worsening condition should always be documented; for example:

An Arizona woman had surgery to remove a peritoneal dialysis catheter. When the surgeon removed the catheter from the scar tissue that surrounded it, he observed some bowel tissue attached to the cuff and a tear in the bowel, which he repaired. He admitted the patient to the hospital for observation. The patient complained of abdominal pain after being admitted, and the doctor responded with a phone order for an increase in pain medication. When the nurse called him again, he was informed that the patient had a tender, distended abdomen, no bowel sounds, and a fever of 102.8° F. The doctor ordered Tylenol (acetaminophen).

The patient subsequently underwent 16 months of enteral feeding and five operations, including an ileostomy. She alleged that both the surgeon who placed the peritoneal dialysis catheter and the surgeon who handled her care when she was placed in the hospital for observation were negligent. The jury awarded $2.3 million, with 65% of the fault attributed to the first surgeon. Thirty-five percent of the fault was apportioned to the second surgeon, and no fault was assigned to the nurse who contacted the doctor about the patient's symptoms (Laska, 1997f).

The way this case is reported makes it clear that the nurse was able to reconstruct, most likely by referring to the nurses notes, what the physician was told about the patient's condition. The importance of precision in this type of documentation cannot be overestimated. Years after an incident occured, the medical records are often viewed as the most reliable source of information about the communication between the nurse and the healthcare team.

DOCUMENT TELEPHONE TRIAGE OR ADVICE

Telephone triage nurses are increasingly used by managed care organizations to answer patient's questions and avoid unnecessary use of medical resources. The telephone triage nurse should record the date and time of the call, names of the callers, and the substance of the conversation. If advice was given to someone for whom no patient chart exists, a record of the call should be made in a log book. The absence of a record creates a situation where the word of one person is pitted against the word of another (Sullivan, 1996).

> Both nurses and physicians should exercise caution in giving any advice or prescribing any treatment over the telephone without seeing the patient. In any telephone conversation in which advice is given or a drug refill is prescribed, the substance of the conversation should appear in the chart (Creighton, 1987a, p. 15).

The following case reveals the difficulties associated with offering medical advice over the phone:

A pregnant 32-year-old woman contacted her obstetrician complaining of swollen glands, a sore throat, and a low-grade fever. The nurse diagnosed the patient as having a cold, but she did not consult with the doctor. She advised the woman to gargle with salt water and take over-the-counter medications to relieve her symptoms. Six days later, the woman again contacted the doctor's office because she still felt ill. While speaking to the same nurse, the patient said she still had swollen glands in her neck. The nurse

did not speak to the doctor, and she diagnosed a virus and recommended that the patient keep her scheduled appointment in 5 days. The patient called the next day, reporting vomiting and flulike symptoms. A different nurse instructed her to call back if she continued to vomit. When the patient called back, the original nurse took the call and consulted with the doctor. The doctor prescribed Phenergan (promethazine) suppositories. The woman continued to vomit, experienced abdominal pain, and began to have vaginal bleeding. When she called the office, she was asked to come to the office. A diagnosis of gastroenteritis was made, and she was admitted to the hospital.

At the time of her admission, her color was purplish and her skin was mottled. She suffered an arrest 6 hours after her admission and died. The cause of death was sepsis. The plaintiff claimed that the doctor and the nurse at his office were negligent and that the nurse had diagnosed and treated the woman in violation of the Indiana Nurse Practice Act. The case was settled for $725,000 (Laska, May 1997i).

This case illustrates the perils of offering medical advice over the phone and stepping outside of the role of the nurse. The phone calls made by the patient should have been referred to the doctor, and the substance of the calls should have been documented in the patient's medical record.

CHART ONLY CARE YOU PROVIDE OR SUPERVISE

Sign only those notes describing care that has been given or supervised. Unlicensed personnel, such as nursing assistants, are not usually involved in writing progress notes. However, nursing assistants may document the completion of tasks on flowsheets. Chart only what is observed. Sometimes other nurses or other personnel will provide a nurse with information about patients; for example:

11:00 AM: Care provided by K. Early, NA, who stated that patient moaned when being turned.—L. French, RN

Think about your potential liability of such a statement. Suppose you chart what the other nurse told you as if you'd heard or seen it yourself, but the other nurse misinterpreted the patient's response or made an inaccurate assessment. Your credibility would suffer if you were forced to admit on the witness stand that you didn't actually see the patient. And what if the other nurse is also called to the stand and denies telling you anything? That certainly wouldn't help your credibility either (Mandell, 1987, p. 46).

Cosigning others' notes is occasionally necessary; for example, student nurses' notes are frequently cosigned by the instructor. Cosigning implies that the instructor approved the care given and assumed responsibility for it. Cosigning an entry on a medication record means that the instructor is accepting the responsibility for the patient having received the correct medication. If an instructor signs an entry without reading it or overlooks a problem raised by the entry, he or she could share liability for any injury that results (Bergerson, 1988). Lawsuits in which student nurses are named are rare. However, if a plaintiff initiates a suit against a student, the instructor, school, agency, physician, and other nurses may be included as well.

Before cosigning another person's entry the nurse should review it carefully to ensure that it clearly identifies who gave the care. If someone else's care results in injury to the patient, the cosigner could share in liability (Maher, 1997).

The recommended procedure for cosigning follows: (1) The student writes the note and signs it with his or her first initial and last name, SN (for student nurse), and the name of the school; (2) After reading the note, the instructor draws a slash and signs the note with his or her first initial, last name, and RN (for example, S. Jennings, SN, U. of Penn./B. Schultz, RN).

Although student nurses provide nursing care, the healthcare facility's nursing personnel are ultimately responsible for the patient. The fact that a student nurse was assigned to the patient does not absolve the nursing staff from its obligation to document important observations or nursing interventions. A nurse should not sign the note of a student nurse if it is apparent that the student has done something clinically wrong. After evaluating the patient the nurse should report the problem to the charge nurse and the student's instructor (Horsley, 1994).

DO NOT TAMPER WITH RECORDS

Healthcare professionals have tampered with medical records in many ways. Because tampering is among the most serious of all documentation issues, it will be discussed in detail, with cases to illustrate the consequences.

Tampering with the record involves the following:

- Adding to the existing record at a later date without indicating the addition is a late entry
- Placing inaccurate information into the record
- Omitting significant facts
- Dating a record to make it appear as though it was written at an earlier time
- Rewriting or altering the record
- Destroying records
- Adding to someone else's notes

Fraudulent additions to a record for the purposes of covering up an incident can be detected by current technology. Expert document examiners have many sophisticated techniques to detect altered records, including chemical analysis, ultraviolet and infrared examination, spectrophotometry, and chromatography. They can date ink samples using a piece of paper the size of a pinprick. Many companies change the composition of the ink in pens and typewriter ribbons at the beginning of each year, which permits the dating of entries (Nygaard and Deubner, 1988). Box 6-8 illustrates the clues used to detect altered records.

If a record is changed, the insurance company defending the healthcare professional may have to settle the case out of court even if no negligence has occurred. Once the accuracy

---

> ### Box 6-8
>
> #### Clues Used to Detect Altered Records
>
> - Writing crowded around existing entries
> - Changes in slant, pressure, or uniformity (or other differences in handwriting)
> - Erasure or obliteration
> - Use of different pens or typewriters to write one entry
> - Misaligned typed notation
> - Impressions (or lack of impressions) from writing instruments on the following pages
> - Ink offsets or lack of offsets on the back side of the preceding page
> - Additions on different dates written in the same ink, whereas original entries were written in different ink

of the record is challenged, the integrity of the entire record becomes suspect.

In recent years, when plaintiff attorneys have proven that tampering has occurred, they have had some success in getting the statute of limitations for these cases extended. (Each state provides a time limit, or statute of limitations, for the initiation of a lawsuit after the plaintiff discovers that an incident has occurred.) Because tampering with records may be considered fraud, such cases have a longer statute of limitations than "pure" malpractice actions.

When records are destroyed, the plaintiff attorney can request sanctions against the defendants for failure to comply with orders to produce the documents. The plaintiff attorney can argue in court that the records were intentionally altered because of conspiracy or fraud. This charge is called "aggravated or outrageous conduct," and it can result in the granting of punitive damages. Furthermore, healthcare professionals who have been named in a malpractice suit involving altered records may sue the person who falsified the records.

CORRECTLY IDENTIFY LATE ENTRIES

Late entries result when the following occur:

- Important information is added to the medical record after progress notes have been completed.
- The medical record is not available for charting at the time the nurse needs it.
- The nurse forgets to write progress notes on a particular chart.

Asking other nurses to leave blank lines so that progress notes can be inserted should be avoided. This information should be added as a late entry. Late entries should not be squeezed into an existing note or placed in the margins. The late entry should *not* be added in such a way as to appear suspicious. When writing late entries, note the reason why

---

Box 6-9

Guidelines for Adding Late Entries

1. Add the entry to the first available line.
2. Label the entry "Late Entry" to indicate that it is out of sequence.
3. Record the time and date of the entry.
4. In the body of the entry, record the time and the date the entry should have been made; for example:

10/17/99 1400   (Chart not available on 10/16). On 10/16 at 1000 patient stated that she felt faint when getting out of bed on 10/16 at 0800 and fell on the floor. Patient stated she did not hurt herself and didn't think she had to tell anyone until her husband encouraged her to report it. No bruises, lacerations noted. Denied pain. Dr. George examined patient at 1020.
    —L. Wilson, RN

---

the entry is being added to the record. Plaintiff attorneys scrutinize late entries, and they may attempt to prove that the nurse tried to alter a record to cover up an error instead of making an addition. If it seems likely that a lawsuit will be filed over an incident, check with the nursing supervisor and defense attorney before adding late entries; they will advise you on the proper procedure (Tammelleo, 1988). Most healthcare facilities have a procedure for adding late entries. The approach in Box 6-9 is recommended. Nurses often ask, "How late can I add a late entry?" The rule of thumb is the sooner a late entry is added, the better. The longer after the fact it is added, the more the late entry appears to be a self-serving response to the fear of liability, particularly with a bad patient outcome.

Charts may be incomplete for a variety of legitimate reasons, and they may lack signatures, dates, and times. Medical records departments are responsible for obtaining complete records within a short time. Healthcare professionals are commonly asked to fill in the blanks. The practice of adding to a medical record after a patient has been discharged must be viewed with caution. All nurses should be careful about what is added to a record after the fact. Adding a signature to one's own handwritten note is probably safe. Trying to remember and document assessment data, times, or other details can be risky. The added information may be inaccurate or be construed as tampering.

RECORD ONLY ACCURATE INFORMATION

Nothing but the truth should go into the medical record. Sloppy record keeping presents a picture of unprofessional

and suspect care. Falsification of the medical record can result in severe clinical and legal consequences. Decisions of the entire healthcare team are based on the accuracy of the recorded information. Judges and juries are likely to doubt the credibility of the healthcare professionals when falsification is detected, making it more likely that a case will settle out of court or punitive damages will be awarded.

In the following Texas case the evidence of falsification of the records probably contributed to the award of punitive damages:

An 84-year-old Texas woman suffered a series of strokes and was admitted to a long-term care facility. She had vascular disease of her legs, which required close monitoring. Ten months later, her daughter-in-law was attempting to put on her shoes when she noticed that the patient's leg was black. The patient was taken to the hospital, where the patient's leg was amputated below the knee. After sustaining a major myocardial infarction, she died. Falsification of the medical record was detected when it was discovered that medical procedures were charted for times when the patient was not even in the nursing home. Former nurses at the nursing home testified that the home was understaffed, and they cited instances of patient neglect. The jury returned an award for the plaintiff that included $721,000 in compensatory damages and $10 million in punitive damages (Laska, 1998b).

DO NOT OMIT SIGNIFICANT INFORMATION FROM THE CHART

The omission of significant information in the medical record has serious consequences. Remembering or proving years after an event that care was provided is impossible if it was not documented. Juries are skeptical when nurses claim that they can remember what happened with a particular patient 4 years or more ago. Failure to document also raises the question of whether the nurse provided the required care. When omissions of documentation are detected, the jury begins to wonder if other information was intentionally not recorded.

Omitted documentation may result in inappropriate or incomplete treatment, as the following case illustrates:

A Louisiana stabbing victim walked around for several months with a broken knife blade in his shoulder because an ED employee did not document an important piece of information. When the patient was brought to the ED, he told a tall, brown-haired white man wearing green scrubs and a white coat that one of the blades of the knife had broken off during the fight and might still be in his shoulder. This man looked at the knife and returned it to the patient. This mysterious person, who may have been a nurse or a doctor, was never identified. Nothing about the knife blade was documented in the patient's medical record or communicated to the ED physician. The ED physician testified that he would have taken x-rays had he known of the broken blade. The knife piece remained in the patient's back for over 2 months (Tammelleo, 1992a, p. 1).

In the following case, several departures from expected nursing practice contributed to a patient's death:

An Illinois woman voluntarily admitted herself to an inpatient detoxification program. Five days later her condition seemed to worsen. She was oversedated, groggy, and incoherent. At the beginning of the 2300 to 0700 hours shift the patient passed out on the bathroom floor. The nurses carried her to her bed but did not contact a physician. This incident was not documented in the medical records. No progress notes were made from 2300 to 0700 hours. The medication doses to be given at 0100 hours and 0500 hours were not administered. The patient was found dead by the day shift. The autopsy placed the time of death at 4 to 6 hours before 0700 hours. She had died from combined drug toxicity, including Darvocet, the drug on which she was dependent (Tammelleo, 1991, p. 2).

The deviations from the standard of care are numerous in this case. The nurses were faulted for failure to inform the physician of the patient's grogginess, failure to monitor the patient, and, of course, failure to document. The patient's husband received a $4 million verdict.

Never let anyone, including a physician or nursing supervisor, succeed in applying pressure to conceal the truth. When asked to omit crucial information from the record, follow the chain of command in discussing concerns about the request. If the supervisor is the person applying pressure or no nursing supervisor is available, the healthcare facility's administrative personnel or legal counsel should be notified. They should provide the needed support. Nurses who are fearful when something unforeseen happens to a patient exhibit a serious misunderstanding of the law. A truthful record of what happened and what was done to handle the problem is the first step in a good legal defense (Regan, 1982).

In the preceding case, the fraudulent preparation of the records was a major factor in strengthening the plaintiff's case. In the following lawsuit a layperson's involvement during surgery was concealed:

In a surgical case the sales manager of a company that supplies hip prostheses practiced surgery without a license. The episode was covered up on the record with the involvement of the operating room (OR) nursing supervisor. During a hip replacement operation the sales manager removed the new prosthesis when it popped out of the acetabulum, cleaned out the old cement, reapproximated bone fragments, and reinserted the new prosthesis. The OR supervisor's log and the medical record made no mention of these events, nor did they even indicate that the sales manager was in the OR. When the truth became known the nurse and others were indicted on criminal charges of assaulting a patient and concealing the unauthorized practice of medicine by a layperson (Bernzweig, 1985, p. 63).

This case has spurred perioperative units to evaluate their policy regarding the presence at surgeries of persons who are not healthcare providers and to redesign consent forms to specify who may be in the operating room.

Some nurses become panic-stricken when notified of an impending lawsuit and are tempted to review the medical record for completeness. The nurse should remember that the plaintiff attorney has a copy of the record by the time the nurse knows that a suit has been filed. The attorney probably knows the contents of the record so well that any attempt to alter it would be immediately detected. One attorney tells each nurse he defends for malpractice, "When making a final decision in your case, the jurors certainly won't remember all the testimony that was presented. But they'll never forget that you altered a patient's record" (Mandell, 1986, p. 21).

CORRECT MISTAKEN ENTRIES PROPERLY

Attorneys are always looking for alterations in the record that raise questions about the chart's accuracy. Methods that have been used to change mistaken entries have included erasing or obliterating information with correction fluid or black markers. These methods provide the plaintiff attorney the opportunity to suggest that the nurse was covering up a clinical error, and they should *never* be used. The questioning in the following example demonstrates the dangers of obliterating information (Bergerson, 1988, p. 55):

Attorney:	You had something to hide, didn't you?
Nurse:	No, not at all.
Attorney:	You altered the evidence to cover up something incriminating, didn't you?
Nurse:	No, I didn't.
Attorney:	Well then, will you tell us what was there?
Nurse:	I don't remember. It was just some sort of mistake.
Attorney:	If you don't remember, how can you be sure that you didn't erase something incriminating? Something that would have proven the plaintiff's case? I think you covered up the entry for that very reason.

The use of correction fluid was questioned in the following Georgia case and resulted in the radiographing of the chart:

A neonatal nurse used correction fluid to change nurse's notes. The court concluded, after examining the results of the x-ray films of the notes, that the white-out procedure was improper but not done for fraudulent or guilty purposes (Tammelleo, 1985, p. 1).

The agency's policies and procedures usually describe the proper way to correct errors. All entries on the record should be made in ink. One way to avoid the temptation to use correction fluid is to remove it from any areas containing medical records. Ensure that all staff, including unit secretaries, understand why correction fluid cannot be used on medical records. Box 6-10 illustrates the guidelines for correcting mistaken entries.

Box 6-10
Guidelines for Correcting Mistaken Entries

1. Draw a single line through the entry so that it is still readable.
2. Write the word "mistaken entry" above or beside the original words. The use of the word "error" is no longer advised because juries tend to associate that word with a clinical error that affected the patient.
3. Place the date and your initials next to the words "mistaken entry."
4. You can streamline this process by adding "ME" (mistaken entry) to the list of approved abbreviations in use in the facility.

Box 6-11
Clues Used to Detect Substituted or Rewritten Records

- Unnatural order of writing and uniformity of handwriting, ink, margins, and spacing
- Intersecting fountain pen entries of different dates that bleed together
- Differences between pages (e.g., folds, stains, offsets, impressions, holes, tears, and types of paper)
- Forms that were not in use at the purported time of entry
- Use of a later year (1999 for 1998), especially if it has been corrected several times

---

DO NOT REWRITE THE RECORD

When errors occur in charting, the nurse should follow the procedure outlined earlier in this chapter. Nurses may be tempted to rewrite pages of the medical record and discard the originals if the nurse spills liquid on it, accidentally tears a page, or writes an erroneous entry. However, if the record should fall into the hands of a plaintiff attorney, convincing him or her that the record was rewritten innocently may be hard. The destruction of the original gives the appearance that the record has been tampered with. Attorneys often consult specialists to identify records that have been rewritten.

The following procedure is recommended if the page is absolutely unreadable and must be recopied.

1. At the top of the new page, identify that the page was rewritten: "Recopied notes from 11/17/98."
2. Retain the original page in the chart along with the recopied page.

In the following case, nurses came forward to blow the whistle on a physician who rewrote medical records:

A 27-year-old mother of five children sought an abortion from the defendant doctor. At 22 weeks' gestation, she was outside the guidelines for a second-trimester abortion due to the increased risk of bleeding. The executive director of the clinic determined that she should be refused an abortion and referred to a hospital. The defendant then contacted the executive director, stating that the clinic needed the money, and ordered the doctor to perform the abortion. After the procedure the woman suffered an amniotic fluid embolism, retained products of conception, and suffered massive hemorrhage and infection, which ultimately led to her death.

When the emergent nature of her complications became evident, she was moved out of the operating room to a recovery room so that other abortions could be performed in the operating room. No monitoring equipment was available in the recovery room. When the defendant found out an ambulance had been called, he became angry and canceled the ambulance. Later he relented when the patient's bleeding continued. She died after arrival at the hospital.

The defendant was charged with a variety of deviations from the standard of care, as well as committing fraud for attempting to cover-up of the cause of the patient's death. The records were determined to have been falsified. The true original records were brought to the Medical Licensing Board by former employees of the clinic. The records had been partially destroyed and burned by the defendant. A $10 million judgment was entered against the defendant, who did not attend the trial. (This was considered by the judge to be an admission of the truth of the plaintiff's evidence.) (Laska, 1997e)

Box 6-11 describes clues used by attorneys and expert document examiners to detect fraudulent dating of records.

DO NOT LOSE OR DESTROY MEDICAL RECORDS

The information age has made it increasingly difficult to lose medical records. The nurse should be aware of the seriousness of this type of tampering. Juries will assume that the information on the missing document was so damaging that the healthcare professional had to destroy it; for example:

The loss of delivery records was a factor in a New York obstetrical case. The suit was brought by a disabled 12-year-old boy, who claimed that he should have been delivered by cesarean section and that the defendant hospital did not timely treat him for hypoxia and seizures following his birth. He claimed that the delivery records, which were lost before trial, showed fetal distress and that a nurse's note indicated meconium aspiration and staining. The defendant argued that a nurse or a first-year resident in the intensive care nursery incorrectly diagnosed meconium aspiration and the infant's initial Apgars of 7 and 8 belied his claim that hypoxia occurred in utero. The defendant claimed that the brain damage was either genetic or caused by an injury or illness to the boy's mother. The parties settled for $1,850,000 (Laska, 1997k).

The defense of this hospital was complicated by the loss of the delivery records. Juries can be expected to presume that missing records contained information that someone wanted to conceal. It is relatively easy for a plaintiff attorney to determine when a medical record is incomplete. The removal of key parts of the medical record is easily detected. The following case illustrates the consequences of the removal of essential parts of the chart:

A 25-year-old woman was admitted to the hospital in her thirty-sixth week of pregnancy. She required treatment for pregnancy induced hypertension, and her condition continued to worsen. She died 2 weeks after delivery and the baby suffered brain damage resulting in mild left-sided hemiparesis. The plaintiff claimed that the defendants were negligent in failing to diagnose and treat the decedent's preeclampsia and in failing to deliver the infant in a timely manner. The defendants contended that no hospital records were available to prove which of the physicians was responsible for the decedent's care because many essential records, such as physician's progress reports and medication charts, were removed from the decedent's chart. All of the defendants denied responsibility for her care. A $2,250,000 settlement was reached (Laska, 1997n, p. 28).

Nurses should never participate in the deliberate destruction of medical records, no matter what the consequences of disclosure of the record. The possibility always exists that another healthcare provider is planning to tamper with the record. Seeking the assistance of the supervisor or others in the chain of command may be necessary to protect the interests of the patient and facility.

DO NOT ADD TO THE NOTES OF OTHERS

In no situation is it acceptable for someone else to alter the nurse's documentation. Nurses may be tempted to fix a coworker's charting error, but correcting an error jeopardizes the accuracy of the record. The other person may deny in court having made the error that you changed. The jury may view the entire record as suspect. The alteration of records is a true risk-management crisis that needs to be immediately stopped. Incidents involving alteration of nursing progress notes by another healthcare professional should be reported to the nursing supervisor. The incident should be followed through until the problem is corrected. The person altering the notes may simply be unaware of the legal implications of tampering with records.

DOCUMENT NONCOMPLIANCE

Several situations should alert nurses to issues commonly associated with lawsuits. The prudent nurse recognizes dangers and practices defensive charting to prevent charges of fault in the patient's care. The following section discusses *potentially contributing patient acts,* a term used in risk management for patient behaviors that may contribute to an injury or failure to respond to medical and nursing care.

Documentation of these behaviors may assist in the nurse's defense against a malpractice lawsuit.

Just as the nurse has responsibilities to a patient, so does the patient have responsibilities toward the nurse and the rest of the healthcare team. The patient's responsibilities include the following (JCAHO, 1997):

1. *Providing information.* The patient and family must disclose information about symptoms, past illnesses, current or chronic medical problems, previous hospitalizations, medications, and allergies.
2. *Asking questions.* The patient and family are expected to ask questions about information that they do not understand or seek clarification concerning how to provide care.
3. *Following instructions.* The patient and family are expected to follow the treatment plan and adapt the plan to the patient's needs.
4. *Accepting the consequences of not following instructions.* When the patient, family, or both are unable or unwilling to follow instructions, they should be advised of the consequences of failing to follow the recommended treatment plan. This information should be documented in the medical record.
5. *Following hospital rules and regulations.* The patient and family are expected to follow rules regarding patient care and conduct, and to display consideration towards the rights of others. They should refrain from making unnecessary noise, smoking, or causing distractions. The property of others and the facility should be treated with respect.

The following potentially contributing patient acts will be presented:

1. A patient's refusal or inability to provide accurate and complete information
2. Noncompliance with medical and nursing interventions, such as the following:
   a. Not staying in bed
   b. Not adhering to dietary restrictions
   c. Not keeping return appointments
   d. Leaving the facility against medical advice
   e. Refusing to leave the facility
   f. Abusing or refusing of medications
3. Presence of unauthorized personal items at the bedside
4. Tampering with medical equipment

Describe Patient's Refusal or Inability to Provide Accurate or Complete Information

A patient may refuse to give information regarding health status, history, and current medications and treatments for any of the following reasons:

- Too many healthcare providers have been collecting the same data.
- The patient is lacking understanding of the significance of providing certain information.
- The patient has suspicions or secretiveness regarding the need for sharing personal information.

The following is an example of the type of information to be charted when the patient refuses to answer questions:

When patient was asked for a list of current medications, he said, "Why do you want to know? What business is it of yours? I don't know why I have to answer that question."—E. Bognar, RN

The documentation of a patient's omission or refusal to provide significant information can be a factor when the patient is harmed as a result of the omitted information; for example:

Controversy concerning whether a man shared information about his seizure disorder was a component of a malpractice suit filed against a prison health service. The plaintiff was a man who had been placed in jail. He fell from a top bunk during a grand mal seizure, sustaining facial fractures and three herniated lumbar discs, which required two surgeries. He claimed that the booking personnel and nurses were negligent in failing to notify the doctor of his history of seizure disorder, failing to communicate his need for Tegretol (carbamazepine), and failing to locate him in the lower bunk, as directed by the doctor. The defendants claimed that the plaintiff did not inform anyone about his condition. The jury returned a $200,000 verdict for the plaintiff. Fifty percent of the negligence was allocated to the plaintiff, and the other 50% was divided between the prison health service and the sheriff (Laska, 1997a).

Note that this jury award acknowledged the negligence of the plaintiff as contributing to his injuries.

A patient may be unable to provide important historical information because of the following:

- Decreased or altered level of consciousness
- Severe pain or fear
- Certain psychiatric disturbances
- Language barriers
- Disorientation

When any of these occurs, the nurse should attempt to gather the information from other sources and clearly document any difficulties in communicating with the patient.

Report Noncompliance With Medical and Nursing Interventions

Patients have the right to refuse medical and nursing care. The progress notes should describe any behavior that specifically contradicts the instructions given to the patient. If a question arises as to the care the patient received, this documentation will provide important information for the defense.

The types of instructions that may result in harm to the patient when ignored are discussed in the following text.

Not Adhering to Dietary Restrictions

The nurse may observe that the patient is failing to follow dietary restrictions by discovering unauthorized food at the bedside.

Not Staying in Bed

Patients may be instructed to stay in bed or to call for help when trying to get out of bed. Failing to follow this advice is a common example of the type of noncompliance that should be well documented, as shown in the following example:

| 1000 hours | Assisted pt. to bathroom. Pt. weak, unsteady on feet. States she gets dizzy when she stands. Instructed pt. to call for assistance to get out of bed (OOB). Call bell placed within reach. |
| 1130 hours | Found pt. in bathroom. Stated she got OOB by herself. Reminded her to call for assistance. Pt. said she understood.—R. Nelson, RN |

This type of charting shows that the nurse recognized that the patient was at risk for falling and tried to prevent it. This may reduce the chances of a successful lawsuit if the patient falls.

Not Keeping Return Appointments

The patient may be instructed to return to the clinic, ED, or physician's office for follow-up treatment. When a patient is examined and treated, the date of the patient's follow-up appointment should be documented in the record. By recording it immediately on the record, nurses protect themselves, the physician, and the hospital or agency. Because patients often suffer adverse effects as a result of their noncompliance with medical advice, a documented record of missed appointments is quite helpful for the defense if a patient later sues. Where an apparent problem of missed appointments exists, it may be worthwhile to send follow-up letters, return receipt requested, to ensure that the patient is aware of his or her failure to keep medical appointments. Document all attempts to reach the patient and keep copies of records to the patient in the patient's file.

Leaving the Hospital Against Medical Advice

A mentally competent patient has the right to leave the hospital and cannot be forced to stay. Only patients who meet the criteria for involuntary commitment can be held against their wishes. (This is discussed further in Chapter 13.) In any situation where the patient's mental capacity at the time of the departure might be questioned, the degree of competence must be documented (Hill, 1991).

When the patient announces his or her plan to leave the hospital, the nursing supervisor and the patient's physician should be notified after the nurse has determined the patient's reason for wanting to leave. The physician is responsible for informing the patient of the risks involved in refusing further treatment. The warning must be specific: The patient may be informed that the condition may worsen, and the physician may even tell the patient, if it is applicable, that death may result.

The patient and family should be told that the patient is welcome to return to the hospital if the patient changes his or her mind. The nurse should not make any statements indicating that the hospital will refuse to readmit the patient or that the physician will not provide further care for the patient. These statements may be inaccurate and legally inadvisable.

If the patient announces an intention to leave but does not want to wait until the physician has been contacted, the nurse should urge the patient to delay the departure until the doctor can be reached. If the patient refuses to wait, the nurse should document that the patient rejected encouragement to discuss the issue with the physician. The patient should be asked to sign a release form indicating he or she understands the risks of leaving. Documentation should include the circumstances of the patient's desire to leave against medical advice (AMA), an assessment of the patient's mental status, the actions that were taken, and the time the patient left the facility. Some facilities use a specific type of incident report to document the occurrence (Figure 6-3).

Refusing to Leave the Facility

Although a discharge order may be written, the facility remains legally responsible for the patient until the patient is off of the facility's property. In some situations, a patient may be reluctant to leave the facility. This may occur when the patient lacks transportation home or support systems after discharge, does not believe he or she is ready to leave the facility, or has no home to which to return. After identifying the reasons for the patient's reluctance to leave the facility, problem solving must occur to resolve the issue.

Tips for Documentation

The following list includes tips for documentation (Thompson, 1998):

- Describe the patient's reasons for wanting to stay in the hospital.
- Document the steps that were taken to resolve the issue.
- If a disruptive patient refuses to leave, document that the patient was given a statement of the necessity for discharge.
- Provide the patient with a formal written request to leave the facility that has been reviewed by hospital counsel.
- If a patient is sent home in a taxi because of a lack of transportation, document the name of the taxicab

company, time of pickup at the hospital, name and badge number of the driver, and instructions given to the driver to contact the hospital when the patient is safely home.

Refusal or Abuse of Medications

The following incidents should be described in the progress notes:

- Refusal of any prescribed medications, including the reason for refusal (if known)
- Notification of the physician regarding the patient's refusal of the medication
- Accidental discovery of any illegal or nonprescribed drugs at the patient's bedside
- Drug-seeking behavior, including the following: a pattern of losing or spilling prescriptions; asking for frequent refills; asking for a large amount of pills in each prescription; simultaneously filling prescriptions at several pharmacies; obtaining analgesic prescriptions from more than one doctor simultaneously; loitering near the medication cart or medication room on a nursing unit
- Accidental discovery of hoarded drugs, indicating that the patient has been collecting medication instead of swallowing each dose
- Sudden changes in the patient's behavior that might have resulted from the injection of narcotics or street drugs, particularly if these symptoms occurred shortly after a visitor has been in the room. For example:

1100 hours	Visitor present at bedside. Pt. alert, oriented. Fetal monitor strip shows contractions every 2 minutes. IV running at 125 ml/hr.
1125 hours	Upon entering room, pt. found to be lethargic. Pupils were constricted; speech was slurred. Pt. stated, "My friend gave me something to help with the pain." Dr. James notified of lethargy, pinpoint pupils, and slurred speech.
1130 hours	Narcan (naloxone) administered as ordered.—W. Silverstein, RN

Describe Unauthorized Personal Items Found at the Bedside

Unauthorized personal items may include equipment from home, which is normally checked by the biomedical department before its use is permitted in the hospital. (Heating pads, hair dryers, and electric razors fit into this category.) Alcoholic beverages and tobacco (in smoke-free hospitals or for certain patients with respiratory or cardiovascular conditions) are also considered contraband. These substances should be removed or sent home with family

AMA OCCURANCE REPORT
Request for Discharge by Voluntary Patient or Representative

<u>Section 1: (TO BE FILLED OUT BY CLINICAL STAFF MEMBER)</u>

Time of Admission:_____

Stated Reason for Discharge:_____

_____

Staff Name:_____ Date/Time_____

Physical/mental status of patient:_____

_____

<u>Section II (TO BE FILLED OUT BY NURSE/CASE MGR.)</u>   Unit RN:_____

1.   Needs Assessment Staff contacted?

    Name:_____ Time called: _____

2.   Program Administrator / House Supervisor / Administrator on Call Notified?

    Name:_____ Time called:_____

3.   Nursing Supervisor notified?

    Name:_____ Time called:_____

    Summary of action taken by Director of Inpatient Services or Nurse Manager:

    _____

    _____

    _____

4.   Attending Physician notified?

    Name:_____ Time called:_____

    Intervention recommendation:_____

    _____

    _____

5.   Case Manager notified?

    Name:_____ Time called:_____

    Summary of action taken by Case Manager/notification of managed care / insurance referral

    source:_____

    _____

    _____

6.   End result of patient's request for discharge:

    _____ Patient signed AMA Form and is waiting to discuss further with M.D.

    _____ M.D. gave AMA discharge order   _____ Patient agreed to stay

    _____ M.D. gave routine discharge order   _____ 24 hour hold instituted

    _____ Other: Specify:_____

    _____

_____   _____
    Date/Time   Signature

Figure 6-3   AMA occurrence report. (Courtesy Charter Behavioral Health System, Chandler, Ariz.)

members as appropriate. The progress notes should describe what was found and its disposition, for example:

Patient found to be using heating pad from home. Pad removed. Dr. Beede contacted. Stated she did not want patient using a heating pad, and Dr. Beede will be in to discuss this with patient later today.—F. Bell, RN

Document Tampering with Medical Equipment

At times, patients manipulate equipment, often without understanding the consequences. Describe any observations or indications that the patient is changing the IV flow rate, removing traction, adjusting monitoring equipment, or manipulating any other biomedical equipment. The documentation should describe what was done about the problem, such as instructing the patient not to touch equipment or notifying the physician of the problem. When the patient is not directly observed adjusting equipment but is strongly suspected of doing so, the available facts should be documented; for example:

0830 hours	IV flow rate at 80 ml/hr, 1000 ml up in bag.
0900 hours	IV found to be running wide open with 400 ml left in bag. Pt. stated he "turned that little dial" because he wanted to get the IV over with. No change in BP, no evidence of fluid overload. Breath sounds clear bilaterally. Instructed pt. about reasons for not touching IV flow meter.—K. Wils, RN

DO NOT USE MEDICAL RECORDS TO CRITICIZE OTHERS

Finger pointing and accusations of incompetence do not belong in the medical record. The plaintiff's attorney would be happy to discover evidence of fighting among healthcare professionals—this would facilitate the job of developing a case. Speaking to the writer of derogatory comments when they are found in the medical record is vital. The person who made the comments may need to understand the potential consequences of including these criticisms. Examples of inappropriate comments are included in Box 6-12.

Consider the dilemma of the nurse in the following case:

A doctor who sees patients in my unit habitually documents what she calls nurses' "errors" in patients' charts and inserts orders for us to write incident reports about events that aren't really problems. For example one "error" she documented was failure to give an prn laxative. The nurse did not administer it because the patient was not constipated and did not request a laxative. I'm not comfortable writing a report about an event I did not witness or signing an order I cannot follow. How should we handle this? (*Inappropriate orders: getting it write*, 1995).

Box 6-12

Avoid Inappropriate Comments

- 7 AM—Patient's toes on right foot beyond the cast are blue and cold. Night shift apparently never checked the circulation in them (Creighton, 1987b).
- Primary nursing care could not be given because nurse:patient ratio was 1:20 (*Nurse's legal handbook*, 1985).
- Patient in extreme pain because the night staff refused to give prescribed medication (Solberg, 1986).
- The IV infiltrated because the night staff forgot to check it (Solberg, 1986).
- If he doesn't start returning calls, he's going to kill a patient (*Manage nurses' expanding liability with strict policies*, 1987).
- Nurse's note: Patient going into shock. Could not get Dr. Jones to come. We never can!!! (Fox, Imbiorski, 1979).
- Fall due to lax nursing supervision (Davino, 1995).
- If doctors would return our phone calls promptly, we would have a lot fewer deaths around here (Calfee, 1995).
- Patient is obviously a victim of child abuse (Calfee, 1995).
- Physician's note: If nurses around here would read medication orders, we'd have fewer emergencies (Fox, Imbiorski, 1979).
- Physician's order: Head nurse to total intake and output.
- Physician's progress note: Inevitably, the lab did not draw the PTT again this morning.

Data from Calfee B: *Nursing 95* p 71, March 1995; Creighton H: *Nurs Manage* p 14, October 1987b; Davino M: *RN* p 62, September 1995; Fox L, Imbiorski W: *The record that defends its friends*, p 20, Chicago, 1979, Care Communications; Manage Nurses' expanding liability with strict policies, *Hosp Risk Manage* p 33, March 1987; Nurses legal handbook, p 189, Springhouse, Penn, 1985, Springhouse; Solberg P: *Legal implications of patient charting* (seminar handouts), p 13, Fayetteville, NC, 1986, Nursing Business News.

The physician in this situation is drawing attention to concerns that have not resulted in patient harm, and are therefore not incidents. These issues are best discussed in person with education provided on the implications of these types of orders.

DOCUMENT INCIDENT (OCCURRENCE) REPORTS

Definition

An *incident* is defined as an unusual occurrence with the potential for patient injury or liability, often representing a breakdown in the system. Examples of system breakdown can occur when a series of people or processes contribute to an injury or a near miss. Examples can include the following: administering blood to the wrong patient who has the same name as the intended patient; of operating on the wrong leg; or administering a fourfold overdose of a medication over the course of 4 days. Incidents may act as warning signs of serious underlying problems in a facility.

Purposes

Incidents should be reported for a number of reasons, including the following:

1. Federal, national, and state accrediting bodies require documentation and analysis of incidents as part of risk-management efforts.
2. The ANA Code for Nurses (1985) states that the nurse is expected to "safeguard the patient and public when health and safety are affected by incompetent, unethical, or illegal practice of any person." This obligation cannot be fulfilled unless the nurse shares relevant information about an incident. The individual involved in the incident can be a healthcare professional, hospital employee, or any number of outside personnel with access to a healthcare facility or healthcare setting.
3. The healthcare agency and (by extension) other employers of nurses have a duty to inform the patient or the patient's survivors of a known deviation from the standard of care that causes an injury (Peters, 1988). Something is owed to those who have been harmed because caregivers have failed to live up to the terms of the "contract" between healthcare providers and patients. A need for compensation is another possible reason. Treating patients with dignity means being honest about what has happened in treatment (Weber, 1994). In many cases a nurse may be the only person who knows about such an incident. For the agency to fulfill its responsibilities to the patient, the nurse must inform the administration about the incident.
4. Many lawsuits can be averted if the agency takes prompt action following an incident. Studies have shown that only a small number of incidents resulting in patient injury lead to a lawsuit. The use of several strategies can reduce the possibility of a lawsuit, including the following: showing concern for the injured patient, writing off a bill, providing future services at no charge, apologizing, or letting the family know a full investigation will be made. These same strategies may be ineffective or contraindicated in other circumstances, and should be carefully used by administrators skilled in risk management.
5. The incident should trigger an investigation of the circumstances and the changes necessary to prevent recurrences. Recommendations for change may include the following: additional education for employees; discipline; revised policies, procedures, and protocols; purchasing of equipment; or changes in patient delivery systems. Incidents occurring as a result of substance abuse or other types of mental and emotional impairment may lead to the identification of the need for treatment.
6. Incident reports can be helpful in pointing out situations that expose the facility to liability and inefficiencies in the system. Recognition of these problems can result in improvements in the system.

Prevalence of Reporting Incidents

Many healthcare professionals believe that the incident reports that are filed represent the tip of the iceberg of all reportable incidents. Concerns about the current climate in healthcare facilities is increasing doubts about the accuracy of incident reporting. As downsizing, right-sizing, reengineering, mergers, and reorganization create new ways of delivering health care, an air of depression and pessimism may creep into an organization. When employees feel overworked and stressed, morale may sink, leading to an increase in errors. Although system errors may foster and contribute to incidents involving patients, many healthcare professionals believe incident reporting will cause finger pointing. Witness these concerns, which were shared with surveyors of the Joint Commission for the Accreditation of Healthcare Organizations (JCAHO) (Jones, Arana, 1996):

> "I knew I gave him the wrong dose, but I was afraid I'd lose my job."
> "There were so many incidents, we decided we couldn't do them all, so we did nothing. I observed the wrong treatment being administered but was too scared to do anything about it."
> "Incident reports used to be routine, now they are performance continuances."
> "We turned our unit into a place that was so different. We were used to helping each other out and knowing that mistakes or errors happened, and it was dealt with. Now we know, fudge, lie, ignore—then we might stay here."
> "A group of nurses on the critical care unit said that each time the surgeon is written up, the vice president of medical affairs comes to the unit in a tirade to 'get to the bottom of this.' The nurses are reluctant to document errors—'they don't go anywhere and we get yelled at.'"

Admninistrative actions that may result in reluctance to report incidents include withholding promotions, raises, disciplinary action, or firing an employee who reports an incident. While there may be some situations that do warrant these actions, their routine use following an incident may hinder forthright reporting of incidents.

When an incident is not reported the healthcare facility is deprived of the opportunity to investigate the situation. The facility's attorney, risk manager, and insurance carrier need to review the incident report to determine whether a case should be settled out of court or a defense strategy to soothe the patient should be planned. Serious incidents should be reported to the risk manager immediately, and an incident report must be filled out. Failure to fill out an incident report or document an untoward event in the medical record can be construed as a cover-up if and when the incident is revealed.

A long-term care nurse described the following dilemma:

"The state has received several complaints about the long-term care facility where I work, so we've been advised to prepare for an inspection. In response, the director of nursing told the nursing staff that, from now on, we shouldn't allude to minor medication errors or slight injuries in the residents' charts, and we shouldn't document follow-up care after an error. She wants us simply to fill out incident reports. But she's provided no written policy to back up her instructions" (*Keeping mum about mistakes,* 1996).

Clearly these nurses are being placed in an unethical position. By not documenting the follow-up care being provided, the nurses are being asked to participate in a cover-up.

No doubt fueled by concerns about concealment of incidents, the Joint Commission took action in November 1997 to address this issue. In December 1997 the American Society for Healthcare Risk Management (ASHRM, 1997) alerted their membership to a policy change by the Joint Commission concerning sentinel events: "A sentinel event is defined as an unexpected occurrence involving death or serious physical or psychological injury. Serious injury specifically includes loss of limb or function. The event is termed 'sentinel event' because it signals the need for immediate investigation and response." The following types of events are also defined as sentinel:

- Infant abduction
- Infant discharged to the wrong family
- Rape (by another patient or staff)
- Hemolytic transfusion reaction
- Surgery on the wrong patient or wrong body part
- Patient death, paralysis, coma, or other major permanent loss of function associated with a medication error
- Suicide of a patient in an around-the-clock facility
- Suicide of a patient following elopement from a facility
- Any elopement that results in death or major permanent loss of function
- Any intrapartum maternal death
- Any perinatal death unrelated to a congenital condition in an infant weighing more than 2500 grams
- Assault, homicide, or other crime resulting in a patient death or major permanent loss of function
- A patient fall that results in death or major permanent loss of function as a direct result of the injuries sustained in the fall

When a sentinel event occurs, the organization is required to complete a root-cause analysis, which examines systems and processes involved in the event. Risk reduction strategies should be developed and implemented. The organization is encouraged to voluntarily report the event to the Joint Commission within 30 days of the occurrence (or becoming aware of it). The results of the thorough and credible root-cause analysis must be reported to the Joint Commission within 30 days. A risk reduction plan will be submitted as a separate report. The Joint Commission has the option of placing an organization on Accreditation Watch status if the organization does not self-report the sentinel event or fails to submit an acceptable root-cause analysis within 45 days. Site visits by the Joint Commission to the organization may occur if the Joint Commission believes an ongoing threat to patient safety exists. Further action, such as placing the organization on Preliminary Nonaccreditation status, may occur if the flaws in the first root-cause analysis are not corrected with a second one (ASHRM, 1997).

After the announcement of the sentinel event policy, questions were raised about the confidentiality and discoverability of these reports. The reporting deadlines were perceived as being too stringent, and the root-cause analysis format was cumbersome and not applicable to all situations (ASHRM, 1998). Clarification of the policy occurred with some modifications in the Joint Commission's approach.

Filling Out an Incident Report

Many insurance carriers have revised the format of incident reports from a narrative report to one that is computerized. Forms that lend themselves to computerization, such as the example in Figure 6-4, have several coded boxes and a small space for comments. Computerization of incidents permits sorting and tallying to identify trends. If the space provided is not large enough for comments, most facilities permit the attachment of an additional page of narrative remarks. The form should be easy to use, objective, pertinent, and designed to be processed quickly.

Incident reports were at one time protected from review by the plaintiff's attorney. Some facilities attempt to protect an incident report by labeling it as a work product generated in contemplation of litigation, a peer review document, a document protected by attorney-client privilege, or the attorney work product. The discoverability of incident reports varies from state to state (Fiesta, 1994). The probability is currently high that the attorney will be able to obtain a copy. Because it is likely that a plaintiff's attorney will see an incident report, keep in mind the following guidelines:

1. An incident report should be filed when the following occur: an injury to a patient, a medication error, an injury to a staff member or visitor, or any unusual occurrence that warrants documentation. The nurse should also report situations that could lead to injury; for example, two different medications that are packaged in nearly identical boxes. Some facilities use separate forms to document concerns about the behavior of an individual, such as a member of the hospital staff, or to report ongoing problems, such as not being able to receive urgent laboratory results in a timely manner. Follow the agency's policies about when to complete an incident report.

REPORT NO. 0316077

HOSPITAL INCIDENT REPORT

CONFIDENTIAL MEMO TO ATTORNEY

HOSPITAL NAME

1 ☐ INPATIENT   4 ☐ VISITOR
2 ☐ OUTPATIENT   5 ☐ OTHER INCIDENT
3 ☐ EMERGENCY ROOM

Health Care Insurance Company
Princeton Insurance Company

COMPLETE OR USE
ADDRESSOGRAPH
FOR PATIENT

COMPLETE
FOR VISITOR

PATIENT ID:

LAST NAME:

FIRST NAME:

SEX (M/F): _____ AGE: _____ (Y)ears (M)onths, or (D)ays: _____

FLOOR/UNIT/ZONE #: _____ ROOM #: _____

ADM DX.

DATE OF INCIDENT: _____ DAY OF THE WEEK: _____

TIME: _____ DATE OF REPORT: _____

DEPARTMENT INVOLVED

1 ADMINISTRATION
2 ADMITTING
3 AMBULATORY SURGERY
4 ANESTHESIA
5 BUILDING & GROUNDS
6 BURN UNIT
7 BUSINESS OFFICE
8 CAFETERIA
9 CARDIOPULMONARY LAB
10 CARDIOVASCULAR LAB
11 CAST ROOM
12 CENTRAL SUPPLY
13 CLINIC
14 CORONARY CARE UNIT
15 COFFEE/GIFT SHOP
16 DELIVERY ROOM
17 DETOXIFICATION UNIT
18 DIALYSIS UNIT
19 DIETARY
20 EMERGENCY SERVICES
21 ENDOSCOPY UNIT
22 EXTENDED CARE
23 GYNECOLOGY
24 HELIPORT
25 HOUSEKEEPING
26 INTENSIVE CARE UNIT
27 INTERMEDIATE CARE UNIT
28 I.V. THERAPY
29 LABORATORY
30 LABOR ROOM
31 LAUNDRY/LINEN ROOM
32 MAINTENANCE
33 MEDICAL HEALTH
34 MENTAL HEALTH
35 NEONATAL I.C.
36 NUCLEAR MEDICINE
37 NURSERY
38 NURSING ADMINISTRATION
39 NURSING SERVICE/MED/SURG
40 OB/POST PARTUM
41 OCCUPATIONAL THERAPY
42 OPERATING ROOM
43 PEDIATRICS
44 PHARMACY
45 PHYSICAL THERAPY
46 PSYCHIATRY
47 RADIOLOGY
48 RECOVERY ROOM
49 REHABILITATION
50 RESPIRATORY-THERAPY
51 SECURITY
52 SOCIAL SERVICE
53 TRANSPORTATION
54 UTILIZATION REVIEW
55 OTHER
56 UNKNOWN

LOCATION

1 PATIENT ROOM
2 PATIENT BATHROOM
3 NURSING STATION
4 MEDICATION ROOM
5 SHOWER/TUB/ROOM
6 RECREATION AREA/LOUNGE
7 OTHER BATHROOM
8 OPERATING ROOM
9 DELIVERY ROOM
10 INTENSIVE CARE UNIT
11 EMERGENCY ROOM
12 EXAMINING/TREATMENT ROOM
13 OTHER PATIENT SERVICE DEPART.
14 OTHER HOSPITAL DEPARTMENT
15 MOBILE INTENSIVE CARE UNIT
16 COFFEE/GIFT SHOP
17 LOBBY/WAITING ROOM
18 ELEVATOR/ESCALATOR
19 HALLWAY/CORRIDOR
20 STAIRWAY
21 DOORWAY
22 ROOF
23 DRIVEWAY
24 WALKWAY/SIDEWALK
25 PARKING LOT
26 STEPS
27 WINDOW
28 OTHER
29 UNKNOWN

NATURE OF THE INCIDENT
(Check off only one code in only one category)

1 ANESTHESIA RELATED

1 ☐ INCORRECT ANESTHETIC AGENT
2 ☐ ASPIRATION
3 ☐ EQUIPMENT
4 ☐ EXTUBATION
5 ☐ INTUBATION
6 ☐ MONITORING
7 ☐ POSITIONING
8 ☐ TECHNIQUE
9 ☐ OTHER
10 ☐ UNKNOWN

INCORRECT AGENT

2 ARTICLE IN PATIENT

1 ☐ NEEDLE
2 ☐ INSTRUMENT
3 ☐ SPONGE
4 ☐ OTHER
5 ☐ UNKNOWN

3 BURN

1 ☐ CHEMICAL
2 ☐ CIGARETTE, CIGAR, ETC.
3 ☐ ELECTRIC
4 ☐ HEATING APPLIANCE
5 ☐ HOT LIQUID
6 ☐ OTHER
7 ☐ UNKNOWN

4 EMERGENCY DEPARTMENT RELATED

1 ☐ DELAY IN TREATMENT
2 ☐ DISCHARGED WITHOUT BEING SEEN BY MD
3 ☐ DOA WITHIN 7 DAYS OF DISCHARGE
4 ☐ HELD OBSERVED BEYOND POLICY
5 ☐ MONITORING
6 ☐ RETURN FOR SAME PROBLEM
7 ☐ OTHER
8 ☐ UNKNOWN

5 EQUIPMENT RELATED

1 ☐ DISCONNECTED/DISLODGED
2 ☐ ELECTRIC SHOCK
3 ☐ ELECTRIC POWER OUTAGE
4 ☐ IMPROPER USE
5 ☐ MECHANICAL PROBLEM
6 ☐ NOT AVAILABLE
7 ☐ TAMPERED WITH
8 ☐ WRONG EQUIPMENT
9 ☐ OTHER
10 ☐ UNKNOWN

6 FALL

1 ☐ OUT OF BED
2 ☐ OFF CHAIR
3 ☐ OFF BEDSIDE COMMODE
4 ☐ OFF SCALES OR EQUIPMENT
5 ☐ OFF TABLE OR STRETCHER
6 ☐ WHILE AMBULATING
7 ☐ DURING RECREATIONAL ACTIVITY
8 ☐ DROPPED
9 ☐ FAINTED
10 ☐ TRIPPED ON EQUIPMENT
11 ☐ FOUND ON FLOOR
12 ☐ OTHER
13 ☐ UNKNOWN

7 I.V./BLOOD RELATED

1 ☐ ADVERSE REACTION
2 ☐ CROSSMATCH PROBLEM
3 ☐ INCOMPATIBLE ADDITIVES
4 ☐ INFILTRATION
5 ☐ MISLABELED
6 ☐ NOT DOCUMENTED
7 ☐ OMITTED
8 ☐ OUT OF SEQUENCE
9 ☐ OUTDATED
10 ☐ PATIENT IDENTIFICATION
11 ☐ RATE OF FLOW
12 ☐ REPEATED ATTEMPTS TO START
13 ☐ SITE PROBLEM
14 ☐ TRANSCRIPTION ERROR
15 ☐ TUBING-NOT-CHANGED
16 ☐ TUBING-PULLED OUT/BROKEN
17 ☐ WRONG ADDITIVE
18 ☐ WRONG SOLUTION TYPE
19 ☐ WRONG TIME
20 ☐ OTHER
21 ☐ UNKNOWN

INJURIES

1 ☐ HEAD
2 ☐ FACE
3 ☐ EYE(S)
4 ☐ NECK
5 ☐ BACK
6 ☐ ARM(S)
7 ☐ HAND(S)
8 ☐ CHEST
9 ☐ ABDOMEN
10 ☐ BUTTOCKS
11 ☐ LEG(S)
12 ☐ FOOT
13 ☐ MULTI-SITES
14 ☐ NO APPARENT INJURY
15 ☐ OTHER
16 ☐ UNKNOWN
99 ☐ N/A

Site of Injury:

Severity of the injury:

1 ☐ MINOR
2 ☐ SIGNIFICANT
3 ☐ DEATH
4 ☐ UNKNOWN
9 ☐ N/A

Nature of the injury: (Most Serious):

1 ☐ AMPUTATION
2 ☐ BLISTER
3 ☐ BURN/SCALD
4 ☐ CIRCULATORY IMPAIRMENT
5 ☐ CONCUSSION
6 ☐ CONTRACTURE
7 ☐ CONTUSION
8 ☐ CUT/LACERATION
9 ☐ DAMAGED TEETH
10 ☐ DECUBITUS
11 ☐ EXCESSIVE BLOOD LOSS
12 ☐ FRACTURE/DISLOCATION
13 ☐ HYPOTHERMIA
14 ☐ INFECTION
15 ☐ NEEDLE WOUND
16 ☐ NEUROLOGICAL DEFICIT
17 ☐ PERFORATION
18 ☐ PHLEBITIS
19 ☐ POISONING
20 ☐ RASH/HIVES
21 ☐ RETAINED FOREIGN OBJECT
22 ☐ SENSORY IMPAIRMENT
23 ☐ SPRAIN/STRAIN
24 ☐ VISCERA INJURY
25 ☐ WOUND DISRUPTION
26 ☐ OTHER
27 ☐ UNKNOWN
99 ☐ N/A

CIRCUMSTANCES SURROUNDING THE INCIDENT: Patient Condition at the time

1 ☐ NORMAL
2 ☐ CONFUSED
3 ☐ DISORIENTED
4 ☐ SEDATED
5 ☐ UNCOOP.
6 ☐ UNCON-SCIOUS
7 ☐ OTHER
8 ☐ UNKNOWN
9 ☐ N/A

Figure 6-4 Incident report format that can be computerized. (Courtesy of Health Care Insurance Company, Princeton, NJ.) *Continued*

WITNESSES (Include Addresses):

COMMENTS

COMPLETED BY:

Signature   Date

Supv. Signature   Date

PHYSICIAN'S FINDINGS: Date Seen   Time Seen

☐ DOCUMENTATION IN PROG. NOTE

Physician's Signature   Date

8 MEDICATION RELATED
1 ☐ ADVERSE REACTION
2 ☐ DUPLICATION
3 ☐ PATIENT IDENTIFICATION
4 ☐ GIVEN WITHOUT ORDER
5 ☐ GIVEN OUT OF SEQUENCE
6 ☐ IMPROPER ORDER
7 ☐ INCORRECT DOSAGE
8 ☐ INCORRECT DRUG
9 ☐ INCORRECT MODE OF ADMIN.
10 ☐ MEDICATION WITHOUT CULTURE
11 ☐ MEDICATION MISSING
12 ☐ MISLABELED
13 ☐ NOT DOCUMENTED
14 ☐ OMISSION
15 ☐ PT TOOK UNPRESCRIBED MED
16 ☐ PHARMACY DISPENSING ERROR
17 ☐ TIMING
18 ☐ TRANSCRIPTION
19 ☐ OTHER
20 ☐ UNKNOWN
MED _____   DOSAGE _____

9 OBSTETRICS RELATED
1 ☐ APGAR SCORE <5 at 5 MIN.
2 ☐ CONTAMINATION
3 ☐ EQUIPMENT
4 ☐ FETAL/MATERNAL DEATH
5 ☐ MATERNAL INJURY
6 ☐ NEONATAL INJURY
7 ☐ MONITORING
8 ☐ PRECIPITOUS DELIVERY
9 ☐ PROLONGED LABOR
10 ☐ RETURN TO DELIVERY ROOM
11 ☐ UNATTENDED DELIVERY
12 ☐ OTHER
13 ☐ UNKNOWN

10 PATIENT INDUCED
1 ☐ AMA ABSENCE
2 ☐ ATTEMPTED SUICIDE
3 ☐ ELOPEMENT
4 ☐ FIGHT AMONG PATIENTS
5 ☐ PATIENT ATTACKED STAFF
6 ☐ PATIENT REFUSED TREATMENT
7 ☐ SELF-INFLICTED INJURY
8 ☐ OTHER
9 ☐ UNKNOWN

11 SURGERY RELATED   ROOM #
1 ☐ CANCELLED
2 ☐ CONSENT PROBLEM
3 ☐ CONTAMINATION
4 ☐ DELAY IN STARTING
5 ☐ DEATH
6 ☐ EQUIPMENT
7 ☐ PATIENT/SITE ID
8 ☐ MONITORING
9 ☐ PREP
10 ☐ RESPIRATORY/CARDIAC CODE
11 ☐ RETURN/REPEAT SURGERY
12 ☐ SPONGE/NEEDLE/INSTRUMENT COUNT
13 ☐ UNPLANNED REMOVAL OF ORGAN OR PART OF ORGAN
14 ☐ OTHER
15 ☐ UNKNOWN

12 TREATMENT/PROCEDURE RELATED
1 ☐ ADVERSE REACTION
2 ☐ CANCELLATION
3 ☐ CHANGE IN DX
4 ☐ CONSENT PROBLEM
5 ☐ DELAY IN PT ARRIVAL
6 ☐ DELAY IN TREATMENT
7 ☐ DEVIATION FROM PROCEDURE
8 ☐ DIETARY PROBLEM
9 ☐ PATIENT/SITE ID
10 ☐ INJECTION SITE
11 ☐ MISSING SPECIMEN
12 ☐ MONITORING
13 ☐ NOT DOCUMENTED
14 ☐ OMITTED
15 ☐ PATIENT REFUSAL
16 ☐ PREP
17 ☐ POSITIONING
18 ☐ REPEAT PROCEDURE
19 ☐ RESPIRATORY/CARDIAC CODE
20 ☐ REPORTING OF TEST RESULTS
21 ☐ TECHNIQUE
22 ☐ TRANSCRIPTION ERROR
23 ☐ TRANSFER/MOVING OF PT.
24 ☐ UNPLANNED TRANSFER TO CRITICAL CARE
25 ☐ OTHER
26 ☐ UNKNOWN

13 OTHER
1 ☐ ASSAULT
2 ☐ FIRE
3 ☐ FLOOD
4 ☐ FOOD POISONING
5 ☐ GENERAL POWER FAILURE
6 ☐ NATURAL DISASTER
7 ☐ OBJECTS IN FOOD
8 ☐ OTHER ACCIDENT WHILE AMBULATING
9 ☐ OTHER ACCIDENT WHILE IN BED
10 ☐ PROPERTY MISSING OR DAMAGED
   1 ☐ DENTURES
   2 ☐ EYE GLASSES
   3 ☐ HEARING AID
   4 ☐ JEWELRY
   5 ☐ CASH
   6 ☐ OTHER
11 ☐ OTHER
12 ☐ UNKNOWN

Ambulation Privileges:
1 ☐ COMPLETE BED REST
2 ☐ BED REST WITH B.R.P. (Assisted)
3 ☐ BED REST WITH B.R.P. (Unassisted)
4 ☐ UP IN CHAIR/WHEEL CHAIR
5 ☐ AMBULATE WITH ASSISTANCE
6 ☐ AMBULATE WITHOUT ASSISTANCE
7 ☐ AMBULATE WITH APPLIANCE
8 ☐ NOT SPECIFIED
9 ☐ OTHER
10 ☐ UNKNOWN
99 ☐ N/A

MEDICATED IN THE PREVIOUS 4 HOURS?
1 ☐ YES   2 ☐ NO   3 ☐ UNKNOWN   9 ☐ N/A

POSITION OF BED RAILS:
1 ☐ UP   2 ☐ DOWN   3 ☐ UNKNOWN   9 ☐ N/A

RESTRAINTS:
1 ☐ NONE   2 ☐ ORDERED   3 ☐ IN USE
9 ☐ UNKNOWN   ☐ N/A

BED HEIGHT:
1 ☐ HIGH   2 ☐ LOW   3 ☐ UNADJUSTABLE
4 ☐ UNKNOWN   9 ☐ N/A

CALL LIGHT:
1 ☐ ON   2 ☐ OFF   3 ☐ UNKNOWN   9 ☐ N/A

FLOOR SLIPPERY:
1 ☐ YES   2 ☐ NO   3 ☐ UNKNOWN   9 ☐ N/A

DISPOSITION
SEEN BY:
1 ☐ ATTENDING PHYSICIAN
2 ☐ ON CALL PHYSICIAN
3 ☐ EMERGENCY DEPARTMENT
4 ☐ EMPLOYEE HEALTH
5 ☐ RN, MD NOTIFIED
6 ☐ RN, MD NOT NOTIFIED
7 ☐ OTHER
8 ☐ UNKNOWN
9 ☐ N/A

DID PATIENT RECEIVE TREATMENT?
1 ☐ EXAMINED AND TREATED
2 ☐ X-RAY ORDERED
3 ☐ REFUSED TREATMENT
4 ☐ TREATMENT NOT INDICATED
5 ☐ UNKNOWN
9 ☐ N/A

MOST SIGNIFICANT TREATMENT RECEIVED:
1 ☐ ADMITTED TO HOSPITAL
2 ☐ CPR
3 ☐ DRESSING
4 ☐ FOLLOW-UP CARE INDICATED
5 ☐ MEDICATED
6 ☐ SUTURED
7 ☐ DISCHARGED
8 ☐ NO FURTHER TREATMENT INDICATED
9 ☐ OTHER
10 ☐ UNKNOWN
99 ☐ N/A

8/91

Figure 6-4, cont'd   Incident report format that can be computerized.

2. Record the details of the incident in objective terms. Describe exactly what was seen or heard; for example, unless the nurse sees a patient fall, he or she should write, "Found patient on the floor."

3. Do not admit to liability or blame by including statements such as, "I made a mistake when I. . . ," "accidentally, I. . . ," or "somehow I. . . ." Avoid pointing fingers at other healthcare professionals or nursing administrators. Do not document statements such as "Better staffing would have prevented this incident." Do not include explanations as to how the incident could be avoided in the future. (However, verbally share such suggestions with the supervisor and risk manager.)

4. Chart only what is observed firsthand. Each staff member who knows about the incident should write a separate report (Cournoyer, 1985). If a patient injury occurs in another department, that department is responsible for documenting the details of the incident.

   An incident that is reported to the nurse, but is not actually witnessed by that individual, should be documented with as much detail as possible; for example, "Jaime Podrost, NA, stated she observed the patient climb over the raised full length side rails and fall to the floor."

5. Describe the actions taken to provide care at the scene, such as helping a patient get back into bed or assessing for injuries.

6. Do not include the names or addresses of witnesses, even if the form asks for this information. If the hospitalized patient's roommate was involved in reporting the incident, do not refer to that individual by name. (This would violate the roommate's confidentiality rights.)

7. Document the time of the incident and the names of the physician, supervisor, and family members who were notified. Complete the incident report as soon as possible, preferably on the same day the incident occurred. Not only will recollections be clearer, but prompt reporting will also enable the agency to take immediate action. Under the Joint Commission requirements to report sentinel events within 30 days, immediate reporting of incidents becomes even more critical.

8. Send incident reports to the person designated by policy to review them. Incident reports should not be filed with the clinical record, but should instead be retained by the hospital administration, usually in a risk-management department (if one exists).

9. If additional information is found after filling out the incident report, do not cross out, alter, or destroy the original report. An amendment, properly dated and signed, may be attached to the original report. Remember, tampering with the record has serious consequences.

Documenting the Incident in the Progress Notes

1. Progress notes should contain a factual, honest, and objective description of the incident. If the circumstances of the incident are not included in the progress notes, it may seem as though a cover-up has taken place. The time and name of the doctor (e.g., attending, resident, intern, or house physician) who was notified of the incident should be documented along with what the doctor was told. The progress notes should also describe the assessment of the patient, the treatment and follow-up care, and the patient's response. This information will indicate that the patient's condition was closely monitored after the incident. If the case should end up in court, the jury may be asked to determine whether the patient received appropriate care after the incident.

2. Avoid writing "incident report completed" after describing the incident. This destroys any possibility that the incident report can be kept confidential and draws the attention of a plaintiff's attorney. Physicians should not write orders for an incident report to be completed. Inform physicians that written orders to make out an incident report may prompt the attorney to request a copy of the incident report and complicate the defense of a suit.

3. Include any statements made by the patient in the progress notes as well as the incident report. In particular, include any admissions by the patient or family that their actions played a role in the incident; for example: "Patient stated, 'The nurses told me to call before I tried to get out of bed, but I climbed over the rails anyway.'" The defense attorney can use these statements to prove that the patient was guilty of contributory or comparative negligence. *Contributory negligence* is conduct by the patient that contributes to his or her injuries. A plaintiff who is found guilty of contributory negligence may not be able to collect money for injuries. Some states have adopted the doctrine of *comparative negligence,* which involves determining each party's percentage of negligence; that is, the jury may decide that the nurse was 30% negligent and the patient was 70% comparatively negligent.

Documenting the Incident for Personal Records

As an additional safeguard the nurse should write an accurate description of the incident in a personal notebook for future reference (Forward, 1998). Include details of the incident and the names of the people who were involved, particularly if they can back up your information. In the event of a lawsuit the information will help refresh memories and provide the defense attorney with valuable facts. However, the discoverability of this document may vary from state to state.

In the following case the nurse's personal notes were obtained through discovery after a lawsuit was filed:

A 72-year-old man fell down a flight of stairs in his home. He was taken to the ED by the rescue squad, who used full cervical precautions. Shortly after his arrival in the ED, a physician removed the cervical collar. The doctor allegedly refused to order x-ray films to rule out a cervical spine injury, although two nurses asked for them. The patient's complaints of neck pain, weakness, and hand tingling intensified. A physician lifted him into a seated position on the stretcher to examine his cervical range of motion. When his torso was lifted to a forty-five-degree angle, the man screamed in pain and cried, "The bones are breaking in my neck." The defendants immediately laid him down and replaced the collar. Within minutes, the man lost all sensation in his legs, abdomen, and eventually up to his shoulder blades. An MRI demonstrated compression of the spinal cord at C4-C5. The plaintiff was rendered quadriplegic despite emergency surgery. He survived for 18 months on a ventilator before his death from aspiration pneumonia. The nurse caring for the patient in the ED carefully recorded all of the events in the patient's chart and also kept personal notes of all of her conversations with the defendants. Those notes were obtained through discovery. A physician admitted in his deposition that lifting the patient was a mistake and probably caused the quadriplegia. The settlement was for $2.03 million (Laska, 1998c, p. 12).

Further Reporting of an Incident

Early reporting of an incident to the insurance company (carrier) facilitates gathering of complete and accurate facts and results in a better resolution of the situation. If the nurse has malpractice insurance, the carrier's requirements should be followed. The policy may ask the nurse for a written notification of any claim and incident that is likely to result in a claim against the nurse. However, the nurse should not make a copy of the incident report or forward it to the carrier. This would violate the confidentiality of the clinical record.

SUMMARY

Several guidelines affect the legal aspects of charting. Many of the suggestions presented here have evolved from the experiences of nurses in litigation, whereas others are based on common sense. As the nurse incorporates these guidelines into practice, they will become second nature. The nurse should be particularly alert to situations and practices that create difficulties in defending nursing care in a lawsuit. Documentation should demonstrate that appropriate care has been provided. In many cases the chart will be the only source of information years after the patient has been forgotten.

REFERENCES

A failure to communicate, *Nursing 97* p 32, February 1997.

American Nurses Association: *Code for nurses with interpretive statements*, Kansas City, Mo, 1985, The Association.

ASHRM: *Legislative Alert: JCAHO sentinel events*, December 10, 1997.

ASHRM: *Position statement and recommendations: JCAHO sentinel event reporting program*, February 13, 1998.

Bergerson S: More about charting with a jury in mind, *Nursing 88* p 51, April 1988.

Bernzweig E: Go on the record with nothing but the truth, *RN* p 63, April 1985.

Black J: Charting chuckles, *Nursing 97* p 53, December 1997.

Calfee B: Avoiding the charge of defamation, *Nursing 95* p 71, March 1995.

Cournoyer C: Protecting yourself legally after the patient is injured, *Nurs Life* p 20, March/April 1985.

Creighton H: Legal significance of charting (part I), *Nurs Manage* p 17, September 1987a.

Creighton H: Legal significance of charting (part I), *Nurs Manage* p 14, October 1987b.

Davino M: Charges of negligence don't belong on a patient's chart, *RN* p 62, September 1995.

Fiesta J: Incident reports: confidential or not? *Nurs Manage* p 17, October 1994.

Forward D: Managing malpractice insurance, *Am J Nurs* p 16BB, March 1998.

Fox L, Imbiorski W: *The record that defends its friends*, Chicago, 1979, Care Communications.

Hill H: Leaving against medical advice. In Henry G, ed: *Emergency medicine risk management*, Dallas, 1991, American College of Emergency Physicians.

Horsley J: When a student's charting is your responsibility, *RN* p 64, November 1994.

Horsley J: When you go toe-to-toe over doctor's orders, *RN* p 59, November 1997.

Inappropriate orders: getting it write, *Nursing 95* p 26, October 1995.

JCAHO: *1997 Comprehensive accreditation manual for hospitals*, Oakbrook Terrace, IL, 1996, The Commission.

Jones L, Arana G: Is downsizing affecting incident reports? *The Joint Commission Journal* p 592, August 1996.

Keeping mum about mistakes, *Nursing 96* p 22, November 1996.

Kerr A: How the write stuff can go wrong, *Nursing 87* p 48, January 1987.

Laska L, ed: Florida prisoner has grand mal seizure and falls from top bunk in jail, *Medical Malpractice Verdicts, Settlements, and Experts*, p 28, February 1997a.

Laska L, ed: Illinois surgical patient found dead of pulmonary embolisms in hospital room, *Medical Malpractice Verdicts, Settlements, and Experts* p 23, February 1997b.

Laska L, ed: Newborn with respiratory distress given overdose of Theophylline, *Medical Malpractice Verdicts, Settlements, and Experts* p 24, February 1997c.

Laska L, ed: Texas woman develops IV infiltration in hospital, *Medical Malpractice Verdicts, Settlements, and Experts* p 22, February 1997d.

Laska L, ed: Woman died from amniotic fluid embolism and hemorrhage after second trimester abortion, *Medical Malpractice Verdicts, Settlements, and Experts* p 18, February 1997e.

Laska L, ed: Arizona woman suffers infection and ileostomy following removal of dialysis catheter, *Medical Malpractice Verdicts, Settlements, and Experts* p 55, March 1997f.

Laska L, ed: California woman goes into respiratory arrest and dies after neurosurgery, *Medical Malpractice Verdicts, Settlements, and Experts* p 23, March 1997g.

Laska L, ed: Maryland woman with hydrocephalus dies of apparent occlusion of ventricular shunt, *Medical Malpractice Verdicts, Settlements, and Experts* p 25, May 1997h.

Laska L, ed: Pregnant woman claims of swollen glands, sore throat, and low fever, *Medical Malpractice Verdicts, Settlements, and Experts* p 31, May 1997i.

Laska L, ed: California man suffers significant bleeding during laparoscopic cholecystectomy, *Medical Malpractice Verdicts, Settlements, and Experts* p 49, June 1997j.

Laska L, ed: New York boy claims he should have been delivered by cesarean section, *Medical Malpractice Verdicts, Settlements, and Experts* p 33, June 1997k.

Laska L, ed: Infiltration of intravenous therapy required skin graft surgery and debridement, *Medical Malpractice Verdicts, Settlements, and Experts* p 21, July 1997l.

Laska L, ed: Excessive dosage of Haldol blamed for leaving Massachusetts man in semi-vegetative state, *Medical Malpractice Verdicts, Settlements, and Experts* p 40, September 1997m.

Laska L, ed: Massachusetts woman suffered pre-eclampsia during pregnancy, *Medical Malpractice Verdicts, Settlements, and Experts* p 28, September 1997n.

Laska L, ed: Surgeon orders stabilization and transfer to trauma center of young man with multiple gunshot wounds, *Medical Malpractice Verdicts, Settlements, and Experts* p 21, November 1997o.

Laska L, ed: Emergency room doctor's failure to recognize symptoms caused by spider bite blamed for girl's death, *Medical Malpractice Verdicts, Settlements, and Experts* p 13, January 1998a.

Laska L, ed: Leg amputation and death of 84-year-old Texas nursing home resident due to gross neglect of her vascular condition, *Medical Malpractice Verdicts, Settlements, and Experts* p 29, January 1998b.

Laska L, ed: Cervical collar removal, no x-rays taken and man lifted after fall at home, *Medical Malpractice Verdicts, Settlements, and Experts* p 12, March 1998c.

Maher V: Countersigning notes by others, *Nursing 97* p 16, June 1997.

Manage nurses' expanding liability with strict policies, *Hosp Risk Manage* p 29, March 1987.

Mandell M: Charting: how it can keep you out of court, *Nurs Life* p 46, September/October 1987.

Mandell M: Ten legal commandments for nurses who get sued, *Nurs Life* p 18, May/June 1986.

Nurses legal handbook, Springhouse, Penn, 1985, Springhouse.

Nygaard D, Deubner S: Altered or "lost" medical records, *Trial* p 46, June 1988.

Paxman G: Verbal orders, *Nurs Spect* p 15, June 1993.

Peters A: Hospital malpractice: eleven theories of liability, *Trial* p 82, November 1988.

Regan W: Charting: the truth, the whole truth, *Regan Report on Nursing Law* p 1, June 1982.

Roach H, Larson E, Bartlett D: Intravascular site care: are critical care nurses practicing according to written protocols? *Heart Lung* 25(5):401, 1996.

Sansivero G: Taking care of PICCs, *Nursing 97* p 28, May 1997.

Solberg P: *Legal implications of patient charting* (seminar handouts), Fayetteville, NC, 1986, Nursing Business News.

Sullivan G: Is your documentation all it should be? *RN* p 59, October 1996.

Tammelleo A: Missing progress notes: nurse's whiteouts x-rayed, *Regan Report on Nursing Law* p 1, March 1985.

Tammelleo A: Who can change a nurse's notes? *RN* p 75, May 1988.

Tammelleo A: Failure to monitor patient: deplorable nursing care, *Regan Report on Nursing Law* p 2, June 1991.

Tammelleo A: Mystery nurse fails to chart broken blades re stabbing victim, *Regan Report on Nursing Law* p 1, February 1992a.

Tammelleo A: Nursing notes can be worth their weight in gold, *Regan Report on Nursing Law* p 1, August 1992b.

Tammelleo A: Is your patient complaining of pain or burning? *Regan Report on Nursing Law* p 4, October 1992c.

Thompson C: When your patient doesn't want to leave, *Am J Nurs* 28(3):40, 1998.

Weber L: The ethics of withholding information about mistakes, *Health Progress* p 65, October 1994.

ADDITIONAL READINGS

Beffa C: Trouble on the line, *Am J Nurs* p 53, December 1994.

Eggland E: Avoiding incomplete charting, *Nursing 95* p 73, October 1995.

Eskreis T: Seven common legal pitfalls in nursing, *Am J Nurs* p 34, April 1998.

Feutz-Harter S: *Nursing and the law,* ed 4, Eau Claire, Wisc, 1991, Professional Education Systems.

Fiesta J: Duty to communicate—"doctor notified," *Nurs Manage* 25(1):24, 1994.

Fry S: Protecting patients from incompetent or unethical colleagues: an important dimension of the nurse's advocacy role, *J Nurs Law* 4(4):15, 1997.

Gibs L: Personal communication via e-mail.

Grane N: Documenting a "harmless" medication error, *Nursing 95* p 80, April 1995.

Grane N: Documenting a patient incident in your notes, *Nursing 95* p 17, January 1995.

Grane N: Quoting patients for the record, *Nursing 95* p 17, August 1995.

Hall J: No substitute for good practice, *Nursing 94* p 4, December 1994.

Horsley J: How far should you go to contact wayward patients? *RN* p 74, October 1994.

Lowell J, Massey K: Sounds of silence, *Nurs Manage* 28(5):40H, 1997.

Mandell M: Not charted, not done, *Nursing 94* p 62, August 1994.

Roth D: A comprehensive review of blood transfusion therapy, *JVAD* 2(3):17, 1997.

Roth D: A comprehensive review of blood transfusion therapy, *JVAD* 2(4):13, 1997.

Roth D: Adverse blood transfusion effects, *JVAD* p 10, Spring 1998.

Roth D: Infusion nursing: risk management strategies, *INS* p 8, November/December 1997.

Roth D: Infusion nursing: risk management strategies, *INS* p 8, January/February 1998.

Shea M: Personal communication via e-mail.

Stirring up a hornet's nest, *Nursing 97* p 12, March 1997.

Thompson C: Writing better narrative notes, *Nursing 95* p 87, April 1995.

Tranbarger R: A nurse executive's nightmare, *Nurs Manage* p 33, February 1997.

Writing a wrong, *Nursing 97* p 12, March 1997.

7

Charting Systems

Many methods of documenting nursing care have evolved over the years. This chapter reviews several of those methods. The reader will be exposed to creative and innovative approaches to documentation through a brief overview and critique of each system. Additional information about each system may be obtained by consulting the references at the end of the chapter.

NARRATIVE CHARTING

Key Elements

Narrative charting, the most familiar method for documenting nursing care, is a diary or story format used to document patient care events that occur during the shift. The narrative is a simple paragraph describing the patient's status, any interventions and treatments, and the patient's response to the interventions; for example:

Date	Time	Progress Notes
4/22	0730	Alert, oriented, and responsive to verbal stimulation. Breath sounds clear bilaterally. Coughing and deep breathing independently. Hypoactive bowel sounds in R and L upper quadrants. No complaints of discomfort at this time. Intravenous (IV) infusing with #18 angiocath in L forearm.—J. Doe, RN

Before the advent of flowsheets, the narrative note was the only mechanism used to document care. Narrative notes were often lengthy and included routine care and normal assessment findings, along with significant findings and patient problems. No clear way existed to discern which information was most important.

With the development of flowsheets, which captured the routine, repetitive aspects of care, the narrative note could potentially be shorter and more meaningful. However, most nurses continued to document information in the narrative note that was already on the flowsheet because they were accustomed to previous methods. This practice created double documentation.

Today few facilities rely solely on narrative notes for documentation. Most have adopted flowsheets to augment the narrative note in an attempt to save time and avoid duplication of information.

Advantages

The following are advantages of narrative charting:

1. Narrative charting is familiar to many nurses and is the documentation format most nurses learned in nursing school.
2. Narrative documentation can be easily combined with other documentation methods; for example, narrative charting can be combined with flowsheets, and the narrative note can then be used to document the patient's progress.
3. If written correctly, the narrative note contains information on the patient's problems, the interventions, and the patient's response (or lack of response) to interventions. In most narrative charting, however, the patient's response is inconsistently charted.
4. Narrative charting is especially useful in emergency situations. Nurses can quickly and easily document the chronological events of the situation.

Disadvantages and Problems

The following are disadvantages of and problems concerning narrative charting:

1. The primary disadvantage of narrative charting is the lack of structure. Most narrative notes are disorganized,

moving from one issue to the next with no apparent connection. Showing relationships between data in narrative notes is difficult.

2. Narrative notes are task-oriented and time-consuming. Documentation has traditionally been process-oriented with little emphasis on evaluation. Narrative charting does not consistently reflect all of the elements of the nursing process, such as planning and evaluation.

3. Since the content of narrative notes is not uniformly defined, information is difficult to retrieve for quality improvement activities, monitoring, and research. Tracking the patient's current status and current problems is difficult. Problems may not be addressed on each shift, making it difficult to evaluate the effectiveness of care over time.

4. Narrative charting does not always reflect critical thinking, decision making, and the nurse's ability to analyze data and draw appropriate conclusions.

PROBLEM-ORIENTED CHARTING

Problem-oriented charting was introduced in the late 1960s by Lawrence Weed, a physician. His intent was to improve the documentation of patient care in clinic settings by focusing all documentation on the patient's problems. He recommended the use of a problem list and a structured, logical format for each entry in the medical record. Although the system was initially designed for physician documentation, it soon became used for nursing documentation. The format used in problem-oriented charting is called SOAP: *S*ubjective data (what the patient tells the nurse); *O*bjective data (what the nurse observes and inspects); *A*ssessment (what the nurse thinks is going on based on the data); and *P*lan (what the nurse plans to do).

As SOAP charting became more widespread over time, nurses recognized that it reflected certain aspects of the nursing process. However, it failed to address implementation and evaluation of care. Over the years the SOAP format has been modified to reflect the entire nursing process more adequately.

Although some facilities still use the SOAP format, many have changed to the SOAPIE format: *S*ubjective data (what the patient tells the nurse): *O*bjective data (what the nurse observes and inspects); *A*ssessment (the nursing diagnosis); *P*lan (what the nurse plans to do); *I*nterventions (specific interventions implemented); and *E*valuation (the patient's response to interventions). This modification incorporates all the steps of the nursing process into daily documentation.

Key Elements

Problem-oriented charting, as originally designed, has five components: data base, problem list, initial plan, progress notes, and discharge summary.

Data Base

The data base is the primary tool for gathering data at the time of admission. The physician completes a history and physical examination to gather pertinent data on the patient's condition. Likewise, the nurse conducts a nursing history and assessment to gather pertinent data on the patient's condition and to define the patient's nursing needs. The data base (as described in Chapter 2) provides information that helps the nurse determine the patient's priority needs and develop the plan of care accordingly.

Problem List

Once the data base is complete, a problem list is generated to identify the patient's important problems. For the purpose of this discussion, the word *problem* is used interchangeably with the term *nursing diagnosis*. Each problem on the list is numbered to facilitate documentation. In some cases, physicians and nurses use the same problem list. The physician documents medical diagnoses and surgical procedures and the nurse documents nursing diagnoses. In most cases, however, the nurse has a separate problem list, or the problems are numbered and written directly on the care plan, eliminating the need for a separate list. The list is updated as new problems arise and others are resolved.

Initial Plan

A plan of care is developed using the problems identified during the admission process. The physician usually documents the initial medical plan in the progress notes after the history and physical examination have been completed. Nurses document the plan of care using a variety of care plan formats (as discussed in Chapter 3). The nursing plan of care generally includes the nursing diagnoses, expected outcomes, and interventions.

Progress Notes

The progress notes in problem-oriented charting reflect documentation of the identified problems or nursing diagnoses on the problem list or care plan. Each progress note entry is written in the SOAP(IE) format; for example:

Date	Time	Progress Notes
6/12	0800	**S:** "I don't like chocolate Ensure. I want some of my wife's bread pudding."
		O: Weight 148 lb. Consumed half of breakfast. Only drank 45 ml of Ensure.
		A: Significant weight loss of 3 lb. in 3 days.
		P: Request order for dietary consult and speak with wife during visiting hours.
	1200	**I:** Order obtained for dietary consult. Dietitian to visit this afternoon.

1400   **E:** Visited by dietitian who will change menu selections. Wife will bring bread pudding tomorrow.—J. Doe, RN

In an integrated medical record, the nurses, physicians, therapists, nutritionists, and other healthcare professionals document on the same progress record. Although the contents of the note may differ, the format remains constant and provides a running report of the patient's status.

Discharge Summary

The discharge summary, which concludes the problem-oriented record, consists of a brief discussion of each problem on the list and how it was (or was not) resolved. For any unresolved problems, a SOAP(IE) note is written. This summary provides a reference for unresolved problems that require further action and a mechanism for communicating information to other hospitals, referral agencies, and the patient. Although most physicians document the medical discharge summary as a separate document, facilities are moving toward multidisciplinary discharge summary forms.

Advantages

Following are some of the advantages of SOAP(IE) charting:

1. SOAP(IE) charting is well structured. Each entry contains information in a predetermined format. The use of the SOAP(IE) format adds consistency to the documentation of patient care.
2. SOAP(IE) charting reflects the nursing process by encompassing assessment, diagnosis, planning, interventions, and evaluation of nursing care.
3. The problem-oriented approach makes it easier to track particular problems for quality-improvement monitoring.
4. SOAP(IE) charting can be used effectively with standard care plans. The problems on the care plan can be numbered for easy reference in the progress notes. Each active problem on the care plan can be addressed each shift in the progress notes, providing evidence that the plan of care was implemented.
5. SOAP(IE) charting is frequently used in an integrated medical record. An integrated progress note can foster collaboration and enhance communication among healthcare professionals. Settings in which the integrated progress note is commonly used include acute care, long-term care, rehabilitation, and psychiatric care units (where multidisciplinary approaches to care are traditionally used).

Disadvantages and Problems

The following are disadvantages of and problems concerning SOAP(IE) charting:

1. The transition to SOAP(IE) charting requires that the nurse rethink the documentation process. The nurse must determine which pieces of information correspond with each letter in the SOAP(IE) entry. Nurses have experienced some difficulty in determining the most appropriate place in the documentation for certain information. In many cases, one or more letters in the SOAP(IE) format are omitted if the nurse cannot decide where information belongs or if the nurse does not have the information necessary to complete the note; for example, the nurse may implement an intervention but be unable to document the evaluation at the same time.
2. SOAP(IE) charting is seldom implemented in its pure form, and modifications to the SOAP(IE) format can diminish the original goal of structured and logical entries.
3. Considerable redundancy occurs when nurses adopt the SOAP(IE) format; for example, both the problem list and care plan identify patient problems. The plan and interventions are noted both on the care plan and in the progress notes. If the documentation system includes flowsheets to capture interventions and treatments, redundancy will occur among the flowsheets, care plan, and SOAP(IE) note.
4. SOAP(IE) charting is not the most efficient method of documentation for nurses: Each problem requires a separate SOAP(IE) entry. Overlap may occur between several problems and their respective interventions. Writing a separate entry for each problem may involve repeating assessment-data and interventions that apply to more than one problem. To circumvent this, some nurses combine several problems into one SOAP(IE) note. This practice makes it difficult to determine which data and interventions apply to a specific problem. In either case, SOAP(IE) charting may not meet the needs of nurses who are searching for a less time-consuming method of documentation.
5. Finally, the transition to an integrated progress note (as is recommended in the pure form of SOAP charting) has met resistance in the past from other healthcare professionals. However, this is beginning to change as more settings embrace the multidisciplinary approach to care. Furthermore, using an integrated progress note may eliminate the possibility of keeping the progress record at the bedside. Although bedside charting is more convenient for nurses, other healthcare professionals usually prefer to keep the progress record with the rest of the chart in a central location. As more facilities adopt computerized documentation the issue of "who has the chart" will cease to be such a concern.

PIE CHARTING

PIE charting is a format for nursing documentation, developed in 1984 at Craven County Hospital in New Bern, North Carolina, that is similar to SOAP in that both formats are problem-oriented. However, SOAP charting originated from the medical model, whereas PIE charting is based on the nursing process. The acronym PIE represents the documentation of *p*roblems, *i*nterventions, and *e*valuation of nursing care.

The goal of PIE charting, as originally designed, was to eliminate the traditional care plan and incorporate an ongoing care plan into the daily documentation. The purpose was to simplify the documentation process, unify the care plan and progress notes, and provide a concise record of the nursing care planned and provided (Siegrist, Dettor, Stocks, 1985).

Key Elements

The PIE system consists of a patient care and assessment flowsheet and the progress notes.

Daily Patient Assessment Sheet

The daily assessment flowsheet (Figure 7-1) is a 24-hour flowsheet that lists specific assessment criteria under human needs categories, such as respiration and skin, along with routine elements of care, such as activity and hygiene (Siegrist, Dettor, Stocks, 1985). The nurse completes the assessment and initials the findings that apply to the patient. Marking criteria with an asterisk (*) indicates that they deviate from the normal, and the nurse must describe the deviation in the progress notes. In addition to assessment data the flowsheet also provides space to document information regarding IVs, medications, wounds, and procedures.

Progress Notes

After completing and documenting the initial assessment, the nurse documents the specific problems that arise during the shift. The problems are identified in the progress note using (whenever possible) a nursing diagnosis from the approved North American Nursing Diagnosis Association (NANDA) list. If the problem does not correspond to one of the approved nursing diagnoses, the nurse should develop an original problem statement using the format advocated by NANDA (human response and related/risk factors). Use of the medical diagnosis to describe nursing problems is not acceptable. The problem statement is labeled with a "P" and numbered for easy reference; for example:

Date	Time	Progress Notes
4/2	0800	P#1 High risk for trauma related to dizziness.

Once stated, the problem is referred to by number only in subsequent entries. In the pure version of the charting system, no separate problem list is created.

The nurse records the specific interventions used to manage the identified problems. The interventions are labeled with an "I" and numbered to correspond to the problem. Only those interventions actually implemented are documented in the progress notes; for example:

Date	Time	Progress Notes
4/2	0800	P#1 High risk for trauma related to dizziness. IP#1 Instructed patient to call for assistance when getting out of bed. Call bell placed within reach.

The evaluation of the effectiveness of the interventions is addressed and labeled with an "E" and the corresponding problem number in the progress note; for example:

Date	Time	Progress Notes
4/2	0800	IP#1 Instructed patient to call for assistance when getting out of bed. Call bell placed within reach.
	1200	EP#1 Patient consistently calls for assistance before getting out of bed. Still experiencing dizziness.

An evaluation of each problem is made at least once each shift and again at the end of the day. If a problem remains current, it is carried through in the documentation from one day to the next until it is resolved. Once a problem has been resolved, it is no longer addressed in the progress notes (Siegrist, Dettor, Stocks, 1985).

Additional Comments

After 6 months of implementation, nurses at Craven County Hospital strongly preferred the PIE system over traditional narrative charting with a separate care plan. Physicians also liked the system because it provided them with ongoing documentation of current patient problems (Siegrist, Dettor, Stocks, 1985).

Evaluation of information from nurses all over the United States has determined that most facilities adopting the PIE method have modified it in one or more of the following ways:

1. A problem list is generated to serve as a central location for identifying problems.
2. Assessment findings that validate the problem with each PIE entry are consistently documented, making the actual entry "APIE;" for example:

Daily Patient Assessment Sheet

Date _7/26/84_   Post-op date _____

DIET	Type	_Reg_		Amount
	Breakfast	_NPO_		%
	Lunch	_Full liquid_		% 50
	Supper			%
	/ /Self / /Assst / /NG:Gastro			

HYGIENE		7-3	3-11	11-7
	Complete			
	Assist	LMS		
	Partial			
	Shower			
	Self			
	Oral care	LMS		
	PM care			BS
	Foley care			

ACTIV				
	Bedrest			BS
	Turn q 2 hr			
	OOB (Chair)			
	BRP			
	Ambulating	LMS		
	BSC			

ELIM				
	Voiding	LMS	BS	
	Cath			
	Incontinent			
	* Emesis			
	Stool			

PULSE				
	Regular	LMS	BS	
	* Irregular			
	Strong			
	* Weak			

M/S				
	MAE	LMS	BS	
	* Weakness			
	* Paralysis			
	* Paresthesia			

RESPIRATORY	Quality:	7-3	3-11	11-7
	WNL	LMS	BS	
	Shallow			
	Deep			
	Unlabored			
	* Labored			
	Rate: WNL	LMS	BS	
	Slow			
	* Rapid			
	Sounds: Clear	LMS	BS	
	* Moist			
	* Stridor			
	* Cough			

SKIN				
	Temp: Warm	LMS	BS	
	* Hot			
	Cool			
	Turgor: Good	LMS	BS	
	Fair			
	* Poor			
	* Edema			
	Moisture: Dry	LMS	BS	
	Moist			
	* Diaphoretic			
	Color: WNL	LMS	BS	
	Pale			
	Flushed			
	* Ashen			
	* Cyanotic			
	* Jaundiced			
	Dr. Moore	LMS		
	Dr. Jones		BS	

MENTAL		7-3	3-11	11-7
	Alert	LMS	BS	
	Oriented x3	LMS	BS	
	* Disoriented			
	* Lethargic			

BEHAVIOR				
	Cooperative	LMS	BS	
	* Uncooperative			
	* Anxious			
	* Withdrawn			
	* Combative			
	* Depressed			

SPEECH				
	Clear	LMS	BS	
	* Slurred			
	* Rambling			
	Aphasic			
	* Inappropriate			

MEDICATION

Time	Drug	Dose	Rt Site	Init

Shift	Time	Type of wound	Size	Appearance	Sutures and drains	Treatments
7-3	11:30 AM	Arteriogram Site (R) Groin	Puncture wound	Dressing intact No bleeding	Ø	Monitor pulses— 3+ bilateral pedal pulses
3-11	4:00 PM	Arteriogram Site (R) Groin	Puncture wound	Dressing dry & intact	Ø	Pulses monitored 3+ bilaterally— pedal pulses
11-7						

TUBES	Type	Location	Drainage	Irri

PROCED	
	10:30 AM Arteriogram

Shift	Time	Site and cath size	Tubing change	Site appearance	Solution and rate
7-3			N/A		
3-11			N/A		
11-7					

SIGNATURES	Init	Name
	LMS	Linda M. Siegrist RN
	BS	Barbara Stocks RN

*Requires specific documentation

Figure 7-1 Daily patient assessment sheet. (From Siegrist L, Dettor R, Stocks B: The PIE system: complete planning and documentation of nursing care, *QRB*, p 186, June 1985. Copyright © 1985 by the Joint Commission on Accreditation of Healthcare Organizations, Chicago. Reprinted with permission.)

Date	Time	Progress Notes
4/2	0800	A#1 Patient's BP drops 20-30 mm Hg when she stands up. Complains of dizziness when changing positions. P#1 High risk for trauma related to dizziness. IP#1 Instructed patient to call for assistance when getting out of bed. Call bell placed within pt.'s reach.
	1200	E#1 Patient consistently calls for assistance. Still experiencing dizziness and orthostatic changes.

3. Some hospitals maintain individualized or standard care plans in an effort to promote continuity. Each PIE entry is based on problems and nursing diagnoses identified in the care plan.

Advantages

The following are advantages of PIE charting:

1. PIE charting simplifies the charting process by using a flowsheet to capture assessment and routine patient-care data that would otherwise be documented in the narrative progress note. Use of this flowsheet reduces redundancy.
2. As originally designed, PIE charting eliminates the traditional separate care plan. The progress note becomes the plan of care by including the documentation of problems, interventions, and evaluation.
3. PIE charting reflects some aspects of the nursing process, encourages the use of nursing diagnoses to identify problems, and assists nursing in applying and documenting the nursing process in daily practice.
4. Each identified problem is evaluated at least once every shift. PIE charting requires the nurse to document an evaluation of the patient's response to interventions. As a result, the progress note reflects ongoing follow-up on all current problems (Siegrist, Dettor, Stocks, 1985).
5. The originators of the PIE method believed it lends itself well to primary nursing. The primary nurse performs the assessment and initiates the PIE note. The associate nurse then has a current plan to follow and add to throughout the shift (Siegrist. Dettor, Stocks, 1985). According to Menenberg (1995), PIE charting has also proven beneficial in the psychiatric setting. The daily PIE charting unifies the mental health treatment plan with the progress notes and eliminates redundant charting.
6. PIE charting enhances professional credibility. Nurses no longer document basket terms such as "had a good day" in the medical record. As a result, the quality of the progress notes improves, making it easier to identify the nurse's contribution to overall patient care (Buckley-Womack, Gidney, 1987).

Disadvantages and Problems

The following are disadvantages of and problems concerning PIE charting:

1. Because PIE charting eliminates a separate plan of care, patient outcomes may not be prominently addressed. While daily charting promotes documentation of problems, interventions, and evaluation, the nurse's ability to evaluate the patient's progress against predetermined outcomes is limited because the expected outcomes are not readily available.
2. The system assumes that all nurses practice with the same level of sophistication and knowledge, and that all make appropriate decisions regarding problem identification and selection of interventions. Without a plan of care, clinical path, or practice guidelines to outline care, inconsistency may result.
3. Because the PIE system incorporates the plan of care into the progress notes, and planning care is ultimately the responsibility of the registered nurse (RN), the question of how to incorporate licensed practical nurses (LPNs) into the documentation process arises. During the implementation of this system, Craven County nurses noted that LPNs, with limited exposure to the nursing process and nursing diagnosis, had the most difficulty with the system. These nurses required more individualized instruction (Siegrist, Dettor, Stocks, 1985). In light of recent developments in healthcare delivery, assessing the staffing mix before selecting any documentation system is prudent.
4. Nurses using the PIE system have noted that it lends itself well to settings where the patient's status changes frequently, but it may not be as well-suited for patients whose problems remain essentially unchanged from one day to the next, such as with long-term care or care of the terminally ill (Siegrist, Dettor, Stocks, 1985).
5. The requirement to chart the problems every 8 hours and every 24 hours can create lengthy documentation, particularly if the patient has many problems.

FOCUS CHARTING

Focus Charting is a method of documentation developed in 1981 by a committee of staff nurses at Eitel Hospital in Minneapolis. Before adopting Focus Charting the hospital used the SOAP format. The nurses had expressed frustration with the limitations of SOAP charting; therefore a committee was formed to review documentation in the hospital (Lampe, Hitchcock, 1987).

The committee began by determining what information was important and should be included in the progress notes.

They examined the nursing process and specific hospital policies, and they collaborated with physicians and hospital department heads to discuss interdisciplinary requirements for documentation. The committee determined the following to be essential elements of nursing documentation (Lampe, 1988):

- Nursing assessment
- Nursing plan of care for each concern identified
- Nursing care provided
- Evaluation of the patient's response to interventions

To determine whether this information was being documented with the SOAP system, audits were done on 100 randomly selected charts. The findings revealed weaknesses in writing care plans (18% compliance) and charting the patient's response to care (12% compliance). The committee chose to develop a new documentation system that would more adequately meet the needs of the nurses and patients (Lampe, 1988).

Key Elements

Focus Charting is a method of organizing the narrative documentation to include data, action, and response for each identified concern.

Identification of Patient Concerns

Patient concerns are identified from data collected during the admission assessment or reassessment during the hospitalization. In Focus Charting, the identified concern is not labeled as a problem but instead as a focus. *Focus* is the key word used to describe the concerns. The use of this term broadens the scope of identified concerns and eliminates the negative connotations of the word "problem."

Although generally phrased as a nursing diagnosis, the focus may also be any of the following:

Focus	Examples
Current behavior or concern	Anxiety Discharge needs
Signs and symptoms	Fever Nausea
Acute change in status	Cardiac arrest Seizure
Significant patient care event	Chemotherapy Surgery
Nursing diagnosis	Ineffective coping High risk for infection

The use of foci to identify areas of concern makes the charting process more flexible, and the nurse is not limited to identifying only nursing diagnoses or problems (Lampe, 1988).

Organization of the Progress Notes

Focus Charting uses a columnar format to separate the identified concern from the body of the progress note, which permits a quick scanning of the focus column to find information on a specific concern without having to search through an unstructured narrative. All entries in the progress notes are organized using the DAR format: *D*ata (subjective or objective data that supports the focus); *A*ction (nursing interventions); *R*esponse (patient's response to interventions) (Lampe, 1988).

The nursing tasks and assessment data are documented on flowsheets. Therefore the progress notes can reflect analysis and conclusions based on the data; for example:

Date	Time	Focus	Progress Notes
6/7	0800	Pain	**D:** Pt. complaining of pain at incision site. **A:** Pt. repositioned for comfort. Demerol (meperidine) 50 mg IM given.
	0900		**R:** Pt. states a decrease in pain, "feels much better."

Lampe (1988) points out that including information on data, action, and response with each entry may or may not be necessary. However, the use of all three types of information as needed helps to promote complete documentation.

Advantages

The following are advantages of Focus Charting:

1. Focus Charting provides structure for the progress notes by organizing the content into data, action, and response.
2. Focus Charting promotes documentation of the nursing process (particularly evaluation) by prompting the nurse to include the patient's response in the progress notes.
3. Focus Charting increases the ease with which information can be located in the progress notes. The nurse can locate specific information simply by scanning the focus column.
4. Nurses are encouraged to identify patient concerns—not just problems. Sometimes nurses have difficulty identifying problems in a basically healthy patient. For example, a new mother might not be perceived as having any problems, but multiple concerns, such as teaching and discharge needs, must be addressed. Focus Charting allows that flexibility by encouraging the nurse to identify and document the patient's needs.
5. Focus Charting promotes analytical thinking by requiring the nurse to analyze data and draw conclusions regarding the patient's status. Nursing judgment is recognized as an essential element of documentation.

Disadvantages and Problems

The following are disadvantages of and problems concerning narrative charting:

1. If not monitored regularly, Focus Charting documentation can become a narrative note with no record of patient response to interventions. In audits done 8 months after the implementation of Focus Charting, Lampe and Hitchcock (1987) found that compliance in the documentation of patient response had decreased from 67% to 51%. Although the 51% result showed a marked improvement over the original 12% compliance, this finding illustrates the need for continued monitoring.
2. In Focus Charting nurses are required to change their thinking. They must be able to accurately identify the focus and sort the data into the appropriate categories of data, action, and response. In addition, the nurse must evaluate the patient's progress toward outcomes and document the response.
3. Nurses vary in the amount of difficulty they have in constructing accurate and logical focus notes. They tend to leave discrepancies between the focus and the content of the note. Following are two unedited examples of actual focus notes:

Focus	Progress Notes
Mental	**D:** Refuses to have BP and respirations taken at this time.
Attitude	**A:** Patient has a nasty temper.
Anxiety	**D:** 36-year-old female HIV+ made aware of test today.
	A: Patient denies use of drugs. Has severe ulcer/pustules in rectal and vaginal areas.
	R: Severe drainage from ulcers.

In the first example, the action is a value judgment, not a nursing intervention. The second example shows a relationship between the focus of the note and the data collected. However, the action and the response are incongruent with the identified focus. These examples illustrate the need for education and continued monitoring to decrease such difficulties and ensure the successful implementation of Focus Charting.

As the emphasis on patient and family education continues to grow, some facilities have modified the original DAR format to include teaching. The modified version involves *d*ata, *a*ction, *r*esponse, and *t*eaching, or DART. Gropper and DiCapo (1995) report a similar approach using the PART system: (*p*roblem, *a*ction, *r*esponse, and *t*eaching). Both methods highlight the need for documented patient education efforts.

CHARTING BY EXCEPTION

Charting by Exception (CBE) as developed in 1983 by staff nurses at St. Luke's Hospital in Milwaukee, Wisconsin.

Since then, a number of organizations have incorporated CBE into their documentation systems. This section describes the key elements, advantages, and disadvantages of the CBE system.

The motivation for the development of the CBE system included the following: overcoming documentation problems by making trends in patient status more obvious; reducing the amount of time necessary for documentation and change-of-shift reports; and making current information regarding the patient's status readily available.

Key Elements

The CBE system consists of several key elements, including flowsheets, documentation by reference to standards of practice, protocols and incidental orders, a nursing data base, nursing diagnosis-based care plans, and SOAP progress notes. Nurses interested in additional information are referred to Burke and Murphy (1988).

Flowsheets

The CBE system uses several types of forms, including the nursing/physician-order flowsheet, the graphic record, the patient teaching record, and the patient discharge note.

The nursing/physician order is unique among flowsheets. The front of the form (Figure 7-2, *A*) is used to document physical assessments and the implementation of physician and nursing orders. Assessment of specific body systems is dictated by the patient's condition and the protocols (discussed later in this section). The back of the form (Figure 7-2, *B*) outlines the elements of a physical assessment to be completed in point 2. In addition, the normal findings are described in point 4 of the guidelines.

The CBE system uses a specific set of abbreviations, as presented in Figure 7-2, *B:*

✓ The assessment was completed and no abnormal findings were noted.
* Significant abnormal findings are present and are described in the bottom section of the flowsheet.
→ The patient's status remains unchanged from the previous entry with an asterisk.

Figure 7-3 illustrates a completed flowsheet. The translation of the cardiovascular assessment is as follows:

The nurse did a cardiovascular assessment at 0730, 1100, 1530, and 2000 hours. This consisted of an assessment (see Figure 7-2, *B*) of the apical pulse, neck veins, capillary refill time (CRT), peripheral pulses, edema, and calf tenderness. The expected findings would be a regular apical pulse, S_1 and S_2 audible, and neck veins flat at 45 degrees. The CRT should be less than 3 seconds. Peripheral pulses should be palpable with no evidence of edema or calf tenderness. At 0730 hours, the patient had significant abnormal findings that were described in the bottom half of the form. No abnormal findings were observed at 1100, 1530, or 2000

Text continued on p. 121

© 1985
St. Luke's Hospital
Milwaukee, Wisconsin

**NURSING/PHYSICIAN
ORDER FLOWSHEET**
05-937555 Rev. 12/85

Date _____

NRSG DX	NURSING/PHYSICIAN ORDER												

* SIGNIFICANT FINDINGS ▼ NURSE INITIAL ▶

A

NRSG DX#	TIME		INIT

INIT	R N SIGNATURE	INIT	R N SIGNATURE	INIT	R N SIGNATURE

See Reverse Side ↘   **NURSING/PHYSICIAN ORDER FLOW SHEET**   Dist: White-Chart   Yellow-Bedside

Figure 7-2   A, The first page of the nursing/physician order flowsheet. (From Burke LJ, Murphy J: *Charting by exception: a cost-effective, quality approach,* Albany, NY, 1988, Delmar. Reprinted with permission.)

GUIDELINES FOR USE OF THE NURSING/PHYSICIAN ORDER FLOW SHEET

1. Indicate the Nursing Diagnosis which relates to the nursing order in the far left hand column of the category boxes. If the order is a physician order, indicate "D.O." ("Doctor Order") instead of the nursing diagnosis number.
2. Indicate the nursing or physician order. If the nursing order includes an assessment to be completed, use the following protocol:
   a. "NEUROLOGICAL ASSESSMENT" will include orientation, pupils, movement, sensation, quality of speech/swallowing and memory.
   b. "CARDIOVASCULAR ASSESSMENT" will include apical pulse, neck veins, CRT, peripheral pulses, edema, and calf tenderness.
   c. "RESPIRATORY ASSESSMENT" will include respiratory characteristics, breath sounds, cough, sputum, color of nailbeds/mucous membranes, and CRT.
   d. "GASTROINTESTINAL ASSESSMENT" will include abdominal appearance, bowel sounds, palpation, diet toleranceand stools.
   e. "URINARY ASSESSMENT" will include voiding patterns, bladder distention, and urine characteristics.
   f. "INTEGUMENTARY ASSESSMENT" will include skin color, skin temperature, skin integrity and condition of mucous membranes.
   g. "MUSCULOSKELETAL ASSESSMENT" will include joint swelling, tenderness, limitations in ROM, muscle strength and condition of surrounding tissue.
   h. "NEUROVASCULAR ASSESSMENT" will include color, temperature, movement, CRT, peripheral pulses, edema and patient description of sensation to affected extremity.
   i. "SURGICAL DRESSING/INCISIONAL ASSESSMENT" will include condition of surgical dressing and/or color, temperature, tenderness of surrounding tissue, condition of sutures/staples/steri-strips, approximation of wound edges, and presence of any drainage.
   j. "PAIN ASSESSMENT" will include patient description, location, duration, intensity, radiation, precipitating factors, and alleviating factors.
                                    OR
   Specify exactly which parts of assessment should be completed.
3. Top of sheet should be dated. Time should be indicated in the small box in upper right hand corner of each category box.
4. Upon carrying out an order that has no significant findings, a "√" in the appropriate category box is sufficient to indicate it was done. If the order includes an assessment, the following parameters will be considered a negative assessment and constitute the use of a "√."
   a. "NEUROLOGICAL ASSESSMENT" - Alert and oriented to person, place, and time. Behavior appropriate to situation. Pupils equal and reactive to light. Active ROM of all extremities with symmetry of strength. No paresthesia. Verbalization clear and understandable. Swallowing without coughing and choking on liquids and solids. Memory intact.
   b. "CARDIOVASCULAR ASSESSMENT" - Regular apical pulse. S$_1$ and S$_2$ audible. Neck veins flat at 45 degrees. CRT <3 sec. Peripheral pulses palpable. No edema. No call tenderness.
   c. "RESPIRATORY ASSESSMENT" - Respirations 10-20/min. at rest. Respirations quiet and regular. Breath sounds vesicular through both lung fields, bronchial over major airways, with no adventitious sounds. Sputum clear. Nailbeds and mucous membranes pink. CRT <3 sec.
   d. "GASTROINTESTINAL ASSESSMENT" - Abdomen soft. Bowel sounds active (5-34/min.). No pain with palpation. Tolerates prescribed diet without nausea and vomiting. Having BMs within own normal pattern and consistency.
   e. "URINARY ASSESSMENT" - Able to empty bladder without dysuria. Bladder not distended after voiding. Urine clear and yellow to amber.
   f. "INTEGUMENTARY ASSESSMENT" - Skin color within patient's norm. Skin warm and intact. Mucous membranes moist.
   g. "MUSCULOSKELETAL ASSESSMENT" - Absence of joint swelling and tenderness. Normal ROM of all joints. No muscle weakness. Surrounding tissues show no evidence of inflammation, nodules, nail changes, ulcerations, or rashes.
   h. "NEUROVASCULAR ASSESSMENT" - Affected extremity is pink, warm, and movable within patient's average ROM. CRT <3 sec. Peripheral pulses palpable. No edema. Sensation intact without numbness or paresthesia.
   i. "SURGICAL DRESSING/INCISIONAL ASSESSMENT" - Dressing dry and intact. No evidence of redness, increased temperature, or tenderness in surrounding tissue. Sutures/staples/steri-strips intact. Wound edges well-approximated. No drainage present.
   j. "PAIN ASSESSMENT" - If medication alone relieves pain and expected outcome is met, documentation on the Medication Profile is sufficient. No specific problem need be identified in the Nurses' Notes or Flow Sheet.
5. Upon carrying out an order that has significant findings, an asterisk is entered in the appropriate box. An asterisk "*" in the category box indicates to "See Significant Findings Section".
6. If status remains unchanged from previous asterisk entry, current entry may be indicated with an " ➔ ".
7. If an order no longer needs to be carried out, the next unused category box in that row should indicate "order D/Ced", and a line should be drawn through the remaining boxes. Any unused rows can be left blank.
8. Each Flow Sheet is used for 24 hours.

B

Figure 7-2, cont'd B, Guidelines for the use of the nursing/physician order flowsheet are printed on the second page of the form.

© 1985
St. Luke's Hospital
Milwaukee, Wisconsin

**NURSING/PHYSICIAN
ORDER FLOWSHEET**
05-937555 Rev. 12/85

Date ___7/8 to 7/9___

NRSG DX	NURSING/PHYSICIAN ORDER		0730	1100	1530	2000									
1	Cardiovascular assessment	✱	✓	✓	✓										
1	Respiratory assessment	✱	✱	→	✓										

✱ SIGNIFICANT FINDINGS ▼ NURSE INITIAL ▶	M7	M7	MB	MB							INIT

NRSG DX	TIME		INIT
1	0730	+4 pitting edema bilaterally of post-tibial areas, mid-inspiratory rales bilaterally in posterior bases	
		which do not clear c̄ cough	MT
1	1100	Mid-inspiratory rales bilaterally in posterior bases which clear c̄ cough	MT

INIT	R N SIGNATURE	INIT	R N SIGNATURE	INIT	R N SIGNATURE
M7	M. Fummillo RN	INIT		INIT	
MB	M. Baumann RN	INIT		INIT	

See Reverse Side ↘   **NURSING/PHYSICIAN ORDER FLOWSHEET**   Dist: White-Chart   Yellow-Bedside

Figure 7-3   Sample of a completed nursing/physician order flowsheet. (From Burke LJ, Murphy J: *Charting by exception: a cost-effective, quality approach,* Albany, NY, 1988, Delmar. Reprinted with permission.)

hours. The respiratory assessment was completed at the same time, following the guidelines in Figure 7-2, *B*. The abnormal finding of rales was noted at 0730, 1100, and 1530 hours but was resolved by 2000 hours. No note was needed at 1530 hours because the respiratory assessment findings had not changed from 1100 hours.

The nursing/physician-order flowsheet is also used to document the completion of nursing and physician orders that are not included in the standards of practice, as discussed later. The column labeled "Nsg Dx" contains the number of the nursing diagnosis associated with a particular nursing intervention. An ongoing list of nursing diagnoses is maintained on a problem list similar to the type used in problem-oriented (SOAP) charting. The abbreviation "DO" is written in the Nsg Dx column when a doctor's order is documented on the nursing/physician-order flowsheet.

An example of a nursing order that might be included on this flowsheet would be to "assist the patient to walk from the bed to the chair twice a day." The completion of the order is documented using the same symbols described previously.

✓ The order was completed.
* The patient had an abnormal response to the intervention, such as dizziness when ambulating.
→ The same abnormal response occurred the next time the order was implemented.

The rest of the flowsheets, including the patient teaching record and patient discharge notes, are similar to other such forms found in this text. The graphic record is different in that it includes a place for the nurse to check that standards of practice have been followed.

Standards of Practice
In the CBE system, standards of practice are the essential aspects of nursing practice that apply to all clinical areas as well as those that are specific to a particular nursing unit. Adherence to standards eliminates the need for documenting routine nursing interventions, such as oral care, repositioning, on care of the IV, Foley catheter, or nasogastric tube. A check mark is used to document the completion of the standards, and an asterisk indicates that not all standards were followed. Any deviations should be described in the nurse's notes.

Protocols and Incidental Orders
As in the CBE system, protocols/practice guidelines define the nursing interventions that deal with the expected clinical course of a specific patient population, such as preoperative and postoperative patients. The protocols outline nursing interventions, treatments, and the frequency of physical assessments. The nursing/physician-order flowsheet is used to document the implementation of the protocol. Incidental orders are used when a nursing intervention is necessary to continue a specific nursing intervention beyond the protocol deadline date or when any time-limited nursing interventions are required.

Nursing Data Base
The nursing data base has a section devoted to health history and physical assessment. The physical assessment section uses the same normal parameters as the nursing/physician-order flowsheet. The normal findings for each body system are printed in a column down the left side of the page. If the physical assessment for that body system is normal, the nurse checks the appropriate box. Abnormal findings are described on the right side of the page.

Nursing Diagnosis-Based Care Plans
The CBE system uses standard care plans that are individualized for each patient. The standard care plans focus on a specific nursing diagnosis, and they include the following: the related or risk factors, defining characteristics, assessment data supporting the presence of the nursing diagnosis, expected outcomes, and interventions.

SOAP Progress Notes
As described earlier in the section on problem-oriented charting, SOAP and SOAPIE notes document the data in an organized manner in the progress notes section. Because the nursing/physician-order and other flowsheets comprise much of the documentation that ordinarily appears in progress notes, the use of SOAP notes in the CBE system is limited to the following situations (Burke, Murphy, 1988):

• When a nursing diagnosis is identified, reactivated, inactivated, or resolved
• When an expected outcome is evaluated
• When a discharge summary is written
• When a major revision of the plan is written

Advantages
The following are advantages of the CBE system:

1. The most current data are available at the bedside. Information is readily accessible to the healthcare providers who interact with the patient in the nursing unit.
2. The flowsheets eliminate the need for worksheets or other scratch paper to record information about the patient. The data are immediately recorded in the permanent record.
3. Guidelines on the back of the form provide easy reference, which is particularly helpful for nurses who are new to the system.
4. Trends in the patient's status are easily discerned from the flowsheets. The assessment information is organized according to body systems and is easy to find.
5. Normal findings are precisely identified so that agreement exists as to what constitutes a normal assessment.

6. Much of the repetitive narrative charting of routine care is eliminated. Reference to the standards of practice eliminates the need to narratively chart this type of information.

7. Charting time is decreased. Burke and Murphy (1988) found that documentation time decreased by 23% with costs savings of $380,591.

8. Charting by exception is easily adapted to documentation on clinical pathways. Short (1997) reports that a pilot study using CBE and clinical paths yielded a 67% decrease in charting time and decreased the amount of time spent on change-of-shift reports as well. By using CBE and clinical paths together, patient variances can be monitored and changes in practice can be implemented immediately.

Disadvantages and Problems

The following are disadvantages of and problems concerning the CBE system:

1. Duplication of charting occurs in the CBE system; for example, nursing diagnoses that are maintained on a problem list are also written on the care plan. In another example, abnormal or significant findings are described on the nursing/physician-order flowsheet. If these findings warrant intervention by the nurse, a SOAP note must be written. The subjective and objective sections of the SOAP note repeat the information described on the flowsheet. Finally, the assessment and plan of the SOAP note may be the same as the care plan.

    Reducing redundancy would be possible by documenting the progress note on the bedside nursing/physician-order flowsheet. However, this would prevent the use of integrated progress notes (because these are rarely found at the bedside).

2. The CBE system was developed in a facility staffed only with RNs. The physical assessment elements need to be reviewed based on the scope of practice of LPNs. Some facilities that implemented the CBE system without an all-RN staff have changed their nursing care delivery system to accommodate the RNs' responsibility for assessment. Although an LPN may be assigned to care for the patient, an RN must complete a physical assessment once every 8 or 24 hours.

3. Complete implementation of this system requires a major change in the organization's documentation system. Unlike some of the systems described earlier, such as Focus or PIE charting, the CBE system requires changing the format of many documentation tools.

4. A major educational effort is required when implementing the CBE system. Nurses at St. Luke's had the most difficulty learning to document only abnormal findings on the nursing/physician-order flowsheet and adherence to the standards of practice. According to Burke and

Murphy, some of these problems may have involved agency nurses who were not familiar with the charting system.

5. The CBE system may have an impact on reimbursement issues until it becomes more widely accepted. One peer review organization (PRO) in Pennsylvania issued a statement that differentiating between events that simply are not documented and events that did not occur is impossible. They further stated that missing documentation of routine activities during PRO chart reviews may represent a failure to perform the action, which would be recorded as a documentation deficiency (KPRO, 1994). This view may change as efforts are made to educate the reviewers about CBE and the system becomes more accepted in the reimbursement community.

6. The legal basis of the CBE system continues to prompt debate. Although St. Luke's attorney reviewed the system and approved its compliance with legal principles, a judge and jury will ultimately rule on the validity of documentation in each particular case. Tammelleo (1994) reports on a case in which the plaintiff, who developed diskitis following surgery, received a $600,000 award based on the fact that "intermittent charting failed to provide the sort of continuous danger signals that would most likely spur early intervention by a physician" (p. 72). However, the CBE system described in this particular case was not defined clearly enough, nor were standards sufficiently delineated, to provide continuity among caregivers. This case illustrates three points:

    1. The standards for nursing assessment and intervention must be clearly defined.
    2. Policies and procedures for CBE must be followed explicitly.
    3. No documentation system will protect healthcare professionals from poor judgment.

CLINICAL PATHS

As described in Chapter 3, clinical paths provide a multidisciplinary mechanism for predicting the problems, interventions, and expected outcomes for a specific disease process across the continuum of care. The impetus to improve the quality of documentation, while streamlining the process, has led organizations to create a clinical path format that can also be used for daily documentation. This method supports outcome-focused charting and ensures that teaching and discharge planning are documented. Some institutions use the path as a documentation tool in conjunction with CBE. Progress note entries are focused on any deviations (variances) from the path. As clinical paths gain more widespread acceptance, documentation practices will have to respond. The merging of clinical paths and CBE may prove to be a suitable solution.

GENERAL CONSIDERATIONS WHEN SELECTING A DOCUMENTATION SYSTEM

When selecting a documentation system, the nurse should consider the following:

- Staffing mix
- Knowledge and skills of the nursing staff
- Cost of implementation
- Educational time
- Legalities
- Requirements of accrediting agencies

Staffing Mix

The documentation system should complement the facility's staff mix. In recent years, hospitals have changed staffing ratios to include more unlicensed assistive personnel (UAP) and fewer RNs. Workers with multiple skills are providing direct patient care in many settings. Although UAP could chart daily care activities on a flowsheet, the patient assessment, decisions regarding appropriate care, and evaluation of expected outcomes remains the professional responsibility of the RN.

Knowledge and Skills of Staff

When choosing a documentation system the knowledge and skills of the majority of the staff must be considered. Depending on age, educational background, and work experience, nurses have varying degrees of exposure to nursing process, nursing diagnosis, physical assessment skills, computer technologies, and quality improvement processes. Noncompliance with a new documentation system may reflect an imbalance between the sophistication of the system and the knowledge and skills of the staff.

Cost

Determining the financial requirements of a new documentation system is essential. Of the new charting systems presented in this chapter, Focus Charting may be the least expensive to implement because it requires fewer form revisions and may be used with existing flowsheets. Regardless of the system chosen, cost estimates should include planning and preparation time, printed materials, design and development of new forms, and educational time.

Educational Time

Any change in documentation practices requires ample educational time to ensure success. The CBE, PIE, and Focus Charting systems all require significant introductory education programs. Additional sessions will be needed to assist staff members having difficulty, to orient new staff, and to keep skills current. Time spent monitoring activities should also be figured into the educational costs. Strategies for successful implementation of a documentation system change are discussed in more detail in Chapter 9.

Joint Commission Requirements and Legalities

Finally, when selecting a documentation system, the Joint Commission standards, state and federal regulations, and legalities must be considered. With healthcare reimbursement in a state of flux and Joint Commission standards emphasizing outcomes of care, new documentation systems must be designed to meet these changing requirements. Similarly, hospitals must obtain feedback from the risk manager and legal counsel to ensure changes are legally sound.

SUMMARY

Each system has its strengths and limitations. By combining the best aspects of each, a documentation system can be developed for the changing healthcare environment. The goal should be to create a system that efficiently captures the essence of nursing care, supports a multidisciplinary approach, and highlights patient outcomes.

REFERENCES

Buckley-Womack C, Gidney B: A new dimension in documentation: the PIE method, *J Neurosci Nurs* 19(5):256, 1987.

Burke L, Murphy J: *Charting by exception,* New York, 1988, John Wiley Sons.

Cesta T et al: *The case manager's survival guide: winning strategies for clinical practice,* St Louis, 1997, Mosby.

Gropper E, DiCapo R: The PART system: perfecting actual recording talent, *Nurs Manage* 26(4):46, 1995.

KPRO: Charting by exception and documentation review, *KePRO Provider Bulletin* March 16, 1994.

Lampe S: *Focus charting,* Minneapolis, Minn, 1988, Creative Nursing Management.

Lampe S, Hitchcock A: Documenting nursing diagnosis using Focus Charting. In McLane A, ed: *Classification of nursing diagnoses; proceedings of the seventh conference,* St Louis, 1987, Mosby.

Menenberg S: Standards of care in documentation of psychiatric nursing care, *Clin Nurse Spec* 9(3):140, 1995.

Siegrist L, Dettor R, Stocks B: The PIE system: compete planning and documentation of nursing care, *Quality Review Bulletin* pp 186, 189, June 1985.

Short M: Charting by exception on a clinical pathway, *Nurs Manage* 28(8):45, 1997.

Tammelleo D: Charting by exception: there are perils, *RN* pp 71-72, October 1994.

ADDITIONAL READINGS

Merkley K, Nelson N: Computerized charting by exception at triage, *J Emerg Nurs* 21:571, 1995.

Scoates G et al: Health care focus documentation-more efficient charting, *Nurs Manage* 27(8):30, 1996.

Tammelleo D: Court holds "charting by exception" policy negligent, *Regan Report on Nursing Law* 34(12):2, May 1994.

8

Computerization of Nursing Information

The computerization of charting is one of the strongest trends in nursing documentation throughout the United States and Canada. Agencies of all sizes and descriptions are developing or purchasing computerized information systems that support nursing practice. This chapter addresses how the electronic chart has evolved, provides some principles for selecting and implementing a computer information system, and offers some predictions for the future of computer-based patient records (CPRs).

COMPUTER-BASED PATIENT RECORDS VERSUS ELECTRONIC CHARTS

Much confusion surrounds the use of computer terminology. Different groups within the healthcare industry are using computer terminology in various ways. This chapter discusses the CPR and the electronic chart. The CPR is a vehicle for long-term collection of an individual's healthcare information over a lifetime. The electronic chart is used to collect information about a specific patient while that individual is receiving services from an agency. This electronic version of the chart replaces manual documentation.

Forces Promoting CPRs

Computerization of medical records has been driven by the recognition of the following factors:

1. The enormous amount of data that are collected about a person's health must be stored and organized in a more efficient system than the current paper-based system. Finding data in a patient's chart is time consuming. The larger the chart becomes, the harder it becomes to locate key information.
2. Electronic charts manipulate and display information in a way that no paper-based system can. All notes related to a specific aspect of care can be collated and printed out. The paper chart cannot be reorganized in this manner, nor can it be merged with records from another facility or healthcare provider.
3. The use of CPRs could lead to a more efficient transfer of information from one healthcare provider to another. Using manual methods of documentation, duplication of testing and data collection can occur when a patient moves from the care of one provider to a second provider. Cost containment and healthcare reform mandate improving efficiency in the management of healthcare data.
4. CPRs track outcomes of care more effectively. Instead of using ineffective methods of treating health problems, data collected about outcomes can be used to define the most appropriate approach to care.

The benefits of the CPR are clear. Vital information about patients is immediately available to those who need it. Costly duplication of testing is avoided. Errors in care should be reduced, particularly as clinical aids indicate the information that needs to be considered in care. Finally, selected information about the patient is maintained in an accessible manner throughout the patient's life.

Attributes of CPRs

In 1991 a landmark study by the Institute of Medicine described the attributes of the ideal CPR. The group acknowledged that no system was capable of supporting a fully automated electronic record or CPR at that time. Since 1991, components of the CPR have become available. Many systems are in development, but very few are currently operational (Andrew, Dick, 1995b). The following are attributes of the CPR (Andrew, Dick, 1995a):

1. The CPR contains a problem list that defines all of the patient's clinical problems and the status of each. All healthcare practitioners, including nurses, dentists, social workers, and doctors, should update the list.

2. The CPR supports systematic measurement and recording of the patient's health status and functional abilities to promote more precise, routine evaluations of patient care outcomes.

3. The logical basis for all diagnoses or conclusions are contained in the CPR, which documents the clinical rationale for decisions about patient care.

4. The CPR provides linkages with the patient's clinical records from other settings and time periods to provide a lifelong record of health events.

5. The CPR comprehensively addresses confidentiality of data, ensuring that the information is accessible only to authorized people.

6. Authorized healthcare providers involved in direct patient care will have simultaneous and remote access to the CPR. This would allow an emergency department, for example, to access the patient's records from the last inpatient admission, or the nurses at a tertiary hospital to access the patient's records at the home health agency.

7. The CPR allows users to retrieve information selectively and choose from several formats when examining and interpreting it. Using artificial intelligence technology, the CPR will help healthcare providers focus on the most pertinent information needed at a particular moment by creating customized views of the same information; for example, the nurse could review a number of past hospitalizations to see whether the patient had experienced pressure ulcers.

8. Local and remote knowledge, literature, administrative data bases, and systems can be linked with the CPR, which will permit ready access to publications, clinical practice guidelines, and clinical-decision support systems; for example, the nurse could look up a policy on some aspect of nursing care from the patient's bedside.

9. The CPR assists in the process of clinical problem solving by offering the nurse decision analysis tools, clinical reminders, prognostic risk assessment, and other clinical aids; for example, the computer can help identify patients at risk for falls or remind the nurse to evaluate the response to the injection of morphine given 1 hour ago.

10. The CPR supports structured data collection, adequately providing for practitioners' direct entries and storing that information according to a defined vocabulary, for example, the program would permit direct data entry by physicians. Programs will use standardized vocabulary, such as the North American Nursing Diagnosis Association's (NANDA) nursing diagnoses.

11. The quality and costs of care can be evaluated through the use of CPRs. Better data access, faster data retrieval, more versatility in data display, and clinical reminders should improve healthcare delivery.

12. The CPR is sufficiently flexible and expandable to support not only today's basic information needs but also the evolving needs of each clinical specialty and subspecialty. As knowledge bases and sophistication in the use of information grow, so must computer systems.

Prerequisites for CPRs

At least five key underpinnings, including the following, are needed to support a CPR (Andrew, Dick, 1995a):

1. *Clinical data dictionary.* A substantial, flexible clinical data dictionary is needed, which would define all of the data elements for the universe of clinical information that will be stored.

2. *Clinical data repository.* A well-designed architecture for the clinical data repository must be in place to support the needs of all members of the healthcare team. The request for medical information about a specific patient must be fulfilled within a very few seconds.

3. *Flexible input capabilities.* A powerful array of appropriate input capabilities (e.g., mouse, keyboard, voice recognition, touch screen, light pen) must be available.

4. *Ergonomically designed data presentation.* The presentation of the data should be tailored to the needs of the individual. For example, a nurse may want to see all nurses' notes first, whereas a surgeon may want to see the vital signs before accessing any other data.

5. *Automated support.* The system should anticipate and support clinical processes and thinking through the support system. This should include access to expert systems, knowledge data bases, medical literature, outcomes-feedback loops, and cost/quality input, all of which can be brought into the clinical decision-making processes.

Minimum Data Sets and Core Health Data Elements

Much work needs to be done before the use of the CPR becomes a widespread reality. Development of a clinical data dictionary, which is taking place in a number of areas, including the federal and private sectors, is part of defining a minimum data set. The minimum data set is defined as "a minimum set of items of information with uniform definitions and categories concerning a specific aspect or dimensions of the health care system which meets the essential needs of multiple users" (McCormick et al, 1997). The most widely used minimum data sets are the Uniform Hospital Discharge Data Set, the Financial Uniform Minimum Data Set, and the Long-Term Health Care Minimum Data Set. The wide use of these data sets is attributed to the mandate by the Health Care Financing Administration pertaining to Medicare and Medicaid reimbursement. The Health Insurance Portability and Accountability Act of 1996 required the adoption of national standard data sets for a wide variety of financial and administrative health care transactions. Federally recommended data elements exist for home care (OASIS, described in Chapter 13), the emergency department (ED), and ambulatory care (McCormick et al, 1997).

The Nursing Minimum Data Set (NMDS) is a data set that was developed in the private sector with much involvement by a nurse named Helen Werley. The NMDS was patterned after other uniform minimum data sets that had been developed for physicians, hospitals, long-term care institutions, ambulatory medical care facilities, and the Department of Veterans Affairs. The three categories of patient information to be included in an information system are illustrated in Box 8-1. The NMDS has been tested in pilot studies and is being refined. Expectations are that it will facilitate nursing research, education, and administration and serve as a major component of nursing information systems. Additional nursing data sets being refined include the Nursing Intervention Classification and the Nursing Outcomes Classification, which are both the work of researchers at the University of Iowa.

The Patient Core Data Set, developed by nurses at Wright State University College of Nursing in collaboration with Blue Chip Computers Company, is another private sector data base. The 51 data elements provide a longitudinal record of a patient's health history. Detailed information

about this system is available in Benner and Swart (1997), Uddin and Martin (1997), and Song, Ho, and Ho (1997). Additional information about other data sets is found in McCormick and others (1997). Joint Commission for the Accreditation of Healthcare Organizations (JCAHO) standards (1996) encourage the use of uniform data definitions, minimum data sets, codes, classifications, and standardized terminology.

INTRODUCTION OF COMPUTERS TO HEALTHCARE FACILITIES

As the CPR or electronic record represent the vision for the future, the electronic chart is the reality of today in many healthcare facilities. In order to explore the evolution of an electronic record, one must look at how computers are typically introduced into a healthcare facility.

Computers are usually first used in a healthcare facility to track admissions, discharges, and transfers (ADT) of patients. This type of application provides simple demographic information about patients and is tied to the financial and billing functions. For many years the use of computers in healthcare facilities did not evolve beyond this function. In the mid-1980s, software vendors began developing software that could be used in nursing documentation. The last 16 years have been marked by an explosion of programs as vendors race to meet the needs of the healthcare industry. During this time, an increasing number of software companies began developing applications (programs) that provide a variety of nonadministrative or financial services. These applications are used by agencies for many clinical purposes.

One of the early common clinical applications involved computerizing the functions of specific departments within the hospital. Developing a unified computer system within a facility is challenging because the facility must ensure that the systems purchased by individual departments can be tied together. When a department buys software or hardware that is incompatible with other applications within the hospital, frustration and limitation are the results. These systems are referred to as stand-alone systems. Efforts are being made to decrease the incompatibilities in software by having the vendors (software development companies) agree to use a common computer language.

Additional challenges related to the incompatibility of clinical systems result from the rapid pace of mergers and acquisitions in health care. When two hospitals merge, for example, no guarantee exists that they will be able to exchange clinical information if the software and hardware used in each hospital is incompatible. These issues can be time consuming, expensive, and result in difficult decisions about which system will meet the needs of all of the joined facilities.

The reporting of results of laboratory and other tests to the nursing unit's computer terminal occurs early in the

---

Box 8-1
Nursing Minimum Data Set

Nursing Care Elements

Nursing diagnoses
Interventions
Outcomes
Intensity of nursing care

Patient Demographic Elements

Personal identification
Date of birth
Sex
Race and ethnicity
Residence

Service Elements

Unique facility or service agency number
Unique health care and number of patient or client
Unique number of principal registered nurse provider
Admission or encounter date
Discharge or termination date
Disposition of patient or client
Expected payer for most of the bill

Data from Werley H, Lang H, eds: *Identification of the nursing minimum data set,* New York, 1988, Springer.

computerization of the clinical functions of a hospital. Results are obtained from tests then placed into the system. Some systems have the capability of activating a signal, such as a flashing message on the screen of the computer terminal in the nursing unit, when grossly abnormal or panic results need to be addressed. Other less-sophisticated systems rely on the laboratory personnel making phone calls to alert the nursing staff when panic results are found.

Charge capturing is another step toward a fully electronic health record. The charge is the cost that is billed to the patient. Charges are captured when a test or piece of equipment is ordered electronically through a computer terminal on the nursing unit or is scanned using a bar code. Electronic charging systems should lead to more accurate hospital bills.

The next step in computerizing the medical record is typically to add the order entry. Examinations (e.g., laboratory and radiology), diets, and physical therapy are ordered through terminals in the nursing units. Several types of personnel are involved in entering orders, including nurses, clerks, and physicians. Many physicians resist order entry because they are uncomfortable with computer technology, cannot type, or feel that direct order entry is too time consuming. Hospital administrators and nurses are encouraging physicians to take full advantage of the capabilities of computer medical records. Fear of change, indifference, inertia, and lack of involvement in the selection of a software program hold many physicians back from full commitment to a system (Hard, 1993).

Many experts believe the most desirable method of order entry is to have the physician input the orders directly into the computer, which reduces the chances of transcription errors. Such errors are more common when the order is written on paper by a physician and then entered into the computer by a unit secretary or nurse. Orders are most commonly entered by keypad, keyboard, light pen, mouse, or touch-sensitive screens. Most systems are set up to avoid extensive typing because it saves time and because not all healthcare professionals know how to type. Requiring that the nurse verify the accuracy of orders entered by a clerk as a double check is common, as is often done in paper systems. Experience has shown that having another person check the transcribed order, regardless of who entered it, is a valuable safeguard for reducing careless transcription errors that could injure patients.

Healthcare facilities commonly see the value of adding pharmacy systems to their electronic capabilities. Although pharmacy systems can be independent or stand-alone systems, their full integration with the mainframe computer is more beneficial. A pharmacy system that provides a printed medication administration record reduces the risks associated with transcription of orders and provides a clear, legible record. The more advanced pharmacy systems print daily medication records for the nurse to use when signing off the drug, or the system permits the nurse to chart the administration of the drug using a computer in the nursing unit or patient's room.

Systems that permit real-time or concurrent surveillance of medication administration have the greatest potential for reducing patient injury from medication errors. A sophisticated system can do the following:

- Search medication orders for dangerous drug interactions
- Compare allergies reported by the patient with the drugs ordered by the physician
- Alert the physician to inappropriate dosages of medications
- Keep track of automatic stop dates for medications

The pharmacy profile, or list of past or present medications, offers healthcare professionals up-to-date, easily retrievable medication information. An advanced pharmacy system in use at the LDS Hospital in Salt Lake City has resulted in a large increase in the reporting of adverse drug reactions. The system monitors for physicians' orders that suddenly stop the administration a drug and request antidotes to counter the effects of a medication.

ADT, results reporting, charge capturing, order entry, and pharmacy systems are fairly common, early software applications. Although software designed specifically for nursing documentation is not common, it is rapidly becoming more prevalent.

Some facilities computerize medical records in a different sequence than that described above. Adderly, Hyde, and Mauseth (1997) describe the steps undertaken to computerize the VA (Veterans Affairs) Domiciliary in White City, Oregon, a residential treatment center that is not connected to a hospital. The earliest applications were laboratory and pharmacy packages. Electronic progress notes for use by the clinicians came next. The transcriptions of discharge summaries were then added to the record. (These can be verified and edited by the physicians before being finalized.) Next, the dictated history and physical examination was transcribed and added to the medical record, then radiology reports, followed by diet orders using order entry screens. The tracking system for allergies, consultations, and the development of a problem list was implemented next. The Domiciliary then added a scanning system to enter patient information that had not been initiated at the facility. With the implementation of all of these components, only 2% of the patient record was not in an electronic format. At the time of the publication of the article, the Domiciliary was planning to convert existing paper forms to electronic ones to eliminate the last vestiges of the paper system.

BARRIERS TO THE INTRODUCTION OF NURSING INFORMATION SYSTEMS

Nursing is often one of the last departments to purchase software. Several barriers to the development and use of nursing information systems exist, as described in the following:

- Administrators may not be convinced that the computerization of nursing information will yield tangible results. Studies performed by software vendors that proclaim the advantages of computerization are sometimes viewed with a skeptical eye. Few studies contain conclusions that can be generalized to other settings.
- Nurses may lack power within the organization, despite the fact that they make up the largest group of information users. The Joint Commission standards (1996) continue to reinforce the need to involve appropriate clinical and administrative staff in assessing the hospital's information needs. The standards mandate that these individuals be involved in selecting, integrating, and using information-management technology.
- Computer information services departments are sometimes threatened by the need to share information with others, and they worry that their power will be diminished by involving others in the decision-making process. This problem is being resolved as nurses join the computer information services department, building a bridge between nurses and computer specialists. Computerization of nursing information is complex. Nurses interact with every other department in the facility and have unique information requirements.
- Few good software programs were available in the past. Some were designed by nurse computer experts without nursing experience, as evidenced by the fact that these products often did not reflect the way nurses gather and process information. As nurses are hired into key positions in software companies and become specialists in nursing informatics, new and better programs are emerging.
- Many software programs are designed to perform a single function, such as staffing and scheduling, care planning, or patient classification. Unless all these products are produced by the same company, linking them can be difficult or sometimes impossible. The nursing information system may not be linked to the hospital information system or other programs outside of the facility, which hinders sharing of data inside and outside the organization.
- The lack of a unified nursing language is one of the barriers hampering the development and use of nursing information systems. Variations in the naming of nursing diagnoses, interventions, and outcomes can create confusion. Differences in nursing practice impede standardization of software. Nursing language is becoming more standardized, with widespread acceptance of the NANDA list of nursing diagnoses, the Omaha System for Community and Ambulatory Care nursing diagnoses, and the Nursing Intervention Classification from the University of Iowa. The Nursing Outcomes Classification project offers hope for standardization in this area of nomenclature as well.
- Nurses may resist computerization because of fears, including fear that the computer is too complicated, that technology will replace nurses, that the computer will direct and dictate nursing care, and that patient confidentiality will be breached (Bowles, 1997).
- Computerization is costly. Hardware, software, staff education, and additional computer support personnel contribute to the expense of computerization.

These barriers to nursing documentation using computers are slowly being overcome. Regulatory agencies, pressure to contain costs, and recognition of the benefits of computerization have led to more widespread development and the purchasing of nursing information systems.

ADVANTAGES AND DISADVANTAGES OF COMPUTERIZED DOCUMENTATION

Advantages

Computerization of nursing documentation may produce many benefits. The following text addresses generalized benefits of using computers for documentation. The advantages of bedside terminals are addressed later in this chapter.

Legible Records

Computer printouts are completely legible, thereby eliminating the risks associated with guessing at the meaning of handwritten words. Nurses no longer need to ask each other "Can you read this order?"

Readily Available Records

The medical record of the patient is readily available for all to use, and the time spent searching for records is eliminated. The electronic chart can be used and reviewed by as many people as the number of terminals permits. The need to stock multiple copies of specific forms is also eliminated.

Improved Nursing Productivity

Studies have shown that nurses spend up to 50% of their time documenting and communicating patient information (Bowles, 1997). Administrators, supervisors, physicians, and especially nurses would like to reduce the amount of time spent on paperwork, thereby increasing the amount of time available to spend caring for patients. One study (Erb, Coble, 1995) found that after computerization, nurses spent 40% more time communicating with patients and 34% more time on patient hygiene. Nursing information systems can save data entry time in comparison with manual charting through more rapid entry of information using keystrokes, menus, or bar-code scanners. Phone calls to other departments and change-of-shift report time may also be reduced. Some systems even eliminate the need for the nurse to enter certain information by linking to clinical monitoring machines.

Note that reduction in the amount of time spent documenting does not occur immediately when changing to computerized medical records. Bush and Ebel (1996) reported that when their hospital implemented electronic admission assessments, the nurses required an average of 60 to 90 minutes (compared with 15 to 20 minutes for a manual admission assessment), creating budgetary problems and unwanted overtime. Within 2 weeks, however, the time needed to collect and enter patient data was returning to the levels that existed before electronic documentation as familiarity with the system increased.

Reduction in Record Tampering

Tampering with the medical record is much more difficult with an electronic system. Software programs should contain a way to correct mistaken entries, such as an incorrect entry, misspelled word, or typographical error. This process is often accomplished much the same way as is done in paper systems—by bracketing the mistaken entry, adding the correct information, and giving a reason for the change, such as "wrong chart." A clock embedded in the software program indicates the precise time and date of an entry, making impossible the backdating of information to make it look as though it was entered earlier. Furthermore, software programs usually have a regularly scheduled backup time to store data, making it impossible for someone to delete previous entries once they are saved.

Support of the Use of the Nursing Process

A computer documentation system may facilitate individualized assessments of the patient. A branching program is designed to move on to more relevant material based on the responses entered by the nurse. Unnecessary questions can be eliminated once problems associated with particular areas have been ruled out. Software has been developed to recognize certain defining characteristics and then suggest nursing diagnoses to the nurse, who must rule out or accept the diagnosis. Some programs will help the nurse select outcomes and interventions. At the time of discharge, many programs can produce a cumulative care plan consisting of all diagnoses, outcomes, and interventions for the period of service.

Reduction in Redundant Documentation

Computerized documentation supports economical use of the date entry process by reducing or eliminating redundant charting. A piece of information is entered into the program only once, then is sent to all appropriate places; for example, the patient's allergy to Demerol (meperidine) should show up wherever this information is needed, such as in the pharmacy, on the medication administration record, or as an alert in the clinical information system.

Clinical Prompts, Reminders, and Warnings

Priority setting and decision making can be facilitated by warnings, prompts, and reminders. For example, the triage nurse in an ED or the telephone triage nurse in a managed care organization can be prompted to ask a series of questions based on the patient's main complaint (Bradley, 1994).

Categorized Nursing Notes

The software can be designed so that the documentation can be sorted and printed out in ways not possible with traditional paper and pen systems. A nurse could request a list of all entries that describe the patient's skin, or a printout of all the patient teaching notes.

Automatically Printed Reports

The system should be able to produce reports and flowsheets that eliminate the tedious copying of information from the kardex during change-of-shift or assignment reporting. Reports that document the activity of the department, such as the number of patients seen in the ambulatory care clinic, may be created without the time-consuming process of retrieving the data by hand.

Documentation According to Standards of Care

Programs can be designed to include unit-specific and agency-wide standards of care and practice. The effect of these programs is to remind the nurse, through the use of clinical flags, of the essential elements to be documented. If the standard states, for example, that a fall prevention program must be initiated for high-risk patients, the program can remind the nurse of the standard. The nurse will not be allowed to delete required interventions and will be prompted to enter specific interventions and observations.

Peck and others (1997) report that the LDS Hospital's system enabled them to define a broad range of care protocols. They note that the HELP program (the software) assisted clinicians in deciding which antibiotics should be used, keeping alert to potential medication incompatibilities, identifying steps in ventilator weaning, interpreting blood gases values, and pinpointing other similar factors in medical management. The clinician is able to accept or decline the HELP system's recommendations. However, when the clinician chooses to not use the recommended approach, documentation of the rationale for this decision is needed.

Many facilities are also putting their policy and procedure manual on-line, thus they are readily available instead of being contained in huge three-ring binders, making it easier to use the policies and procedures to follow the standard of care and to document accordingly.

Improved Recruitment and Retention of Nurses

Anecdotal information has shown that computers tend to increase nurses' job satisfaction and morale, which is a significant advantage, given the high economic cost of employee turnover.

Improved Knowledge of Outcomes

Analysis of data compiled from several patients' records can lead to conclusions about the outcomes that are being achieved. This information can enhance the quality of clinical decision making and lead to improvements in the system. Outcome data increasingly affects decisions about reimbursement, licensing, accreditation, and reappointment to the medical staff. As outcome data is released to the public, it can even affect the financial survival of the agency. LDS Hospital's HELP system has been invaluable in identifying the best practices and consequentially in lowering costs (Peck, 1997).

Availability of Data

The information compiled from a large number of patient records enhances the use of nursing research and quality improvement to spot recurring systemic issues or to aggregate information about patient outcomes. Consider the large number of people and organizations who have access to computerized medical records, including those in the following list (Dawson, 1997):

- Insurance companies
- Managed care organizations
- Public health reporting systems
- Medical providers
- Medical facilities
- Pharmacies
- Employers
- Governmental agencies
- Researchers
- Educational institutions
- Attorneys

All of these groups have their own priorities and perspectives when analyzing the data contained in medical records.

Prevention of Medication Errors

The software may call attention to inappropriate orders, incorrect dosages, or incompatible medications. A Salt Lake City hospital's information system prevented 249 medication errors during a 3-month period (Randall, 1990). Another study found a 34% reduction in medication errors using a point-of-care data entry system (Cerne, Brennan, 1989).

Facilitating Cost-Defining Efforts

The ability to base charges on the actual care delivered is improved by computer documentation systems.

Printed Discharge Instructions

Many facilities store routine discharge instructions in the computer; these can be individualized and printed out for the patient's use.

Benefits of computerized documentation can be difficult to quantify. A review of the nursing literature yielded few recent studies (i.e., published in the last 5 years), but some articles were published in the last 10 years. Pierskalla and Woods (1988) found a decrease in waiting time for orders, information, and laboratory results to be benefits of computerization. They note an elimination of unnecessary orders and services occurred. Childs (1988) found a significant reduction in phone calls between departments and a saving of between 45 minutes to 2 hours of nurses' documentation time per shift. Minda and Brundage (1994) conclude that the time required for computer documentation was significantly less than handwritten documentation, and the number of observations recorded by computer charting was significantly greater than those that were handwritten. Johnson and others (1987) report a significant increase in legibility of documentation and improved timing of charting. Gross (1989) comments on the significant reduction in overtime occuring during the first year after the computers were installed.

Disadvantages and Issues

Although the advantages of using computers for documentation outweigh the disadvantages, a few areas are troublesome.

Advantages of the Paper Chart

The paper chart has the following five major strengths (Bradley, 1994):

1. The paper chart is familiar to its users. (Exposure to computers soon makes them familiar as well.)
2. The paper chart is portable and can be carried to the point of care. (Bedside and portable computers are also available, which permits data entry at the bedside.)
3. No perceived downtime occurs when using a paper chart. (The search for missing records constitutes downtime, as well as waiting to use a chart that someone else is using at the time.)
4. The paper chart is perceived to have flexibility in recording data, permitting easy recording of subjective data and narrative entries. (Software can be designed to permit free text typing.)
5. The paper chart can be rapidly browsed and scanned. (Depending on the length of a hospitalization or legibility of handwriting, however, finding information can be difficult.)

Problems with Security and Confidentiality of Patient Information

The medical literature contains an increasing number of articles concerning the need for privacy, confidentiality, and security of computerized medical records. (These three terms are defined in Box 8-2.) Long before the advent of

---

computerized medical records, the Code for Nurses defined the nurse's responsibility for safeguarding the patient's rights by protecting information of a confidential nature (ANA, 1985). To keep this issue in perspective, the release of confidential information and the destruction of medical records has always existed with the use of paper-only charts. Faxing of medical information is a key example of this type of risk (Box 8-3). Tampering with the medical record has already been discussed in Chapter 6. Computers offer levels of security that paper charts cannot provide. No password is required to open a paper chart, for example.

Computerized medical records present new challenges to the nurse's ethical and legal obligation to safeguard confidential information. The ability of individuals to access the patient's computerized medical record from distant sites requires rigorous adherence to security measures. The placement of computer screens in relation to the presence of patients and visitors needs to be considered. Devastation of medical records through computer viruses introduced via floppy disks or by downloading files from the Internet is a very real concern.

The consequences of releasing private health information can be severe, including ruined careers, public ridicule, social rejection, and economic devastation of individuals and their families (Milholland, 1994). Breach of security is another serious issue. Several hospitals have fired nurses for giving their passwords to unauthorized individuals. Simpson (1994) reports about a disgruntled nurse in Chicago who acquired a physician's password by looking over the doctor's shoulder. The nurse then prescribed a cardiac medication for a pediatric patient (the order was intercepted), prescribed antibiotics for a geriatric patient, and ordered the discharge of a patient who was not ready for discharge. The nurse was sent to jail.

The importance of maintaining security, even around trusted people, is underscored by the following story. Styffe (1997) described a security breach that occurred when a 13-year-old girl gained access to the phone numbers of former hospital ED patients. She obtained the numbers from the hospital computer when she visited her mother at work. The girl said she later played a prank by calling the patients and falsely informing them that they had tested positive for HIV. The consequences of her actions were not reported in the article.

Some concern exists that patients may withhold critical medical information about their health status because of the fear of breaks in confidentiality. Medical records may contain sensitive data, such as mental health issues, sexually transmitted diseases, sexual preferences, pregnancy and abortion history, cosmetic surgeries, abuse of substances, genetic test results, and HIV status (Lawrence, 1994). A 1993 Equifax study found that 27% of 1000 people surveyed in the United States believed that their own medical records had been improperly disclosed. Fifty-one percent of these people described themselves as very concerned that outsiders might be able to access the computers to obtain medical information for improper purposes (Equifax, 1993).

Witness this solicitation, which was sent to one of the authors of this book via e-mail, part of which is quoted as it appeared:

Dear Web User: DID YOU KNOW THAT with the Internet you can uncover EVERYTHING you ever wanted to know about your EMPLOYEES, FRIENDS, RELATIVES, SPOUSE, NEIGHBORS, even your own BOSS! You can check out ANYONE, ANYTIME, ANYWHERE, right on the Internet. It's no secret that the Internet is a GIGANTIC and POWERFUL SOURCE of information, if you only know WHERE TO LOOK. But one of the best kept secrets in the world right now is probably the amount of PERSONAL INFORMATION other people can find out about YOU and others—right on the INTERNET. EXAMPLE! INFORMATION AVAILABLE ABOUT YOU: Right now, with just your name and address, I can almost instantly find out what you do for a living, name and age of your spouse and children, the make and color of your car, the value of your home (and probably how much you paid for it), credit information, your employment records, family tree, military records, which web sites you visit, etc., etc., etc. I can even find that long forgotten drug bust you had in college. AND THAT'S JUST THE BEGINNING, but you get the idea. . . . " (unsolicited e-mail, source will remain anonymous).

It is no wonder with messages like this that a certain amount of paranoia exists concerning confidentiality of medical information.

Many computer systems are designed to require two levels of security to enter the computer system. Passwords, keys, badge readers, and biometrics are used to gain access to the system. Biometrics refers to the use of physical traits, such as voice, blood vessel patterns in the eye, shape of the hand, and fingerprints, to identify the user of the computer. Although this technology is expensive and presently beyond the reach of most purchasers of systems, it is expected to become more widespread in the future. Suggestions for confronting the issue of confidentiality are listed in Box 8-4.

Disruptive Computer Downtime

An additional disadvantage of computerized medical records relates to the disruption of a system on which many functions depend. *Downtime* is defined as any time when the computer is not working because of routine servicing or sudden, unexpected failure. During this time the nurse may need to revert to paper for operations that are normally computerized. When paper systems are not used routinely, the opportunity for mistakes to occur increases. Critical patient information may be lost when the computer crashes or unexpected downtime occurs. Many healthcare professionals find it difficult to return to manual documentation after becoming skilled at using the computer.

Size of the Record

Hospital policy or software requirements may result in thick charts filled with daily printouts of data. The disadvantages of voluminous charts may be offset by the fact that the nurse will have the benefit of reading a perfectly legible record when charts become completely automated.

Erroneous Acceptance of Computerized Information

The adage "garbage in, garbage out" applies to computer medical records just as it does to other aspects of computer programming. Incidents in which clearly inaccurate information is included in the medical record may increasingly occur, but this has not been questioned by healthcare professionals because computerized information is perceived to be infallible. No machine can replace a healthcare professional who can critically evaluate patient data and question information that does not make sense. Healthcare personnel must guard against deification of the computer. A psychiatrist reminds us that "Diagnoses are made by people and not machines and are as useful as the criteria used and the knowledge and experiences of the people who use them. Validity and precision are not necessarily related" (Viederman, 1995). Computers are simply tools that help qualified people get jobs done.

Box 8-4

Strategies for Protection of Confidential Healthcare Information

Suggestions

The following suggestions come from Styffe (1997):

- Make nursing managers responsible for developing and reinforcing policies that address breaches in confidentiality.
- Training of new users must include explanation of the organization's policies and procedures on information security.
- Ask employees and physicians to sign a confidentiality policy on a yearly basis.
- Reward individuals who report security breaches.
- Periodically perform surveillance to monitor compliance with policies.
- Provide passwords with sufficient complexity to avoid accidental discovery.
- Immediately delete the password of an individual who resigns or is terminated.
- Use a mechanism for an audit trail that shows access to the medical record.

Additional Suggestions

- Employees should be prohibited from bringing in disks with software or files from other computers, because these disks may contain viruses (Gilham, 1996).
- Facilities should have a separate backup system to protect from failures in the primary system (Gilham, 1996).
- Install software that locks out anyone who repeatedly attempts to access the system with an improper password or code. Some software can be programmed to sound an alarm at the terminal when this occurs (Gobis, 1994).
- Periodically change passwords (Gobis, 1994).
- Investigate the feasibility of having the software log off after a fixed period of inactivity so that the terminal does not remain open and active (Gobis, 1994).
- Instruct employees to not walk away from a terminal without signing off. This breaches the security system and allows unauthorized access to the computer (Fiesta, 1996).
- Control the distribution and discarding of printouts. Staff nurses, for example, should discard computer generated worksheets in specific containers in the facility and should not bring them home at the end of the shift.
- Provide stiff consequences for those who share passwords.
- Post signs reminding staff to maintain confidentiality of information.

Data from Fiesta J: *Nurs Manage* 27(9):12, 1996; Gilham C: *Health Prog* p 18, May/June, 1996; Gobis L: *J Nurs Adm* 24(9):15, 1994; and Styffe E: *Nurs Adm Q* 21(3):21, 1997.

Limitations in the Format of Charting

Nursing information software that limits the use of free text may force the nurse to omit key information about the patient. Important observations of the patient that do not fit neatly into a category may be left out of the medical record. Dr. Viederman commented on this issue when discussing a bedside pen-entry computer system that consisted of 102 items to be checked off:

> The 102 bits of data in the portable database systems become a theory that in its own right organizes and significantly limits our "freedom" in understanding the text. Deprived of context, associations, emotional correlates, reactions, and so forth, they offer a confining and at times misleading view of the patient's experience. The capacity to read (hear) the text of patient-as-person will therefore be partially formed by a preexisting structure that potentially distorts and perhaps worse, falsely affirms the consultant in his conviction that he has captured the essence of the patient's difficulty.

Resistance

Resistance to change is a potent force that can affect the acceptance of computers. Strategies for dealing with resistance to change are discussed in Chapter 9.

Inadequate Number of Terminals

Nursing stations designed before the introduction of healthcare computerization are often too cramped for each nurse to have a computer terminal.

Computer Lag During Peak Usage

A nursing information system can quickly use up the capacity of the mainframe, requiring expansion of the system.

Nurses' Difficulty in Giving Up Worksheets

Rather than entering the data directly into the terminal, some nurses will continue to write information on the worksheet first and enter it later, decreasing the efficiency of the system.

Cost

Costs include the purchase of hardware and software, the education of the nursing staff, licensing fees, and changes that need to be made in the hardware or software to accommodate the purchaser. An Australian intensive care unit removed their computers when they lacked the funds to upgrade software and hardware. They did not perceive an increase in efficiency from using their system and were stymied by the lack of interfaces with ventilators, infusion pumps, the radiology and pathology departments, and the hospital computer information system (Marasovic et al, 1997).

BEDSIDE TERMINALS

Point-of-care (bedside) terminals are becoming more common. Although estimates of the number of hospitals with bedside terminals are imprecise because this area is changing so rapidly, Hughes (1996) found that 3% to 5% of all hospitals in the United States have in-depth patient care documentation and bedside computer terminals. Bedside systems using standard keyboards, touch-sensitive screens,

hand-held units, palm-sized terminals, and other devices allow nurses to document vital signs, intake and output, medication administration, progress notes, admission assessments, care plans, and a variety of other functions. In bedside-terminal systems, the terminals are located in patients' rooms, at the nurses station, and possibly at other key locations such as physicians' offices. The terminals are linked to each other and to the agency's mainframe computer.

Advantages of Bedside Systems

In addition to the benefits associated with computerizing documentation, ideal bedside systems have the following benefits.

Improved Timeliness, Completeness, and Quality of Nursing Documentation

Charting is done at the point of care (the patient's bedside), which reduces the chances that the nurse will overlook data. Worksheets, which contain handwritten information that is later entered into the record, can be eliminated. As Peck (1997) notes, "The nurse is able to enter data in real time; that is, as the nurse has interactions in the patient's room or later at a computer station outside the patient's room. We prefer real-time charting that makes patient data available to everyone caring for or interacting with the patient."

Readily Available Test Results

In some computer software systems, nurses can be notified of any abnormal test results for their assigned patients when they use a terminal in any patient room. This permits the nurse to notify the physician more expediently when critically abnormal test results are obtained.

Reduction of Medication Errors

Orders can be checked at the bedside immediately before medications are administered, reducing the risk of medication errors.

Enhanced Patient Perception of Nurses

Patients tend to perceive that the nurse is spending more time with them when documentation occurs at the bedside. Most patients have either neutral or positive reactions to having terminals in their rooms.

Less Clerical Work

Several studies have shown that bedside systems can eliminate 30 to 90 minutes of clerical work, allowing nurses to spend more time in patient care (Korpman, 1991).

Better Organization and Greater Work Efficiency

Using bedside terminals should reduce or eliminate the risks of omissions in charting and improve the accuracy and quality of charting. Care can improve because the computer presents prompts about what to look for and the type of care to provide.

Better Nurse Recruitment Possibilities

The presence of bedside terminals in a hospital may be a significant factor in recruiting nurses. Improved morale, retention, and recruitment may give the hospital a competitive edge.

Reduction in Overtime

Charting at the bedside using a terminal may reduce overtime associated with documentation. A study sponsored by TDS Healthcare systems found overtime savings of nearly one half hour per nurse per shift. Hospitals trying to justify the costs of a bedside system often cite this point (Meyer, 1992).

Better Accessibility

The bedside computer system provides a record that is immediately accessible to the nurse, and it also allows the physician to access the record from the nurses station. Access to the chart by personnel other than nurses, such as therapists, is simplified because the nurse no longer needs to have the physical record to chart. The central nursing station becomes quieter and less congested (Brennan, 1991). Time spent walking through the corridors to reach a medical record is reduced.

Disadvantages of Bedside Systems

Cost

Cost is one of the major obstacles to investing in bedside systems. Depending on the number of beds in a facility, the cost can be prohibitive. In an attempt to address this issue, some vendors have suggested the use of portable computer devices, such as modules or pen pads, to enter information at the bedside. These devices are attached to a terminal at the nursing station, and the information in the portable unit is then downloaded into the terminal to update the patient's record.

Possible Increase in the Volume of Paper

The printing schedule and the layout of the pages may create a medical record that is twice as thick as with paper-based systems. Charts may need to be more frequently thinned by storing documentation.

Less Resting Time for Nurses

At many hospitals using bedside terminals, nurses say they had to become accustomed to not having an opportunity to sit down. Previously they were able to sit down when they charted, but now they were up all day (Knickman, 1992).

Physician Objections

Some physicians object to bedside terminals because they like to review the clinical record before entering the room.

This objection can be overcome by using bedside systems that incorporate a terminal at the nursing station, which can be used to review the record of any patient in the unit.

SELECTION OF A COMPUTER INFORMATION SYSTEM

Many factors need to be considered when a nursing department decides to move toward selecting a nursing information system, as noted in Box 8-5. Chapter 9 presents information on the process of change and the factors that must be considered when making changes in a documentation system. Selection of a computer system has far-reaching consequences affecting virtually every department. For example, Town (1993) reports that a change in nursing documentation in her hospital affected the following groups and departments: the information systems, the intravenous therapy team, nurse specialists, the peer review organization, the quality assurance group, the education department, nursing students and professors, nursing agencies, finance specialists, staffing coordinators, the radiology department, the risk management teams, infection control nurses, patients and their families, the utilization review board, ancillary departments, medical records, the administrative staff, and physicians. One is hard-pressed to think of an area that will not be affected by a change in nursing documentation.

Typical Sequence in the Selection Process

The selection of a computer information system is influenced by a number of factors, including the familiarity of the personnel with various options, alliances with other healthcare facilities, cost, and ease of use. The groundwork may be laid for selection of a system in the following manner:

1. Nursing and administration staff recognize the need to implement a computer information system.
2. A task force is established consisting of nurses, information management specialists, other care providers, and possibly a consultant. The nursing representative should have veto power.
3. A committee of clinical nurses is created to voice opinions, suggestions, and reactions regarding the possible use of a computer system. This group will act in an advisory capacity to the task force.
4. The task force may review the literature, attend conferences, talk with vendors at exhibits, request literature from vendors, talk with or visit other organizations that use computerized systems, or send out questionnaires to users of nursing information systems.
5. The task force identifies the essential features that must be present in the system to be purchased. (Although some organizations decide to develop

---

Box 8-5

Selection of a Computer System

- How much does the system cost? (Include the cost of hardware, software, supplies, repairs, consultation, and education upgrades.)
- Can the system be modified by the user, or do all changes need to be made by the vendor?
- What will additional changes cost?
- Does the vendor employ nurses in the software development area, or are people who are not nurses writing the programs?
- How long has the vendor been in business? Will the vendor be available to service the product in the long run?
- How many facilities have purchased the software? Can the vendor give you the names of facilities that are satisfied with the product, as well as those that have experienced problems?
- Does the system support the nursing process? Can information be manipulated in ways that are not possible using paper-based systems?
- How sophisticated is the system? Does it simply automate manual documentation, or does it maximize the power of the computer?
- Is the system compatible with other systems in use at the facility? For example, will the system be able to interface with the mainframe computer system, the pharmacy, and the laboratory?
- How is security managed in the system? Are passwords, code numbers, keys, or cards used?
- How is the confidentiality of information protected?
- How reliable is the system? What backup method is used? Will data be lost if the system unexpectedly shuts down (crashes)?
- What type of support does the vendor offer? Is support available 24 hours a day, 7 days a week?
- What type of training is provided by the vendor? Does the vendor have personnel who will be available on-site when the system is activated?
- How fast is the system? When the system is being used by the maximum number of users, how long will it take to access information?
- What type of screen displays are available? Are colors used? How large are the numbers and the letters that appear on the screen? What type of input devices are used by the system?

---

their own software, most choose to buy a system that has been developed by a vendor.)

6. The task force sends the vendors Request for Information forms that consists of specific questions about the product.
7. Certain vendors may be invited to the facility to present information on their systems and to present a demonstration to the task force. A formal Request for Proposal asks for estimates of the cost of the software and associated services. Sometimes the Request for Information and the Request for Proposal are combined.
8. Members of the task force may visit facilities that use the software of vendors who are under serious consideration.
9. Extensive negotiation and development of a contract occurs once the facility has made the final selection.
10. A nurse project coordinator is hired or assigned to oversee the implementation of the system. (Look for an individual who is organized, is computer literate, and has good communication skills.)
11. The software is customized to the needs of the agency.
12. The computer terminals are installed.
13. Users receive education on the system, including hands-on experience. Training manuals and learning resources should be prepared as well.
14. Either one unit is activated at a time, or the entire facility begins using the program at the same time.
15. Resource personnel are typically available in the unit for extensive periods of time in the initial phases of implementation.

Pitfalls in the Selection of a Computer Information System

Although undertaking a purchasing decision of this magnitude without making a few false moves is impossible, Box 8-6 points out common pitfalls to avoid.

Recommendations on System Selection

Rapid changes in health care are changing some of the old rules related to selection of systems. According to Pasternack (1998), these six rules have changed:

1. *Old rule:* look for big client lists; *new rule:* big does not mean better. Bigger does not necessarily mean better when it comes to how many users a vendor claims are using their product. A long list could mean that the products were developed long before hospitals began forming integrated health systems. A long list of users might also mean that new customers end up receiving less attention.
2. *Old rule:* buy software in bulk; *new rule:* buy only what you need. One type of software may not fit every component of a healthcare system. Software vendors must recognize that diverse cultural issues may affect the components of a healthcare system. A healthcare enterprise is not a collection of pieces that are alike.
3. *Old rule:* go for what is new and hot; *new rule: what is hot may not stay hot.* Between 1992 and 1996, many cutting edge healthcare software companies reaped windfalls, but as the pool of early adopters dried up, many saw their stock prices and performance plummet. A greater emphasis is now placed on the stability of the vendor.

Box 8-6

Pitfalls to Avoid When Selecting a Computer Information System

- *Not knowing in advance how the system will interface with other hospital computer systems.* Incompatible hardware or software will create expensive headaches.
- *Not clearly defining terms or definitions in the Request for Proposal.* For example, if the vendor is asked if the system handles acuity or patient classification, the question may be too broad and not give enough information to judge the product.
- *Not obtaining adequate information and support from the medical staff when selecting a system.* Failure to involve practicing physicians in the system's design or selection can lead to mutiny when the system is implemented. Physician resistance tends to decrease when the software is customized to the way physicians want to see the information displayed and when influential physicians are part of the task force that selects the computer system.
- *Failing to recognize that the process of selecting a system is time-consuming and costly.* Meeting time, trips to other facilities, and attending conferences consume resources.
- *Believing that there is one system that will meet all needs.* Some compromises are inevitable. Determine what absolutely must be included in a system and what is not really necessary.

4. *Old rule:* buy the best, then integrate; *new rule: stick with a few vendors.* In the old scenario, buyers bought specialized software for each department and then attempted to link them together. This approach does not work well for a health system (as opposed to a single facility). Now buyers are looking for a set of related software products from one supplier to avoid integration problems.

5. *Old rule:* buy what's available and let the vendors take care of you; *new rule:* find a vendor who will share the risks and rewards. Today's healthcare systems can easily spend $30 million to $50 million on a major software project, a dramatic increase from the $5 million it cost 5 years ago. As a result, healthcare systems are becoming more aggressive about sharing the risks and rewards of complicated installations. Mergers and partnerships between healthcare organizations and software companies are beginning to occur.

6. *Old rule:* when shopping for software, high price equals high function; *new rule:* shop for value. As the quest for system-wide efficiency focuses on how work flows across departments, some vendors are marketing their programs as enablers for change and reengineering. Newer functions in software, such as Windows operating systems or the Internet, may promise improved function, but many facilities have not invested in the type of computers needed to use these systems.

The purchasing rules are changing, requiring consideration of a whole new set of issues and priorities. Nursing documentation systems cannot be purchased without considering how the software affects other factors, including hardware, compatibility, functionality, and cost.

IMPLEMENTATION AND EDUCATION

Sabo (1997) notes that a complete multidisciplinary team, which includes representation from all departments and disciplines that will be impacted by the system, is needed to guide the implementation process. Strong support from the highest levels of management is needed for successful implementation. Today education about computers often starts in kindergarten, so tomorrow's nurses will likely have a greater knowledge about computers. A good possibility exists that today's nurse has a home computer and will use his or her knowledge, experience, and comfort with computer technology when computers are placed in the work site. For the nurses who do not have home computers, part of the challenge of introducing a computer documentation system is recognizing that anxiety about the computer system may affect the learning process. The fear of doing something wrong that will cause the computer to crash must be reckoned with. Bush and Ebel (1997) note that time, patience, and effort were required by the managers to reassure their staffs that they would not harm the system if they made an error. Involving users in the selection and modification of software is essential.

One of the earliest steps in the implementation of computers is ensuring that a level of comfort and computer knowledge exists among those who will be responsible for teaching or problem solving in the units, such as the educators and shift supervisors. Staff-development educators can obtain this knowledge by attending conferences, reading books on nursing and computers, and talking with the computer information management personnel and vendor.

Many vendors provide educational programs to assist the facility in introducing the software. Training programs typically contain simulated patient scenarios. After receiving some didactic instruction in the form of a lecture, videotape, or self-learning module, learners are asked to perform computer functions using fictitious patients. Classes are typically limited in size to maximize learning and to permit the instructor to give personalized attention. A computer laboratory located away from the nursing unit permits nurses to better concentrate on learning. Classroom learning is usually followed by guided or supervised practice in the nursing unit under the direction of an experienced user. Many facilities put log books on the unit to encourage nurses to document comments or suggestions about the program. A hotline for answering questions can provide useful support during the transition to a new system.

The more complex the system, the more gradual introduction and training should be. A gradual training process may result in some temporary decreases in productivity and efficiency, but in time the gains from computerizing the nursing documentation should offset the initial investment. Development of a tool to measure documentation before and after the implementation of the software is helpful for identifying gains achieved by the change. Of course, additional training will be needed as the software is updated.

SUMMARY

Many exciting developments in computer programs are taking place. The Institute of Medicine has promoted the vision of fully automated medical records in hospitals by the end of the decade, but no current system is capable of supporting a completely computer-based record. Its recommendations are based on a far-reaching concept of a fully integrated medical record that acts as a repository of lifelong medical information. Much work needs to be done to develop software programs for functions that are not currently automated before nurses will see the complete computer-based medical record.

REFERENCES

Adderly D, Hyde C, Mauseth P: The computer age impacts nurses, *Comput Nurs* 15(1):43, 1997.

American Nurses Association, *Code for Nurses,* St. Louis, MO, American Nurses Association, 1985.

Andrew W, Dick R: Applied information technology: a clinical perspective; feature focus: the computer-based patient record (part II), *Comput Nurs* 13(3):118, 1995a.

Andrew W, Dick R: Applied information technology: a clinical perspective; feature focus: the computer-based patient record (part III), *Comput Nurs* 13(4): 176, 1995.

Benner A, Swart J: Patient core data set: standard for a longitudinal health/medical record, *Comput Nurs* 15(2):S7, 1997.

Bowles K: The barriers and benefits of nursing information systems, *Comput Nurs* 15(4):191, 1997.

Bradley V: Innovative informatics: CPR-computerized patient record, *J Emerg Nurs* p 230, June 1994.

Brennan M: Computerization is possible in rural hospitals, *Nurs Manage* 22(5):56, 1991.

Bush A, Ebel C: Testing an electronic documentation system, *Nurs Manage* 27(7):40, 1996.

Cerne R, Brennan P: Study finds bedside terminals prove their worth, *Hospitals* 63:72, 1989.

Childs B: Bedside terminals: status and the future, *Health Care Commun Comput* (5):12, 1988.

Dawson E: Confidentiality and computerized medical records, *Nursing Connections* 10(1):49, 1997.

Equifax, Inc: *Health care information privacy: a survey of the public and leaders,* New York, 1993, Louis Harris and Associates.

Erb P, Coble D: Vital signs measured with nursing system, *Computers in Healthcare* 10:32, 1995.

Fiesta J: Legal issues in the information age, part 2, *Nurs Manage* 27(9):12, 1996.

Gilham C: Legal implications of computerized medical records, *Health Prog* p 18, May/June 1996.

Gobis L: Computerized patient records: start preparing now, *J Nurs Adm* 24(9):15, 1994.

Gross M: The potential of information systems in nursing, *Nursing Health Care* (9):477, 1989.

Hard R: Hospitals increase medical staff use of IS, *Hospitals,* p 43, January 5, 1993.

Hughes L: Choices of nursing systems. In Mills M, Romano C, Heller R, eds: *Information management in health care,* Springhouse, Penn, 1996, Springhouse.

Johnson D et al: Evaluation of the effects of computerized nurse charting. In *Proceedings of the Eleventh Annual Symposium on Computer Applications in Medical Care,* Washington, DC, 1987, IEEE Computer Society Press.

JCAHO: *1997 comprehensive accreditation manual for hospitals,* Oak Brook Terrace, Ill, 1996, The Commission.

Knickman et al: *Appendix for an evaluation of the New Jersey nursing incentive reimbursement awards program: final report,* New York, 1992, The Health Research Program of New York University.

Korpman R: Patient care automation: the future is now: does reality live up to the promise (part VI) *Nurs Econ* 9(3):175, 1991.

Lawrence L: Safeguarding the confidentiality of automated medical information, *J Qual Improve* 20(11):639, 1994.

Marasovic C et al: A comparison of nursing activities associated with manual and automated documentation in an Australian intensive care unit, *Comput Nurs* 14(4):S20, 1997.

McCormick K et al: The federal and private sector roles in the development of minimum data sets and core health data elements, *Comput Nurs* 15(2):S23, 1997.

Meyer C: Beside computer charting: inching toward tomorrow, *Am J Nurs* p 38, April 1992.

Milholland D: Privacy and confidentiality of patient information: challenges for nursing, *J Nurs Adm* 24:19, 1994.

Minda S, Brundage D: Time differences in handwritten and computer documentation of nursing assessment, *Comput Nurs* 12(2):277, 1994.

Pasternack A: Six new buying rules, *Hosp Health Netw* p 35, February 20, 1998.

Peck M et al: LDS Hospital: a facility of Intermountain Health Care, Salt Lake City, Utah, *Nurs Adm Q* 2(3):29, 1997.

Pierskalla W, Woods D: Computers in hospital management and improvement in patient care: new trends in the United States, *J Med Systems* (12):411, 1988.

Randall A: It's time for the next generation of patient care systems, *US Health Care* 6:54, 1990.

Sabo D: Clinical information system: a "gateway" to the 21st century, *Nurs Adm Q* 21(3):68, 1997.

Simpson R: Ensuring patient data, privacy, confidentiality, and security, *Nurs Manage* 25(7):18, 1994.

Song L, Ho J, Ho S: The integrated patient information system, *Comput Nurs* 15(2):S14, 1997.

Styffe E: Privacy, confidentiality, and security in clinical information systems: dilemmas and opportunities for the nurse executive, *Nurs Adm Q* 21(3):21, 1997.

Town J: Changing to computerized documentation-PLUS! *Nurs Manage* 24(7):44, 1993.

Uddin D, Martin P: Core data set: importance to health services research, outcomes research and policy research, *Comput Nurs* 15(2):S38, 1997.

Vierderman M: The computer age: beware the loss of the narrative, *Gen Hosp Psychiatry* 17:157, 1995.

Werley H, Lang H eds: *Identification of the nursing minimum data set,* New York, 1988, Springer.

SUGGESTED READINGS

Andrew W, Dick R: Applied information technology: a clinical perspective, feature focus: the computer-based patient record (part I), *Comput Nurs* 13(2):80, 1995.

Bliss-Holtz J: Computerized support for case management, *Comput Nurs* 13(6):289, 1995.

Bliss-Holtz J: Using Orem's theory to generate nursing diagnoses for electronic documentation, *Nurs Sci Q* 9(3):121, 1996.

Brown S et al: Evaluation of the impact of a bedside terminal system in a rapidly changing community hospital, *Comput Nurs* 13(6):280, 1995.

Conrad S, Rensink Y: Using internet technology in ICU, *Nurs Manage* 28(7):34, 1997.

Eggland E: Using computers to document, *Nursing 97* p 16, January 1997.

Fiesta J: Legal issues in the information age (part I), *Nurs Manage* 27(8):15, 1996.

Gabrieli E: Longitudinal electronic patient records: a challenge of our time, *Comput Nurs* 15(2):S48, 1997.

Grobe S: The nursing intervention lexicon and taxonomy: implications for representing nursing care data in automated patient records, *Holistic Nurs Pract* 11(1):48, 1996.

Hendrickson G et al: Implementation of a variety of computerized bedside nursing information systems in 17 New Jersey hospitals, *Comput Nurs* 13(3):96, 1995.

Johnson D, Martin K: Preparing for electronic documentation, *Nurs Manage* p 43, July 1996.

Lower M, Nauert L: Charting the impact of bedside computers, *Nurs Manage* 23(7):40, 1992.

Rhodes A: The need for security with computerized records, *MCN* 20:299, 1995.

Tallon R: Computer-based patient records: hype versus reality, *Nurs Manage* 27(3):53, 1996.

9

Implementing Changes in Documentation Systems

IMPLEMENTATION OF CHANGES IN DOCUMENTATION SYSTEMS

Today's emphasis on reducing healthcare costs by performing only work that is essential to patient care makes documentation a prime candidate for reorganization (Smeltzer et al, 1996). In addition, hospital mergers and acquisitions have created the need to standardize documentation practices within multiple-hospital systems. The successful implementation or revision of a documentation system requires thoughtful, deliberate planning. This chapter provides information on identifying the need for change, addressing problems within the system, and developing strategies to implement documentation changes efficiently and effectively.

Classic Change Theory

According to Kurt Lewin (1961), the originator of classic change theory, change is a three-phase process used to obtain the desired behavioral change: unfreezing, moving, and refreezing.

The unfreezing phase involves disrupting the balance or equilibrium within the system. As long as balance is maintained, change will not occur. However, when people become dissatisfied with the status quo, the equilibrium is disrupted. Dissatisfaction with healthcare practices in general, and documentation practices specifically, provides the impetus for change. During this phase, initial data is collected, both formally and informally, to identify strengths and limitations in the current documentation system.

The second phase of change involves moving toward the new goal. The forces for change conflict with the forces to maintain the status quo, and resistance to change occurs.

Development and implementation of new ideas and practices also develop during this phase. Committees are formed, goals are established, systems are redesigned, and pilot programs are successfully implemented to introduce the new practices to the staff. As one might suspect, this phase is the longest in the change cycle.

The final phase of Lewin's theory is refreezing, which is characterized by consolidation and adoption of the new ideas. The hallmark of this phase is monitoring and evaluating the changes. Providing resource people and materials during this phase is essential to ensure continued compliance and increased knowledge. As the staff becomes more comfortable with the revised documentation practices, acceptance of the change will increase and resistance will fade.

Tips for Promoting Successful Change

O'Brien and Landstrom (1994) highlight the following success factors when redesigning documentation systems:

1. Gain top-level administrative support early in the process to minimize barriers.
2. Obtain financial and human resource commitment for the project from the nurse executive.
3. Survey the needs of the healthcare team involved in the change.
4. Develop a team that is committed to the project's success and respectful of one another's opinions and expertise.
5. Form nursing committees to generate ideas, collect and communicate feedback, and support the change.
6. Maintain communication with all levels of the nursing department (and other departments).

7. Consult informally with the Medical Records staff and incorporate their requirements into the process.
8. Incorporate nursing staff input into revisions, education, and implementation to give the staff a measure of control over the change.
9. Undertake pilot programs to implement the changes on all the units that will use the new system. Make necessary adjustments, but never rescind a pilot and return to the old system because of pressure from the staff.

Barriers to successful change may exist if the following circumstances are present:

1. Large numbers of committees are required to approve the change.
2. The nursing care planning and documentation system has been in place for a long time and is outdated.
3. The hospital's documentation system has recently been changed.

All of these situations may create resistance to change among the staff who will be affected by the proposed revisions.

ESTABLISHING A TASK FORCE

To initiate changes in a documentation system, a task force is formed to examine the options. Their discussions will focus on the selection and composition of the task force, its purpose, goals, and responsibilities, and the cost of change.

Selection and Composition

The overall composition of the task force and selecting the appropriate members affect the outcome. Task force members should be chosen for their interest in documentation and their ability to contribute to the work of the group. The best guideline is to have the smallest number of the most appropriate people. Selection should be based on the following criteria (Haynes, 1988):

- Knowledge of the subject area (expertise to help develop a viable solution to the problem)
- Commitment to solving the problem (participant should have a vested interest in the success of the change)
- Enough time to participate in the task force
- Diversity of viewpoint (to avoid patterned thinking or "group thinking")
- Expressiveness (freedom and ability to express facts, opinions, and feelings)
- Open-mindedness (willing to listen to others)

The majority of the representatives are usually from clinical nursing, management, and staff development. However, as healthcare embraces a more multidisciplinary

---

> ### Box 9-1
> #### Suggested Meeting Ground Rules
>
> 1. The meeting will begin and end on time.
> 2. Attendance and participation is expected and encouraged.
> 3. Members respect one another's right to express opinions.
> 4. Conflict is normal and should be handled professionally.
> 5. Decisions will be made by consensus.

> ### Box 9-2
> #### Purposes of a Documentation Task Force
>
> - Explore the current documentation system to identify strengths and limitations.
> - Gather data from a variety of sources, including the literature, other institutions, and nursing staff.
> - Develop strategies to institute changes.

---

approach, including personnel from other departments, such as medical records, risk management, utilization review, social services, discharge planning, materials management, and the medical staff, becomes necessary.

The chairperson of the committee should be selected and clearly identified to provide needed guidance and ensure that the committee's objectives are met in a timely manner. A consultant with expertise in documentation systems can be a valuable facilitator of the ad hoc committee.

Establishing Ground Rules

To promote effective meetings and efficient use of time, ground rules should be established and followed during each meeting. Setting ground rules helps clarify expectations of acceptable group behavior. The ground rules may be established by the group leader, or they may be discussed and decided on by the full membership. The latter approach promotes a more participative atmosphere and gives the participants ownership of the process. Suggested ground rules are listed in Box 9-1. Attendance at meetings should be expected. To prevent delays in the decision process, one multiple-hospital system adhered to a policy stipulating that if a hospital was not represented at a work meeting, decisions would be made without that hospital's input (O'Brien, Landstrom, 1994).

Purpose and Goals

To provide direction and enhance productivity, the task force must clearly define its purpose and goals. The purposes of the task force are shown in Box 9-2. The goals of the task force vary depending on the organization's needs

---

Box 9-3

Criteria for an Optimal Documentation System

- Reflects all aspects of the nursing process
- User-friendly
- Improves reimbursement from third-party payers
- Saves time
- Integrates with patient classification system
- Computer applicable
- Cost-efficient
- Patient-focused
- Multidisciplinary

Box 9-4

Responsibilities of a Documentation Task Force

- Establishing priorities when several aspects of a documentation system require change
- Defining the purpose of the change
- Brainstorming possible solutions
- Developing an operational plan
- Assigning tasks leading to the achievement of the outcomes
- Establishing the criteria for judging accomplishments
- Communicating the plan and implementation strategies to others
- Monitoring the progress of the project
- Reviewing and updating the objectives of the change process
- Evaluating the success of the project

---

and the nature of the documentation changes. However, Krause (1996) articulated the following goal, which effectively addresses current healthcare practices: "To develop an effective, efficient, user-friendly documentation system that reflects a patient-focused, interdisciplinary, and collaborative process of care" (p. 25).

Regardless of the specific goal, the expected outcomes must be clearly delineated to ensure that task force members work toward the same end result. Box 9-3 lists outcome criteria for an optimal documentation system.

Responsibilities

Membership responsibilities include those listed in Box 9-4. Specific responsibilities that can be delegated to task force members include the following: researching the most current regulatory agency requirements for documentation; promoting pilot programs in specific units, communicating with ancillary departments affected by the changes, developing audit and evaluation tools for use during the pilot programs; and preparing educational materials.

CHANGE PROCESS

Many institutions generate creative ideas for improving nursing documentation practices. However, organizations that understand change theory and develop a plan to implement change have a greater chance of success. The remainder of this chapter provides details for changing documentation systems structured according to the nursing process.

Assessment

Individuals involved in change must perceive the need for change and recognize the value of the proposed idea for the change process to continue. During the assessment step, concentrating efforts on raising awareness within the group and explaining the need for the change is key. Assessment includes gathering data from nursing staff, current literature reviews, educational programs, and quality improvement activities to pinpoint problem areas.

A number of reasons for changing documentation practices exist, and many factors affect the decision to change documentation practices. Among them are regulatory agency requirements, financial reimbursement concerns, legal issues, and changes in care delivery.

Regulatory Agency Requirements

Accrediting and regulatory agency standards play a major role in motivating nursing departments to change documentation practices. The Joint Commission for the Accreditation of Healthcare Organizations (JCAHO) standards are framed in broad terms that outline the desired outcomes of a documentation system. In recent years the focus has shifted from process to patient outcomes, and the standards now include recommendations for establishing a multidisciplinary approach to care that ultimately impacts documentation systems.

Financial Reimbursement

Documentation can have an adverse effect on reimbursement by third-party payers. In many cases, reimbursement is denied because of inadequate nursing documentation. When this occurs, the hospital or home care agency should examine the documentation system to determine what changes will enhance reimbursement.

Legal Issues

Sometimes an unfortunate incident prompts the nursing department to examine its documentation practices. If a malpractice suit is brought against the facility, the chart will be scrutinized for evidence that the standard of care was met. If little or no evidence exists in the record, the case may be difficult to defend. The legal counsel may suggest changes in the documentation practices to avoid future problems.

Changes in Care Delivery

The ripple effect occurs when one change in a system necessitates other changes. Changes in nursing care delivery may lead to revisions in forms or systems. For example, the increased use of unlicensed assistive personnel, and fewer registered nurses (RNs) may require a change in documentation practices. The move toward multidisciplinary, patient-focused care, use of integrated clinical pathways, and computerized nursing records will have a significant impact on nursing documentation.

Other Sources of Assessment Data

Learning about new innovations from colleagues is one way to gain information about what to change in a documentation system. Site visits to facilities known for their innovation and creativity may also provide the stimulus for change. Researching the literature, attending workshops and seminars, and anticipating future innovations in nursing will help to decide what changes need to be made now.

Diagnosis

Developing a diagnosis involves pinpointing the nature of the documentation problem. During this stage, quality improvement tools are helpful in determining the root cause of the problem. The use of flowcharts and fishbone diagrams helps to illustrate each step in the documentation process and to uncover problems (Martin, 1992).

Potential causes of the documentation problem include poorly designed forms, an outdated documentation system, and inadequate staff compliance.

Poorly Designed Forms

Changing the forms may involve creating a new form or simply revising an existing one. New or revised forms should complement the existing expectations for care, reduce duplication of information, and meet accreditation requirements. (Designing forms is addressed in Chapter 4.) Once a form is revised or created, education and continued monitoring is necessary to enhance compliance.

Outdated Documentation System

Many facilities operate with outdated charting practices and systems. Knowledge of the new system may be obtained through education. However, incorporating new behaviors evolves over time. Introduction of clinical pathways and computerized charting to replace outdated practices is a huge undertaking. Such a project should be divided into manageable segments to ensure successful implementation.

Inadequate Staff Compliance

If the forms are determined to be adequate and the documentation system supports the care delivery in the organization, then the source of the documentation problem

---

Box 9-5
Questions That Help Define Staff Nurse Utilization

- Is it possible to reduce the time nurses spend performing duties outside the realm of nursing?
- Do the job responsibilities and performance expectations need to be revised?
- Do "gray" areas exist surrounding the documentation responsibilities for licensed practical nurses (LPNs) and unlicensed assistive personnel (UAP)?
- Are the professional responsibilities of RNs versus the technical responsibilities of LPNs well defined?
- What are the logistics of charting?
- Do the nurses have to write notes on a worksheet and then copy them into the medical record?
- Would bedside charting be more efficient?

---

may be the people using the system. Compliance issues generally fall into one of the following three categories:

1. Lack of knowledge
2. Improper utilization of staff
3. Lack of desire to comply

Lack of Knowledge. In some cases a lack of knowledge regarding the form or system contributes to noncompliance. Many institutions educate the full-time staff, inadvertently neglecting the part-time, weekend, per diem, and agency staff. Education efforts should cover all shifts to ensure consistency. Some hospitals have requested that a nursing representative from each agency attend an educational offering designed to explain documentation practices. The agency representative is then responsible for educating other agency personnel. To facilitate this process, self-learning modules are prepared and distributed to the agencies. The cost of educating the staff is minimal compared to the potential cost of a lawsuit that hinges on nursing documentation.

Utilization of Staff. If lack of knowledge is not the problem, perhaps the utilization of the nursing staff should be explored. Box 9-5 lists some questions that help define how staff nurses are utilized. If these issues are interfering with the outcomes of the documentation system, they must be addressed.

Lack of Desire to Comply. The source of the problems in a documentation system may be a lack of willingness by nurses to comply. If nurses do not value documentation as a primary, essential professional responsibility, they may not adhere to documentation standards. Discussing the importance of documentation in today's healthcare environment may increase awareness and improve compliance.

Some nurses are noncompliant because they have no reason to comply. They are not rewarded for documenting well, and no consequences result from documenting poorly, which implies that documentation is not valuable. To combat this problem, documentation expectations should be clearly stated from the time of initial employment, and documentation must be made part of the performance standards. The staff should be evaluated on their ability both to provide and to document care according to the organization's expectations.

Finally, some nurses are noncompliant because the documentation system is cumbersome. The requirement to chart information in several places often results in nurses not filling out one or more forms completely. Analyzing the reason for noncompliance objectively is beneficial. To move ahead with quality improvement strategies, managers must move away from blaming the individual and focus energy on changing the system.

Plan

Establishing a plan to manage the documentation change provides the organization with a clear understanding of the changes. The planning stage requires collaboration and communication between managers, educators, staff, physicians, and other departments to develop a workable plan for changing the documentation system.

Breaking the documentation project down into manageable segments and creating a timeline for project management is essential. Establishing goals and time frames for completion helps to maintain the productivity of the group and keep the project moving.

Documentation Policies

Begin by examining the existing documentation policies, which are the governing rules of the organization. Whereas professional practice standards developed by specialty nursing organizations tend to be broad, institutional policies and procedures are usually more specific. Box 9-6 provides guidelines for documentation policies.

The Role of Staff Development in Planning

Staff development is very important in planning and implementing changes in documentation. Educators contribute to the planning process in the following ways:

- Prioritizing which parts of the system to change
- Developing surveys and leading focus groups to gather input from the staff
- Establishing timelines for project management
- Recommending the most effective teaching methods for implementing change
- Serving as facilitators
- Providing guidance and support for the staff

An integral part of the planning phase is communicating about the process and pending documentation changes. Staff development instructors specialize in "getting the message

---

Box 9-6

Guidelines for Documentation Policies

1. Documentation policies should reflect professional organization standards and accrediting agency requirements. It is equally important that the organizational policies reflect the resources (both capital and human) required to achieve the standard. Realistic expectations for care delivery and accurate documentation are essential.
2. Policies must address the differences in the roles and responsibilities of RNs and LPNs. The state practice act should be reviewed when documentation policies are defined for different categories of nurses. Accountability must be clearly identified for the admission assessment, development of the plan of care, and periodic reassessments. Documentation by unlicensed personnel must also be defined in the policies.
3. Documentation policies should be determined based on patient acuity. For example, hospitalized patients who are in stable condition and awaiting nursing home placement do not require the same frequency or detail of documentation as those recovering from surgery, even though they may be in the same nursing unit. The methods of charting will generally be different in a medical-surgical unit than in a critical care unit. Nurses who work in long-term care units usually chart less often than nurses who work in acute care. (The documentation of home care and long-term care are discussed in Chapters 13 and 14.)
4. Policies should include realistic time frames for completing the admission assessment and initiating the plan of care. In addition, the policy should clarify what portion of the admission data collection can be delegated to nurses other than RNs.
5. Policies should clearly articulate not only the minimum frequency for charting but also the expected content. Risk-management personnel or legal counsel should be consulted to provide feedback when the legal aspects of a documentation policy are examined. For example, a strictly written or unrealistic policy should be reviewed.
6. Before new documentation policies or procedures are adopted, they should pass through the appropriate steps for approval. The nursing staff should be notified of the new policy or procedure and the rationale for the change. Sharing such information at a staff meeting is an excellent strategy. For those not in attendance, information can be placed in a communication book that all staff must read. After reading the book, staff members sign or initial to verify that they received the information.

---

out." The strategies presented here represent several approaches for communicating about change and educating the staff.

Questionnaires. When change is first undertaken, obtaining input from those using the current system is essential. Developing and distributing a questionnaire may elicit such information. Questions should be developed to obtain data on the strengths and limitations of the current documentation system. In most cases, some parts of the documentation system are effective and need not be changed. Identification of these areas through a questionnaire will assist the task force in setting priorities for which aspects to change and which to retain.

Newsletters. Many nursing departments have a monthly newsletter designed to publicize their activities, accomplishments, and other interdepartmental news. The newsletter can be an excellent vehicle for describing upcoming documentation changes. As the implementation process continues, the newsletter can be used to publish the results of questionnaires, the progress of pilot programs, the accomplishments of quality improvement activities, and praise for excellent charting. Printing the newsletter on the back of the education calendar and distributing it with the paychecks is an effective strategy that is not costly. Staff members benefit from increased awareness of the change, and they appreciate being kept informed and having their accomplishments recognized.

Posters. Another low-cost strategy involves placing posters in the nursing units, which provides the staff with visual cues to augment discussion and inservice education. Posters can be used to announce upcoming changes and pilot programs and to illustrate how documentation should be performed. The poster remains in the unit as a reference during charting activities and can be used during orientation to acquaint new staff members with the system.

Inservices. Inservice education is the traditional strategy for implementing changes. At the beginning of a documentation change project, an inservice program generally is presented throughout all shifts and on weekends to reach as many staff members as possible. The program should list specific objectives and content to be addressed. Time should always be provided for questions and answers. In many organizations, more than one person is responsible for inservice presentations on documentation changes. To enhance consistency among speakers, detailed outlines of each program should be developed. The speakers can meet before presentations to discuss any ambiguous areas needing clarification. Although personal presentation styles may vary, the content should be consistent. After the general inservice program has been completed, nurse managers, preceptors, instructors, or clinical specialists often follow up with a unit-based program that reinforces the information provided at the general program and addresses the specific needs of a particular unit. If a documentation change affects only one unit, general inservice programs are not necessary.

Workshops. If a form is being revised or introduced, or other minor changes are being implemented within the documentation system, the inservice format will often address the educational needs adequately. However, when more extensive changes in documentation are proposed, the workshop format is beneficial because it not only provides information but also provides hands-on learning.

Case studies also facilitate the learning process. Having been given a case study, nurses are instructed to document the necessary information using the new system. Most adult learners, and particularly nurses, want to apply new knowledge immediately. The use of case studies in workshops allows the learners to participate in the educational process and helps to identify individual strengths and limitations.

Self-Learning Modules and Videotapes. Despite best efforts, some staff members will not be able to attend the inservice programs and workshops. In such cases, self-learning modules provide a suitable alternative. A self-learning module contains the objectives, content, and activities necessary to learn new methods. An evaluation tool must be included to determine whether the learner has met the objectives. Self-learning is an excellent strategy when specific information must be repeated and reinforced.

When developing self-learning modules, limit the time needed to complete the module to 30 to 45 minutes. If the changes are complex or generate questions, self-learning modules may not be a reliable method of teaching. Follow-up completion of the module with a face-to-face discussion to clarify any misconceptions. Offer continuing education credit for completion of the self-study as incentive and recognition for the staff.

Videotaping is another strategy used to instruct staff members who are unable to attend scheduled inservice programs. Many organizations videotape the program and use the tapes as an instructional tool for ongoing education and orientation.

Other Creative Strategies for Implementing Changes

Other creative strategies for implementing changes include the following:

- Use the computer screen to communicate daily tips on documentation.
- Plan a "Documentation Month" to focus attention on the documentation system, any changes, and the results of those changes.
- Offer recognition for excellent charting.
- Use e-mail for receiving and responding to questions about documentation changes. Route responses to appropriate subgroups (Krause, 1996).
- Use humor, music, skits, games, buttons, slogans, and anything else necessary to get the staff involved.

Implementation

Implementation translates the plan into action. This step involves organizing and implementing pilot programs to familiarize the staff with the changes in documentation and identifying problems that may need to be corrected before full implementation. Many of the strategies used during the pilot program may then be employed when implementing the documentation changes throughout the organization.

Pilot Programs

Pilot programs are an excellent approach to implementation, allowing the changes to be implemented on a small scale to detect problems and limitations. The pilot program is like a dress rehearsal, and any concerns or limitations can be addressed before the revision is implemented throughout the institution.

Units chosen to implement the pilot programs should exhibit high enthusiasm, a stable staff, supportive management, and moderate-to-high tolerance for change. Depending on the size of the hospital and the type of form being tested, a cross section of units (e.g., medical-surgical, intensive care, pediatrics) may be used for the pilot to gain different perspectives. If the change affects only one or two units, the cross-section approach is not necessary.

The pilot program should be discussed with all departments affected by the proposed changes to maintain open communication. Effective strategies include the following:

1. Communicate with the chairperson of the medical records committee. Explain the new form(s) or changes in documentation practices and obtain approval to use the new form(s) temporarily so that nurses will not have to duplicate charting by using both the new and old forms during the pilot.
2. When interacting with physicians, do not assume that they understand nursing documentation. Provide basic explanations of the proposed changes. To enhance physician acceptance, explain the benefits of the change for the physician, nurse, and patient.
3. Find out what other hospitals in the area are doing in regard to this form or documentation change. Be prepared to answer the question, "Who else uses this approach?" or "What does that hospital do?"

Once these things have been done and the inservice programs have been completed, the pilot program can begin. Most pilot programs are conducted over a 4- to 6-week period, enabling the staff to become familiar with the changes and detect any problems with the new forms and charting techniques. However, it may take 4 to 6 months for the nursing staff and ancillary departments to acknowledge and accept the changes.

During the pilot program, having resource people available to assist the staff with the new system is essential, particularly during charting times. Staff development personnel, preceptors, and clinical specialists should be on the unit during the shift and at changes of shift to answer questions about the new system. The literature supports the use of resource people 24 hours a day for the first 3 days of the pilot, followed by weekly meetings to discuss progress. Additionally, communication books are used to share concerns, solutions, and feedback (Wong, Budgell, 1994; Mosher et al, 1996).

Feedback from the staff is a key element in the success of pilot projects. Staff meetings should have some time allotted for the discussion of the pilot program. Managers and educators should communicate with other pilot units to determine whether common problems that must be addressed exist. The expectations for staff regarding documentation must be constantly reinforced. Surveys can be distributed to elicit comments about the strengths and weaknesses of the proposed changes.

During the pilot program monitoring should be used to determine whether the new system is being used appropriately and consistently, and whether the new forms need to be revised. Results from the studies should be shared with the staff. Adjustments in the system should be based on the results of the pilot program, comments from the staff, and feedback from others affected by the change.

Once the pilot program has been completed and areas of concern have been identified and modified, the program can be fully implemented. Many of the strategies used during the pilot program can also be used to facilitate full implementation. Communication and follow-up are key elements in the success of implementation.

Evaluation

Monitoring and evaluation are essential to determine whether the established objectives are being met. Many different objectives can be achieved by monitoring documentation, including those listed in Box 9-7. Most organizations diligently monitor and evaluate documentation during the pilot programs; however, once the program is finished and the change is fully implemented, monitoring activities diminish. Monitoring and evaluation activities are essential in determining not only the degree of compliance, but also any specific problems hindering compliance. If the desired outcomes of the documentation change are not being achieved, the task force must investigate until the root cause is discovered.

Bernick and Richards (1994) suggest the use of peer auditing to bolster the success of documentation changes.

Box 9-7

Objectives of Monitoring Documentation

- Tracking patient outcomes as part of a quality improvement program
- Monitoring the quality of nursing care being delivered
- Measuring nurses' awareness of documentation policies
- Identifying individuals with charting strengths or weaknesses
- Evaluating the design of the form
- Evaluating the success of a change in the documentation system

Registered nurses, functioning as documentation team leaders, reviewed coworkers' documentation and provided clarification, immediate feedback, and recognition for the nurses' achievements. The staff nurses reported that the auditors' feedback fostered a spirit of mutual support and assistance. The peer auditors were able to identify group trends and difficulties, and then address these effectively during staff meetings.

SUMMARY

This chapter addresses documentation revisions within the framework of change theory and the nursing process. Revising a documentation system is a major change, involving strategic planning and implementation. Furthermore, such changes require an understanding of internal documentation standards, current (and evolving) external regulatory requirements, legal implications, utilization review criteria, and information system capabilities and potential. Input from staff, management, educators, and other departments helps to ensure success. Ongoing education and monitoring helps maintain compliance.

REFERENCES

Bernick L, Richards P: Nursing documentation: a program to promote and sustain improvement, *J Contin Educ Nurs* 25(5):203, 1994.

Haynes M: *Effective meeting skills,* Menlo Park, Calif, 1988, Crisp Publications.

Krause C et al: Forming an integrated documentation system, *Nurs Manage* 27(8):25, 1996.

Lewin K: Quasistationary social equilibria and the problem of permanent change. In Bennis et al, eds: *The planning of change,* New York, 1961, Holt, Rinehart, and Winston.

Martin CA: Improving the quality of medical record documentation, *J Healthc Qual* 14(3):16, 1992.

Mosher C et al: Documenting for patient-focused care, *Nurs Econ* 14(4):218, 1996.

O'Brien K, Landstrom G: Using system integration to revise documentation, *Nurs Manage* 25(2):56, 1994.

Smeltzer C et al: Streamlining documentation: an opportunity to reduce costs and increase nurse clinician's time with patients, *J Nurs Care Qual* 10(4):66, 1996.

Wong C, Budgell L: Documentation redesign, *Can Nurs* p 38, June 1994.

ADDITIONAL READINGS

Bhola HS: The CLER model: thinking through change, *Nurs Manage* 25(5):59, 1994.

Burke L, Murphy J: *Charting by exception applications,* Albany, NY, 1995, Delmar.

Corpuz L, Conforti C: Organizing and documenting clinical standards, *Nurs Manage* 25(5):70, 1994.

Fitzhenry F, Snyder J: Improving organizational processes for gains during implementation, *Comput Nurs* 14(3):171, 1996.

Kim I, Kim M: The effects of individual and nursing-unit characteristics on willingness to adopt an innovation: a multilevel analysis, *Comput Nurs* 14(3):183, 1996.

Muoio R et al: A win-win situation: the pilot program, *J Contin Educ Nurs* 26(5):230, 1995.

Scharf L: Revising nursing documentation to meet patient outcomes, *Nurs Manage* 28(4):38, 1997.

Tiffany C: Analysis of planned change theories, *Nurs Manage* 25(2):60, 1994.

10

Maternal-Child Documentation

OBSTETRICAL DOCUMENTATION
Joanne McDermott, RN, BSN, MA

As in other specialty areas of nursing, Labor and Delivery (L&D) has its own criteria for documentation. The Association of Women's Health Obstetrical and Neonatal Nursing (AWHONN) has developed guidelines to assist the nurse in identifying areas that need to be documented. The American College of Obstetrics and Gynecology (ACOG) and American Academy of Pediatrics (AAP) publications also provide recommendations. Hospital policy and procedures, which are developed based on the recognized standards, should delineate the obstetric nurse's role in documentation. Nurses hear about documentation at conferences, meetings, inservices, and evaluations. Nurses wake up at night remembering something they should have documented. Nurses sometimes resent all the time they have to spend doing the documentation, because they would rather be delivering nursing care. But there is no avoiding it. Nurses must document, and they must do it well.

The AWHONN's *Standards and Guidelines* (1998) recommend that documentation follow the nursing process, and they stress that relevant data should be documented in a retrievable form. Diagnoses are to be documented in a way that facilitates the determination of the expected outcomes and plan of care. Outcome measures are to be documented as measurable goals, and the plan, interventions, and patient's response to interventions are to be documented as well. Revisions to the diagnoses, plan of care, and outcomes should also be documented.

ANTENATAL TESTING

When caring for a patient undergoing antenatal fetal surveillance, documentation will need to include criteria specific to the type of testing utilized. The review of the tracing from any antenatal testing procedure needs to be done in a systematic manner, incorporating the baseline, variability, accelerations, decelerations, and periodic or episodic patterns. The types of accelerations and decelerations, as well as any interventions, need to be recorded. The nurse should document the conversation with the physician and the plan of care (Murray, 1997). Table 10-1 indicates documentation criteria for specific antenatal tests. The form utilized to document antenatal testing, patient observation, and discharge instructions should be suitable for incorporation into the patient's prenatal records. This will help to facilitate continuity and ensure appropriate follow-up. An example of discharge instructions appropriate for use after antenatal evaluation is illustrated in Figure 10-1.

LABOR AND DELIVERY DOCUMENTATION
Admission

At the time of admission to L&D, a full assessment should be performed and documented. The admission form should flow in order as the assessment is completed. Whenever a pregnant woman is evaluated for labor, the factors shown in Box 10-1 should be assessed and recorded (ACOG, AAP, 1997; Simpson, Creehan, 1996).

A key function of the initial nursing history and physical is identifying risk factors that will influence ongoing care (Chagnon, Easterwood, 1986). The nursing admission/assessment form should incorporate all of the areas described above to facilitate the process of risk identification, resulting in appropriate nursing diagnoses, plan of care,

TABLE 10-1   Antenatal Test Documentation

Antenatal Test	Documentation
NST (nonstress test)	1. Identifying information 2. Expected date of delivery (EDD) 3. Physician's name 4. Date, time monitor applied 5. Reason for test 6. Vital signs 7. Maternal position 8. High-risk conditions 9. Systematic review of tracing 10. Any interventions 11. Patient teaching 12. Notification of physician of the test results 13. Documentation of conversation and plan of care 14. Identification of person reviewing tracing 15. Discharge instructions, including plan for follow-up, and monitoring of kick counts or fetal movement; test results recorded as "reactive" or "nonreactive"
FAD (fetal activity acceleration determination)	Document 1-15 as above; test results also interpreted as "reactive" or "nonreactive." Mark fetal movements (or have patient do so) on monitor tracing. Document fetal activity in record. Document results with description of fetal accelerations (e.g., baseline 140-150; spontaneous acceleration $\uparrow 170 \times 40$ sec.).
BSST (breast stimulation stress test, nipple stimulation)	Document 1-15 as above, plus informed consent, explanation of procedure, palpation of uterine resting tone and uterine activity. Describe criteria for test results. Document whether criteria was met and whether test was positive, negative, suspicious, or unsatisfactory. Record meeting criteria (e.g., three contractions in 10 minutes). Describe FHR pattern in relation to contractions (Murray, 1997).
CST (contraction stress test)	Document 1-15 as above. Document 20-minute baseline tracing, IV initiation, IV fluid type and amount, dosage of Pitocin (oxytocin), type of fluid, type of infusion equipment. Document informed consent, vital signs, indication for test, maternal position, and initiation. Document dosage of Pitocin (mU/min), times of increments, and time discontinued. Document intake and output and name of person interpreting test. Document results as reactive negative, nonreactive negative, positive, equivocal, hyperstimulation, or unsatisfactory. Document uterine activity (UA) and resting tone before discharge. Indicate criteria used to interpret test (Murray, 1997).
FAST (fetal acoustic stimulation test)	Document 1-15 as above, plus indication for testing, order and communication from physician. Document the number and duration of stimulations and the type of device used to stimulate the fetus. Chart the systematic review of tracing before and after stimulation. Document reaching criteria according to institutional protocol (e.g., two accelerations $\uparrow 15$ beats above BL and lasting for 15 or more seconds, returning to BL between accelerations, within a 20-minute period). Describe the interpretation as reactive or nonreactive (Murray, 1996).
BPP (biophysical profile)	Document the indication for test and results with parameters (e.g., amniotic fluid index [AFI] 2, tone 2, breathing 2, fetal movement 2, reactive NST 2; score: 10/10).

Data from Murray M: *Antepartal and intrapartal fetal monitoring,* ed 2, Albuquerque, 1997, Learning Resources International.

◆ **COLUMBIA**
Katy Medical Center

5602 Medical Center Drive
Katy, Texas 77494
FAX (281) 392-0483/Phone (281) 392-1111
COLUMBIA's home page is *http://www.columbia-hca.com*   **OBSTETRICAL DISCHARGE INSTRUCTIONS**
You have been seen and possibly treated for one of the conditions below:

Decreased Fetal Movement:
If you feel your baby is not moving as much as usual, do the following:
1. Drink a large glass of water.
2. Lie on your left side and count the baby's movements.
3. You should have at least 5 movements per hour
4. If you have less than 5 movements, repeat the above steps.
5. If at the end of the second hour you still do not feel at least 5 movements, call you doctor.

Urinary Tract Infections:
1. Drink plenty of fluids, at least 10-12 glasses of water daily.
2. Have your prescription filled today.
3. Take all of the medication-even if you are feeling better.
4. Empty your bladder often-at least every couple of hours.
5. Be sure to wipe from front to back after urinating.
6. Notify your doctor if:
   a. You have a fever of 101 F orally after taking it twice, 4 hours apart.
   b. You see blood in your urine.
   c. You are unable to urinate.
   d. You have severe pain when you urinate.
7. Avoid alcoholic beverages, soft drinks, or caffeinated beverages during this treatment.

Bleeding:
1. It is normal to have spotting after a vaginal exam.
2. Spotting is not unusual, especially later in the pregnancy.
3. However, if bleeding is as heavy as a period:
   a. Note the amount with the number of pads saturated.
   b. The color of the bleeding.
   c. Any pain associated with the bleeding.

Preterm Labor:
1. Drink at least 10-12 glasses of water daily.
2. When resting or sleeping, stay off of your back as much as possible - use pillows for extra support.
3. Be sure to empty your bladder frequently-at least every couple of hours
4. Notify your doctor if you have more than 6 contractions per hour and the above steps have not helped.
5. No sexual intercourse or orgasm until checking with your doctor.
6. No tampons or douching until checking with your doctor.

Signs of Preterm Labor:
1. Tightening of the uterus-more than 6 per hour.
2. Period-like cramping.
3. Low back pain.
4. Pelvic pressure and/or aching thighs.
5. Abdominal cramping with or without diarrhea.
6. Vaginal spotting or bleeding with any of the above symptoms.

Call your doctor if:
1. Contractions become regular (every 5-6 minutes) for at least one hour after walking and drinking a large glass of water.
2. Your bag of water breaks
   a. If you are not sure if it has broken, go to the bathroom, empty your bladder.
   b. Put a pad on. If it is wet within ½ hour- call your doctor.
   c. Note the color and odor of the fluid.
3. Elevated oral temperature of 101F twice 4 hours apart.

MEDICATIONS:

NEXT DOCTOR'S VISIT:

I understand the above instructions:

Patient:_____

Date:_____

Nurse:_____

obdis

Figure 10-1   Obstetrical discharge instructions. (Courtesy Columbia Katy Medical Center, Katy, Texas.)

Box 10-1

Documentation Guidelines for Admission of the Patient in Labor

- Temperature, pulse, respiration
- Blood pressure
- Frequency, intensity, duration of uterine contractions, time of onset
- Fetal heart rate (FHR)
- Clinical estimation of fetal weight by physician
- Urinary protein and glucose
- Cervical dilation and effacement (unless contraindicated)
- Presenting part and station (unless contraindicated)
- Status of membranes
- Date and time of the patient's arrival
- Notification of care providers of the patient's arrival
- Record of previously identified risk factors (from the prenatal record)
- Presence or absence of bleeding
- Fetal movement
- History of allergies
- Time and amount of most recent food or fluid ingestion
- Use of any medications (prescribed or over the counter)
- History of smoking, illicit drug use, or alcohol use
- Psychosocial status
- Identity of the physician who will be caring for newborn
- Childbirth education preparation, breastfeeding assessment

---

intervention, and evaluation. Figure 10-2 shows an example of an admission form.

Documenting Labor

Labor and delivery nurses can be extremely creative when it comes to documentation forms. Nurses have used paper towels, scrub attire, pillowcases, gauze packets, examination glove packets, and even their own skin. Of course, the data written on these "forms" is then later transcribed by the nurse into the hospital-approved forms. (Hopefully the bedding has not been stripped, trash removed, and so forth.) Nurses engage in these bizarre charting rituals because they know that accurately noting the time of key events is necessary; therefore they do so in any way they can without taking critical time away from delivering needed care in emergency situations. Nurses know that charting ideally should be done in a concurrent manner. Realistically, when the fetal heart rate (FHR) drops, the level of documentation sometimes does as well—right to the bottom of the list of priorities. The nursing process takes place in a dynamic and expeditious manner. In emergency situations action takes precedent over the written word. Thus retrospective charting is better than no documentation at all (Simpson, Creehan, 1996). As soon as possible, the nurse should record the nursing process accurately. Late entries following a bad

outcome are often controversial in litigation (Simpson, Creehan, 1996). However, the story needs to be told, and someone reading the notes at a later date should be able to understand the course of events as they occurred.

Frequency of Documentation in Labor and Delivery

The ACOG and AAP have published guidelines describing how often maternal and fetal assessments should be made (and therefore documented). If risk factors are present, the FHR should be evaluated at least once every 15 minutes in stage I of labor. During labor stage II, the FHR tracing should be evaluated once every 5 minutes. If no risk factors are present, evaluation of the FHR should be documented at least once every 30 minutes in labor stage I and at least once every 15 minutes in labor stage II. The frequency may be increased, particularly as active labor progresses, according to clinical signs and symptoms (ACOG, AAP 1997). Other parameters for assessment and recording include maternal temperature and pulse (once every 4 hours or more often if indicated). Assess the frequency, duration, and quality of contractions regularly. During oxytocin induction or augmentation, assess blood pressure, FHR, and uterine contractions before every dosage increase (at a minimum) (Simpson, Creehan, 1996).

Additional parameters to be assessed and documented include the data shown in Box 10-2. Other documentation may include the presence of physicians or nurses and maternal position changes. Labor notes should also reflect the support person's interactions, breathing, relaxation, and massage techniques used, and patient teaching and response.

Certain events that occur in labor and delivery require that specific criteria be documented. Table 10-2 illustrates some of these events and the corresponding areas that need to be addressed in the nurse's documentation.

Labor Flow Records and Narrative Notes

The L&D flowsheet (Figure 10-3, pp. 155-158) should include all areas that are necessary to assess, reflective of the recognized standards of care. The flowsheet should not force the nurse to use specific intervals; instead, it should ideally accommodate the time when the assessment was actually made. If standardized increments are used (e.g., every 15 minutes, every 30 minutes), the narrative notes should be used to delineate the specific times of the assessment, interventions, evaluation, and so forth.

The abbreviations used should be defined on the form or in the institution's policies and procedures; for example, define terms like US (ultrasound), LW (left wedge), or LTV (long-term variability). The facility's policy on specific parameters of care can also be indicated on the form; for example, when a patient is at low risk, the form identifies that the FHR and uterine assessments should be done once

WEST HOUSTON MEDICAL CENTER
12141 RICHMOND AVENUE
HOUSTON, TEXAS 77082

LABOR AND DELIVERY ADMISSION ASSESSMENT

DATE	TIME	AGE	LMP	EDC	PARITY

ALLERGIES

PAST OB HX	YEAR	PLACE	MODE	GEST	WT.	SEX	OUTCOME	COMPLICATIONS
1st Preg								
2nd Preg								
3rd Preg								
4th Preg								
5th Preg								
6th Preg								

PRENATAL HX: Complications: ❑ PIH ❑ Gest DM ❑ Bleeding ❑ Infections
  Describe _____

MEDICAL PROBLEMS ❑ Yes ❑ No Describe _____

SURGERIES ❑ Yes ❑ No Describe _____

HOSPITALIZATIONS ❑ Yes ❑ No Describe _____

SEXUALLY TRANSMITTED DISEASES ❑ Yes ❑ No _____
DRUG ABUSE ❑ Yes ❑ No Type/Amount _____
SMOKE ❑ Yes ❑ No Amount _____ ALCOHOL ❑ Yes ❑ No Amount _____
ANTENATAL LABS: Blood Type _____ RPR _____ GC _____ PAP _____

PLANS FOR ANESTHESIA

Obstetrician: _____ ❑ Local ❑ Epidural
Pediatrician: _____ ❑ Other: _____

PRENATAL EDUCATION
❑ Prepared Childbirth
❑ C-Section Class
❑ Other: _____

PATIENT PLANS	PATIENT HAS
Room Preference:	❑ Vision Impairment
❑ Private	❑ Glasses
❑ Semi-Private	❑ Hearing Impairment
Early Discharge: ❑ N/A	❑ Prosthesis
❑ 24 hr. ❑ 48 hr. ❑ 36 hr.	❑ Dentures
❑ 72 hr. Post C/S	❑ Contacts
❑ Other: _____	❑ Sent Home
Person Present For birth _____	❑ Kept With Patient
Feeding: ❑ Breast ❑ Bottle	Language Spoken
❑ Post Partum BTL	
❑ Circumcision	

DATE	TIME	DATE	TIME	DATE	TIME

MODE OF TRANSPORT	MODE OF TRANSPORT	MODE OF TRANSPORT
T- P- R- BP-	T- P- R- BP-	T- P- R- BP-
FHR —┼— EGA	FHR —┼— EGA	FHR —┼— EGA
CHIEF COMPLAINT	CHIEF COMPLAINT	CHIEF COMPLAINT

CONTRACTIONS	TIME OF ONSET	CONTRACTIONS	TIME OF ONSET	CONTRACTIONS	TIME OF ONSET

MEDICATIONS PRESENTLY TAKING	MEDICATIONS PRESENTLY TAKING	MEDICATIONS PRESENTLY TAKING
URINE Protein _____ Ketones: _____ Glucose _____	URINE Protein _____ Ketones: _____ Glucose _____	URINE Protein _____ Ketones: _____ Glucose _____
LAST ORAL INTAKE (TIME) Fluids _____ Solids _____	LAST ORAL INTAKE (TIME) Fluids _____ Solids _____	LAST ORAL INTAKE (TIME) Fluids _____ Solids _____
CURRENT WEIGHT	CURRENT WEIGHT	CURRENT WEIGHT
CERVIX Dil _____ Eff _____ Station _____ Position _____ Examiner _____	CERVIX Dil _____ Eff _____ Station _____ Position _____ Examiner _____	CERVIX Dil _____ Eff _____ Station _____ Position _____ Examiner _____
MEMBRANES ❑ Intact ❑ Ruptured Fern: ❑ Pos ❑ Neg ❑ NA Nitrazine: ❑ Pos ❑ Neg ❑ NA	MEMBRANES ❑ Intact ❑ Ruptured Fern: ❑ Pos ❑ Neg ❑ NA Nitrazine: ❑ Pos ❑ Neg ❑ NA	MEMBRANES ❑ Intact ❑ Ruptured Fern: ❑ Pos ❑ Neg ❑ NA Nitrazine: ❑ Pos ❑ Neg ❑ NA
VAGINAL BLEEDING ❑ None ❑ Show	VAGINAL BLEEDING ❑ None ❑ Show	VAGINAL BLEEDING ❑ None ❑ Show
R.N. SIGNATURE	R.N. SIGNATURE	R.N. SIGNATURE

Figure 10-2 Labor and delivery admission assessment. (Courtesy West Houston Medical Center, Houston, Texas.)

Box 10-2

Documentation Guidelines for the Patient in Labor

- Maternal bladder status and voiding at least every 3 hours
- Cervical status (e.g., dilation, effacement, consistency)
- Fetal position, station, molding, caput
- Character and amount of bloody show (mucous discharge) and vaginal bleeding
- Intake and output
- Maternal affect and response to labor
- Level of maternal discomfort
- Effectiveness of pain management and pain relief measures
- Labor support person's abilities
- Valsalva efforts

every 30 minutes, and once every 15 minutes in a high-risk patient. The flowsheet should reflect the nursing process at all times. An abnormal assessment in one area should trigger further evaluation. For example, if the nurse checks the patient's blood pressure and it is documented as elevated (e.g., 160/100) on the flowsheet, the nursing process would appear as illustrated in Figure 10-4, p. 159.

The corresponding narrative notes may appear as follows:

1240 hours: BP↑, repositioned to left side. Dr. Smith informed of patient's status per flowsheet. Orders received. (These would be reflected on the physician's orders.) Plan of care explained to patient and significant other, verbalizes understanding.—N. Nurse, RN.

1255 hours: BP↓, maintained on left side, on-going assessments continue. Blood drawn by lab tech for Chem 22. Darkened, quiet environment provided.—N. Nurse, RN.

If the flowsheet being used does not reflect all the assessment parameters, the narrative notes should be used. The flowsheet should ideally allow for a concise, accurate, time-saving method of documentation. If the flowsheet is deficient in this respect, consideration should be given to improving the forms to better incorporate all the necessary information (AWHONN, 1996). However, be careful to keep the forms user-friendly. If the forms require manuals to explain their use, a third-party reviewer will most likely be unable to develop a true picture of the patient's clinical course. If a jury were ever required to review these records in a medical malpractice case, the nurse defendant would need to explain how the information is all included. As the record reflects the patient's "story" unfolding, the jury will have a clear picture of the nursing process and how it reflects the standard of care.

The following is an example of the nursing process reflected in the nurse's notes:

Scenario: The patient is dilated 4 cm, contractions every 3 minutes, and receiving Pitocin at 8 mU/min. The electronic fetal monitor shows decelerations down to 70 beats per minute, lasting 30 seconds, having no relationship to contractions.

Documentation: FHR ↓ 70 × 30 sec., not related to UA: episodic variable decelerations. Patient turned to left side. No further variable decelerations noted. Dr. Smith informed of variable decelerations and response with position change. Continue to observe. FHR BL 120-130, ave. LTV, STV+, spont. accel. ↑ 155 × 20 sec.—N. Nurse, RN

The nursing documentation reflects an ongoing care plan, assessments, interventions, and evaluation.

Lack of documentation may be inferred as a lack of the required clinical skills. Nurses are legally accountable for their practice. The following is an actual case example that illustrates this point:

A patient's blood pressure on admission to L&D was 140/100, and no urinalysis was obtained. Her blood pressure was not rechecked for another 6 hours. At delivery, her blood pressure was still elevated, but it was not taken for another 10 hours, when it was found to be 192/110. No further action was taken, and 5 hours later, the patient began to have seizures. Although medical care was obtained, the patient died about 24 hours later. In the subsequent lawsuit the court found that the obstetrical nurses should have acted, "because a reasonably prudent obstetric nurse should recognize the signs of preeclampsia, should know the importance of checking and recording vital signs regularly, and should generally know how to manage the patient" (Chagnon, Easterwood, 1986).

Also consider the following example:

A woman who was observed to be gravida 2 para 1 was admitted in active labor. Her first child was delivered by cesarean birth because of cephalopelvic disproportion (CPD). On this occasion her labor was allegedly monitored for 5 hours by licensed practical nurse (LPN) who did not understand the progress of labor and did not recognize that the baby was in fetal distress. The heart rate of the fetus subsequently dropped precipitously, and an emergency cesarean birth was performed. The apgar scores were low, and the infant's deficits include cerebral palsy and severe mental retardation. A settlement was made for $1,000,000 (Laska, 1997j).

"A chart is the witness that never dies and never lies" (Chagnon, Easterwood 1986, p. 308). Nursing documentation must show that the standard of care was met and that the nurse followed the appropriate institutional policies and procedures. Documentation and communication of observations are important defenses against litigation (Eganhouse, 1991).

The following case involves a patient with a preterm gestation at 28 weeks and a history of pinkish discharge and cramping:

A fetal monitor was not ordered, but the nurse was instructed to observe and notify the doctor of any change in bleeding or cramping. The woman started labor that

TABLE 10-2 Documentation of Obstetrical Events

Event	Documentation
Abruptio placenta	Identify risk factors; complaints of uterine pain, tenderness, irratability, tone, rigidity; vaginal bleeding; systematic review of the tracing; signs of fetal well-being; interventions and evaluations (AWHONN, 1996).
Amnioinfusion	Document time of intrauterine pressure catheter (IUPC) insertion, person inserting, zeroing times; resting tone, baseline; type of fluid used for amnioinfusion; use of blood or fluid warmer (if applicable); bolus initiation time, amount, completion time; continuous maintenance infusion initiation time, rate, and completion time; perineal care or underpads changed; fetal response; changes in the FHR pattern and uterine activity pattern following amnioinfusion; changes in meconium consistency (if applicable), fluid color, amount, odor every 30 minutes; uterine activity assessments; uterine resting tone every 30 minutes; any interventions; total volume infused every 8 hours; patient teaching and support; communications with physician or midwife (Murray, 1997; Simpson and Creehan, 1996).
Brethine (terbutaline sulfate)	Record informed consent; maternal pulse, ECG, blood pressure before administration; explanation of side effects; patient's response to medication and any side effects; frequent pulse, vital signs per institution's protocol and before subsequent dosage; systematic review of tracing with indications of fetal well-being; strict intake and output; breath sounds; maternal position, activity; and patient teaching and support.
Cervical ripening agents	Record informed consent; vital signs; cervical examination; risk factors; indication; estimated gestational age; uterine activity, tone, contractions, irritability; fetal status included in systematic review of the tracing; indications of fetal well-being; person inserting agent; explanation to patient; and response to procedure.
Cord blood gases	Chart time drawn, source, time samples went to lab, results (Murray, 1997), and person who drew the sample.
Diabetes	Document diabetic history of patient; method of treatment and control; fetal surveillance; systematic review of tracing, indicating signs of fetal well-being; urine glucose and blood levels as appropriate estimated fetal weight (EFW).
Epidural anesthesia/analgesia	Record hemoglobin and hematocrit results; bolus amount; time procedure began; time of test dose; time medication administered; time procedure completed; initiation of continuous infusion pump (if applicable); person performing procedure; patient teaching; informed consent; tolerance of procedure; systematic review of EFM tracing before and after procedure; blood pressure, pulse, and FHR before procedure; vital signs and FHR per institution protocol (e.g., every 5 minutes × 30 minutes, then every 15 minutes upon completion of procedure), patient response (e.g., pain relief); position of patient during and after procedure; use of hip rolls; any adverse outcome; intervention; and evaluation of effectiveness in detail. Also record status of bladder (NAACOG, 1993).
Fetal scalp electrode (FSE)	Document time FSE was inserted; person inserting FSE, fetal heart rate before and after insertion; patient teaching.
HELLP (hemolysis elevated liver low platelets) syndrome	Assessments and documentation are the same as for pregnancy induced hypertension (PIH) (AWHONN, 1996).
Induction/augmentation of labor	Evidence of fetal well-being should be documented before initiation of Pitocin (oxytocin). Record should reflect who the responsible physician is because he or she needs to be readily available (ACOG, 1997). Document blood pressure and FHR noted before all Pitocin increases; uterine contraction pattern and resting tone documented with no evidence of hyperstimulation. Document discontinuation of Pitocin for any adverse assessments; patient teaching and informed consent; amount of Pitocin/fluid type and amount and method of infusion, dosage increments in mU/min; strict intake and output, progress of labor, communications with physician, ongoing systematic review of EFM tracing, interventions, and evaluations.
Intrauterine pressure catheter (IUPC)	Document insertion time; person who performed insertion; time zeroed; maternal tolerance of procedure; uterine frequency, duration; peak intrauterine pressure; montevideo units (MVUs); resting tone on left side, right side, and in semi-Fowler's position (Murray, 1997).

Continued

TABLE 10-2 Documentation of Obstetrical Events—cont'd

Event	Documentation
Magnesium sulfate	Document per protocol to include dosage, concentration, delivery mode, maternal effect and tolerance; fetal effect with systematic review and assessments of fetal well-being; Deep tendon reflexes (DTRs), strict intake and output, breath sounds and respiratory rate; any complaints of chest pain, times for loading dose, maintenance dose initiation; explanation of side effects; and blood pressures (ACOG, 1994; Murray, 1997).
Malpresentations	Document exact position of fetus; cervical examination and diagnostic testing findings (e.g., ultrasound); systematic review of the tracing, including indicators of fetal well-being; status of membranes; presence of meconium; patient teaching and support; communications with physician; and interventions and evaluation.
Meconium	Record time meconium is first noted; systematic review of the tracing, notification of physician; consistency, color, odor, amount of meconium in fluid; and notification of nursery personnel.
Multiple gestation	Document uterine tone, irritability; positions of both fetuses; record BL rates for both twins; evaluation of fetal well-being for both twins; and maternal position, activity. Document on the tracing "twin A" and "twin B" from time to time; document locations of twins and their FHRs (Murray, 1997). Use the same criteria for triplets, quadruplets, . . . even septuplets.
Placenta previa	Document uterine tone, contractions, irritability; assessments of bleeding; pad counts, intake and ouput, maternal position, activity status, patient teaching and support, systematic review of the tracing, assessments of fetal well-being, interventions and evaluations.
Preeclampsia toxemia (PET)	Documentation should be the same as for PIH.
Pregnancy-induced hypertension (PIH)	Record blood pressure frequency as ordered or per institutional protocol; maternal position during blood pressure assessment; rollover test (if applicable); urine protein assessment; reflexes, clonus, headaches; visual disturbances; epigastric pain; intake and output; maternal position, weight, activity, edema, breath sounds; assessment of fetal well-being; communications with care provider; gestational age and fundal height; systematic review of tracing (NAACOG, 1993; AWHONN, 1996).
Preterm labor	Record presence and frequency of uterine contractions, activity, tone and irritability; risk factors; cervical status; vaginal discharge; communications with healthcare providers; fetal status through systematic review; notification of nursery personnel; patient teaching and support; reevaluation of gestational age (ACOG, 1994).
Rupture of membranes	Record date, time; spontaneous or artificial; color, consistency, quantity, odor; FHR before and immediately after rupture of membranes; notification of physician after membranes rupture; maternal temperature every 2 hours (Simpson, Creehan, 1996; Murray, 1997).
Trial of labor after cesarean (TOLAC)	Note rate of cervical dilation and fetal descent, being alert to abnormal progress; note any complaints of abdominal pain or referred pain (e.g., shoulder pain); record uterine activity assessments every 15 minutes and prn, including resting tone; note any uterine hypertonus; document interventions and evaluations; and continued ongoing assessments.
Vaginal birth after cesarean (VBAC)	Document whether uterine exploration was done; fundal consistency; position; amount of lochia; patient's complaints of pain.

Data from ACOG: *Precis V: an update in obstetrics and gynecology,* Washington DC, 1994, Author; AWHONN: *Standards and guidelines for professional nursing practice in the care of women and newborns,* ed 5, Washington DC, 1998, The Association; Murray M: *Antepartal and intrapartal fetal monitoring,* ed 2, Albuquerque, 1997, Learning Resources International; NAACOG: *Core curriculum for maternal-newborn nursing,* Philadelphia, 1993, WB Saunders; and Simpson K, Creehan PA: *AWHONN's perinatal nursing,* Philadelphia, 1996, JB Lippincott.

evening, and the cramps became worse about 2 hours later. The doctor was soon called, but he did not come to the hospital. Instead, he instructed the nurse to call when the contractions were 5 minutes apart. The doctor was called ½ hour later because the contractions were 5 minutes apart. He arrived at the hospital ½ hour after this, and the patient's cervix was dilated 4 cm. Tocolysis was then ordered. Labor progressed until the cervix was dilated 5 cm, tocolytics were stopped, and a cesarean section was performed. Apgar levels were 1 at 1 minute and 6 at 5 minutes. The child suffered from RDS, apnea, and mild retrolental fibroplasia. The plaintiff claimed that the nurse had failed to properly notify the physician of a change in the mother's condition, and that the doctor had failed to order proper monitoring and to begin tocolytic therapy in a timely manner. A jury awarded a $13,639,000 verdict (Laska, 1997e).

Text continued on p. 159

DATE: _____ PATIENT: _____

VITAL SIGNS				FETAL HEART RATE							UTERINE CONTRACTIONS					OTHER		OB	
TIME	TEMPERATURE	B.P.	PULSE / RESP.	MONITOR MODE	BASELINE	LTV / STV	ACCELERATION	DECELERATION	DESCRIPTION	INTERPRETATION	MONITOR MODE	FREQUENCY	DURATION	INTENSITY	RESTING TONE	MATERNAL POSITION	MATERNAL ACTIVITY	DILATION	EFFACEMENT

Figure 10-3 Labor and delivery flowsheet. (Courtesy West Houston Medical Center, Houston, Texas.)

Continued

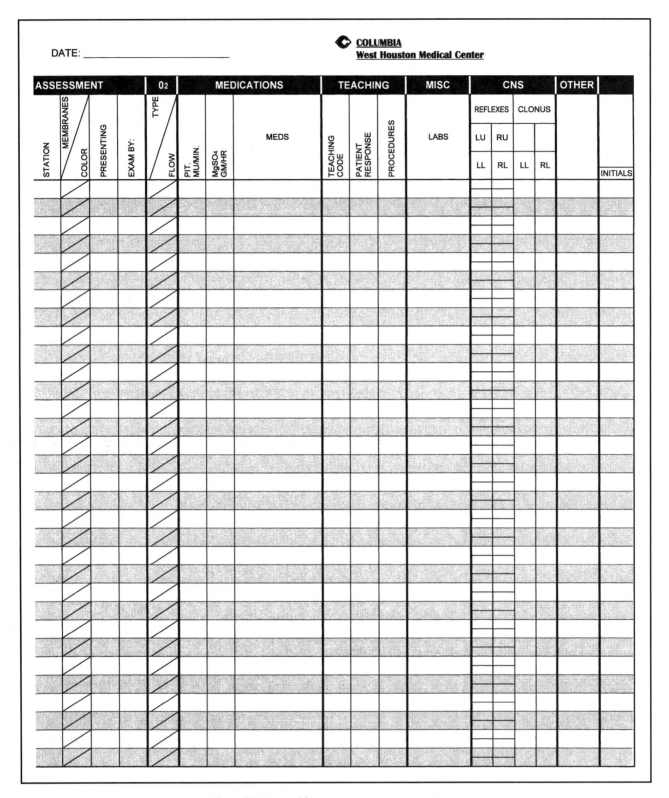

Figure 10-3, cont'd   Labor and delivery flowsheet.

MATERNAL ACTIVITY CODES

SQ	- Squatting
P	- Pushing
RC	- Rocking Chair
AMB	- Ambulatory
ST	- Sitting
B	- In Bed
SL	- Sleeping
BRP	- Bathroom Privileges

STANDARDS OF CARE

ACTIVE LABOR

1st STAGE

*1. BP, P, R $\bar{q}$ 1 - FHR evaluated $\bar{q}$ 15-30 minutes

2. Temp. $\bar{q}$ 2 $\bar{c}$ ruptured BOW
   Temp. q 4 c intact BOW

2nd STAGE

*1. FHR evaluated $\bar{q}$ 5 min. until delivery

2. BP, P $\bar{q}$ 15 min.

INDUCTION/AUGMENTATION (PITOCIN)

*1. BP, P, R $\bar{q}$ 60 min.

2. FHR eval. $\bar{q}$ 15 min.

3. Temp. as in Active Labor

PREG. INDUCED HYPERTENSION IN LABOR

*1. BP, P, R $\bar{q}$ 15 min. until stable, then $\bar{q}$ 30-60 min.

2. Reflexes hourly.

---

3. Albumin check $\bar{q}$ void.

4. Hourly urine output if MgSO4 infusing, otherwise $\bar{q}$ shift.

TERBUTALINE

1. BP, P, R & FHR $\bar{q}$ 5 min. x 3, then $\bar{q}$ 30 min. until required dose is reached, then $\bar{q}$ 1 hr. (HOLD MHR>120; FHR >170)

2. Assess breath sounds when counting respirations.

3. Strict I & O.

MgSO4

*1. BP, P, R $\bar{q}$ 5 min. during loading dose, then $\bar{q}$ 15 min. until stable, then 1q 30-60 min.

2. Strict I & O.

3. Reflexes/clonus $\bar{q}$ 1 hour.

ACTIVE LABOR/LOW RISK

1st STAGE

*1. BP, P, R, $\bar{q}$ 1 hr. - FHR evaluated q 30 minutes.

2. Temp. (same as High Risk)

2nd STAGE

1. BP, P, R & FHR $\bar{q}$ 15 min.

TEACHING CODES

1. Orient to Room
2. Orient to L/D
3. Fetal Heart Monitoring
4. Plan of Care
5. Breathing/Relaxing
6. Positions of Labor
7. Analgesia

---

8. Anesthesia
9. Medications
10. Induction/Augmentation
11. Positions for Pushing
12. Postpartum Care
13. Breastfeeding
14. Bottlefeeding
15. Newborn Care (immed.)
16. Transfer
17. Discharge
18. NCST/BSST/OCT
19. Ultrasound
20. Labor Warnings
21. Meconium
22. Preterm Labor
23. Diabetes
24. IUFD
25. Chronic HTN
26. PIH
27. Nursery Orientation
28. Cesarean Birth
29. Pre-op
30. Post-op
31. Ambulation with Intermittent Monitoring
32. Telemetry
32. Stages of Labor
33. Hydration

RESPONSES

V	- Verbalizes Understanding
R	- Reinforcement Needed
*	- See Nursing Notes
D	- Demonstrates

PROCEDURES

40. Doppler
41. Sterile Speculum Exam
42. Cultures

---

43. Sterile Vag Exam
44. Permits
45. Prep
46. Enema
47. Shower
48. Ultrasound
49. Ext. Monitors
50. AROM
51. SROM
52. FSE
53. IUPC
54. Catheterization
55. Medication
56. Epidural
57. Epidural Reinject
58. Fluid Bolus
59. C.V.P.
60. BSST
61. NST
62. OCT
63. ECV
64. Prostin
65. Amnio
66. Bed Bath/Linen Change
67. Amnioinfusion
68. Induction-Pit IOU/Pla 1000cc
69. Augmentation-Pit IOU/Pla 1000cc
70. Jacuzzi
71. Report to M.D.
72. Orders Received & Noted
73. M.D.'s Visit
74. Cord Gases
75. IUPC Zero Flush
76. Stirrups
77. Pedi Notified
78. Scalp Stimulation
79.
80.

ASSESSMENT CODES

UTERINE CONTRACTIONS

Monitor Mode

T	- Tocodynamometer
IUPC	- Intrauterine Pressure Catheter
P	- Palpated

Intensity

MI	- Mild
M	- Moderate
F	- Firm
(IUPC)	- mmHg at peak

Resting Tone

| PS | - Palpated Soft |
| (IUPC) | - mmHg |

OB ASSESSMENT

Membranes

I	- Intact
IB	- Intact Bulging
AR	- Artificial Rupture
SR	- Spontaneous Rupture

Presenting

Vtx	- Vertex
Br	- Breech
T	- Transverse
U	- Undetermined

Fluid

C	- Clear
M1	- Thin Meconium
M2	- Moderate Meconium
M3	- Thick Meconium
NS	- None Seen
BL	- Bloody

FETAL HEART RATE

Monitor Mode

A	- Auscultation
U/S	- Ultrasound
FSE	- Fetal Scalp Electrode
STV	- Short Term Variability
Ab	- Absent (0-2 bpm)
M	- Minimal (3-5 bpm)
Mod	- Moderate (6-25 bpm)
Mk	- Marked (>25 bpm)
NA	- When Using External Mode
LTV	- Long Term Variability
P	- Present
Ab	- Absent

Acceleration

| + | - Present (15 bpm in baseline x 15 sec. duration) |
| Ø | - Absent |

Deceleration (Description in Notes)

E	- Early
MV	- Mild Variable
V	- Mod. Variable (<70 bpm)
L	- Late

Interpretation

R	- Reassuring
RR	- Reassuring, needs review
NR	- Non-reassuring*
*	- Requires documentation in Nursing Notes regarding description, interventions and evaluations.

EPIDURAL VITAL SIGNS

B/P, P, FHR $\bar{p}$ ea. test dose and loading dose:

$\bar{q}$ 1 min. x 5
$\bar{q}$ 5 min. x 3
$\bar{q}$ 15 min. x 3
q 30 until delivery.

OXYGEN

FIO2/Flow
  % O2 or Liters per minute

Type

n/c	- Nasal Cannula
M	- Mask
O	- Other (describe)

MATERNAL POSITION

R Lat	- Right Lateral
R T	- Right 45
L Lat	- Left Lateral
L T	- Left 45
S	- Supine
SF	- Semi Flowler's
HF	- High Flowler's
TR	- Trendlenburg
KC	- Knee Chest
L	- Lithotomy
SQ	- Squat

CNS

Reflexes

0	- Absent
1+	- Minimal
2+	- Normal
3+	- Greater Than Normal
4+	- Hyperactive, may exhibit clonus

Clonus
  # of beats counted

Other

E	- Epigastric Pain
H/A	- Headache
V	- Visual Disturbances
*	- See Nursing Notes

INIT.	SIGNATURE	TITLE	SHIFT

ADDRESSOGRAPH

Figure 10-3, cont'd Labor and delivery flowsheet. (Courtesy West Houston Medical Center, Houston, Texas.)

Continued

PATIENT NAME _____

ASSESSMENT SUMMARY	Date	Time			
✓ - yes, within normal limits					
—— - not applicable or not assessed					
NN - see nurses' notes/flow sheet	Initials				

SAFETY
Call bell in reach					
Bed in low position					
Siderails up (note "all" "Ø" or "# of rails up)					
Informed of Advanced Directives					

PSYCHO-SOCIAL
Understands, accepts situation, coping well with minimal anxiety					
Significant other is present, supportive					
Feels rested					

NEURO
Alert, oriented X 3, appropriate behavior, speech clear					
No weakness or c/o dizziness					
Denies headache or visual disturbances					
DTR's 1+ to 3+, no clonus					

INTEGUM-ENTARY
Skin color within patient's norm					
Skin warm and intact					
Mucous membranes moist, good skin turgor					

MUSCULO-SKELETAL
No joint swelling or pain					
Normal ROM of all joints					
No muscle weakness					

CARDIOVASCULAR
SBP ± 30mm Hg of early/pre-pregnancy value					
DBP ± 15mm Hg of early/pre-pregnancy value					
Skin warm and dry					
Skin pink. Peripheral pulses normal					
Afebrile					
Heart rate regular with no irregularities, 60-100BPM					
No c/o chest pain or discomfort					
No edema of extremities					
No facial or presacral edema					
Edema: 1+ = 0-¼", 2+ = ¼-½", 3+ ½-1"					
IV site(s): No puffiness, redness, or tenderness					
IV containers, tubing, sites, current per hospital policy					

RESPIR-ATORY
Breathing easily. Respirations regular, normal depth					
Respiratory rate 12-22/minute					
Lungs clear bilaterally w/good breath sounds to bases					
No rhinitis, nasal stuffiness or cough					

GI
Taking ≥ 50% of diet					
No nausea or vomiting					
No epigastric pain resistant to antacids					
No diarrhea or constipation. Last BM					

GU
Voiding without c/o difficulty or discomfort					
Foley catheter					
Urine clear, not dark. No strong odor					
≤ trace protein on urine dipstick, when appropriate					
Urine output ≥ 120cc/4hrs (estimated/measured)					

MISC.
Total fluid intake at least 2000cc/24hrs					
Maintaining fluid restriction of ≤ cc/24 hrs					
Intake and output appropriate					
Daily weight ± .5 lb of previous day (or ± .25kg)					
Labs reviewed, normal for pregnancy					

OB
No vaginal bleeding					
Uterus non-tender					
Fetus active					
Amniotic membranes intact					
Ruptured, fluid clear (note amount in NN periodically)					
Ruptured, no odor to fluid					

Membranes ruptured: ____ / ____ _____   **AROM / SROM**

NURSE'S NOTES

FREQUENT VITAL SIGNS

TIME	BP	P	TIME	BP	P	TIME	BP	P

ADDRESSOGRAPH   959-201-001 9/96

Figure 10-3, cont'd Labor and delivery flowsheet.

Flowsheet example		
Time	1240	1255
BP	160/100	138/84
Headache	∅	∅
Edema	1+/LE	1+/LE
Visual disturbances	∅	∅
DTRs	2-3+	2+
Clonus	∅	∅
Maternal position	SF, to LL	LL
Urine pro/gluc/ket	tr/N/N	-
Lab Work	/	Chem 22

Figure 10-4 Flowsheet example.

OBSTETRICAL NURSING LIABILITY

The following types of nursing negligence consistently appear in medical records of cases that come to litigation (Chagnon, Easterwood, 1986):

- Incomplete initial history and physical examination
- Failure to assess and take appropriate action
- Incomplete or inadequate documentation
- Failure to use or interpret fetal monitoring appropriately

The following case highlights an example of a failure to assess and take appropriate action in the interpretation of electronic fetal monitoring. The allegations included that the hospital staff knew or should have known of the likelihood of complications resulting from the onset of nonreassuring and ominous fetal heart rate tracings. This case was settled for $250,000.

> The patient, who was in the twenty-seventh week of gestation, was admitted for weight loss and other nutritional problems. A Doppler check of the FHR identified a deceleration. No other tests had been ordered for fetal well-being. Five hours later the mother was sent to L&D for nonstress test (NST) and observation. The strip was nonreactive and nonreassuring. A biophysical profile (BPP) was done later that evening and a score of 8 was assigned, but the physician believed that the amniotic fluid was low. Immediately after the BPP was done, several severe decelerations appeared and a sinusoidal pattern developed. Beat-to-beat variability disappeared around 12:45 AM, and the strip remained flat until delivery at 5:45 AM. A BPP had been performed at around 3:30 AM, and a biophysical profile score of 2 was assigned. The child was born with evidence of severe intracranial bleed and died later that day (Laska, 1997d).

Many more cases that illustrate the above areas of nursing negligence have been recorded in the literature. Avoidance of liability encompasses the following: documenting an assessment of a thorough initial history and physical assessment, appropriate practice of the nursing process through ongoing assessments, interventions and evaluations, documenting accurately and thoroughly, and proficiency in electronic fetal monitoring (EFM) interpretation.

DOCUMENTATION AND ELECTRONIC FETAL MONITORING

Documentation and EFM often promote lively discussions among L&D nurses because many different viewpoints are held on what, where, how, and when to document when using fetal monitoring. Documentation would not be complete or accurate if a failure to identify any component of the FHR pattern occurs. Bear in mind that malpractice suits often involve the interpretation of electronic fetal monitor strips (Eganhouse, 1991). Complete consensus on what nomenclature should be used and documented has not been reached in this country (Simpson, Creehan, 1996). The National Institute of Child Health and Human Development (NICHHD) has recently developed guidelines for the standardization of fetal monitoring terms. Because documentation is a form of communication, common nomenclature should be established among the members of the same perinatal healthcare team. This ensures that all members comprehend the meaning of patterns and appropriate standards of care are followed. Documentation, whether on the tracing or in the medical records, reflects the standard of care provided (Murray, 1997).

Documenting on the Fetal Monitor Tracing

When beginning electronic fetal monitoring, placing identifying information on the first page of the tracing is important. This would include the patient's name, medical record number, physician's name, and the date and time initiated. During monitoring, times should appear on the tracing, as well as events related to the patient's care. Refer to Box 10-3 for recommendations on what to document on the tracing.

Documentation on Fetal Monitoring Tracing

- Gravida, parity
- High-risk conditions
- Scalp or acoustic stimulation
- Purpose of monitoring (e.g., NST)
- Vital signs
- Medications
- Anesthesia/analgesia (beginning and ending times)
- Fetal movement
- Pushing
- Auscultated FHR
- Maternal heart rate
- Infant's gender
- Number of strip in series (e.g., 1, 2, . . .)
- Expected date of delivery (EDD)
- Monitor mode (i.e., external, internal)
- IV fluid bolus
- Status of membranes; time of rupture; amniotomy or spontaneous; color, amount, consistency, or odor of the fluid
- Maternal movements (e.g., turned to left side, out of bed [OOB] to bathroom, bedpan)
- Vaginal examinations (e.g., dilation, effacement, station, position, examiner)
- Delivery time
- Apgar score
- Other interventions that might affect the FHR or UA tracing (e.g., Foley catheter insertion, emesis, coughing, effluerage, maternal position)

Data from Murray M: *Antepartal and intrapartal fetal monitoring*, ed 2, Albuquerque, 1997, Learning Resources International; Eganhouse DJ: Electronic fetal monitoring: education and quality assurance, *JOGNN* pp 16-22, January/February 1991.

Attention should *not* be drawn to any part of the tracing, such as a deceleration, by circling, initialing, or in any way marking it. This could adversely affect objectivity in the review of the tracing and, in a retrospective study, appear to be damaging.

Writing only on the tracing does not satisfy documentation requirements necessary to meet standards recommended by the AWHONN, ACOG, and AAP, and it also would not meet requirements set forth by the Joint Commission for the Accreditation of Healthcare Organizations (JCAHO) and specific institutional policies and procedures. In emergency situations, nurses will depend on the tracing and will record many key events there. However, anything documented on the tracing must also be recorded in the medical record. No doubt, nurses will double chart at times, which is time consuming (Eganhouse, 1991; Murray, 1997).

The nurse's notes or flowsheet must illustrate the interpretation of the actual fetal monitor tracing. Instances have occurred in which tracings could not be found. (The loss of tracings is invariably viewed with suspicion by those involved in a lawsuit.) However, the record should describe the FHR and UA in such a manner that the tracing could actually be reproduced freehand from the description. Good documentation can tell the story, and it can discount the belief held by many that, if the strip is lost, so is the potential medical malpractice suit. Accurate documentation is the best defense for the nurse to demonstrate that a strip was used.

Many L&D nurses have been instructed to place their initials on the strip at regular intervals. However, current literature disagrees with this premise. "Placing one's initials on the strip only reflects one's ability to write one's initials" (Murray, 1997, p. 13). Some have argued that initialing the tracing does not prove the nurse's presence at the bedside, and it does not reflect assessments or care given (i.e., the nursing process). This action does not prove the nurse or physician actually analyzed the tracing. The flowsheet and narrative notes are the place where it is important to record data, and they are better places for initialing.

Documenting the Interpretation of the Electronic Fetal Monitor Tracing

Nurses are accountable for documenting the FHR, the contraction data, and the actions taken when changes occur in the FHR (Murray, 1997). The appropriate utilization of a comprehensive flowsheet can accurately reflect the interpretation of the fetal monitor tracing.

Uterine Activity

Uterine activity should be documented according to the mode of monitoring (e.g., palpation [abbreviated as "P"], external transducer [abbreviated as "ext," "e," or "toco"], or intrauterine pressure catheter [abbreviated as "IUPC" or "int"]). The labor flowsheet should define the abbreviations to be used on the form. Even with the use of EFM, palpation of uterine resting tone is an important parameter that should be documented periodically. The uterine resting tone is assessed in the absence of contractions (AWHONN, 1996, p. 211). The usual manner would be to record the uterus as either "soft" or "firm" between contractions. "Rigid" has also been utilized (Simpson, Creehan, 1996). Palpated contractions are usually recorded as mild, moderate, or strong. Symbols have also been utilized (e.g., +, ++, +++). Whatever method is used should be defined on the flowsheet and used universally in that unit. An example of documentation of uterine contraction activity using a labor flowsheet is given in Figure 10-5.

Documenting the Fetal Heart Rate

The systematic review of the fetal monitor tracing has to encompass both the UA and FHR. Specifics related to the FHR include the BL, assessment of variability, periodic or episodic patterns, other decelerations, and accelerations. Any abnormalities, such as a fetal heart rate arrhythmia, would need to be described in detail.

Uterine Contraction Documentation		
Mode	ext	IUPC
Frequency	2-3	2-2½
Duration	50-60	55-65
Intensity	mod	65-75 mm HG*
Resting tone	soft (P)	5 mm Hg
MVU†	-	260

Figure 10-5 Uterine contraction documentation. *When using an IUPC, uterine tone is documented in terms of mm Hg of intramniotic pressure (AWHONN, 1996, p. 211). †Calculation of MVUs is done by subtracting the resting tone from the peak IUP and then adding these values for all the contractions in a 10-minute period. The sum total equals the MVUs for that point in time.

Fetal Heart Rate Documentation		
Mode	ext	int
Baseline	125-135	130-140
LTV	ave.	ave.
Decels	∅	variables
Accelerations	+	+
Pattern	reassuring	compensatory

Figure 10-6 Fetal heart rate documentation.

An example of the use of a flowsheet in recording the FHR appears in Figure 10-6. The narrative note would describe the variable deceleration (e.g., "var. decel. ↓ 100 × 30 seconds with contraction. Spontaneous accel. noted ↑ 150 × 25 seconds with return to 140 BL with average variability. Turned to right side. Dr. Jones informed of FHR pattern, will continue to observe at this time. —N. Nurse, RN.").

Appropriate intervention (e.g., the position change) would need to be recorded, as well as its effect, with evidence of ongoing assessment.

Documenting signs of fetal well-being is imperative (Murray, 1997); this includes reports of fetal movement or palpated movement. When EFM is in progress, document the presence of FHR accelerations, including the duration and height of the largest acceleration (Murray, 1997). When a change in the FHR has been noted, documenting a subsequent return to reassuring findings is important. The ACOG and AAP guidelines (1997) recommend using terms that describe the FHR patterns (e.g., early, late, variable decelerations, accelerations, and beat-to-beat variability) in chart entries as well as in verbal communications.

Standardization of terminology in interpretation of FHR patterns is needed. Toward this effort, the National Institute of Child Health and Human Development (NICHHD) Research Planning Workshop met between May 1995 and November 1996 to develop standardized and unambiguous definitions for FHR tracings. Many nurses believed that a major impediment to progress in the evaluation and investigation of FHR monitoring was the lack of agreement in definitions and nomenclature for FHR patterns, despite

the large number of publications on the subject (NICHHD Research Planning Workshop, 1997). The patterns to be defined are categorized as either baseline, periodic, or episodic. Periodic patterns are patterns associated with uterine contractions, and episodic patterns are those patterns not associated with uterine contractions. Periodic patterns are distinguished by wave form, currently accepted as abrupt (versus gradual) onset of the deceleration (NICHHD Research Planning Workshop, 1997).

An important determination resulting from the NICHHD workshop is that no distinction is made between short-term variability (or beat-to-beat variability) and long-term variability, because in actual practice they are visually determined as a unit. With the exception of the sinusoidal pattern, the definition of variability is based visually on the amplitude of the complexes (NICHHD Research Planning Workshop, 1997).

The NICHHD reports that good evidence exists that many characteristics of FHR patterns are gestational age-dependent, so gestational age must be considered in the full description of the pattern. They also indicate that any FHR pattern must be evaluated in the context of the maternal medical condition, previous results of fetal assessment, medications, and other factors. The individual components of the FHR patterns do not occur alone and generally evolve over time. The NICHHD therefore supports the idea that a full description of an FHR tracing requires a qualitative and quantitative description of the BL rate; BL FHR variability; the presence of accelerations, or periodic or episodic decelerations; and changes or trends in the FHR patterns over time (NICHHD Research Planning Workshop, 1997).

Fetal Heart Rate Baseline

The FHR baseline is defined by the NICHHD as the approximate mean FHR rounded to increments of 5 beats

TABLE 10-3 NICHHD FHR Variability Classification

Amplitude Range	Variability
Undetectable	Absent
>Undetectable but ≤5 bpm	Minimal
6-25 bpm	Moderate
>25 bpm	Marked

per minute (bpm) during a 10-minute segment. This would exclude any periodic or episodic changes, as well as periods of marked (or greater than 25 bpm) variability. Evaluation of baseline should be done in 10-minute windows, with the minimum baseline duration being at least 2 minutes, or the baseline for that period would be indeterminate (NICHHD Research Planning Workshop, 1997). Variability is a characteristic of the FHR baseline (Murray, 1997; AWHONN, 1996). Variability categorization should be defined on the L&D flow chart. The current practice is to separately record both short-term variability (STV) and long-term variability (LTV) (Murray, 1997). However, the NICHHD standardization may become recognized as the standard in the obstetrical community. Baseline variability was defined as fluctuations in the baseline FHR of 2 cycles per minute or greater with irregular amplitude and frequency. They are visually quantified as the amplitude of the peak-to-trough, measured in bpm. Table 10-3 provides the NICHHD definition of ranges for documenting FHR variability.

Short-Term Variability. Individual institutions may still utilize the differentiation between short- and long-term variability. Electronic fetal monitoring technology has advanced over the years. However, first-generation monitors exaggerated FHR variability when a US transducer was used (Murray, 1997). As a result, nurses were taught that STV cannot be assessed when recording the FHR with a US transducer. Murray (1997) asserts that even if the STV could not be visually assessed, it could have been conceptually present; therefore it should still be documented as being present. When a spiral electrode is in use, one can visually assess the baseline. The STV would appear bumpy, rough, or "grass-like" (Murray, 1997). When using an external US transducer, STV is conceptually present only when the baseline is stable, appearance chaotic, and a reactive acceleration is present. Short-term variability can be then documented as "+" (present). The STV can be documented as absent when monitoring with either a spiral electrode or a US transducer. Labor and delivery nurses are familiar with the phrase "If it looks bad on external, it's worse on internal" (Murray, 1997). With absent STV, the FHR baseline will be flat (or almost flat). The FHR could also exhibit a sinusoidal or wandering baseline, and no accelerations would be present. Beat-to-beat variability (BTBV) and STV

are sometimes used interchangeably, although STV should not be recorded as BTBV. The BTBV is the difference in time intervals between consecutive heartbeats. The STV is actually calculated from the BTBV (Murray, 1997).

Long-Term Variability. Long-term variability has been defined as "the fluctuation of the FHR around the baseline mean over the course of 1 minute (Murray, 1997). Whereas STV is recorded as either present or absent, LTV is documented according to the identification of the amplitude of these fluctuations. Terminology includes the following: absent (0 to 2 bpm), minimal or decreased (3 to 5 bpm), average (6 to 10 bpm), moderate or average (11 to 25 bpm), and marked or increased (greater than 25 bpm). (Simpson, Creehan, 1996). The L&D flowsheet needs to define the classification system to be used in documenting variability.

Accelerations

The NICHHD has defined acceleration as a visually apparent, abrupt increase in the FHR above the baseline. (Abrupt is defined as the onset of acceleration to peak in less than 30 seconds.) The peak (acme) of the acceleration is greater than or equal to 15 bpm above the baseline, the length of the acceleration is greater than or equal to 15 seconds, and the time from the onset to the return to the baseline is less than 2 minutes. In preterm gestation before 32 weeks, the NICHHD considers an acceleration to have an acme of greater than or equal to 10 bpm above the baseline and have a duration of greater than or equal to 10 seconds. A prolonged acceleration is greater than or equal to 2 minutes, but less than 10 minutes in duration. An acceleration that lasts for 10 minutes or longer is described as a baseline change (NICHHD Research Planning Workshop, 1997).

Most L&D flowsheets should have room to note the presence or absence of accelerations. The acceleration should be identified as either spontaneous or uniform (periodic). Other criteria for documenting the acceleration include the baseline and the length of the acceleration before returning to the baseline (e.g., BL 140-150 bpm, spontaneous acceleration ↑ 160 × 25 seconds).

Decelerations

Decelerations should be identified when documenting in the nurses notes or flowsheet based on their recognition criteria (Murray, 1997). Examples of decelerations, recognition criteria, and charting are provided in Table 10-4. Other types of abnormal FHR decelerations (e.g., spontaneous deceleration, prolonged deceleration) should be documented in descriptive terms and described in relation to the uterine activity. A prolonged deceleration has been described by the NICHHD as a decrease from the baseline that is greater than or equal to 15 bpm, lasting 2 minutes or less, but greater than 10 minutes from onset to the return to baseline. A prolonged deceleration that lasts 10 minutes or longer is considered a change in baseline. Decelerations are documented as recurring if they occur in conjunction with 50%

TABLE 10-4 Documenting Early, Late, and Variable Decelerations

Type	Recognition Criteria*	Recognition Criteria†	Document
Early	Gradual onset; nadir usually ≤18 seconds after the peak; gradual offset, usually is not greater than 25 bpm; duration similar to contractions; shape similar, uniform; stable BL; STV+, LTV+, accelerations+	Gradual decrease (defined as onset of deceleration to nadir that is ≥30 seconds) and return to baseline FHR associated with a uterine contraction; nadir of deceleration occurs simultaneously to the peak of contractions	Early deceleration; quantify the depth of the nadir in bpm below the BL and the duration in minutes and seconds from the beginning to the end of the deceleration
Late	Onset is after the ctx begins and reaches nadir in ≥30 seconds; peak to nadir lag time is >18 secs; nadir may reach a depth of 60 bpm; similar shape; BL may be bradycardic, tachycardic, or WNL; STV + to absent, LTV + to absent; acceleration may be present in fetus who is not acidotic	Gradual (defined as onset of deceleration to nadir that is ≥30 seconds) decrease and return to baseline FHR associated with a contraction; nadir of deceleration occurs after the peak of the contraction	Late decelerations; quantify the depth of the nadir in bpm below the BL and the duration in minutes and seconds from the beginning to the end of the deceleration
Variable	Abrupt onset; depth varies; shapes: U, V, or W; may have shoulder or overshoots	Visually apparent, abrupt decrease (defined as onset of deceleration to the beginning of nadir that is <30 seconds) in FHR below the baseline; decrease in FHR is ≥15 bpm, lasting ≥15 seconds, and <2 minutes from onset to return to baseline	Variable deceleration; quantify the depth of the nadir in bpm below the BL, and the duration in minutes and seconds from the beginning to the end of the deceleration; indicate if shoulders or overshoots are present

*Data from Murray M: *Antepartal and intrapartal fetal monitoring,* ed 2, Albuquerque, 1997, Learning Resources International.
†Data from NICHHD Research Planning Workshop: *JOGNN* 26(6):637, 1997.

or more of uterine contractions (NICHHD Research Planning Workshop, 1997).

L&D nurses should be able to recognize the different types of decelerations noted on the EFM tracing, and they should label them in their notes accordingly. If terminology such as mild, moderate or severe is used to describe variable decelerations, then hospital protocol, the chart form, or both should identify recognition criteria to maintain consistency. Otherwise document a description of the deceleration, including the BL, variability, duration, depth and return to BL, along with any "shoulders" or "overshoots" observed.

Sinusoidal

The two types of sinusoidal patterns are benign (pseudo, false) and pathologic (true). Nurses often do not label a benign pattern as sinusoidal in their nurses notes, but they should document a description of the rhythmic undulations and identify the etiology (e.g., after narcotic administration) (Murray, 1997). Pathologic patterns can either be described (e.g., BL 120-130, regular undulations with intermittent flat areas) or labeled as a sinusoidal pattern. Proficiency in interpretation of EFM tracings, including sinusoidal pattern

identification, should be validated and documented for all L&D nurses.

Interpretation of EFM Tracing

Once the nurse has performed the systematic review of the tracing, the interpretation is then documented as either reassuring, compensatory, nonreassuring, or ominous. Appropriate interventions (e.g., patient placed in lateral position, oxygen given via face mask at 10 L/min, IV fluid bolus given, physician notified, further evaluation made of fetal well-being) should be described in the nurses notes. Ongoing assessments and evaluation of patient outcomes needs to be documented. Documentation of communication should include who was told what and what their response was (Murray, 1997). Any lack of response should also be documented, as should the nurses' follow-up action and the initiation of the chain of command (if applicable).

Communication was an issue in the following case:

The patient was observed to be gravida 2 para 1, had previously undergone a cesarean section, and was given Pitocin (oxytocin) to speed up labor. The defendant doctor testified that after 11 hours of labor, a cesarean section was recommended, but the plaintiff declined. The plaintiff said no suggestion of a cesarean section was made. While labor continued, the defendant doctor went home. After he left, the fetal monitor strip, which had shown no problems up to that point, began to show periodic variable decelerations, and at one point the FHR dropped below 100 bpm for 5 minutes. The defendant doctor was called, and he prescribed medication. When the FHR continued to fall, he was called again. He rushed to the hospital and performed an immediate cesarean. At the time of delivery, the baby was found in the abdomen with a completely ruptured uterus and an 80% abruption. The child sustained permanent brain damage, including cerebral palsy and severe developmental delays. The parents sued the doctor and the hospital for not performing a cesarean section sooner. The doctor claimed that the nurse did not fully inform him of the decrease in the baby's FHR. The hospital claimed that he was fully informed. The jury verdict of $18.4 million was reduced to $4.5 million pursuant to state law (Laska, 1997i).

Documentation of the communication between the nurse and physician would be a vital component of this case; the assessments of the uterus during labor could be at issue as well.

After communicating a concern about an area of the patient's care to the physician, many times the nurse will not be comfortable with the physician's actions, or inactions, related to his or her concerns. If the physician and nurse cannot resolve their differences, and the nurse feels unable to carry out the physician's plan of care, the nurse should invoke the chain of command (Mahley, Beerman, 1998). In each care setting, the identified administrative chain of command should be clearly identified to help resolve conflicts involving the management of patients (Mahley, Beerman, 1998). The nurse's actions in this regard should be clearly documented. Many nurses do not want to write these occurrences in the record because they do not want to "point fingers." Even worse, the nurse could have a real fear of retribution from the physician or the institution itself. However, the nurse will be accountable for his or her own action or inaction and thus should do the right thing (Murray, 1997). The nurse must provide an accurate description of the course of the events that occurred. In the event of a lawsuit this documentation could be the cornerstone of the nurse's defense.

A primary area of conflict between physicians and nurses is the failure of physicians to respond to nurses' report of a nonreassuring FHR pattern (Mahley and Beerman, 1998). The nurse is still responsible for initiating intrauterine resuscitation in the presence of a nonreassuring tracing, and he or she should pursue further assistance regarding the inaction of the physician to her report. In a case described by Mahley and Beerman (1998) the nurses testified that they were unfamiliar with the chain of command policy. Furthermore, they believed that as long as the physician was aware of the FHR pattern, the nurse was no longer legally obligated to take action to protect the patient's safety. Invoking the chain of command can provide protection for the nurse against a claim of negligence. The nurse has a duty, independent of that of the physician, to protect patients from harm. The nurse expert who reviewed this case found that the nursing care contributed to the proximate cause of the outcome, and the hospital reached a settlement in favor of the plaintiff (Mahley, Beerman, 1998).

VAGINAL DELIVERY

Nursing documentation of a vaginal delivery should include information such as that illustrated in Figure 10-7. Other information that is often recorded includes the presence of a support person and evidence of the use of personal protection equipment. Any other occurrences that warrant further explanation should be described in detail in a narrative form. See Table 10-2 for some illustrations of information related to deliveries that require special consideration when documenting.

CESAREAN SECTION

Preoperative documentation should include full admission assessment, documentation of the EFM tracing, patient teaching, nothing by mouth (NPO) status, a record of intravenous fluids given, informed consent, the shave and other prep, Foley catheter insertion (include amount and color of the urine), medications that were ordered, transport mode, and the time the patient went to the operating room (OR) (Simpson, Creehan, 1996).

Intraoperative nursing documentation should reflect recommendations by Association of Operating Room Nurses (AORN) (AWHONN, 1998). Documentation should include the patient's position on the OR table (e.g., hip wedge in place) and results of any EFM, if applicable. The following information also should be noted (Simpson, Creehan, 1996):

- Abdominal preparation
- Skin condition before incision
- Grounding pad site
- Patient's emotional status
- Maternal vital signs
- Presence of support person
- FHR
- Sponge, needle, and instrument counts
- Maternal and newborn status before transfer to postanesthesia care unit (PACU)

POSTANESTHESIA CARE UNIT

Postanesthesia documentation needs to reflect recommendations by American Society of Postanesthesia Nurses (ASPAN) (AWHONN, 1998). Documentation in the record for patients in the obstetric PACU should be done according

※ Hollister

Labor and Delivery Summary
Hollister Maternal/Newborn Record System   **Page 1 of 2**
To order call: 1.800.323.4060   Re-order No **5712**

Labor Summary

G	T	Pt	A	L	Type and Rh	EDD
						/ /

Prenatal Events ☐ **None**
☐ No Prenatal Care
☐ Preterm Labor (≤ 37 Weeks)
☐ Postterm Labor (≥ 42 Weeks)
☐ Previous Cesarean
☐ Prenatal Complications
☐ _____

Intrapartal Events
Maternal
☐ Febrile (≥ 100.4°F/38°C)
☐ Bleeding—Site Undetermined
☐ Preeclampsia (mild) (severe)
☐ Seizure Activity
☐ Medications ☐ **None**

Date	Time	Medication	Dose	Route

☐ Transfusion _____ units
☐ Blood Component _____
☐ _____

Amniotic Fluid
☐ SROM ☐ AROM Date _____ Time _____
☐ Premature ROM ☐ Prolonged ROM
☐ Clear
☐ Meconium-Stained (describe) _____
☐ Bloody
☐ Foul Odor
  ☐ Cultures Sent _____ Time _____
☐ Polyhydramnios
☐ Oligohydramnios
☐ _____

Placenta
☐ Placenta Previa
☐ Abruptio Placenta
☐ _____

Labor
☐ Precipitous Labor (< 3 hrs)
☐ Prolonged Labor (≥ 20 hrs)
☐ Prolonged Latent Phase
☐ Prolonged Active Phase
☐ Prolonged 2nd Stage (> 2.5 hrs)
☐ Secondary Arrest of Dilatation
☐ Induction   ☐ **None**
  ☐ AROM   ☐ Oxytocin ☐ _____
☐ Augmentation   ☐ **None**
  ☐ AROM   ☐ Oxytocin ☐ _____

Labor Summary (Cont'd.)
Fetus
Gestational Age (Wks) _____ By Dates
                      _____ By Ultrasound

Presentation	**Position**

☐ Vertex
☐ Face/Brow
☐ Breech ☐ Frank   ☐ Complete
         ☐ Single Footling
         ☐ Double Footling
☐ Transverse Lie ☐ Back-up ☐ Back-Down
☐ Compound
☐ Unknown
☐ Cephalopelvic Disproportion (CPD)
☐ Cord Prolapse

Monitor ☐ **None**   FHR   UC
            External ☐   ☐
            Internal ☐   ☐
☐ STV ☐ Present ☐ Absent
☐ LTV _____
☐ Fetal Bradycardia
☐ Fetal Tachycardia
☐ Sinusoidal Pattern
☐ Accelerations ☐ Spont.   ☐ Uniform
☐ Decelerations ☐ Early   ☐ Late
               ☐ Variable ☐ Prolonged
☐ Scalp pH ≤7.2
☐ _____
FM Discontinued _____ Time _____
FHR Prior to Delivery _____ bpm Time _____

Delivery Data
Support Person Present ☐ Yes   ☐ No
Delivery Location
         ☐ LDR ☐ LDRP ☐ DR
         ☐ Birthing Room ☐ OR
         ☐ _____

Method of Delivery
☐ Vaginal ☐ VBAC
         Number Previous Cesareans _____
☐ Vertex
  ☐ Spontaneous
  ☐ Assisted [   ][   ] to [   ][   ]
  ☐ Manual Rotation
  ☐ Forceps (type _____)
     ☐ Outlet ☐ Low ☐ Mid
  ☐ Vacuum Extraction
☐ Breech (type _____)
  ☐ Spontaneous
  ☐ Partial Extraction (assisted)
  ☐ Total Extraction
  ☐ Forceps Assist
    ☐ Piper ☐ _____
☐ Cesarean
  ☐ Scheduled   ☐ Emergency
  ☐ Primary   ☐ Repeat (x _____)
  ☐ Other
Operative Indication
  ☐ Previous Uterine Surgery
  ☐ Failure to Progress

Method of Delivery (Cont'd.)
Operative Indication (Cont'd.)
☐ Placenta Previa
☐ Abruptio Placenta
☐ Fetal Malpresentation _____
☐ Non reassuring FHR Pattern _____
☐ Other _____
Uterine Incision
☐ Low Cervical, Transverse
☐ Low Cervical, Vertical
☐ Classical
Hysterectomy   ☐ No ☐ Yes
Tubal Ligation ☐ No ☐ Yes
Skin Incision
☐ Vertical
☐ Pfannenstiel

Episiotomy ☐ **None**
☐ Midline
☐ Mediolateral L R
Laceration/Episiotomy Extension ☐ **None**
☐ Periurethral
☐ Vaginal
☐ Cervical
☐ Uterine
☐ Perineal ☐ 1° ☐ 2° ☐ 3° ☐ 4°
Repair Agent Used _____

Placenta
☐ Spontaneous
☐ Expressed
☐ Manual Removal
☐ Adherent (type _____)
☐ Uterine Exploration
☐ Curettage
Configuration
☐ Normal
☐ Abnormal _____
Weight _____ gms
Disposition _____

Cord
☐ Nuchal Cord (x _____)
☐ True Knot Length _____ cms
☐ 2 Vessels
☐ 3 Vessels
Cord Blood ☐ To Lab ☐ Refrig ☐ Discard
Lab ☐ Type + Rh ☐ Cultures ☐ Coombs
    ☐ pH ☐ _____

Surgical Data
Sponge Counts Correct
☐ N/A ☐ Yes ☐ No _____
Needle Counts Correct
☐ N/A ☐ Yes ☐ No _____

                          Date
_____ Completed __/__/__
(Signature)

Figure 10-7 Labor and delivery summary. (Courtesy Hollister Incorporated, Libertyville, Ill.)

Continued

Hollister™

Labor and Delivery Summary
Hollister Maternal/Newborn Record System   **Page 2 of 2**
To order call: 1.800.323.4060   Re-order No **5712**

Delivery Data (Cont'd.)

Surgical Data (Cont'd.)
Vaginal Pack Count Correct
☐ N/A ☐ Yes ☐ No _____
Estimated Blood Loss _____ ccs

Delivery Anesthesia   ☐ **None**
☐ Local   ☐ Pudendal   ☐ General
☐ Epidural   ☐ Spinal

Date	Time	Medication	Dose	Effect

Complications ☐ **None**

Delivery Medications   ☐ **None**

Date	Time	Medication	Dose	Route Site	Init

Chronology

	Date	Time		
EDD				
Admit to Hospital				
Membranes Ruptured				
Onset of Labor		Total Time Hrs/Min		
Complete Cervical Dilatation			I	
Delivery of Infant			II	
Delivery of Placenta			III	
			Total Labor	

Infant Data   ☐ Male ☐ Female
ID/Band No. _____
Condition ☐ Alive
          ☐ Stillbirth   ☐ Antepartum
                         ☐ Intrapartum
          ☐ Neonatal Death
Birth Order _____ of 1 2 3 4
Repeat Apgar every 5 min until score ≥ 7

Apgar Score	1 min	5 min	10 min
Heart Rate			
Respiratory Effort			
Muscle Tone			
Reflex Irritability			
Color			
Total			

Scored by _____

Infant Data (Cont'd.)

Airway
☐ Bulb Suction
☐ Suction Catheter   Size _____ Fr
   ☐ Mouth   Pressure _____ mm Hg
   ☐ Nose   ☐ At Delivery
   ☐ Pharynx
☐ Endotracheal Tube Size _____ Fr
   ☐ Meconium Below Cords Times _____

Breathing
☐ Spontaneous
☐ O₂ _____ # Liters
   ☐ Free Flow   Time Init. _____
   ☐ PPV
      ☐ Bag/Mask   Time Init. _____
      ☐ ET Tube Size _____ Fr Time Init. _____
      ☐ CPAP _____ mm
_____ minutes to First Gasp
_____ minutes to Sustained Respiration

Circulation
☐ Spontaneous
☐ External Cardiac Massage
   Time Initiated _____ Time Completed _____
   _____ minutes for HR>100
   Heart Rate (bpm)
      _____ Time _____
      _____ Time _____
      _____ Time _____

IV Access
☐ Umbilical Catheter
☐ Peripheral Line
Person Managing Resuscitation:
_____

Neonatal Medications ☐ **None**

Date	Time	Medication	Dose	Route Site	Init

Lab Data ☐ None   Time _____

Blood Gases	Sent	Umb Art	Umb Vein
pH			
pO₂			
pCO₂			
HCO₃			

Test	Result
Dextrostix	

Initial Newborn Exam
Weight _____ gms _____ lbs _____ ozs   ☐ Deferred
Length _____ cms _____ ins   ☐ Deferred
Head _____ cms _____ ins   ☐ Deferred
Chest _____ cms _____ ins   ☐ Deferred
Abdomen _____ cms _____ ins   ☐ Deferred
Temp _____ ☐ Rectal ☐ Axillary
AP _____ Resp _____ BP _____
☐ No Observed Abnormalities

Initial Newborn Exam (Cont'd.)
☐ Abnormalities Noted
☐ Meconium Staining   ☐ Cephalhematoma
☐ Petechiae   ☐ Other
Describe _____
_____

Intake ☐ **None**
   Breast Fed ☐ Yes ☐ No
Output ☐ **None**
   ☐ Urine ☐ Stool (type _____)
   ☐ Gastric Aspirate _____ ccs
Examined By _____
Transfer   ☐ With Mother
           ☐ To Newborn Nursery
           ☐ To NICU
           ☐ _____
Date ___/___/___ Time _____
Mode of Transport _____

Delivery Personnel
RN (1) _____
   (2) _____
Anesthesiologist/CRNA _____
CNM _____
Physician—Attending _____
Physician—Assist (1) _____
            (2) _____
Pediatric Provider _____
   ☐ Notified   ☐ Present at Birth
Remarks _____

_____ Date
(Signature)   Completed ___/___/___

Figure 10-7, cont'd   Labor and delivery summary. (Courtesy Hollister Incorporated, Libertyville, Ill.)

Box 10-4
Documentation Guidelines for the PACU

- Rate, quality, and depth of respirations
- Breath sounds
- Oxygen saturation via pulse oximetry
- Blood pressure
- Pulse and ECG findings, if applicable
- Skin color and condition
- Orientation
- Response to verbal, tactile, and painful stimulation
- Uterine fundus and contraction (involution)
- Abdominal dressing
- Bladder status
- Lochia (i.e., amount, color, type, odor)
- Maternal-newborn attachment
- Condition of the maternal breasts
- Breast-feeding, if applicable
- Intake and output
- Perineal condition
- Pain and comfort levels (e.g., patient's desires, medications given, effect of medication)

Data from Simpson K, Creehan PA: *AWHONN's perinatal nursing,* Philadelphia, 1996, JB Lippincott.

to the institution's PACU policies and procedures, and it should include the information in Box 10-4.

POSTPARTUM DOCUMENTATION

Documentation in the postpartum period also encompasses the area of clinical assessment, nursing diagnosis, interventions, and evaluation. The focus during the postpartum period is on the physiological and physical changes that return the woman's body to a nonpregnant state of function (NAACOG, 1993). Health education is a vital component during this period, as are psychosocial assessment, support, and intervention.

The AWHONN recommends that postpartum checks be done every 15 minutes for the first hour, every 30 minutes for the second hour, and then every 4 hours for the first 24 hours. More frequent assessments should be performed if indicated (Simpson, Creehan, 1996). After 24 hours, assessments can be made every 8 hours (NAACOG, 1993). These assessments should include vital signs and BP, as well as some of the areas described in Box 10-5. Hospital protocol should provide guidance as to the frequency of assessment parameters and documentation.

Nursing diagnoses should include pertinent information such as impaired tissue integrity, altered urinary elimination, alteration in comfort, potential knowledge deficit in care of self and newborn infant, and individualized care parameters needed (NAACOG, 1993). All interventions should be documented as they are performed. These areas of the postpartum nursing process are conducive to flow charting with checklists. Narrative notes should be used to report

Box 10-5
Postpartum Documentation

Abdomen and Bowel Function

Abdominal muscle tone, bowel sounds, bowel movements, hemorrhoids

Bladder and Urine Output

Fullness before and after voiding, voiding pattern and amounts voided, bladder distention, pain or burning

Breasts and Chest

Soft, filling or firm, engorged, reddened, or painful; nipples (e.g., erectility, cracks, redness); description of breath sounds

Cesarean Section Incision Site

Dressing and incision, drainage, edema, color changes, redness, ecchymosis

Extremities

Deep tendon reflexes, clonus, varicosities, edema, Homans' sign, width of calf as measurement of redness, tenderness, warmth, activity tolerance

Health Education

Care of self, activities, nutritional needs, exercise, emotional responses, signs of complication, rubella and Rhogam status

Lochia

Type (e.g., rubra, serosa, alba) and amount (i.e., scant, less than 2.5 cm on menstrual pad in 1 hour; light, less than 10 cm on menstrual pad in 1 hour; moderate, less than 15 cm on menstrual pad in 1 hour; heavy, saturated menstrual pad in 1 hour; excessive, menstrual pad saturated in 15 minutes); presence of odor or clots

Perineum, Labia, and Rectum

Episiotomy site condition, lacerations, hemorrhoids, bruising, hematoma, edema, drainage, loss of approximation, reddened areas (indicative of infection)

Psychosocial

Maternal-infant bonding, postpartum depression signs, support systems, inappropriate behavior, any needs identified from health history or social history

Uterus

Consistency and tone, position, height, size

Data from ACOG, AAP: *Guidelines for perinatal care,* ed 4, Washington, DC, 1997, Author; NAACOG: *Core curriculum for maternal-newborn nursing,* Philadelphia, 1993, WB Saunders; and Simpson K, Creehan PA: *AWHONN's perinatal nursing,* Philadelphia, 1996, JB Lippincott.

information not included in the flowsheet (as well as all abnormal parameters). Documentation of the nurse's evaluation of the care given should be recorded.

Given the "drive-through" atmosphere of today's deliveries, they can be very overwhelming for the patient, who

---

Box 10-6

Documentation of Newborn Care

Abdomen

Shape, symmetry, consistence, bowel sounds; palpate liver and kidneys

Back

Spine curvature, dimple or sinus, anal patency, sphincter response, fissures, even gluteal folds, trunk incurvation reflex

Behavioral

Sleeping patterns (e.g., deep sleep, light sleep, drowsiness), activity patterns (e.g., quiet alert, active alert, crying), response to stimulation, feeding and elimination patterns, sucking

Cardiovascular Status

Rate, rhythm, sounds, pulses, cyanosis, BP

Chest and Respiratory Status

Circumference, retractions, shape, symmetry, grunting, breast enlargement or engorgement, equal and bilateral breath sounds, rate, rhythm, apex at left third or fourth intercostal space

Ears

Position, formation, pinna, cartilage, response to loud noise, startle reflex

Eyes

Edema of lids, color of iris, presence of red reflex, pupil reactivity, absence of tears, presence of scleral hemorrhages, following and fixation, drainage, jaundice

Genitalia

Female

Labia, clitoris, edema, hymenal tag, urethral meatus, vaginal discharge (whitish or blood-tinged)

Male

Scrotum (e.g., size, edema), palpable testes, urethral opening position, adherence of foreskin, presence of hydrocele

Gestational Age

Scoring of the characteristics of skin, lanugo, breasts, ears, genitalia

Head

Molding, symmetry, swelling, movement, size, shape, consistency of fontanelles, sutures, circumference, bruising

Health Education

Maternal teaching in the care of the newborn, breast- or bottle-feeding, developmental stages, follow-up instructions, phenylketonuria, jaundice

Kidneys

Palpable; urine (amount, color, odor, consistency)

Mouth

Mucous membrane color; intact palate; midline uvula; normal frenulum of tongue and upper lip; little or no salivation; suck, root, and gag reflexes; infections

Musculoskeletal

Symmetry, range of motion, clavicles, hip abduction, muscle tone, scarf sign, creases on the anterior two thirds of the sole, brachial and femoral pulses present and equal

Neurologic

Newborn reflexes (e.g., rooting, sucking, swallowing, palmar and plantar grasps, Moro, Babinski's), posture, tone, tremors

Nose

Nasal patency, discharge, flaring, sneezing, sense of smell

Posture

General flexion, extremity flexion onto the chest and abdomen

Psychosocial

Maternal-infant interactions, social services needs, maternal health problems or addictions, support systems

Sensory

Hearing (turning head towards sound), vision (focusing on close objects), taste, smell, touch

Skin

Texture, vernix, lanugo, color, acrocyanosis, mottling, rashes, jaundice, discolorations, bruising, petechiae, nails, drying, peeling, edema, milia, abrasions, lacerations, temperature regulation

Umbilical Cord

Three vessels; consistency, redness, drainage, meconium staining, hernia

---

Data from NAACOG: *Core curriculum for maternal-newborn nursing,* Philadelphia, 1993, WB Saunders; *Lippincott's manual of nursing practice,* ed 6, Philadelphia, 1996, JB Lippincott; and Simpson K, Creehan PA: *AWHONN's perinatal nursing,* Philadelphia, 1996, JB Lippincott.

has to deal with her physiological, physical, and emotional changes, as well as caring for a newborn infant. Documentation of these parameters is essential.

DOCUMENTATION OF NEWBORN CARE

A thorough and systematic assessment should be documented for all newborns. Measurements of weight, length, head circumference, and chest circumference are recorded initially and as needed. Weight should be documented daily. Vital signs should be recorded as indicated in the institutional protocol. Information that should be documented in the examination of newborns is discussed in Box 10-6.

Newborn documentation forms can provide a system where checkmarks or initials can indicate expected findings and the narrative notes reflect abnormal findings (as well as follow through of the nursing process). Documentation of parental education is an important area, and it should provide evidence of their understanding. Documentation of the expected follow-up and participation in homecare programs is also needed.

SUMMARY

Many institutions are adopting complete documentation systems that integrate physician orders, nursing assessments, diagnoses, interventions, and the expected outcomes. Any deviations from the expected outcomes, or "falling off the path," should be addressed. These types of documentation methods vary from one institution to another and are called by many different names (for example, critical pathways, integrated plans of care, collaborative carepaths, integrated clinical pathways, and clinical maps). Computer charting has been instituted at many hospitals, and it is purported to follow the pathways and identify deviations.

No matter what type of documentation system is used by individual institutions, the documentation should provide the record of the nursing process followed in the delivery of nursing care to each individual patient. The documentation should be individualized to reflect each patient's "story." Nurses are the "authors" of a vital record. If that record should ever be scrutinized to hold nurses to the standard of care, the nurse should be able to show how each patient's story begins, continues, and ends—with contributions from all care providers.

NEONATAL DOCUMENTATION

Barbara Ashley, RN, BSN, MSN

Occurrences of neonatal nurses being sued used to be rare. However, this is not true any more. Attorneys are advertising on television: "If your child suffers from specific conditions, such as brain damage or seizures, maybe the neonatal care was inappropriate. Come see us." For this reason alone the neonatal nurse must determine how to focus on providing and documenting care appropriately. The purpose of this chapter is to assist the nurse in performing a more patient-focused assessment of the newborn and neonate and in documenting this assessment accurately.

REACTION TO THE DELIVERY PROCESS

At the time of delivery the following series of changes in the infant's vital signs and clinical appearance take place if the infant is reactive to the birthing process:

1. Period of reactivity
2. Relative unresponsive interval or sleep period
3. Second period of reactivity

For example, a normal infant with an Apgar score of 7 to 10 is usually very vigorous during the first 15 to 30 minutes after birth. Then the second phase (sleep period) occurs, followed by the third phase (Klaus, Fanaroff, 1993). The nurse should understand the physiological process that is occurring; if this is not understood, the nurse cannot accurately assess any abnormalities that might be present. Failure to recognize an abnormality prevents the nurse from reporting it to the physician. If the infant suffers damages as a result of this failure, the nurse's chances of being sued increases. Later in this chapter, case studies are presented.

PHYSICAL EXAMINATION OF THE NEWBORN INFANT

Serial examinations are more valuable than a single physical examination. With each serial evaluation, determining the infant's physical condition occurs. The ideal scenario would involve a delivery room examination, a first-day examination, and a detailed examination after the infant's first day of life. The initial examination should include a concise history, a complete developmental assessment, and a thorough physical examination. The nurse must separate normal anomalies related to intrauterine positioning from more serious abnormalities that may require early intervention and treatment (Alexander, Kuo, 1997).

Nursing school instructors often teach that each assessment should "paint a picture of the patient by itself." Unfortunately, neonatal medical records are sometimes filled with incomplete or contradicting assessments. Reconstructing the picture from incomplete fragments can be difficult. To assist the healthcare provider, the following section deals with painting that picture and focuses on assessment and evaluation documentation.

Delivery Room Examination

The Apgar score is used to evaluate the infant in five categories at 1, 5, and 10 minutes after delivery: heart rate, respiratory effort, muscle tone, responsiveness, and color (Korones, Bada-Ellzey, 1993). Apgar scores are assigned to every infant born in a hospital. They are not always accurate. In addition, some individuals attempt to use the scores to substantiate claims (Letko, 1996). After the delivery room appraisal, a time period may pass before a pediatrician sees the infant. Detecting any problems not apparent in the delivery room therefore becomes the responsibility of the nursing personnel (Klaus, Fanaroff, 1993). This is why understanding the transitional process is essential for the nurse. The nurse must have knowledge of the delivery room evaluation and maintain an ongoing evaluation of the infant during the first 24 hours so that he or she can report any abnormalities to the physician.

Guideline for Physical Examination of the Newborn

First, the nurse must understand the purpose of the newborn assessment. The assessment should establish whether a congenital anomaly exists, determine the gestational age category, and detect any other abnormalities that might affect the neonate. The assessment is performed using a systemic approach, except that the observations requiring a quiet infant are done first. Since the infant may be under the influence of maternal anesthesia and analgesia, reexamination when the infant is 24 hours old may reveal new findings that were not evident during the first day (Klaus, Fanaroff, 1993).

Box 10-7 is a tool that is organized according to the anatomy of a neonate. Box 10-8 provides key documentation points by body systems. Frequently used neonatal equipment is listed in Box 10-9. After each main topic, suggestions for documentation are provided.

The initial baseline assessment is extensive but imperative. It allows the nurse to be aware of any changes that occur during the transitional state, as well as any abnormalities. Vital signs, which are first recorded in the delivery room, are monitored until the infant's condition stabilizes. (This should be performed according to institutional policy.) When the nurse notices a deviation from the normal transitional period, he or she must report it to the physician in a timely manner for further evaluation.

If an abnormality is reported to the physician, the nurse should record the orders that were given (if any), what measures were taken, and what the outcome was. By providing appropriate care for the newborn or neonate, the legal rights of the patient, nurse, physician, and institution are ensured. Thus the nursing process requires that the nurse constantly evaluate and reevaluate the patient. Appropriate monitoring of a neonate's condition is essential. Detecting changes and preventing of complications is imperative, as the following case illustrates:

Box 10-7

Guidelines for Physical Examination of the Neonate

In addition to what has been discussed previously, the following information about neonates should be documented.

Cardiovascular System

- Umbilical artery catheter/umbilical venous catheter: Patent, blood return (e.g., quality), distance in cm from insertion site, toes (e.g., pink), blanch (e.g., well)
- Type of ventilator
- Humidification
- Chest drainage: Type and volume
- Chest physical therapy (CPT) schedule: For example, every 2 hours, 4 hours
- Suction: Color, consistency, amount
- Chest tubes

Gastrointestinal System

- Feedings: Parenteral, oral, nasogastric (NG), nasal jejunal (NJ)
- Gavage/NJ feedings: Check placement of tube, residual, consistency, amount
- Formula: Type, amount, frequency
- Suck: Present, absent, quality
- Stools: Color, size, consistency, guiac
- NG drainage: Suction, amount of output, appearance
- Palpation: Liver edge

Genitourinary System

- Voiding: Specific gravity

Neuromuscular System

- State of arousal
- Response to stimuli
- Sedation: Medication, response

Extremities

- Restraints: Reason, type, location, duration

Integumentary System

- Wound: Type, location, drainage, color, odor
- Dressing change: Type, frequency

Psychosocial

- Bonding: Present, absent

The plaintiff was born 6 weeks premature and required resuscitation at the time of birth. She had good Apgar scores, indicating that, although born early, she was normally developed and suffered no injury before birth. Shortly after midnight on the day of her birth, she was transferred to neonatal intensive care unit (NICU) for close monitoring because of difficulty in breathing. In the NICU the plaintiff was placed under the care of a resident and a fellow. Another physician in training was present and was deemed to be the

Box 10-8

Key Documentation Areas

Head

- Fontanelles: Sunken, soft, tense, bulging, size (i.e., anterior or posterior)
- Sutures: Overlapping, separated (in cm), fused, softness
- Scalp: Cephalohematoma, caput, lacerations, bruising, scalp electrode placement, head circumference (i.e., frontal occipital circumference)
- Face: General appearance, color, forceps marks, birthmarks, edema, symmetry, paralysis, malformations, eye spacing, skin tags
- Eyes: Fused, conjunctivitis, description of drainage, edema, size, pupil reaction, red reflex, sclera hemorrhage
- Ears: Vernix, degree of recoil, form, positioning, tags
- Nose: Patent, degree of nasal flaring
- Mouth and lips: Palate (i.e., cleft lip, cleft palate), teeth, suck reflex, chin size, mucous membranes (i.e., color, moisture), lesions
- Neck: Supple, crepitus, palpable glands and masses, neck lag, tracheal alignment

Cardiovascular System

- Point of maximal impulse: Location (e.g., fifth left intercostal space)
- Rate and rhythm: Regular, irregular, sound (e.g., distant)
- Murmurs: Description, location, intensity
- Vital signs: Apical and radial heart rate, blood pressure in upper and lower extremities
- Capillary refill: Less than 3 seconds
- Peripheral pulses: Equal in all four extremities, strong, weak, bounding, thready
- Edema: Location, degree, pitting or nonpitting

Respiratory System

- Chest circumference: Usually smaller than the frontal occipital circumference
- Rate and characteristics: Shallow, rapid, symmetrical
- Movement and description of breath sounds: Equal, clear, audible in all lobes, wheezes, rales, rhonchi
- Grunting and nasal flaring: Present or absent
- Cyanosis: Location, degree
- Retractions: Substernal, intercostal, supraclavicular
- Apnea: Present or absent
- Breathing pattern: Regular, Cheyne-Stokes respirations
- Chest: Shape (e.g., barrel), placement and number of nipples, breast development

Gastrointestinal System

- Abdominal circumference
- General appearance: Round, distended, ascites, flat, scaphoid
- Umbilical cord: Appearance, number of vessels
- Palpation: Masses, organomegaly, tenderness, rebound
- Bowel sounds: Hypoactive or hyperactive, audible in all four quadrants
- Anus: Patent or imperforate
- Stool: Passage of meconium

Genitourinary System

Male

- Testes: Canal or scrotum
- Scrotum: Edema, masses, amount of rugae on scrotum, herniation
- Penis: Obvious or questionable, presence of edema, circumcision, hypospadias

Female

- Gender: Obvious or questionable
- Vaginal: Discharge (e.g., blood-tinged, frank)
- Clitoris: Size (e.g., abnormally large)
- Labia: Size of majora and minora
- Edema
- Masses: Type, location
- Herniation

General

- Voiding: Time, amount, frequency, color, consistency

Neuromuscular System

- General activity: Active, lethargic, paralyzed
- Posture: Tremulousness, jitteriness, seizures
- Reflexes: Sucking, rooting, grasping, Babinski's, Moro
- Range of motion: Limited
- Tone: Quality

Extremities

- Gross abnormalities: Congenital
- Simian creases
- Skin tags: Quantity, location
- Digits: Number, webbing, clubbing, cyanosis
- Symmetrical movement of limbs
- Fractures: Location, type
- Paralysis: Location
- Hips: Clicks, gluteal fold symmetry, thigh length
- Feet: Sole creases, rocker-bottom feet

Integumentary System

- Color: Pink, dusky, cyanotic
- Turgor: Good, poor
- Anomalies: Mongolian spots, birth marks, forceps marks
- Lacerations or abrasions: Location, degree
- Petechiae: Location
- Rashes: Milia, heat, erythema toxicum
- Vernix: Location
- Lanugo: Amount, location
- Skin temperature

Psychosocial

- Mother's marital status: Single, married, divorced, separated, widowed
- Primary caregiver: Mother, father, grandparents
- Feeding: Breast, bottle
- Siblings: Number
- Financial: Caregivers employed or unemployed
- Dwelling: Lives with parents or grandparents

Box 10-9

Frequently Used Neonatal Equipment

- Type of bed: Warmers, isolette or crib, temperature, position
- Cardiac/respiratory monitor: Type, alarms with set high or low limits
- Ventilator: Type, settings, other equipment
- Suction: Functioning, pressure limits
- Bag and mask at bedside: Functioning
- Blood pressure transducer: Zeroed, wave form, quality
- Phototherapy: Lights, eye patches in place, skin exposed
- Chest tubes: Location, patent, functioning, type of apparatus, wall-suction setting
- Intravenous fluids/pumps: Type of fluids, fluid levels, infusion rate, site, time of last tubing change, intravenous fluids
- Isolation: Type, precautions, reason
- Protocols: Minimal stimulation

---

supervisor. When the infant was admitted to the NICU, tests were performed. The arterial blood gas (ABG) values revealed the infant was not receiving an adequate supply of oxygen. About 2 hours later the infant was placed on oxygen delivered by mask or continuous positive airway pressure (CPAP) and a machine that was supposed to record the percentage of oxygen in her blood through a patch placed on her skin. Blood testing using the capillary route (through the infant's heel), was performed during this time. The oxygen levels were abnormal, but the defendant argued that capillary blood tests do not accurately measure the oxygen percentage in the blood. A chest x-ray examination was performed because of concerns about pneumonia. A diagnosis of pneumonia was never clinically confirmed, but the defendants maintained that they were treating the infant for it because the pneumonia was the cause of the patient's breathing problems. The newborn's condition continued to deteriorate, and at 3:45 AM, she was intubated and placed on a ventilator. At 5:00 AM the infant was eliminating only a scant amount of urine. The capillary blood tests continued to show problems with the patient's oxygen level as did the transcutaneous carbon dioxide (TcPO$_2$) monitor. The only documentation from this period was an admission note written by the resident, who had the least amount of medical training. The supervising physician came to the hospital around 7:00 AM but did not provide any further testing or intervention. At 11:00 AM another ABG test was performed, which confirmed the problems with the infant's oxygen levels. A second team of doctors-in-training then assumed care of the infant. No documentation was proved by either physician on the second team relative to the infant's condition. The documentation was mainly from the nursing staff, who failed to record any BP measurements. Throughout the evening, further testing confirmed problems that included a drop in hematocrit levels, a continued decrease in urine output, low blood oxygen percentages, and a mottling in skin color. The infant ultimately suffered brain damage and cerebral palsy. A $1.7 million verdict was returned with interest added (Laska, 1997k).

In this case the nurse should have been aware of the deteriorating condition of the neonate and thoroughly communicated this to the physicians. If their response was inappropriate, then the nurse should have followed the chain of command. The nurse had a duty to properly evaluate and monitor the neonate, which would include an assessment, evaluation, documentation of vital signs, and a report of any abnormalities.

BILIRUBIN THERAPY

Hyperbilirubinemia is a regular occurrence in all neonates, but jaundice occurs in only one half of all affected neonates because the serum bilirubin levels must exceed 4 to 6 mg/100 ml before it becomes visible as jaundice in the skin. At any bilirubin level, the appearance of jaundice during the first 24 hours of life or its persistence beyond the normal age limit usually indicate a pathologic process (Korones, 1986). The nurse should know the normal bilirubin lab values and be aware of the values of the infant.

If the physician has standing orders regarding when the bilirubin levels should be drawn, then the nurse is responsible for overseeing the completion of these tests. Depending on the institution's policy, the nurse may be the individual responsible for reporting abnormal laboratory values to the physician, which is why it is critical that nurses know the institution's policy and procedures.

> The infant's bilirubin level was to be checked every 24 hours. The level had been rising, and the physician was contemplating performing an exchange transfusion. However, the nurse failed to verify that the 6:00 PM bilirubin level had been checked. The blood sample allegedly was not drawn. The next morning, when the 6:00 AM results were evaluated, they were extremely elevated. The parents claimed that the infant suffered brain damage from elevated bilirubin levels. The parents allege that if the 6:00 PM level had been evaluated, the staff would have noticed it to be rising, and the physician would have performed the exchange transfusion sooner, thus preventing the infant's brain damage. The nurse was charged with failing to perform the bilirubin test as ordered, and failing to monitor the bilirubin levels, which caused the infant to suffer brain damage caused by kernicterus (anecdotal report).

One form of treatment for an infant suffering from hyperbilirubinemia is phototherapy. The nurse needs to know the untoward side effects of phototherapy, including increased metabolic rate, hyperthermia, loose stools, and increased loss of water through the skin (Korones, 1986; Korones, Bada-Ellzey, 1993). In caring for an infant receiving phototherapy, the nurse needs to ensure that the infant is wearing eye patches. They should be removed and changed daily, and an eye examination should be performed to observe for conjunctivitis. Failure to change the eye patches can result in severe purulent conjunctivitis leading to blindness. The nurse should document that this procedure was performed and should include the results of the eye examination. If a problem occurs and the physician is notified, then the nurse should document the orders (if any) and the outcome. The eye patches can be secured by a stockinette or with a bilirubin mask. Before applying the eye patches, the nurse should verify that the infant's eyes are closed and ears are flat.

While the infant is receiving phototherapy, its intake and output should be monitored. The physician may order an increase in fluid intake, supplements, or IV fluid rate. Specific gravity tests should be performed by the nurse every day to assist in monitoring the infant's hydration status.

The nurse should monitor the infant's temperature at least once every shift (or more often, depending on the results). In an open crib an infant's temperature may be low, whereas an infant in an isolette may require a lower temperature because the phototherapy lights increase the heat of the isolette and thus the temperature of the infant.

During phototherapy the gastrointestinal transit time may be decreased; therefore the nurse should realize that the infant could pass loose, green, seedy stools. The number of stools should be documented to maintain an accurate record of the infant's intake and output. The nurse should monitor the infant's skin and provide appropriate care. The phototherapy lights should be kept at an appropriate distance from the infant to prevent burns, and this distance should be recorded in the nurse's notes. Again, the nurse should know the institution's procedure for administering phototherapy.

Lawsuits often arise from laboratory tests that allegedly were not performed as the infant's condition would have warranted. Because the nurse obtains the medical history of the patient at the time of admission, he or she should be aware of possible complications. The following case illustrates this point; the L&D nurse should have known that a pregnancy complicated by Rh blood-factor incompatibility could result in a hemolytic blood disorder in the infant.

> Early in the plaintiff's pregnancy she learned that her blood was incompatible with that of her husband. Shortly before delivery the mother was tested by U.S. Army doctors for problems caused by the incompatible blood. After the birth (at Womack Army Medical Center), the infant was not tested for any of the blood diseases normally associated with pregnancies complicated by Rh blood-factor incompatibility—even though the plaintiff's chart allegedly indicated the mother was at high risk for delivering an infant with hemolytic blood disease. Six days after birth the infant was taken to the emergency room at Womack with severe jaundice. The infant was transferred to another hospital, where he developed seizures and had difficulty breathing. According to published accounts, the $1,399,140 settlement placed $1,279,140 in trust for the infant and awarded $120,000 to the parents (Laska, 1997a).

In many institutions, the nurse receives the laboratory results. The nurse needs to be aware of the normal or abnormal blood levels that are reported and what further actions are required. The nurse is primarily responsible for follow-up and notifying the physician of any abnormal laboratory result.

The following medical negligence case involved hypoglycemia:

> The plaintiff was diagnosed at the time of birth with intrauterine growth retardation, resulting in borderline hypoglycemia. The defendant doctor was responsible for the plaintiff's care during the first four days of his life. After discharge from the hospital, the plaintiff's hypoglycemia became worse, resulting in seizures and eventually brain damage. The plaintiff contended that the doctor was negligent in caring for the child because he failed to closely monitor the condition and did not ensure that blood glucose levels were adequate. The defendant contended that the plaintiff's injury was the result of cerebral microdysgenesis and negligent care by the mother. A $15.75 million verdict was reached in favor of the plaintiff (Laska, 1997g).

INTRAVENOUS ISSUES

The nurse is responsible for knowing the institution's neonatal policies and procedures regarding documentation of IVs and the administration of IV fluids and medications. The nurse should know specifically what should be documented when an abnormality arises. In addition, the nurse must be aware of the policies and procedures for mixing IVs and IV additives. Since newborns and neonates can suffer severe injuries from rapid fluid overload, an IV pump should be used to administer most IV fluids.

At the beginning of every shift, or whenever an adjustment is made, the nurse should record all types of IV fluid, the rates, the sites, and the condition of the sites. Documentation of the details of IV therapy entails recording the type of IV pump, the alarm limits, and whether the alarms were functioning. If a particular unit utilizes flowsheets that indicate the IVs are to be monitored once every hour, then this assessment must be performed and recorded every hour.

When administering a medication via any route, the nurse is responsible for knowing the implications of the use of the medication, and for knowing the "Five Rights" for administering medications. (The five rights are right medication, right dose, right time, right route, and right patient.) The nurse should document the outcome of the medication administered (e.g., analgesic: relieved the pain; sedative: infant resting, not fighting ventilator; antipyretic: decreased fever). If the medication failed to work as expected, then the nurse should reevaluate the situation and follow up with the appropriate individual. The following case provides an example of a medication error:

> The plaintiff was a premature baby who had been hospitalized in a level 3 NICU since birth. At the time of the incident he was 9 months old and was suffering from

bronchopulmonary dysplasia. Although the patient was developmentally delayed, he was progressing and was eating rice cereal and baby foods. In December of 1988 the patient's heart rate dropped, and he was placed back on a ventilator. On the same day the patient had a seizure and was treated with Valium (diazepam) and phenobarbital. That night the patient's potassium level dropped below the normal level. The defendant nurse notified the resident physician, received an order for 2 mEq of potassium chloride, and administered this medication by IV push. Early in the morning of the next day, the resident ordered an additional dose of 3 mEq of potassium chloride to be administered by IV bolus. The nurse mistakenly administered 12 mEq, and the infant went into cardiac arrest within 1 hour. Vital signs were reestablished almost 50 minutes later. The child exhibited profound brain damage following the incident and remained in a persistent vegetative state. A potassium blood level drawn almost 2 hours after the administration of the potassium chloride showed the level to be higher than normal. The nurse did not come forward and admit to the overdose until 2 days later, at which time an incident report was written. The neonatologist wrote in the incident report that the potassium chloride administration might have been the cause of the cardiac arrest. The defendant's experts contended the following points: the prolonged CPR had no impact on the child's brain damage; the seizure the day before the overdose caused the brain damage; children can tolerate high levels of potassium chloride without ill effect; and 3 mEq of potassium chloride can be given over 1 to 2 minutes. The defense conceded that an overdose had occurred. During discovery it was uncovered that potassium chloride was not on the hospital's list of drugs that could be administered IV by nurses, and that the hospital had no method by which to verify a nurse's competency to give medications by the IV route. The plaintiff's cardiology expert testified that the potassium chloride injection was the cause of the cardiac arrest. A settlement agreement of $2.75 million was reached (Laska, 1995).

This case had an interesting additional twist: the child survived until age 7, but a few days before the family received the settlement check, the child died at home while under the care of an LPN. When the child went into respiratory distress, the nurse had been instructed to call the emergency medical services (EMS). The plaintiff alleged that the LPN called the child's father instead. Her documentation was unclear as to the timing and sequence of events. When the child's father arrived home, he found the child in a state of cardiopulmonary arrest. The EMS was called, but the child did not survive. This malpractice case was settled for approximately $500,000 (*Ballon v. Nursing Care,* unpublished verdict).

The following case involved failure to properly monitor a neonate which culminated in a $2.1 million verdict.

A woman arrived at the defendant hospital and delivered her child at the twenty-eighth week of gestation. About 6 hours after birth, the infant was transferred to the neonatal unit of the second defendant hospital. The mother claimed that the defendants failed to properly monitor the infant, resulting in clogging of the endotracheal tube, which lead to brain damage and cerebral palsy. She also claimed that the defendants failed to adequately manage the infant's hematocrit levels, either causing or contributing to a ventricular hemorrhage. The defendants argued the child's injuries were related to the extreme prematurity of the delivery and had nothing to do with a lack of care on their part (Laska, 1997c).

INTAKE AND OUTPUT

Because most neonatal body systems are immature, a slight fluid overload could have devastating results. Therefore the nurse should monitor the infant's intake and output hourly or as ordered by the physician. Many units have standing orders requiring that the nurse monitor the infant's intake and output hourly. The NICU flowsheet is unique in that it has a section for recording the hourly intake and output for IV fluids, feedings, output, and other information. These hourly recordings are totaled at the end of every 8-hour shift to determine whether the balance is positive or negative. Another way in which the infant's fluid status can be monitored is by daily weight (unless otherwise specified). The nurse should record the weight every day and whether it has increased or decreased from the preceding day. All of these measures assist the physician in evaluating the infant's fluid and electrolyte status. If the nurse fails to record the intake and output, then the 24-hour total will be inaccurate. If this occurs, the physician cannot monitor and maintain the infant's nutritional, fluid, and electrolyte requirements.

BONDING

Parents need the support of the nursing staff to help them with their feelings of guilt, anxiety, fear, grief and frustration resulting from dealing with an ill infant. If the mother was hospitalized before the birth, especially for an extensive time, the nursing staff should anticipate potential problems with maternal-infant bonding (Vestal, McKenzie, 1983). The parents should be introduced to a caring supportive staff member and encouraged to ask questions and express their feelings and concerns. The mother should be permitted to see her infant as soon as possible (Jones, Gleason, Lipstein, 1991). Whenever it is feasible, she should be encouraged to touch and hold her infant. Until a mother sees her infant, she may envision the worst case scenario.

The necessary information should be conveyed to the parents by the staff as soon as possible. The nurse needs to provide information at a level the parents can understand. Documentation should summarize the information provided as well as the parents' responses.

A primary care nurse should be assigned with whom the parents can form a bond and develop trust, which will hopefully decrease the parents' anxiety and increase the bonding between the parents and the child or ill infant. The parents should be encouraged to name their infant, and the staff should call the infant by that name. As the infant's condition stabilizes, the parents should be encouraged to provide as much of the care as possible. Documentation should include the nurse's evaluation of the parents' capabilities for providing care.

Breast-feeding is an excellent way to encourage mother-infant bonding; if impossible, the mother should be encouraged to pump her breasts, which will allow her to feel like she is participating in her infant's care. In order to provide consistency and aid in parent-infant bonding, the nurse should document the interactions that transpire between the parents and infant. The nurse should be nonjudgmental and offer encouragement. Documenting these interactions in the medical record will allow the other staff members to focus on the issues and concerns of the parents. A study at the University of Oklahoma concludes that parents experience the most stress from alterations in their parenting role and changes in their infants' behavior and appearance. Parents considered problem-focused coping more helpful than appraisal- or emotion-focused coping (Watson, Corff, Young, et al, 1997).

KEY DOCUMENTATION POINTS

The nurse should document a baseline assessment on admission. This should include vital signs (heart rate [HR], respiratory rate [RR], BP, temperature [T]), measurements (weight, height, frontal occipital circumference, chest circumference, abdominal girth), and a physical assessment (systemic review, as discussed). Next the nurse should document an ongoing baseline assessment at least every 8 to 12 hours, dependent on the institution's policy. This assessment is typically performed at the beginning of every shift and should include documentation about the environment, all equipment functions, a review of systems, observations of drainage, and information on IV fluids.

The nurse should chart and report changes in the infant's condition (e.g., deterioration in vital signs). Such charting is to be performed at the time of occurrence, not later. This situation requires the use of nursing judgment and a knowledge of nursing standards and the nursing process. The standard of care requires that the nurse determine whether the physician needs to be notified of a change in the patient's condition, unless specific physician's orders have been given as to when the physician is to be notified. In this case the nurse is required to adhere to these orders and to document that they were carried out. Many nurses are named in lawsuits for failing to notify a physician when a patient's condition changes even though orders were given that specify when the nurse was to call the physician.

If the nurse informs the physician about the infant's change in condition and the physician does not respond or implement changes, the nurse has a duty to go up the chain of command, if the situation warrants such action. The first step is usually for the nurse to notify his or her supervisor. The supervisor now knows about the situation and has a duty to intervene. Documentation should include the name of the supervisor and the specific information conveyed.

The primary care nurse needs to chart objectively and factually. This documentation should include the following:

- What is seen
- What is heard
- What is smelled
- What is felt
- Effects and actions taken
- What was done and why

Documenting what was seen and heard is vital. If the nurse documents based on someone else's rendition of events, then this fact should be recorded; otherwise the nurse who did the charting will be held accountable for the record.

Consider the following scenario:

Nurse A was at lunch when an incident occurred with the infant she was caring for in the NICU. She documented what transpired based on Nurse B's rendition of the event and signed her name. However, she failed to document the fact that this rendition was told to her by Nurse B. Later it was learned that Nurse A was not present when the event occurred, but had charted the incident as if she had been. Both nurses were being sued and accused of falsifying a record. They were also accused of failing to monitor the infant, to record a change in the patient's condition, and to notify a physician in a timely manner.

Nurse A should have documented that she was going to lunch, the time she left, who was providing care to the infant, the condition of the infant, and any other necessary information at the time she left the unit. Nurses should not document or sign anything they do not have personal knowledge of or have not witnessed (anecdotal report).

DISCHARGE SUMMARY

Because most neonates are transferred to a transitional nursery before discharge, the nurse should summarize what care has been provided for the infant. The nurse examines each problem on the infant's problem list and explains whether it was resolved (or not resolved) and how. The discharge summary, which should highlight the problems, serves as a reference for recurring or new problems, a means to convey information, and a way to communicate health information to the family.

If the institution has a printed discharge summary form, ensure that it has places for all the information needed. Although nurses commonly overlook the vital signs section, it is an important section to complete. Many lawsuits have been filed regarding patients who were discharged when their condition was unstable or they were febrile (and thus should not have been discharged). Unfortunately the nurses failed to record the patient's vital signs at the time of discharge in many cases, which hampers the defense of the nurse because they cannot prove the patient was stable for discharge. The status of the neonate at the time of discharge was an issue in the following case:

> The plaintiff's child was born in the very early morning of June 1, 1995 and was discharged the next day around 10:00 AM. The defendant doctor, a family practitioner, had examined the baby on each day. The baby slept after being brought home, with the exception of one breast feeding around 1:00 PM. The plaintiffs' checked the child's temperature around 8:00 PM and found it to be below normal. They brought the child to the emergency room. The emergency room physician thought the problem was a lack of recent feeding and the father began giving the baby glucose and water from a bottle. The baby coughed, gagged, and then looked blank. The baby had arrested and could not be resuscitated. The coroner determined that the child died from a genetic metabolic disorder, but could not specify which one. Further testing revealed a diagnosis of medium-chain acytyl-CoA dehydrogenase (MCAD), a genetic disorder. The plaintiff's expert neonatologist claimed the baby had exhibited abnormal symptoms before discharge and that testing should have been performed before the infant was discharged. The expert maintained that testing for hypoglycemia and bilirubin would have resulted in a diagnosis of hypoglycemia, and frequent feedings would have been ordered, which would have saved the infant's life. The defendant's experts maintained that the infant had been normal, that testing for hypoglycemia was unnecessary, and the discharge was proper. A defense verdict was returned (Laska, 1997b).

Even though the case referenced above was not a nursing case, the nurse's duty would be to teach the parents to observe for abnormal findings in the newborn. The parents would have been taught when to notify their physician. This information would be documented on the discharge summary as well as the patient/family education sheet.

The position of the National Association of Neonatal Nurses is that in order for the neonate's specialized needs to be met, broad guidelines must exist for such discharge. Discharge preparations and follow-up care must be performed by knowledgeable and experienced neonatal nurses who can determine whether the infant is ready for discharge and home care and can assess follow-up needs. All discharge and teaching criteria must be met to ensure positive neonatal and family outcomes (NANN, 1997).

SUMMARY

Nurses should realize that we live in a litigious society. To help reduce the number of lawsuits, nurses should follow the nursing process, document accurately and appropriately, and know their institutional policies and procedures. This chapter presents information and issues relevant to the nurse for use in documenting. Remember: When in doubt, document.

PEDIATRIC DOCUMENTATION

Joyce Hamlin, MSN, RNC, CS

Gail Coplein, BA, JD

The role of the pediatric nurse focuses on assisting children in attaining their optimal level of health. Current U.S. statistics indicate that the population of children under the age of 21 is more than 63 million. Approximately 30% of the population of the United States is made up of children (U.S. Bureau of the Census, 1997).

Children experience unique healthcare problems, depending on their level of growth and development. The leading causes of death during the first month of life include congenital anomalies and respiratory distress syndrome. In children between the ages of 1 and 9, leading causes of death include unintentional injuries, such as motor vehicle accidents, drowning, burns, and falls.

Pediatric nurses in acute care settings work not only with the child, but also with the family unit. The concept of family-centered health care takes family values and dynamics into consideration. When planning care, the pediatric nurse should assess the health of children and their families. The nursing care provided attempts to incorporate the family's routines to better support the family unit.

FACTORS IN CARING FOR THE PEDIATRIC CLIENT

Pediatric patients provide special challenges to nurses. Many pediatric clients are unable to communicate their needs or verbalize pain. Nurses must be keenly sensitive to forms of nonverbal communication, such as cries, body positioning, and eye contact. The infant's inability to communicate means that the nurse must anticipate the child's needs.

Physiologically, children differ from adults. Children exhibit more rapid metabolic rates. Vital signs ranges change as the child matures. Infants demonstrate faster heart and respiratory rates and lower arterial pressures. Fluid requirements, especially for infants, are smaller. Although daily fluid requirements of a child are greater per kilogram of body weight, the amount of fluid required is smaller than that required by adults. Excessive fluid administration must therefore be avoided through careful monitoring and documentation of fluid intake. Urine volume is also less in children, and it also requires careful measurement. Infants have relatively more body water (approximately 75%) when compared with an adult. This fluid mainly comprises the extracellular fluid. When the extracellular fluid balance is altered, rapid dehydration results. Numerous body organs and systems do not develop during the infancy and early childhood period. Furthermore, some diseases, such as meningitis, are more likely to occur in the pediatric population. Children are generally more susceptible to infectious diseases, particularly respiratory and viral infections, because of the immaturity of their immune systems.

In pediatric settings a medication error may be life-threatening. Standard pediatric dosages do not exist, and in pediatric patients the functioning of immature body systems can alter the pharmacokinetics of drugs. Children's immature livers often metabolize drugs ineffectively, especially during the first year of life. The risk of drug toxicity increases with immature liver function. The slight difference between the therapeutic and toxic serum concentrations of certain commonly prescribed children's drugs necessitates the monitoring of serum concentration levels. These include medications such as digoxin and phenytoin (Dilantin).

Disturbances in the acid-base balance or electrolyte balance and dehydration can alter the effects of medication. Because these alterations occur in the pediatric population, monitoring children for adverse reactions is a critical nursing responsibility.

Accidents are a leading cause of mortality and morbidity in childhood. Children are at greater risk for injury as a result of burns or falls. The level of mobility related to a child's developmental stage is a vital assessment when defining the potential for injury. A toddler who has recently acquired walking skills is at greater risk for injury from a fall. Nurses must continuously monitor infants for potential hazards in their environment.

COMMUNICATING WITH CHILDREN AND FAMILIES

Because the family acts as the support system for the child, they must be treated as a unit. Establishing communication with all family members is therefore essential. Effective communication is clear, consistent, and frequent. Rapport established with the family should be based on concern for the child and his or her support system. The establishment of trust must be accomplished quickly in acute care settings. Information needed to formulate the child's plan of care should be gathered and documented in an efficient, yet comprehensive, manner. The initial interview is the means for establishing a professional relationship with the family. The following strategies can be used to facilitate taking a nursing history and establishing a therapeutic relationship with the family:

- Before an interaction, determine who should be interviewed. Nurses must be careful not to assume that an adult accompanying the child is the parent. Determine whether the child needs to be interviewed separately.
- Provide a private, quiet setting in which to conduct the interview. This ensures that the interview will be the sole focus of attention for the entire time that the interaction is taking place.

- Begin the interview with the nurse introducing himself or herself to the child and family. The nurse's name, title, and role should be shared. Determine the name each family member prefers to use.
- Explain the reason for and length of the interview, and obtain verbal permission to proceed.
- Employ the open-ended questioning technique to direct the focus of the session. Close-ended questions should be used to elicit specific information.
- Engage the child by using age-appropriate questions to demonstrate interest in the child. Provide the child with quiet activities to occupy him or her while the caregiver is being interviewed.
- Use therapeutic techniques of communication (e.g., silence) and active listening.
- Convey empathy, genuineness, and concern to aid in establishing trust.
- Observe nonverbal cues, such as facial expressions, body posturing, and a hesitancy to answer questions.

Communication with children must reflect their developmental stage. Box 10-10 provides tips related to communication with children.

Even as early as in the first years of life, infants can communicate through a two-way form of interaction. The infant's needs are made known through vocalizations and non-verbal behaviors. By the end of the first year of life, the child speaks several words.

Box 10-10

Guidelines for Communicating with Children

Age: 0-1 Years Old
- Hold, rock, and talk to infant, especially when he or she is upset or frightened.
- Use a soft, low-pitched voice.
- Approach the infant in a slow manner and avoid frightening movements.

Age: 2-5 Years Old
- Provide short, clear instructions.
- Allow the child to participate in the decision-making process (if appropriate).
- Be honest and tell the child when a procedure is likely to hurt.

Age: 6-12 Years Old
- Include the child in discussion with the parents.
- Provide opportunities for the child to participate through role-playing and storytelling.
- Allow the child to select a reward after the procedure.

Adolescent
- Provide an opportunity to interview the child without the parents.
- Maintain a nonjudgmental attitude.
- Use open-ended questions and restating techniques.

In toddlerhood, there is rapid growth of language skills through the use of word imitation and speech intonation. The nonverbal method of communication is used, including gestures such as pointing or pounding the feet during temper tantrums. Preschoolers' vocabularies increase to over 2000 words. However, they often misinterpret what they are told because their grasp of meaning is often literal. A classic example is that during immunization, the nurse describes a "stick" in the arm, which is interpreted by the child to mean a tree branch.

School-aged children are capable of self-care, and at this age children are able to take an active role in their own health care. Adolescents may be interviewed without the presence of the parents. However, privacy and confidentiality must be ensured to gain the adolescent's trust.

LEGAL RISKS OF PEDIATRIC CARE

Nurses caring for pediatric patients may be held to a higher standard of care and skill because very young patients require more attention (Calloway, 1986). "Because these patients cannot fend for themselves, they rely on [nurses] to anticipate, detect, document, and communicate even the most subtle signs of impending illness or complication. [Nurses'] willingness and ability to fulfill the patient advocacy role may mean the difference between a positive and a negative outcome" (DiCostanzo, 1996, p. 57). For nurses, in terms of self-protection, this means "the smaller the patient, the bigger the risk" (Greve, 1990). In the last few years a trend has been to bring criminal charges against nurses, particularly those caring for the elderly or the very young, for deviations that were not intentional but constituted gross negligence. Within the last 2 years, three nurses working together were charged with criminally negligent homicide in the death of an infant injected with 10 times the prescribed dose by the wrong route of administration (Ventura, 1997).

Statutes of Limitation

Exposure for malpractice liability is significantly greater with the pediatric population, because most states require an adult to file a medical malpractice suit within a few years from the date or discovery of injury. There is no such time requirement, called the statute of limitations, for minors in many states. The statute of limitations is tolled (suspended) for our youngest citizens until the date on which they reach their majority and then the adult limitations period begins to run. For that reason, a 2-year-old child who is injured while under your care may have 20 years to sue you, 16 years until she reaches 18 and 2 to 4 more years for the limitations period. This extended period of liability involving pediatric patients underscores the necessity of thorough documentation, for the chart may be all you have to rely on when that 2-year-old is a 22-year-old plaintiff.

Moreover, even when a suit is filed, trial may not be reached for 2 to 5 years under our court system.

Even when the patient's parents bring suit while the patient is a minor, courts commonly defer trial of a pending suit until the child reaches an age at which neurological milestones can be evaluated. In one case, for example, the Court elected to delay trial against a nurse who had injected a newborn with ampicillin diluted with potassium chloride—causing permanent brain damage—until the child reached age 7 and could undergo a complete neuropsychological evaluation (Kessler, 1993).

Nurses caring for pediatric patients outside the hospital setting and without direct supervision may have even more liability exposure. In 1990 the first case of a school nurse being held independently liable was reported (in this case, for failure to provide adequate care to a high school student who suffered an asthma attack) (Weitzman, 1990). Consider the following case:

> A recent New York case was reported in which a nurse in a pediatrician's office gave poor advice to the parents of a 6-month-old baby who had been diagnosed with an inner-ear infection the day before. After treating the child with Ceclor (cephaclor) and Tylenol (acetaminophen), the parents called the doctor's office to report that the baby was no better. His temperature was 104° F, and he had vomited four times. Because the doctor was unavailable, the nurse told the parents to continue with the prescribed medications. The baby actually had meningitis and suffered severe neurological sequelae requiring that he be institutionalized. He died at age 3 (Laska, 1971).

The case does not report whether the nurse was sued independently, but it would be surprising if that did not occur.

Pediatric nurses may also be sued for improper delegation. Consider the following case:

> A 14-year-old was admitted for observation after receiving a head injury during a soccer game and then vomiting in the locker room. He stopped breathing after 7 hours in the hospital and suffered permanent brain damage because nursing assistants who had been assigned to monitor him did not know the neurological tests they were supposed to perform to evaluate his condition. The charting was haphazard, inconsistent, and done at the end of the shift. Additionally the institution had no written procedure for monitoring head injuries (*Reidmiller et al v. Suburban Hospital Assn. Inc.,* 1978).

You should also be aware that the financial settlements or verdicts in pediatric injury lawsuits are likely to be catastrophic because an injured child will require many more years of care because of his or her potentially greater life expectancy. For instance, in a 1986 trial, a normal infant admitted for a lumbar puncture was rendered a spastic quadriplegic because he was improperly restrained by a nurse. The plaintiff obtained a verdict of $27.5 million (Weitzman, 1997c). The nurse must therefore protect himself or herself with thorough documentation while giving young patients the best care possible.

Nevertheless, the purpose of documentation is not simply to fulfill legal requirements and serve the institution. A flowsheet serves the patient when used as an organizational tool and assessment outline for the nurse. A flowsheet for a particular care issue, such as restraints, can incorporate institutional guidelines in a readily available form and serve to remind the nurse that to document something is to be reminded to *do* it.

DOCUMENTATION DEFENSE STRATEGIES TO MINIMIZE LEGAL RISK

To plan and individualize the child's nursing care, a nursing admission history must be obtained. This is achieved most often during the initial visit with the child and family. Although a pediatric admission assessment tool is often organized in a format similar to that of an adult, several areas, such as developmental and psychosocial issues, must be further explored. The tool must be flexible enough to accommodate its use for a range of ages: infancy through adolescence (Figure 10-8). Another option is to design assessment tools aimed at specific age groups: 0 to 3 years old, 4 to 12 years old, and 13 to 18 years old. Pediatric admission tools contains a health history, physical and psychosocial assessments, and sections related to daily routines, diet, motor and sensory development, and education or discharge needs.

Information that should be documented in the pediatric health history includes an account of the details of the primary reason (chief complaint) for seeking health care. The nurse should document the direct quotations of the family member or child who provided the information. Previous hospitalizations and coping strategies of the child should be discussed. The nurse should note whether a delay in seeking medical intervention occurred and whether the child's current condition is consistent with the history or the child's developmental level. The section for the history of present illnesses may also provide information that could be used in determining the possibility of neglect or abuse (to be discussed later in this chapter).

In addition, the past medical history of young children requires detailed information. Topic areas often include birth history, dietary history, immunizations, and developmental milestones. Information must be gathered concerning the mother's prenatal care, labor and delivery, the newborn's condition, and any perinatal problems. Many of the problems encountered in childhood may be explained by events in the antenatal or perinatal periods. These areas (except for immunizations) are usually deleted in the history of older children or adolescents.

Information regarding medications currently being given to the child must be obtained. The method by which the child is being given medications is critical when planning

appropriate care. Medication, latex, and blood-product allergies must be documented.

A dietary history must include data related to allergies and the ages at which feeding milestones were achieved, such as the introduction of solid foods. Actual or potential problems, such as failure to thrive or iron deficiency anemia, may be revealed through the information obtained in a detailed dietary history. Food preferences are important when planning the child's hospital diet. An infant's formula should be noted if the child is being bottle-fed, as well as the feeding style and frequency.

The immunization record reveals whether the child is up-to-date on immunizations. The Advisory Committee on Immunization Practice and the Center for Disease Control periodically issue updated guidelines for immunization. Therefore an updated copy of these standards should be available in all units where children are assessed. The rationale for delayed immunizations should be explored with parents.

Information regarding growth and development is an essential part of the child's past history. The ages at which developmental milestones, such as head control, crawling, walking and speech, were achieved must be obtained from the parents. Safety issues, such as the need for a safety crib or jacket, should be discussed with parents to minimize the possibility of injury. (This conversation should be documented.) Hospital units where children are assessed should have a list of developmental milestones, according to age, to screen the child for developmental delays.

Habits such as sleep patterns, toilet training, thumb sucking, and rituals must be explored. This information may be vital to the safety of children in acute care settings, and it may provide opportunities for health teaching and anticipatory guidance. Home routines of the child are reviewed to promote an easier transition to the hospital setting. Special toys or security objects, siblings, and friends are other topics to be covered at admission. All spaces on the nursing admission history form must be completed. If any information is missing, the nurse must note the reason for the omission. Box 10-11, p. 186, summarizes charting tips related to the hospital admission of a pediatric patient.

Ongoing communication with the child and family is vital to building a trusting relationship. A child's illness is a stressful crisis for all members of the family. Establishing an effective rapport with the child and family helps to establish trust between the nurse, child, and family. In doing so, the nurse may decrease the likelihood of a future lawsuit.

DOCUMENTATION TOOLS USED IN THE PEDIATRIC SETTING

Because flowsheets are easily adapted to address the unique needs of a healthcare setting, they can be adapted to the needs of the pediatric population. These forms are especially

Text continued on p. 186

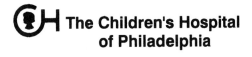 **The Children's Hospital
of Philadelphia**

Department of Nursing

NURSING DATA BASE

(PATIENT PLATE IMPRINT)

SECTION I: INTAKE INTERVIEW (Complete on admission)

Name _____ Nickname _____

Time of Arrival _____ Unit _____ Accompanied by (Name) _____

Person interviewed/Relationship to patient _____

English speaking ☐ Yes ☐ No _____

Admitted from: ☐ Admissions ☐ Clinic ☐ ED ☐ Transfer from _____

Diagnostic Studies Completed Prior to Admission _____

VITAL SIGNS   T _____   P _____   R _____

BP: Cuff Size _____ RUE _____ LUE _____ RLE _____ LLE _____

Height/length (cm) _____ Wt (Kg) _____ Scale # _____ Birth Wt (if needed) _____

Head Circumference (cm) _____ Abdominal girth (cm) _____

HEALTH PERCEPTION/MANAGEMENT

History of Present Illness _____

What have you been told about why your child is in the hospital _____

Previous Hospitalizations   ☐ No   ☐ Yes   Explain _____

Other Health problems   ☐ No   ☐ Yes   Explain _____

Allergies   Drug   ☐ No   ☐ Yes   Explain _____

       Food   ☐ No   ☐ Yes   Explain _____

       Blood Products   ☐ No   ☐ Yes   Explain _____

       Latex   ☐ No   ☐ Yes   Explain _____

       Other: Explain _____

Immunizations:

       Where does your child receive immunizations _____

       When / what was their last immunization _____

Recent Exposure to Communicable Disease ☐ No   ☐ Yes, Explain _____

Medications   ☐ None

Name	Dose	Schedule	Last Dose

Form of Medication Preferred   ☐ Pills   ☐ Crushed   ☐ Chewable   ☐ Liquid   ☐ Other _____

Figure 10-8   Pediatric admission sheet. (Courtesy The Children's Hospital, Philadelphia.)

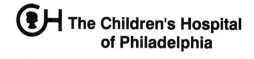

The Children's Hospital of Philadelphia

Department of Nursing

NURSING DATA BASE

SECTION I: INTAKE INTERVIEW (continued)

GENERAL INFORMATION

Has parent/guardian/patient completed admission paperwork ☐ Yes ☐ No - Sent to admissions ☐ No - Needs to go

Admission Consent signed ☐ Yes ☐ No

☐ Patient wearing ID band ☐ Parent wearing ID band Family Handbook received by _____

Advanced Directives Verification Form ☐ N/A (<18 yrs) ☐ N/A (>18 yrs: incompetent) ☐ Completed ☐ Needs to be done

Newborn Screening ☐ N/A (>30 days) ☐ Complete ☐ Not Complete: Date due _____

Admission Education per Patient/Family Education Standard 21:1:a - Admission

Orientation to: ☐ Unit environment ☐ Food ☐ Hospital Policies ☐ Safety Measures ☐ Hospital Staff ☐ Unit care routine

Signature of staff completing section I. _____ Date/Time _____

SECTION II: PHYSICAL ASSESSMENT (Reflects admission status, Complete on shift of admission)

NEUROLOGIC (Choose 1 answer per category)

LOC: ☐ Alert ☐ Depressed ☐ Stuporous ☐ Comatose

Pupils Size: Right _____ Left _____ • 2 • 3 ● 4 ● 5 ● 6 ● 7 ● 8 ● 9

Reactivity to light: Right: ☐ Brisk ☐ Sluggish ☐ None Left: ☐ Brisk ☐ Sluggish ☐ None

Eye Opening: ☐ Spontaneous ☐ To Voice ☐ To Pain ☐ None:

Verbal Response: ☐ Oriented ☐ Confused ☐ Inappropriate words ☐ Incomprehensible words ☐ None ☐ Artif. Airway

Motor Response: ☐ Obeys commands ☐ Localizes (pain) ☐ Withdraws (pain) ☐ Flexion (pain) ☐ Extension (pain) ☐ None

Glascow Coma Score (if applicable) _____

Reflexes: Gag ☐ Present ☐ Absent Swallowing: ☐ Present ☐ Absent

For Infant: Suck: ☐ Strong ☐ Weak ☐ Absent

Anterior Fontanel (less than 18 mo): ☐ Soft ☐ Bulging ☐ Sunken ☐ Closed   Nuchal Rigidity: ☐ Absent ☐ Present

Seizure Activity: ☐ Absent ☐ Present, Describe _____

Other pertinent data _____

PAIN

Child having pain: ☐ No ☐ Yes, Description/Management _____

HEAD/NECK/FACE

Check if present and describe: ☐ Lesions ☐ Drainage ☐ Swelling ☐ Tenderness ☐ Mass(es) ☐ Deformity ☐ Loose teeth

☐ Other _____

Description: _____

Figure 10-8, cont'd   Pediatric admission sheet.   *Continued*

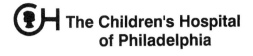

The Children's Hospital
of Philadelphia

Department of Nursing

NURSING DATA BASE

(PATIENT PLATE IMPRINT)

SECTION II: PHYSICAL ASSESSMENT (continued)

RESPIRATORY

Rhythm: ☐ Regular   ☐ Irregular   ☐ Periodic/apnea   ☐ Artificial ventilation   Depth: ☐ Deep   ☐ Shallow

Respiratory effort: ☐ Nonlabored   ☐ Retractions   ☐ Dyspnea   ☐ Accessory muscle use   ☐ Grunting   ☐ Nasal flaring

Breath Sounds: ☐ Clear   ☐ Rhonchi   ☐ Stridor   ☐ Crackles   ☐ Diminished

Location of abnormal breath sounds _____

Wheezing: ☐ None ☐ Expiratory ☐ Inspiratory   Cough: ☐ Absent   ☐ Infrequent   ☐ Frequent   Productive of _____

Secretions (color/amount) _____   Artificial Airway (type/size) _____

Other pertinent data: _____

CARDIOVASCULAR

Rhythm: ☐ Regular   ☐ Irregular   Peripheral pulses (Key: S-strong, W-weak, A-absent)_____ RUE _____ LUE _____ RLE _____ LLE

Capillary refill time _____   Murmur ☐ None ☐ Present _____

Pacemaker ☐ No ☐ Yes Type _____   Settings _____

Other pertinent data _____

GI/GU/ELIMINATION

Abdomen: ☐ Nontender   ☐ Tenderness/pain: Location _____

☐ Nondistended   ☐ Distended   Bowel Sounds: ☐ Present   ☐ Absent   ☐ Hypoactive   ☐ Hyperactive

Stoma/appliances/tubes/catheter (type and size) _____

Other pertinent data _____

MUSCULOSKELETAL

Gait: ☐ Steady   ☐ Unsteady   Describe _____   ☐ Unable to walk

Passive ROM   ☐ Full   ☐ Limited   Describe _____

Muscle Strength: (Key: S-strong, W-weak, A-absent) _____ RUE _____ LUE _____ RLE _____ LLE

Muscle Tone: ☐ Normal   ☐ Flaccid   ☐ Rigid   ☐ Spastic _____

Involuntary Movements: ☐ None   ☐ Twitching   ☐ Tremors   ☐ Spasms _____

Other pertinent data _____

SKIN

Color: ☐ Acyanotic   ☐ Pale   ☐ Flushed   ☐ Cyanosis   ☐ Acrocyanosis   ☐ Jaundice   ☐ Mottled

Mucous Membranes: ☐ Moist   ☐ Dry   ☐ Cracked   ☐ Ulcers

Temperature: ☐ Warm   ☐ Cool   ☐ Hot   ☐ Diaphoretic

Turgor: ☐ Elastic   ☐ Tented

Check if present and describe: ☐ Edema   ☐ Scaling/Dryness   ☐ Bruises   ☐ Rash   ☐ Petechiae   ☐ Scars   ☐ Stoma   ☐ Umbilical Cord

☐ Birthmark   ☐ Lesions   ☐ Breakdown

Vascular Access/site _____

Other pertinent data _____

RN Signature (completed physical assessment) _____   Date/Time _____

Figure 10-8, cont'd   Pediatric admission sheet. (Courtesy The Children's Hospital, Philadelphia.)

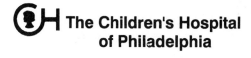

The Children's Hospital of Philadelphia

Department of Nursing

NURSING DATA BASE

SECTION III: HISTORY/PATTERNS (Complete within 24 hours)
ACTIVITIES OF DAILY LIVING/ROUTINES

Any problems with: Hearing ☐ No ☐ Yes, explain _____

Vision ☐ No ☐ Yes, explain _____

Assessment of Dependence Level (reflects status prior to admission) ☐ Infant: Less than 1 Year (May skip dependence scoring)

Dependence Scoring: 4 = Independent   2 = Requires help or a person for assistance, supervision or teaching
3 = Requires use of equipment or device   1 = Requires help from another person and equipment or device
0 = Dependent - does not participate in activity

Category	Score	Describe if score other than 4
Feeding	___	
Toileting	___	
Dressing	___	
Grooming	___	

Recent changes in assistance required with ADLs ☐ No   ☐ Yes _____

Mobility Needs: (assessment of pre-admission status)

Walking ☐ Independent ☐ N/A ☐ Needs Assistance _____

Transfers ☐ Independent ☐ N/A ☐ Needs Assistance _____

Bed Mobility ☐ Independent ☐ N/A ☐ Needs Assistance _____

Recent changes in mobility needs: ☐ No ☐ Yes _____

Safety Needs: ☐ Siderails ☐ Safety Crib ☐ Safety jacket ☐ Supervise with ambulation ☐ Slippers

☐ Special safety needs _____

Daily Routines: Diet: Foods/formula/schedule _____

Bottle/Nipple/Cup/Assistance with Feeding _____

Difficulty eating ☐ No ☐ Yes, explain _____

Recent weight gain/loss ☐ No ☐ Yes, explain _____

Other pertinent data _____

Toilet: Voiding/diapers/toilet trained _____

Words Used _____

Other pertinent data _____

Stool (pattern/description/date last stool) _____

Sleep: Bedtime/routines/naps _____

Bath: Habit/ointments _____

Other pertinent data _____

DEVELOPMENT

What changes have you seen in your child's development recently _____

Development appropriate for age as per nursing assessment ☐ Yes ☐ No Parent's perception of development consistent with nurses. ☐ Yes ☐ No

Comments: _____

Figure 10-8, cont'd Pediatric admission sheet.   *Continued*

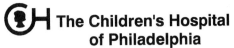 **The Children's Hospital
of Philadelphia**

Department of Nursing

NURSING DATA BASE

(PATIENT PLATE IMPRINT)

SECTION III: HISTORY PATTERNS (continued)

SEXUAL/REPRODUCTIVE

Sexually Active ☐ No ☐ Yes ☐ Not applicable

History of: ☐ Pregnancy/fathering a child ☐ Sexually transmitted diseases _____

Currently using birth control ☐ Yes, Method _____ ☐ No ☐ Not applicable

Last menstrual period _____ Change in flow: ☐ No ☐ Yes, explain_____

Other pertinent data _____

PSYCHOSOCIAL ASSESSMENT

Family Assessment:

What is the best way to reach you? Day _____ Evening _____ Other_____

Who participates in the child's care _____

Primary caregiver _____

Where does the child spend the day? ☐ Home ☐ Day Care ☐ Babysitter ☐ School ☐ Other _____

Grade/Name of School _____

Who lives with you at home _____

Child Care arrangements for siblings _____

Other parent/adult involvement (custody, visiting) _____

What is your plan for visiting _____

Would you like to participate in care ☐ No ☐ Yes, How _____

Is there any other information that would be important for us to know? _____

Cultural assessment

Cultural beliefs/needs that may affect care that you would like considered during hospitalization _____

Spiritual resources desired for self and/or child _____

Current Stresses and Coping Strategies

Have there been any stressful events in the family recently _____

Who helps you in times of stress _____

What worries you about being in the hospital _____

What worries your child _____

What would make your child more at ease while in the hospital _____

_____

_____

RN Signature (completed Section III) _____ Date/Time _____

Figure 10-8, cont'd   Pediatric admission sheet. (Courtesy The Children's Hospital, Philadelphia.)

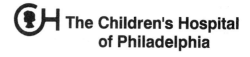

The Children's Hospital of Philadelphia

Department of Nursing

NURSING DATA BASE

SECTION IV: EDUCATION/DISCHARGE NEEDS (Complete within 24 hours)

EDUCATIONAL NEEDS

Identify learners (include patient if appropriate) _____

Do the learners need education in the following areas:

Disease Physiology	☐ No ☐ Yes _____
Tests & Labs	☐ No ☐ Yes _____
Diet	☐ No ☐ Yes _____
Treatments	☐ No ☐ Yes _____
Medications	☐ No ☐ Yes _____
Discharge Criteria	☐ No ☐ Yes _____
Other	☐ No ☐ Yes _____

Limitations/Barriers to Learning No Yes Identify learner/problem

	No	Yes	
Sensory	☐	☐	_____
Physical	☐	☐	_____
Cognitive	☐	☐	_____
Social/Cultural	☐	☐	_____

Readiness/Motivation to Learn _____

Best time for Teaching Sessions _____

Other Pertinent Data _____

DISCHARGE NEEDS

Anticipated home care needs: No   Yes

	No	Yes	
Home Nursing care	☐	☐	_____
Long Term Care Facility	☐	☐	_____
Equipment (Suction, O2 equipment, pumps, chairs)	☐	☐	_____
Medications/IV infusions/Parenteral nutrition	☐	☐	_____
Transportation Availability	☐	☐	_____
Car Seat	☐	☐	_____
Tutor/contact with school	☐	☐	_____
Immunization Follow-up	☐	☐	_____
Other			_____

Presently involved with:

Home Care Agency ☐ No ☐ Yes, Name _____

Contact Person _____ Number _____

Social Worker ☐ No ☐ Yes, Name _____ Number _____

Primary Physician: Name _____ Number _____

Other Pertinent Data: _____

RN Signature (Completed Section IV) _____ Date/Time _____

Figure 10-8, cont'd   Pediatric admission sheet.

Box 10-11

Charting Tips Related to the Hospital Admission of a Pediatric Patient

The following information should be documented when admitting a pediatric patient:

- Name of the family members present and their relationship to the child
- Family's orientation to the inpatient unit (e.g., location of phones, visiting hours, and location of kitchen and hospital cafeteria) and to the child's room (e.g., call light, bed or crib rails)
- Application of identification band
- Explanation of unit routines, including meal times, bed times
- Completion of the nursing admission history form
- The child's exact weight, age, and any food or medication allergies
- Detailed assessment of the child's condition at the time of admission
- Vital signs and growth measurements (e.g., height or length, head circumference)
- Any written materials given to the family
- Response of the child and family to the admission process and orientation
- Any findings shared with the family regarding laboratory examination results, dietary needs, and procedures
- Reasons for any information deleted from the admission history
- Phone numbers of persons to contact in any emergency
- Special toys left with the child

---

useful in situations where frequent monitoring is essential. Activity flowsheets are often used in pediatric settings. Activities such as feeding, hygiene, and respiratory or neurological status are periodically monitored using these sheets (Figure 10-9).

Another type of flowsheet used in pediatric settings is the specialty flowsheet, which focuses on one primary care area. An example of this would be the "Comprehensive Bone Marrow Transplant Documentation Tool" described by Tesno (1995) and used at St. Louis Children's Hospital (Figure 10-10). This tool was designed to address the specific issues when a pediatric bone-marrow transplant patient is being hospitalized. Topics addressed in this form are unique to the transplant patient and include assessment of mouth care regimen, central line care, and perirectal care history. The tool also includes a specialized teaching sheet for the family that focuses on tasks related to the care of the child undergoing bone marrow transplants.

CRITICAL DOCUMENTATION ISSUES IN THE PEDIATRIC SETTING

Use of Restraints

The use of restraints in any and all settings is currently controversial. Documentation of the application of restraints should be done with extreme care. According to a recent study, a review of the literature revealed no empirical support for this intervention with children. Furthermore, the Joint Commission guidelines requiring "the least restrictive safe and restrictive restraint" are not helpful in designing policy for pediatric patients because the guidelines are limited to emergency situations and dangerous behaviors (JCAHO, 1996; Selekman, and Snyder, 1997).

The restraint standards are written so that individual policies can be formulated, but they must address the following points (Selekman, Snyder, 1997):

1. Protection of the patient's rights, dignity, and well-being during use
2. Use based on patient's assessed needs
3. Decisions about the least-restrictive methods
4. Safe application and removal by competent staff members
5. Monitoring and reassessment of the patient during use
6. Time limit of the orders
7. Documentation

The standards also permit the ordering of restraints by an independent licensed practitioner, not just physicians (JCAHO, 1996).

Restraints are often necessary in the pediatric setting for the patient's protection during a procedure, to restrict body movement, protect a site, or keep equipment from becoming dislodged. The nurse is therefore called upon to use his or her judgment about the necessity of restraints in this setting. Decisions often must be made on a case-by-case basis (Calloway, 1986). Nevertheless, the nurse should be aware that the improper or careless use of restraints or restraining techniques can have devastating consequences. Consider the following scenario:

> A 6-year-old boy admitted for eye surgery suffered neurological damage to his arm, which had been restrained so that he could not touch his dressings (Fiesta, 1983).

A written institutional policy should govern the use of restraints in general and especially for use with pediatric patients. Joint Commission standards allow as-needed (prn) orders in medical settings (JCAHO, 1996). Documentation should include compliance with institutional policy. If a restraint flowsheet does not exist at the institution, the nurse may want to develop one, because the appropriate use of restraints requires assessment and consideration of a number

Text continued on p. 192

The Children's Hospital of Philadelphia
Department of Nursing
NURSING FLOW SHEET

FOUNDED 1855

(PATIENT PLATE IMPRINT)

DATE	DIET / FORMULA	PO	NG/GT HRLY / CUM		INTAKE TOTAL	URINE	URINE TESTS	STOOL	STOOL TESTS	COMBO	EMESIS			OUTPUT TOTAL
06														
07														
08														
09														
10														
11														
12														
13														
14														
TOTAL														
15														
16														
17														
18														
19														
20														
21														
22														
TOT														
23														
24														
01														
02														
03														
04														
05														
06														
TOT														

Figure 10-9   Nursing flowsheet. (Courtesy The Children's Hospital, Philadelphia.)

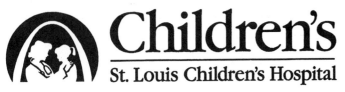

Children's
St. Louis Children's Hospital
Bone Marrow Transplant Program
Teaching Flow Sheet

Patient Stamp

VIRAL STATUS: Patient: CMV_____ EBV_____ HSV_____ VZV_____ Donor: CMV_____ EBV_____ HSV_____ VZV_____

ASSESSMENT

MOUTH CARE
▼ Mouth care protocol currently being followed and perceived compliance with protocol

▼ Outline plan for oral care negotiated with patient and family (identify staff/family responsibilities and plan options when oral care becomes difficult)

CENTRAL LINE CARE
▼ Current home central line care

▼ Plan for central line care while in unit (identify staff/family responsibilities and dressing to be used)

PERIRECTAL CARE
▼ History of perirectal breakdown and treatment that has worked in the past

BATHING
▼ Plan for bathing routine while in unit (identify staff/family responsibilities and AM or PM routine)

TRANSFUSIONS
▼ Outline transfusion history and requirements for pre-medication

▼ Antibiotic/Antifungal medication history (allergies, reaction to Amphotercin)

Figure 10-10 Comprehensive bone marrow transplant documentation tool. (Courtesy St. Louis Children's Hospital, St. Louis.)

Bone Marrow Transplant Program

Teaching Flow Sheet

Patient Stamp

Initial Education	Ongoing Education	TEACHING	
INITIAL/DATE	INITIAL/DATE	Task	Comments
		UNIT GUIDELINES	
		Visiting policy	
		Use of yellow gowns	
		Patient's clothing	
		Parents' clothing	
		Handwashing (1 minute scrub/septisol)	
		Use of Wexcide	
		Dirty floor concept	
		Use of nurse server	
		Airhandling system	
		Use of lounge	
		Low bacteria diet	
		Nursing/Unit Tech Roles	
		▼ Weights	
		▼ Blood draws	
		▼ I & O	
		Child Life/Physical Therapy/Social Service	
		Prophylactic antiviral and antibacterial therapy	
		MOUTH CARE	
		Importance of mouth care	
		Unit protocol (expected frustrations)	
		Medications	
		Alternative to Nystatin (troche, popsicle)	
		Pain control	
		CONDITIONING THERAPY	
		Purpose of therapy (ablation of bone marrow/irradiate tumor cells)	
		Specific protocol to be followed	
		High dose chemotherapy reviewed: Specific Drugs: _____ _____ _____ _____	
		Total body irradiation	
		▼ transportation	
		▼ length of procedure	
		▼ skin care	
		▼ anticipate jaw pain	
		▼ diversional activities	

Figure 10-10, cont'd   Comprehensive bone marrow transplant documentation tool. *Continued*

Bone Marrow Transplant Program

Teaching Flow Sheet

Patient Stamp

Initial Education INITIAL/DATE	Ongoing Education INITIAL/DATE	TEACHING	
		Task	**Comments**
		SIDE EFFECTS OF CONDITIONING THERAPY	
		Mucositis	
		Nausea/vomiting (Ondansetron/Ativan)	
		Diarrhea	
		Alopecia	
		Changes in skin condition	
		Anorexia and use of TPN	
		Infections	
		TEMPERATURE SPIKE	
		What is a temperature spike	
		Cultures (blood, urine, mouth, lesions, nasal)	
		Antibiotics	
		Amphotercin	
		BLOOD PRODUCT TRANSFUSIONS	
		Indications for	
		CMV status/irradiation/leukopoor	
		Need for pre-medication	
		TRANSPLANT DAY	
		Pre-medication	
		Marrow administration	
		Immediate complications (fluid overload, pulmonary edema, nausea, vomiting, red urine if autologous)	
		ENGRAFTMENT	
		What is engraftment (ANC 500 x 3 days)	
		Use of colony stimulating factors	
		GRAFT-VS-HOST DISEASE	
		Cause	
		Organs involved and staging system	
		Prophylactic medication	
		Treatment	
		Acute GVHD vs. chronic GVHD	
		CHILD LIFE SERVICES	
		Transplant Process (Calendar)	
		Transplant Day (Medical Play)	
		Mouth Care (Incentive Chart)	
		Pan Control (Pain Scale)	

Figure 10-10, cont'd Comprehensive bone marrow transplant documentation tool. (Courtesy St. Louis Children's Hospital, St. Louis.)

Bone Marrow Transplant Program

Teaching Flow Sheet

Patient Stamp

Initial Education INITIAL/DATE	Ongoing Education INITIAL/DATE	TEACHING	
		Task	Comments
		DISCHARGE EDUCATION	
		INFECTION CONTROL	
		Crowd control at home	
		Bathing	
		Handwashing	
		How to deal with pets	
		Allowed activities	
		When to call for help (fevers, bleeding, rash)	
		NUTRITIONAL ISSUES	
		Low bacteria diet	
		Fluid intake	
		Eating out	
		SKIN CARE/MOUTH CARE	
		Skin protection from sun	
		Care of dry skin	
		Use of toothbrush/toothettes	
		Oral care program	
		CENTRAL LINE CARE	
		Dressing charge demonstration	
		Return demonstration of dressing change	
		Central line irrigation demonstration	
		Central line irrigation return demonstration	
		HOME MEDICATIONS	
		List dose, administration and side effects	
		SPECIAL INSTRUCTIONS/FOLLOW-UP	

INITIALS	SIGNATURE	INITIALS	SIGNATURE

Figure 10-10, cont'd Comprehensive bone marrow transplant documentation tool.

of items. These items should be documented according to the nursing process, as follows:

1. Assessment should include the necessity of restraints, a consideration of the least restrictive method available for use, and what has been tried previously. Restraints are not a substitute for observation; rather, they require heightened observation and detailed assessments. Assessment must be ongoing until the restraints are removed. Observations should include airway, skin integrity, neurological status, circulation, range of motion, and limb alignment.

2. The nursing diagnosis should support the choice for using or not using restraints. This should be done with the utmost care because the choice of whether to use restraints should be the result of the weighing of competing concerns.

3. Parent teaching should include explanation of restraint use. An informed consent must be obtained for the use of the restraint. A developmentally appropriate explanation should be offered to the child. Documentation should include the nurse's advising of the parent and child to "tell me if it feels too tight." A documented teaching plan not only reduces the risk of injury; it enhances cooperation to the highest possible degree.

4. Documentation of implementation must include the type of restraint, who applied the restraint, the time of application, how the restraint was employed (e.g., whether a knot was tied for quick release), and that the restraint will not tighten as the patient moves (Selekman, Snyder, 1997). Document the explanation to the nonprofessional staff and parents about restraints so they do not release them out of misplaced compassion for the child.

5. Documentation of evaluation should include whether the restraints are accomplishing the purpose for which they were ordered, progress toward goals or behavioral outcome, whether a continued need for restraints exists as a result of medical condition, and a justification for their continued use (AAP, 1997).

Child Abuse and Neglect

In 1991 the New Jersey Division of Youth and Family Services received 53,750 reports of abuse and neglect, 36% of which were substantiated. Forty-three percent of these cases were related to physical abuse and 48% were related to neglect (Hansen, 1993). Injuries from child abuse are one of the leading reasons for childrens' hospital admissions, particularly in the emergency department. Malpractice claims in the emergency department are one of the fastest growing claim categories. Nearly 38% of the records of an emergency department in one large metropolitan pediatric hospital were subjected to legal review because of outside requests for copies of the records (Schoenfeld, 1991).

Following the theory that the reporting of child abuse as it was occurring would lead to early intervention and treatment plans for abusers, the federal Child Abuse Prevention and Treatment Act of 1973 (42 U.S.C.A., sect. 5101-5106 [1973]) required that individual states pass laws providing for reporting of abuse to the appropriate county or state social services agency. Failure to report is often a misdemeanor, so the nurse should be familiar with his or her state's requirements. The report does not have to be made only in cases of *proven* child abuse—only cases in which a reasonable suspicion exists of its occurrence. One author suggests that physicians reporting only those cases of proven child abuse are underreporting (Clayton, 1997).

Healthcare providers have been wrongly sued for not releasing children to their parents while awaiting the investigation of a government agency. In one case parents sued a hospital for retaining their 5-month-old baby who had suffered an unexplained fractured femur. Although criminal charges were never proven against the parents, the hospital won the case because it was complying with the law and acting under a reasonable belief that its actions were warranted to prevent further imminent harm to a child that had already been abused (*Sager v. Rochester General Hospital*, 1996).

All nurses who come into contact with the pediatric population, including emergency department nurses, community health nurses, school nurses, and pediatric floor nurses, may discern abuse or neglect. Failure to act to protect a young client may be criminal; therefore knowing one's state reporting requirements and institutional procedures (e.g., who may report, the criteria for reporting) is very important. Because a nurse may be criminally liable for failing to report and liable in a civil action for any injuries sustained by a child injured after release when abuse was suspected, the nurse should be able to distinguish between injuries with a low index of suspicion for abuse and injuries that do not generally occur in the absence of abuse.

Injuries with a low index of suspicion include foreign bodies in the ears and noses, sprains in children aged 15 and older, dog bites, isolated digit injuries, corneal injuries, and isolated head lacerations (Boyce, Melhorn, Vargo, 1996). All fractures (especially those of the ribs and temporal and posterior bones of the skull, and any spiral fractures, which do not occur in the absence of a twisting motion), bruises, burns, injuries to the chest or abdominal organs, and bleeding in the retina should have a high index of suspicion (Hansen, 1993).

Nurses should be aware of the risk factors for abuse when an injury is reported or observed. If two or more factors are present, consider reporting your concerns. The most important signs should be documented in the medical record. A review of the chart and observation of the patient may reveal the following (Boyce, Melhorn, Vargo, 1996):

- Differing accounts over time or from one examiner to another as to how the injury occurred—whether from the actions of either the child or the custodian

- Conflicting accounts from child and parent as to how the injury occurred
- Delay in seeking treatment
- History of unexplained or suspicious injury
- Injuries inconsistent with the child's history or developmental level
- Injuries older than the stated time of occurrence
- Detached parent or one who makes no attempt to comfort the child
- Diagnosis of mental retardation or other developmental delay

An extremely upset parent whose toddler was injured during a momentary inattention can be easily identified (Hansen, 1993). Institutional policies often include other factors to assess. The following are risk factors for neglect (Helberg, 1983):

- Delay in seeking treatment
- Diagnosis of mental retardation or other developmental delay
- Lack of knowledge of the child care by the primary caregiver
- Unusual responses of the child to parent-initiated contact or unusual response of parent to child-initiated contact
- Inability of the child to perform age-specific developmental tasks
- Weight of the child that is out of proportion to height or head circumference, which indicates nutritional neglect
- Child under age 10 left home alone

Documentation should include detailed assessment for risk factors. Conflicts in the reporting of injuries to different examiners should be charted by each professional and communicated by members of the healthcare team to each other. Documentation should also include descriptions of the relationship between the child and the person presenting the child for treatment. Relatives and caregivers other than parents can also be responsible for abuse. Furthermore, the unit should keep an instant camera to take color photographs of injuries. Long after injuries have healed, the photographs will explain to anyone who investigates what the nurse saw. Two photographs should be taken of each injured site. On the back of each photograph, write the date taken, the name of the patient, the hospital's name, and the title of the photographer. Without this information, the photographs will not be admissible in court.

Consent and Privacy Issues

Pediatric patients are legally minors who cannot consent on their own behalf to medical, surgical, or diagnostic treatment. Their parents or legal guardians must therefore sign a written consent for treatment on their behalf. In emergency situations verbal consent may be obtained by telephone from an absent parent or guardian. However, if no person is *in loco parentis* (i.e., "standing in place of the parent"), healthcare providers should be aware of and comply with state law and institutional policy. The age of majority is prescribed by statute (generally age 18, but it may vary).

Nurses should be aware that certain situations exist in which a minor can consent on his or her own behalf, without the knowledge of a parent or guardian. In the first situation a teenager may be an emancipated minor, one who by having achieved a certain status may make his or her own decisions. Emancipated minors include those who are married or in the armed forces, are responsible for their own financial affairs, or have one or more children of their own. State law may vary greatly on the definition of an emancipated minor, so the nurse should be informed about the state's legal requirements. The decision to treat a child as an emancipated minor should include documentation of the examination of written proof of marriage, service records, or any other document proving emancipation, including a court order. Photocopies should be appended to the chart.

The second situation in which an adult's consent is unnecessary, in which the minor does *not* have to be emancipated, involves the kind of treatments sought by teenagers, such as treatment for venereal disease, sexual assault, birth control, abortion, prenatal care, drug or alcohol addiction, or counseling. State law also varies here, and again the nurse should know state law.

Some states recognize the mature minor doctrine in special situations in which parental consent cannot be obtained and the minor appears to understand and consent to the treatment, or cases in which a minor has suffered a life-threatening injury. Consider the following scenario:

> A 17-year-old accompanied her mother to the hospital for the mother's surgery. After the mother went into surgery, the daughter caught her finger in a door and needed emergency treatment. Because the parents were divorced and the father was 200 miles away, a surgeon repaired the finger. The mother sued for lack of informed consent. The courts in Kansas agreed that consent was generally required, but that an exception can be made for an emergency or situations in which the parent is remote. In this case the teenager raised no objection to the repair to her finger, and she was seen to be intelligent and capable (*Younts v. St. Francis Hospital and School of Nursing, Inc.*, 1970).

The mature minor doctrine has limited application factually and from one state to another. The previous case was decided in the 1960s; today, with the advent of cellular phones and fax machines, it might be of little practical value. Nevertheless, if a nurse practices in any state where the mature minor doctrine is commonly invoked for treatment, careful documentation should be made of the fact that the parents are unavailable, of attempts made to reach them, and of the demeanor and words of the minor.

Divorced parents can present a special need for documentation in pediatric cases. Two types of custody arrangements exist: sole custody, in which only one parent has legal control of the child, including the right to make major medical decisions; and joint legal custody, in which the child has a parent of primary residence. The second type is more common today. In both types, either parent can probably consent to treatment in emergencies. For non-emergency treatments, however, only the sole custodian, in cases in which one parent has been granted that privilege by court order, may determine which course of treatment will be followed when more than one alternative exists (e.g., with cancer treatments).

Minors have privacy rights similar to adults. Do not be tempted to discuss a child's care with anyone other than the custodial parent without his or her permission. The identity of those people who are permitted to give or receive information about the child's care or make decisions on the child's behalf should be recorded in the chart. Some state laws allow the healthcare provider to withhold information from the parents, guardian, or spouse of a minor seeking treatment for an exempt treatment classification related to the child's sexuality or drug or alcohol use. The law may also allow the provider to inform the parent, guardian, or minor's spouse over the minor's express refusal. The nurse also is responsible for keeping a child's HIV or AIDS status confidential. Only direct caregivers have a right to know the diagnosis, which should not be displayed anywhere but in a carefully guarded chart (Greve, 1990).

DOCUMENTATION AND COMMON PEDIATRIC NURSING DEVIATIONS

Nurses are commonly sued for a number of routine pediatric care measures when a child is injured, primarily medication errors, IV errors, and burns. The injuries, which can include severe brain damage or death, are often catastrophic. As stated in this chapter, a nurse can face criminal charges for reckless disregard of the standards of practice. No substitute exists for common sense, coupled with continuing education and an ability to focus on the task at hand. Documentation tools should be designed to assist nurses with the organization of tasks, including medication administration and the monitoring of sites and equipment, as prescribed by institutional policies.

Medication Errors

One piece of information must be on all pediatric charts, Kardexes, and medication cards: the patient's weight at the time of admission, which should be updated as ordered or needed. Without this information nurses increase the risk of administering the wrong amount of medication. The nurse should weigh the patient, ask the parent, or calculate the dosage himself or herself, particularly for digoxin, insulin,

heparin, and chemotherapeutics. "If your calculation is different than the order, check the Physicians' Desk Reference or with the pharmacist first, then check the order. . . . It's your legal duty to defer carrying out any order that's unclear or contraindicated. . . . It's never safe to assume that because a doctor ordered it, it's correct" (Greve, 1990). Consider the following case:

A 1-year-old child died after a surgical repair of a congenital heart defect, and the ICU nurses were held liable because they administered the prescribed doses of 0.1 mg. of digoxin with two follow-up doses of 0.55 mg each. The nurses were negligent because they failed to recognize a digoxin overdose by correlating body weight with the dose ordered. (*Brosseau v. Children's Mercy Hospital*, 1984). In another case, nurses were found negligent for administering an adult dose of insulin to a child (*Peterson v. Fairfax Hospital*, 1992).

If nurses must question an order, they should document all the steps taken to question the physician or use their chain of command.

The crash cart in the emergency department should contain readily available information on pediatric emergency drugs in dosages for weights from 1 to 50 kg, approved and signed by a pediatrician (Leifer, Brown, 1997). Nurses are "floated" more often today, and deadly consequences can occur when dosages and medications are unfamiliar. An often-cited pediatric case involved a nurse supervisor who was helping out in a pediatric ward. Instead of giving an elixir of Lanoxin (digoxin) orally based on an unclear order, she injected it, and her 3-month-old patient died (*Norton v. Argonaut Insurance Co.*, 1962). Nurses must know all the existing forms of pediatric medications: pills, elixirs, suspensions, and parenterals.

Administering a prescribed amount is not enough under current standards of care. Nurses who have fought for professional status on the healthcare team now find that their status as independent professionals creates a standard that does not allow them to blindly carry out their orders if a child is injured. The stakes are too high for the child (and the nurse, also). A nurse was recently prosecuted for administering medication by the wrong route and at the wrong dosage—even though the dosage was sent up by the pharmacist (Ventura, 1997). Fifty percent dextrose was given instead of 10% dextrose as ordered. The 50% dextrose concentration was erroneously sent up by the pharmacy. The baby suffered severe brain damage and her parents obtained an $11 million verdict (Weitzman, 1997b).

Nurses must document on the chart in detail both when and why a medication was held or omitted. If the cause was signs of patient toxicity, document what was done to report the signs and symptoms to the physician. Document the results of laboratory tests that influenced the judgment. (Documentation tip: document not only who *gave* an injection but also who *assisted*.) Because the recognized standard is for two persons to administer an injection, given the possibility that a child will move, the nurse should document whether he or she received assistance from a parent or nursing aide. Numerous cases exist in which claims of tissue necrosis and nerve damage from injections were made.

Intravenous Therapy

Because infants and children are composed of a higher percentage of water than adults (newborns are composed of 75% body water, which decreases to 45% by adulthood), children can suffer greater injury from sudden fluid shifts and fluid overload (Whaley, Wong, 1995). Overload can happen rapidly, with disastrous consequences. Consider the following case:

> A child with type I diabetes was admitted with ketoacidosis for rehydration. Nurses assessed and completed documentation on the child's status on an hourly basis. However, in a 15-minute period, the child was incontinent of 400 ml of urine. One-half hour later, the child's neurological status was altered and he suffered a cerebral edema and infarct. He is now in a persistent vegetative state (Weitzman, 1996).

A child's more delicate skin and tissues are exposed to greater injury from IV infiltration and extravasation because a bigger percentage of skin surface is likely to be involved. Remember that a child's muscles and tissues are still developing, and injury may retard or prevent the growth process.

The standard of care now requires the use of an infusion pump because "even a small fluid overload can have alarming consequences" (Greve, 1990). The pump setting should always be recorded contemporaneously, which will assist the nurse in reviewing that the setting is correct. In one case a 3-month-old in respiratory distress was overdosed with Ativan (lorazepam). She was supposed to receive 4 mg per hour, but the pump was programmed in error so that she received 24 mg in 1½ hour. She suffered seizures and permanent neurological injury because of an overdose of propylene glycol, the diluent in which the Ativan was suspended (Laska, 1997h).

Nurses must also carefully monitor the IV site and line. Institutional policy may guide how often the nurse must check the site. Young patients may not be able to communicate symptoms of soreness and pain at the site. One author recommends site inspections every hour (DiCostanzo, 1996); another, every half hour, and more often if a vesicant is used (Greve, 1990). However, if the nurse comes on duty in a unit where the lines are normally checked every 15 minutes, but the nurse checks every ½ hour, and a child is injured, the nurse may be liable for deviating from the standard created by the unit. Reviewing a chart or flowsheet for how often monitoring is to be done on the unit is important (Figure 10-11).

Consider the following scenario:

> A 4½-month-old retarded infant admitted with dehydration had a limb amputated because of the nurse's failure to monitor the IV site. The verdict was for $1.2 million (Weitzman, 1987c). In another case, a 3-year-old suffered second- and third-degree burns, which required skin grafting, from a vitamin solution (Zarin, 1980).

Monitoring of the site should be hands-on. Any bandages covering the site should be removed for inspection, or clear dressings should be used. Documentation at the time of inspection should describe the appearance of the site and whether any redness, swelling, excessive warmth, coolness, or discoloration is present. Thereafter, the nurse may chart "site unchanged" or use a similar code on a flowsheet. If an abnormality is apparent, the nurse should monitor and document more often.

Once the nurse has a reason to believe that infiltration has occurred, he or she should immediately discontinue the IV and notify the medical provider because measures, such as injections of certain medications and (if necessary) a fasciotomy, can be taken to limit the damage if the nurse does not delay. The nurse should document all steps taken to limit the damage. Infiltrations are not uncommon and may not be caused by negligence. However, the nurse may be liable for failing to limit the damage after infiltration. Consider the following case:

> A 10-month-old girl suffered third-degree burns and ulcerations when a nurse applied scalding hot compresses to decrease the swelling in her IV-infiltrated foot. She needed surgery to repair the scar tissue and settled the case on an annuity basis for the principal sum of $367,000 (*Roman v. St. Elizabeth's Hospital,* 1984). In another case, a 2-year-old girl suffered an extravasation from an IV in her arm. The pediatrician and nurses used only warm soaks and elevation after the discovery of the extravasation. The girl suffered Volkmann's ischemic contracture and obtained a verdict of $385,000 against the physician and nurses (Weitzman, 1987a). It should be noted that legal awards have increased exponentially in the last decade.

Burns

The nurse can rarely avoid liability when a child is burned. Most burn injuries to pediatric patients are caused by the nurse's unfamiliarity with the equipment, using the equipment improperly, and failing to heed warnings or directions for use. Consider the following case:

> A 3-month-old suffered second- and third-degree burns on the buttocks from a heating pad—even though the manufacturer's label stated it was not to be used with an infant or a sleeping person (*Smelko v. Brinton,* 1987).

Halogen lamps, infrared lamps, light bulbs, vaporizers, heating pads, hot water bottles, and feeding bottles are

**The Children's Hospital
of Philadelphia**

Department of Nursing

NURSING FLOW SHEET

(PATIENT PLATE IMPRINT)

| DATE | IV SOLUTION | | | | IV SOLUTION | | | | IV SOLUTION | | | | SITE | IV FLUSH | MEDS | |
	BUR	PUMP	HR/CUM	RATE	BUR	PUMP	HR/CUM	RATE	BUR	PUMP	HR/CUM	RATE				
06																
07																
08																
09																
10																
11																
12																
13																
14																
14																
15																
16																
17																
18																
19																
20																
21																
22																
22																
23																
24																
01																
02																
03																
04																
05																
06																

Figure 10-11 Hourly intravenous therapy record flowsheet. (Courtesy The Children's Hospital, Philadelphia.)

just some of the equipment that may cause severe injury to young children in the hospital. Consider the following case:

> A nurse detached a temperature-probe monitor for an infrared lamp warming a premature infant. The baby suffered second- and third-degree burns, resulting in a leg amputation at the knee. A $4.5 million verdict was returned against the nurse. Because other alternatives were available, the lamp should have been used only as a last resort—and with careful monitoring (Weitzman, 1995).

Nurses must ensure that the equipment is working by testing it first, stay with the patient long enough to determine that it is not malfunctioning, and monitor frequently to observe that the patient is not being harmed. This means a careful inspection of all body surfaces. Nurses should document everything done to test the equipment, how long they observed its operation, and the appearance of the patient's skin each time it was monitored.

Other types of medical equipment that have caused serious injuries include respirators, traction weights and pulleys, cardiac monitors, and pulse oximeters, to name a few. Equipment can malfunction, be used improperly, or be overused. Equipment use should be monitored at frequent intervals with a hands-on observation and documented according to the type of equipment used. The pulse oximeter's sensor should be moved to a different digit at frequent intervals. A child in traction must have frequent neurovascular checks. A child on a respirator should be wearing a pulse oximeter with a visible display, and alarm bells must be answered immediately. Do not assume that the alarm is going off without a malfunction. In one case a respirator alarm sounded three times because of disconnection. The fourth time the respirator alarmed, the 17-year-old patient suffered severe brain damage and went into a coma (*Blolbaum v. St. Louis Children's Hospital,* 1982). The nurse should evaluate all equipment to look for alarms malfunctioning or to detect early changes in the child's condition.

Siderails and Falls

Another area of possible injury to children and potential liability to nurses involves the supervision of children in the playroom. Unaccompanied children should never visit the playroom because of the possibility of falling, fainting, vomiting and aspiration, or injury from another child. Document when the child goes to the playroom and with whom.

Children can easily fall from bed. Active children in particular must be monitored. If the child is too young to understand why he or she should remain in bed, the child should be in a hospital crib. The nurse must assess and document what type of bed a toddler or preschooler sleeps in at home and provide the same kind of bed. Consider these well-known cases:

> The mother of a 3-year-old admitted for a tonsillectomy and adenoidectomy (T & A) told the nurse her child slept in a crib at home. However, he was placed in a bed with siderails. During the night, he put his head between the rails and was strangled (*St. Luke's Hospital Association v. Long,* 1952).

> A hospital was found liable when a 2-year-old fell from a hospital bed after climbing over the side. The child's parents had told the nurse that the child was very active and would climb (*Pierson v. Charles Wilson Memorial Hospital,* 1946).

How often nurses must chart siderails as up or down may be a matter of institutional policy. Every time a child is returned to the room or to the bed, the position of the siderails should be charted. The family should be asked to cooperate in the use of the rails for the child's safety. The nurse should document any instances in which the family fails to cooperate with this or any other aspect of care because the family's contributory acts to an injury can be a defense against a charge of nursing negligence. The nurse should also document any instances of tampering with medical equipment, removing the child from bed against the staff's instructions, or feeding the child when the child's diet is restricted.

Emotional Distress

Whenever a child is injured, not only is it possible that a lawsuit will be filed on the child's behalf, but the parents may also have an independent right of action to claim damages for their emotional distress. Parents can sue for emotional distress in two ways. First, the parents can sue because their distress was caused intentionally or recklessly, with outrageous conduct on the part of the nurse. Consider the following case:

> Two parents had a nasty exchange of comments with a triage nurse who had assessed their sick baby in the emergency department. The parents insisted that the baby receive immediate medical care. The nurse raised her voice and yelled at them. Then she assured the parents that their son was "doing okay" and they left after being reassured. The baby died several hours later. The parents recovered $1.85 million against the hospital employing the nurse. The court found the nurse's conduct outrageous under the circumstances (*South Fulton Medical Center v. Poe,* 1996).

The second way parents can recover for emotional distress is by claiming that they themselves suffered while witnessing their child's death or deterioration, even if the healthcare provider was only negligent. Usually the death in such cases was protracted and the provider did not respond to the parent's pleas for help. Although courts formerly were reluctant to allow damages for emotional injuries, the occurrence of these cases, like malpractice cases, is on the rise. Nurses should document who was with the child at the time of death or crisis for their own protection. In one claim against a hospital for a child's death, it was discovered that no parental relationship existed between a child and her father, with whom she had never lived, and who never visited her in the hospital (Weitzman, 1991).

An emerging type of malpractice claim, referred to as the "lost chance of survival," is related to emotional distress claims. In this type of case a very sick patient is admitted to the hospital with very little chance of survival. If the healthcare providers choose to stand by and do nothing on the theory that the patient could not be saved anyway, they may be subject to a suit for lost chance of survival. A court can determine through expert testimony whether the patient had a 20% or 40% chance of surviving. Then the court will calculate the damages, which can normally be predicted based on the child's condition and the provider's negligence, and multiply that amount by the survival percentage. This amount can still be very high, given that juries can feel enormous sympathy for the bereaved family of a child who had been sick for an extended period. Even in a seemingly hopeless case, nurses should document everything that was done to save the patient, the time the patient was brought to the emergency department or coded in the unit, any drugs and the dosages used, and the resuscitation efforts. A well-documented record may be the only defense against a lost chance of survival claim.

Communication Issues

Documentation is one way of communicating important information about the patient to other members of the healthcare team. Communicating effectively with young patients and their families and building trust are equally important, forming the foundation for all the other tasks the nurse must perform to improve or maintain the child's health. The more trust built between the nurse and the patient's family, the less likely a family is to file a lawsuit.

Monitoring and documentation go hand in hand. To protect themselves, nurses must document what they observe when they monitor. Nurses cannot document what they have not observed. Therefore scheduled observations must be made. That fact will impress no one when a child under a nurse's care is seriously injured. The rapidity with which pediatric patients can suffer fluid overload, overdose from a medication, or be injured by a burn or fall can not be overstated. Negative outcomes can be avoided if "appropriate nursing observations [are] made and significant information communicated to providers in a timely manner" (DiCostanzo, 1996).

Documentation is a written communication record; not only should it be a record of the nurse's assessments and interventions, it should be a record of what the nurse reported orally about the patient to other members of the healthcare team. The same principles apply to oral communication as to written. Be clear and factual in this context.

Nurses are frequently sued for failing to timely and adequately report changes in the patient's condition to the medical provider. Significant events, such as seizure, accidents, or changes in condition, signaled by abnormal vital signs or laboratory values, must be reported immediately to the physician.

A classic case of failure to report is reported in *Ramsey v. Physicians Memorial Hospital* (1977). Consider the following scenario:

> The mother of a feverish child brought to the emergency department reported to the nurse taking the history that she had found a tick on her child shortly before the illness. The nurse never reported this to the physician; as a result, the child died from untreated Rocky Mountain spotted fever. An autopsy disclosed the disease, and the child's sibling was saved with treatment. The plaintiff's expert in the case testified that "it is incumbent upon an emergency room staff . . . to record significant medical data. . . . The knowledge by a nurse that ticks were removed from a patient in the spring . . . represents significant data. If this were not passed on I would consider that a failure to apply an adequate level of conformance as to standards. . . . " (Aiken, Catalano, 1994).

According to DiCostanzo (1996), nurses must document the time and content of all nurse-provider interactions. "Be precise about when you called or paged, when a response was obtained, what information you related and any subsequent instructions or orders. This is a correct entry: 'Dr. M. informed of poor feeding and lethargy.' This is an incorrect entry: 'Dr. M. informed of infant's condition'" (DiCostanzo, 1996, p. 52). Failure to chart a telephone call to a physician raises credibility and character issues when testimony of an uncharted telephone call is given under oath. A nurse failed to win a case because she testified that she had a telephone conversation with a physician years earlier, which she had not charted (*Morse v. Flint River Community Hospital,* 1994). Conversely, a case was reported in which a nurse was able to defeat a claim by a physician—that he had told her something she never charted—because her charting was so exemplary. The patient's care was recorded in such detail that the only thing missing was what the doctor claimed to have told the nurse. The jury apparently had enough evidence to conclude that, had the conversation occurred, the nurse would have recorded it (*Dent v. Perkins,* 1992). There is no better way to win a case.

A nurse will be held liable if a patient reports something significant and the nurse fails to act upon it. For instance, an experienced mother told her nurse that her new baby gasped for air, gagged, and pulled its head away from the breast when being fed. The nurses documented the mother's statement, but failed to report it to the physician or take any other action. The baby subsequently aspirated and died (Weitzman, 1987b).

What happens when the nurse has reported and gets no response (or a response that he or she believes would be dangerous to the patient if followed)? A recent case highlights the complex problems faced by nurses today. Consider the following case:

A baby was admitted for repair of a diaphragmatic hernia. Surgery was successful, and the baby was placed on a ventilator after the operation. The nurse on the 3 PM to 11 PM shift noticed a high potassium value in the laboratory studies and called the physician to find out whether she should give the potassium that had been ordered. The doctor told her to give the maximum dose as ordered, which she did. The nurse on the 11 PM to 7 AM shift called the intern on duty in the early morning (it was a holiday) to report an increase in the respiration rate, a temperature of 104° F and no urine output. The intern gave no immediate response, and the night nurse gave the baby acetaminophen and a sedative. The nurse on the 7 AM to 3 PM shift came on duty and called the night nurse to clarify that there had been no urine output. The monitor alarms then sounded. The baby suffered permanent brain damage. The verdict against the caregivers totaled $24,000,000 with interest (Weitzman, 1997a).

What should these nurses have done? The nurse who knew enough to call the physician when she first noticed the high potassium value should have followed chain of command if she doubted the physician's order to give the maximum dose. Physicians—even with their extensive training—can make errors in judgment or make a mistake because they're tired. However, if the nurse decides to contact his or her supervisor when continuing to question an order, again the nurse should document who he or she contacted, the time, and the information relayed. The night nurse in the preceding case should have also followed the chain of command when she saw the baby was becoming sicker and received no response from the intern.

Cases like the preceding one illustrate the changing status of nurses, particularly those who care for helpless patients. Nurses who ignore their own training and experience when following doctor's orders may be found to have deviated from the standard of nursing care. Consider the following case:

A 7-month-old infant was admitted with a diagnosis of toxic megacolon. A Fleet Enema was ordered and administered. Thereafter the child exhibited several signs and symptoms of dehydration. The child later arrested and died. A jury found the nurses liable because the *Physician's Desk Reference* says that a Fleet Enema is contraindicated with megacolon and no dosage schedule is established for a child under age 2 (*Doerr v. Hurley,* 1985).

In another enema-related case involving a child in the hospital for an elective barium enema study, a physician ordered nonsaline enemas until clear without any restrictions on osmolality or volume. The standard for a child of the patient's weight (55 lbs.) was two enemas. The nurses gave between six and eight enemas, and the child died from water intoxication. No consultation occurred as to why the child's stool was still not clear (*Peters v. Missouri Delta Community Hospital,* 1979). These cases illustrate the idea that even if a doctor ordered a treatment or a medication, the nurse who administers it can be equally liable. Remember: No substitute exists for one's own professional judgment.

SUMMARY

Children rely on nurses to anticipate, detect, and communicate their unique needs. Astute monitoring and documentation are essential aspects of pediatric care that help protect the young client from injury and minimize liability risks for nurses in the pediatric setting. This chapter examines cases associated with nursing negligence in the pediatric setting and reviews defensive strategies for protecting pediatric nurses.

REFERENCES

ACOG: *Precis V: an update in obstetrics and gynecology,* 1994, Author.

ACOG, AAP: *Guidelines for perinatal care,* ed 4, Washington, DC, 1997, Author.

AAP Committee on Pediatric Emergency Medicine: The use of physical restraint interventions for children and adolescents in the acute care setting, *Pediatrics* 99(3):497, 1997.

Aiken TD, Catalano JT: *Legal, ethical and political issues in nursing,* Philadelphia, 1994, FA Davis.

Alexander M, Kuo KN: Musculoskeletal assessment of the newborn, *Orthop Nurs* 16(1):21, 1997.

AWHONN: *Standards and guidelines for professional nursing practice in the care of women and newborns,* ed 5, 1998, The Association.

Blolbaum v St Louis Children's Hospital, 25 ATLA Law Reptr, Washington, DC, 1982.

Boyce MC, Melhorn KJ, Vargo G: Pediatric trauma documentation, *Arch Pediatr Adolesc Med* 150:730, 1992.

Brent NJ: *Nurses and the law: a guide to principles and applications,* Philadelphia, 1997, WB Saunders.

Brosseau v Children's Mercy Hospital, 27 ATLA Law Reptr, 473, 1984.

Calloway SD: *Nursing and the law,* Eau Claire, Wis, 1986, Professional Education Systems.

Chagnon L, Easterwood B: Managing the risks of obstetrical nursing, *Matern Child Nurs J* 11:303, 1986.

Clayton EW: Potential liability in cases of child abuse and neglect, *Pediatr Ann* 26(3):173, 1997.

Dent v Perkins, 598 So 2d 1101, La, 1992.

DiCostanzo CD: Legal issues in neonatal nursing, *J Perinat Neonat Nurs* 10(3):47, 1996.

Doerr v Hurley, 28 ATLA Law Reptr, 42, 1985.

Eganhouse DJ: Electronic fetal monitoring: education and quality assurance, *JOGNN* pp 16-22, January/February 1991.

Fiesta J: *The law and liability: a guide for nurses,* New York, 1983, John Wiley.

Greve P: Legally speaking, *RN* 53(2):77, 1990.

Hansen CM: Child abuse and neglect in New Jersey: an overview, *Trends Health Care Law Ethics* 8(2):54, 1993.

Helberg JL: Documentation in child abuse, *Am J Nurs* 83(2):236, 1983.

JCAHO: 1997 comprehensive accreditation manual for hospitals, Oak Brook Terrace, Ill, 1996, The Commission.

Jones Jr C, Gleason A, Lipstein S: *Hospital care of the recovering NICU infant,* Baltimore, 1991, Williams and Wilkins.

Kessler BM, ed: Liability alleged against defendant hospital for negligence of employee nurse in injecting minor plaintiff with antibiotic improperly diluted with potassium chloride, *New Jersey Jury Verdict Review and Analysis* 14(5):25, 1993.

Klaus M, Fanaroff A: *Care of the high-risk neonate,* ed 4, Philadelphia, 1993, WB Saunders.

Korones S, Bada-Ellzey E: *Neonatal decision making,* St Louis, 1993, Mosby.

Korones S: *High-risk newborn infants,* ed 4, St Louis, 1986, Mosby.

Laska L, ed: Neonatal nurse gives overdose of potassium chloride to infant, *Medical Malpractice Verdicts, Settlements and Experts,* p 18, February 1995.

Laska L, ed: Neonatal nurse gives overdose of potassium chloride to infant, *Medical Malpractice Verdicts, Settlements and Experts,* p 18, February 1995.

Laska L, ed: Army doctors fail to test infant for blood diseases caused by Rh blood incompatibility, *Medical Malpractice Verdicts, Settlements and Experts,* p 26, Ocrtober 1997a.

Laska L, ed: Child dies twelve hours after discharge on day after, *Medical Malpractice Verdicts, Settlements and Experts,* p 25, October 1997b.

Laska L, ed: Clogging of endotracheal tube causes brain damage and cerebral palsy in premature newborn, *Medical Malpractice Verdicts, Settlements and Experts,* p 24, May 1997c.

Laska L, ed: Delivery of child not timely performed after fetal heart rate deceleration noted, *Medical Malpractice Verdicts, Settlements and Experts,* p 30, January 1997d.

Laska L, ed: Failure to assess fetus and start tocolytic drugs, *Medical Malpractice Verdicts, Settlements and Experts,* p 29, January 1997e.

Laska L, ed: Failure to diagnose and treat meningitis, brain damage and eventual death, $1 million dollar verdict in New York, *Medical Malpractice Verdicts, Settlements and Experts,* p 43, April 1997f.

Laska L, ed: Failure to monitor and timely treat hypoglycemia blamed for child's brain damage, *Medical Malpractice Verdicts, Settlements and Experts,* p 26, October 1997g.

Laska L, ed: Infant overdosed with Ativan, Propylene Glycol causes seizures, $750,000 settlement in Virginia, *Medical Malpractice Verdicts, Settlements and Experts,* p 21, February 1997h.

Laska L, ed: Maryland obstetrician blamed for infant's brain damage after failing to recognize signs of fetal distress, *Medical Malpractice Verdicts, Settlements and Experts,* pp 29-30, July 1997i.

Laska L, ed: Missouri hospital nurse monitors labor but fails to recognize fetal distress, *Medical Malpractice Verdicts, Settlements and Experts,* p 29, July 1997j.

Laska L, ed: Newborn suffering from lack of oxygenation not properly treated: brain damage and cerebral palsy, *Medical Malpractice Verdicts, Settlements and Experts,* p 32, March 1997k.

Laska L, ed: Two-month-old suffers potassium overload in hospital after surgery for congenital diaphragmatic hernia, cardiorespiratory arrest causes brain damage, blindness and need for constant care: $16 million Massachusetts verdict, *Medical Malpractice Verdicts, Settlements and Experts,* p 42, April 1997l.

Leifer G, Brown M: Pediatric codes: a cheat sheet, *RN* 60(4):30, 1997.

Letko MD: Understanding the Apgar score, *JOGNN* 25(4):299, May 1996.

Lippincott's manual of nursing practice, ed 6, Philadelphia, 1996, JB Lippincott.

Mahley S, Beerman J: Following the chain of command in an obstetric setting: a nurse's responsibility, *J Legal Nurs Consult* pp 7-13, January 1998.

Morse v Flint River Community Hospital, 450 S E 2d, 253, Ga, 1994.

Murray M: *Antepartal and intrapartal fetal monitoring,* ed 2, Albuquerque, 1997, Learning Resources International.

NAACOG: *Core curriculum for maternal-newborn nursing,* Philadelphia, 1993, WB Saunders.

NANN: Position statement: early discharge of the high risk neonate, *Neonatal Netw* 16(6):67, 1997.

NICHHD Research Planning Workshop: Electronic FHR monitoring: research guidelines for interpretation, *JOGNN* 26(6):635, 1997.

Norton v Argonaut Insurance Co, 144 So 2d, 249, La App, 1962.

Peters v Missouri Delta Community Hospital, 22 ATLA Law Reptr, 137, 1979.

Peterson v Fairfax Hospital, 35 ATLA Law Reptr, 24, 1992.

Pierson v Charles Wilson Memorial Hospital, 78 N Y S 2d, 146, 1946.

Ramsey v Physicians Memorial Hospital, 373 A 2d, 26, Md App, 1977.

Reidmiller et al v. Suburban Hospital Association, Inc, 21 ATLA Law Reptr 39, 1978.

Roman v St Elizabeth's Hospital, 27 ATLA Law Reptr, 375, 1984.

Sager v. Rochester General Hospital, 647 N Y S 2d, 408, NY Sup, 1996.

Schoenfeld PS: Documentation in the pediatric emergency department: a review of resuscitation cases, *Ann Emerg Med* 20(6):641/67, 1991.

Selekman J, Snyder B: Institutional policies on the use of physical restraints on children, *Pediatr Nurs* 23(5):531, 1997.

Simpson K, Creehan PA: *AWHONN's perinatal nursing,* Philadelphia, 1996, JB Lippincott.

Smelko v Brinton, 740 P 2d, 591, Kan, 1987.

South Fulton Medical Center v Poe, 480 S E 2d, 40, Ga, 1996.

St Luke's Hospital Association v Long, 240 P 2d, 917, Col, 1952.

Tesno B: A comprehensive pediatric bone marrow transplant documenta-tion tool, *Oncol Nurs Forum* 22(5):841, 1995.

US Bureau of the Census, Current Population Reports, pp 25-1095; and Population Paper listings, 5-7, pp. 10-64 cited in Statistical Abstract of the United States, 1997, p. 15.

Ventura ML: Are these nurses criminals? *RN* 60(12):26, 1997.

Vestal KW, McKenzie CA: *High-risk perinatal nursing,* Philadelphia, 1983, WB Saunders.

Weitzman LB, ed: Verdict following negligent failure of defendant pediatrician to timely diagnose and treat compromised circulation, a complication resulting from administration of IV fluids, *National Jury Verdict Review and Analysis* 2(2):21, 1987a.

Weitzman LB, ed: Failure to monitor infant following incidents of gagging and gasping upon feeding, *National Jury Verdict Review and Analysis* 2(4):20, 1987b.

Weitzman LB, ed: Negligence of defendant pediatrician and defendant hospital in selecting improper site for IV induction results in cut off of sufficient blood supply to leg of 4½ month old retarded infant, *National Jury Verdict Review and Analysis* 2(9):23, 1987c.

Weitzman LM, ed: Verdict for failure to perform nursing assessment of student with history of asthma exhibiting breathing difficulties, *National Jury Verdict Review and Analysis* 5(3):9, 1990.

Weitzman LM, ed: Wrongful death of four-year-old child institutionalized with multiple congenital anormalities, *National Jury Verdict Review and Analysis* 6(2):29, 1991.

Weitzman LM, ed: Failure to properly monitor preemie being warmed under infrared lamp, *National Jury Verdict Review and Analysis* 10(4):7, 1995.

Weitzman LM, ed: Failure to adequately monitor rehydration of minor, *National Jury Verdict Review and Analysis* 2(1):9, 1996.

Weitzman LM, ed: Toxic potassium overload results in infant suffering cardiac arrest and brain damage, *National Jury Verdict Review and Analysis* 12(5):2, 1997a.

Weitzman LM, ed: Negligent administration of incorrect concentration of dextrose to premature infant, *National Jury Verdict Review and Analysis* 12(7):2, 1997b.

Weitzman LM, ed: 27.5 million dollar medical malpractice, *National Jury Verdict Review and Analysis* 12(9), 1997c.

Whaley LF, Wong DL: *Nursing care of infants and children,* ed 5, St Louis, 1995, Mosby.

Young S et al: Parent stress and coping in NICU and PICU, *J Pediatr Nurs* 12(3):169, 1997.

Younts v St Francis Hospital and School of Nursing, Inc, 669 P 2d, 330, 1970.

Zarin IJ, ed: $107,200 verdict, medical malpractice, *New Jersey Jury Verdict Review and Analysis* 1(6):3, 1980.

11

Critical Care Documentation

EMERGENCY DEPARTMENT DOCUMENTATION

Mary Kathryn Sadler, RN, BSN, MBA, CEN

Patricia Meadows, RN, BSN, CEN

EMERGENCY NURSING

Emergency nursing is by nature intense and fast-paced, and it demands a high level of critical thinking. Emergency nurses must rapidly assess their patients and plan interventions while collaborating with emergency physicians, consulting specialists, admitting physicians, and ancillary departments. Furthermore, they must implement treatment plans, evaluate the effectiveness of treatment, and revise the plan within very narrow time parameters. These things present a huge challenge to the nurse, who must also provide an accurate record of care through documentation.

Throughout the patient's emergency care experience, the patient expects that the registered nurse (RN) will be competent enough to skillfully perform all aspects of the nursing process under intense pressure.

Equally as important as competence, communication, and timeliness is the emergency nurse's responsibility to act as a patient advocate by knowing the applicable standards of care for specific conditions. These standards are the measure by which the patient and community view nursing performance and hold the nurse accountable.

In the emergency setting, lives are saved or lost within minutes. The emergency nature of some of these cases brings the contribution of nursing to patient outcomes into sharp focus, and it underscores the necessity of nurses recording their professional contributions. This chapter addresses the importance of accurate documentation, provides some tips on how to accomplish it, and considers some of the consequences for those who do not do it.

Standards of Care

The standard of care is the level of conduct to which a nurse is held accountable, and it is defined as the way in which a reasonably prudent nurse would render care under the same or similar circumstances. In 1983 the Emergency Nurses' Association (ENA) developed standards of care for all professional nurses functioning in emergency settings. These standards remain the foundation for clinical emergency nursing practice today (Selfridge-Thomas, Shea, 1994). Thus they serve as the benchmark for determining whether an individual emergency nurse negligently caused or contributed to a patient's adverse outcome.

The responsibility of every licensed professional nurse is to be familiar with hospital policies or internal standards regarding patient care. Examples of internal standards include the following:

- Emergency department job descriptions for staff nurses and nonlicensed caregivers
- Policies regarding treatment of patients
- Descriptions of how to perform procedures
- Protocols for the management of specific clinical scenarios

Following of policies and procedures of the institution may not relieve the RN of the responsibility to function at a higher level than that set forth by that institution. Nursing professionals are held to standards set by specialty organizations, periodic journals, and published research as applied to practice settings. Review of the facility's policies and procedures is at least a starting point in the nurse's understanding of what documentation is appropriate, because internal standards detail specific expectations to be met by the RN. By comparing institutional policies with national standards of care pertaining to a specialty, nurses may improve practice at their facilities through professional collaboration and policy revision or development.

Purposes of Medical Records

The patient's medical history consists of information of paramount importance for the patient and healthcare provider alike. The data is used to preserve health or promote quality of life by systematically evaluating the patient and comparing historical facts with current findings. Medical records are used for many reasons; therefore accuracy and comprehensiveness are imperative. The emergency medical record has three primary uses:

1. The emergency medical record is a record of patient information pertinent to diagnosis and treatment.
2. The emergency medical record is used to secure reimbursement for the institution. To accomplish this, the record must reflect what treatment was indicated, what the results were, and that further intervention was justified. The Joint Commission for the Accreditation of Healthcare Organizations (JCAHO) uses nursing documentation to evaluate the quality of care when accrediting facilities. Furthermore, Joint Commission opinions directly affect the viability of healthcare institutions and the livelihoods of hundreds of employees.
3. The emergency department record is a legal record for the patient. Some information may be vital in matters unrelated to the clinical course, such as forensic investigations involving victim statements, mechanisms of injury, wound patterns, and gunpowder residue patterns, to name a few.

Importance of Documentation

Accurately documenting in the medical record is one of the best ways for the clinical nurse to defend against lawsuits alleging negligent healthcare delivery. Documentation flowing from policies that reflect national standards will serve as a powerful risk management tool for the emergency nurse. It will allow an objective reviewer to conclude that the nurse was appropriately monitoring and communicating the patient's progress (or lack thereof) to the treatment team.

Nurses' understanding of their professional responsibilities, which is attained by learning national specialty standards, enhances their appreciation of the value of documentation as a means of proving that the clinical nurse met his or her obligations to patients. Charting, whether by computer, narrative note, or flowsheet, must demonstrate that the emergency nurse assessed and communicated, planned and collaborated, implemented then evaluated the care provided, and reported important findings to the

physician as often as necessary during a serious situation. Furthermore, it must show that the emergency nurse acted as a patient advocate when disruptions of the standards of care threatened the patient's safety or a positive outcome.

Human Worth and Nurse Advocacy in the Emergency Department

Human worth is the fundamental idea behind the emergency nurse's role as patient advocate. Demonstration of respect for human dignity, autonomy, and individuality in emergency care settings is increasingly evaluated in customer satisfaction studies and Joint Commission surveys as both an ethical and a risk management concern. In no other healthcare specialty do nurses interact with so many people, such a variety of medical specialties and ancillary departments, or such a large cross section of humanity, as they do in the emergency department. Patients of all ages need rapid treatment for every conceivable type of affliction.

Respecting human worth is only one aspect of the emergency nurse's duty as patient advocate. Protecting patient confidentiality and patient safety after discharge comprise a large part of this responsibility, as does protecting patients from unsafe medical practices, such as dangerous orders and inappropriate medical response time. The opportunities and responsibilities of nurses in these areas have become pivotal in many hospital negligence claims, and they serve, during a very trying time for the profession, as powerful justification for keeping licensed professional caregivers at the bedside. A distinct section must be added to the nursing process approach in order to address ENA standards and documentation issues affecting emergency nurses on this topic: the role of nurse as patient advocate.

Use of Nursing Diagnoses in the Emergency Department

The often dramatic symptoms of emergency department patients, the volume of patients (sometimes as many as 80 or 90 for busy facilities in a 24-hour period), and the rapidity with which physiologic and psychosocial needs change during the critical period all serve to increase the challenges to the forming of nursing diagnoses.

In recognition of the fact that nursing diagnosis is a component of the nursing process, the list of diagnoses approved by the North American Nursing Diagnosis Association (NANDA) was incorporated into the ENA Core Curriculum in 1987. Emergency nurses are encouraged to keep this list in their departments for reference and become familiar with its use. As computer nursing documentation becomes more prevalent, NANDA diagnoses will become more readily available, and consistency in the application of nursing diagnoses will increase. An example of a nursing diagnosis in the emergency department follows:

A 65-year-old patient's symptoms include shortness of breath with a history of congestive heart failure. The nurse's assessment includes crackles and wheezes, tachycardia, coughing frothy sputum, and anxiety with restlessness. The patient's skin is pale.

Nursing diagnoses:

1. Ineffective airway clearance related to pulmonary congestion
2. Impaired gas exchange related to pulmonary congestion

Chapter Format

This chapter follows the nursing process as it relates to the care of emergency patients and ENA practice standards, which are summarized under appropriate components of the nursing process.

Assessment and communication are emphasized throughout a patient's course of treatment because, without relaying critical information to the physician and other key team members, nursing assessments are isolated and meaningless to the patient and a comprehensive plan of care can not be developed or implemented.

Included at the end of nursing process components are examples of legal issues in which nursing documentation plays (or should play) a major role, with relevant charting tips included. In some cases the nurse's actions as patient advocate actually prevented the hospital from being named in the action or resulted in a defense verdict for the hospital—even when physicians were found liable. In other scenarios the lack of documentation punctuates the fact that emergency nurses failed all of their duties to the patient according to the established standards of emergency nursing. It should be emphasized that the costs associated with going through the legal system, such as attorney fees, time spent away from work giving depositions and attending trials, and the emotional trauma of being accused of negligence, are not reflected in settlement amounts or jury awards.

The practicing emergency nurse will readily appreciate the human cost of failure to adhere to the prevailing standards of this complex specialty area. The examples make it clear that disastrous patient outcomes often result from the failures of nurses to properly utilize more than one element of the nursing process. Furthermore, these examples illustrate the value of nursing's contribution to outcomes and the need for professional accountability, as reflected in nursing documentation.

ASSESSMENT AND COMMUNICATION

Triage

According to ENA practice standards, "Emergency nurses shall triage every patient entering the emergency department and determine priorities of care based on physical and psychological needs, as well as factors influencing patient flow through the system" (ENA, 1995b).

The Importance of Triage

The importance of an effective triage process and the significance of nursing skill in triage cannot be overemphasized. The use of RNs in this role is inherent in successful triage design. Triage nurses must be very experienced in general nursing practice and highly skilled in rapid assessment. This enables the nurse to correctly evaluate the urgency of a patient's symptoms and rapidly determine who among several acutely ill patients most needs immediate medical treatment. Nurses must be capable of dealing with the stress caused by ringing telephones and repeated interruptions by visitors, family members, and other patients arriving for service. Emergency RNs must demonstrate outstanding communication skills, compassion, and patience because the interaction between the triage nurse and the patient sets the tone for this individual's entire emergency department experience.

The Triage Process

The triage process includes documentation of the following:

- Time and means of arrival
- Chief complaint (i.e., "What brings you here today?")
- Designation of care priority or acuity
- Determination of the appropriate healthcare provider
- Placement in the appropriate treatment area (e.g., cardiac versus trauma, minor care versus critical care)
- Initiation of interventions (e.g., sterile dressings, ice, application of splints, diagnostic procedures such as x-ray examinations, electrocardiograms [ECGs], or arterial blood gases [ABGs])

The triage process begins when the patient walks through the door. The triage nurse should begin by introducing himself or herself, then obtaining a brief history and assessment. For example, this might include taking a brief look at an ambulance patient on a stretcher before directing the crew to an appropriate treatment bay. This collection of subjective and objective data must be performed very quickly—requiring no longer than 5 minutes—because it is not intended to be as inclusive as the primary nurse's assessment. The triage nurse is responsible for assigning patients to the appropriate area of treatment; for example, a trauma bay with specialized equipment, a bay with cardiac and blood pressure monitors for cardiac complaints, or a rapid treatment area for minor complaints, such as sore throats without fever, toothaches, or minor sprains. Regardless of where a patient is first placed after triage, each patient should be reassessed by the primary nurse at a minimum of once every 60 minutes. For those who have been categorized as "urgent" or "emergent," reassessment every 15 minutes or more may be necessary. Each reassessment should be documented on the medical record. New information about the patient's condition may change the acuity categorization and thus the patient's location in the treatment area. For instance, the need to move a patient who initially presented for minor treatment to a monitored bed is obvious if the patient becomes nauseated or develops shortness of breath, syncope, or diaphoresis.

The Ideal Triage Interview

The ideal triage interview and documentation includes the following:

- Name, age, gender, and mode of arrival
- Chief complaint
- Brief history (including onset, degree of intensity, previous occurrence of the same condition, and previous medical problems)
- Medications
- Allergies
- Date of last tetanus immunization
- Date of last menstrual period for women of childbearing age (include gravida, para, and abortions, as appropriate)
- Assessment of vital signs and weight
- Patient classification and acuity level

Acuity Priorities

Certain cues should be recognized by the triage nurse that indicate the need for a high priority classification. These include the following:

- Severe pain
- Active bleeding
- Stupor or drowsiness
- Disorientation
- Emotional disturbance
- Dyspnea at rest
- Extreme diaphoresis
- Cyanosis
- Vital signs outside the normal limits

Patient Classification Systems

When a nurse accepts the role of triage nurse, he or she must have a complete understanding of the system in use by that institution. Some systems in use are Traffic Director, Spot Check, and Comprehensive. Each system differs in staff qualifications, acuity classifications, and documentation requirements.

In the Traffic Director system, the nurse identifies only the chief complaint and then chooses between "urgent" or "nonurgent" status. Based on this classification the patient is sent to the waiting room or the acute care area. No preliminary diagnostic tests are ordered and no further evaluation is performed until the time of treatment.

In the Spot Check model, the nurse obtains the chief complaint along with limited subjective and objective data, and the patient is categorized in one of three treatment priorities: "emergent," "urgent," or "delayed." Some preliminary diagnostic tests may be selected, and the patient

is placed in a specific care area or in the waiting room. No planned reevaluation occurs until treatment.

The Comprehensive system is the most advanced, using physicians as well as nurses in the triage role. A data base is initiated, including educational and primary healthcare needs, chief complaint, and subjective and objective information. Preliminary diagnostic tests are selected and the patient is placed in the acute care or the waiting room. If placed in the waiting room, the patient should be reassessed every 15 to 60 minutes (Rea, 1987).

Acuity levels range from I to V, with the least serious having the lowest number, as shown in Box 11-1.

Reassessment in Triage

Keep in mind that all acuity classifications have required reassessments. Documentation of reassessments should include times, vital signs, and changes in the acuity categorization. For example, consider the plight of the triage nurse who has to defend assigning an acuity level of nonurgent for a patient who suffered an unwitnessed myocardial infarction while waiting for 4 hours in the waiting area with no reassessment and no communication by the nurse with the physician during that time. The nurse will be very uncomfortable if an investigation determines that the history and symptoms taken at the time of arrival would have clued a reasonable nurse to rank the patient as emergent. Likewise, a patient whose symptoms include shortness of breath is incorrectly classified in triage as nonurgent will be denied the opportunity for testing, such as ABG evaluation or chest x-ray studies, or interventions, such as oxygen or potential medications for serious medical

---

Box 11-1

Acuity Levels

Class I

Routine physical examination (e.g., minor bruising); can wait indefinitely without harm

Class II

Nonurgent (e.g., rash, cold symptoms); can wait indefinitely without harm

Class III

Semi-urgent (e.g., cystitis, otitis media); can wait up to 2 hours for treatment

Class IV

Urgent (e.g., fractured hip, severe lacerations, asthma); can delay care for 1 hour

Class V

Emergent (e.g., cardiac arrest, shock); no delay in treatment can occur; life-threatening situation

conditions (e.g., congestive heart failure). (This could occur if the triage nurse fails to consider the history and symptoms carefully.) Similarly a patient with a broken leg could lose a limb if he or she is detained in triage after being categorized as nonurgent when appropriate assessment would have revealed swelling, discoloration, and the absence of a pulse.

Triage Is the Gateway to Treatment

The triage nurse should realize that arrival by emergency medical services (EMS) should not automatically guarantee immediate access to the treatment area because many patients misuse ambulance transport. Equally as many gravely ill or injured patients arrive through the front door of the emergency department. Effective triage nurses assess and determine clinical status to ensure that the sickest patients are seen and treated first.

Triage nurses facilitate patient flow in the emergency department and communicate relevant information to the appropriate healthcare providers, the patient, and family or friends. Patient acuity determines how quickly a patient is evaluated by the physician, as well as the patient's priority for nursing care. Triage nurses can contain much of the chaos in the waiting room by soothing nonurgent patients while facilitating the evaluation of urgent and emergent patients. By ordering minor x-ray studies on limbs and ECGs as appropriate, the triage nurse also can increase patient flow while obtaining information that primary nurses can use to further prioritize acuity. The primary nurse is the RN assigned to patient care after triage occurs. During the time a patient spends in the emergency department, his or her acuity may change quickly, and interventions should be adjusted appropriately to any changes in condition. At the time of disposition, acuity should be reassessed by the primary RN. Patients should not be discharged with a higher acuity categorization than the one with which they arrived.

Charting tips: Fill in all blanks on the emergency department record, including medications, allergies, temperature, pulse, blood pressure, oxygen saturation (as indicated), weight, last menstrual period (if appropriate), immunizations, history, time of arrival, time of triage, and especially the time that the primary nurse or physician received notification of potentially critical symptoms. If the waiting room time is extended because of a lack of available beds in the treatment area, the following information should be clearly documented:

- Vital signs and assessments timed and repeated as often as clinically appropriate
- Time and content of communications with charge nurse and physician regarding the patient's status
- Interventions performed in the triage area, including the patient's response

Excessive rushing or excessive delay in processing patients is not worth the cost of inappropriate evaluation and treatment or the consequences of being held responsible for depriving a patient of treatment.

Consider the following hypothetical scenario:

A normal infant boy was born at the thirty-fifth week of gestation because of premature rupture of the membranes of his mother, a young, unmarried woman. He experienced uneventful, routine growth until age 4 months, when he developed a cough and runny nose without fever. This illness occurred after he began attending a new child care facility. He was examined at his pediatrician's office, and the mother was instructed in the use of a decongestant. Three days later, during the late evening hours, the infant developed a fever of above 103° F, measured rectally, that would not respond to Tylenol (acetaminophen) at home. The pediatrician did not respond to two pages from the mother, so she brought her son to the emergency department after trying to lower the temperature for 7 hours. The mother and child waited for 2 hours in the waiting room before they were seen by the triage nurse. During the triage the RN noted the child had a temperature of 102.4° F (rectal), a pulse of 140 beats per minute, and a respiration rate of 40 per minute, and she documented "sleeping" as the level of consciousness. A history of previous congestion and runny nose was not elicited, nor was the fact that the baby had required medical evaluation 3 days earlier. The baby's pediatrician was not notified, and the triage classification was nonurgent.

The baby was discharged after 45 minutes in the emergency department without investigation of the fever and without antibiotics. He had continued to "sleep" throughout his brief emergency department stay. Ten hours later, he returned (via EMS) in cardiac arrest and died as a result of overwhelming streptococcal sepsis, clinically diagnosed by a different emergency department doctor and later confirmed by blood cultures.

Charting tips: The triage nurse set the stage for tragedy by failing to document the pertinent history. No note was made stating "report given to primary nurse" or of communication with the physician, and no evidence was shown of reassessment or recategorization to expedite care. Although documenting all conversations with staff for all emergency department patients may not be necessary, a wise nurse will document what he or she communicated and to whom when the clinical outlook is potentially serious.

Assessment

According to ENA practice standards regarding assessment, "Emergency nurses shall initiate accurate and ongoing assessments of physical and psychosocial problems of patients in the emergency department" (ENA, 1995b).

Variety of Presenting Specialties and Symptoms

A state of readiness exists in the emergency department at all times. At any moment, individuals of any age can arrive who are experiencing difficulty in any or all body systems.

Emergency nurses must be prepared to recognize abnormalities in any system and to participate in medical management appropriate for general medicine and surgery as well as pediatric, adolescent, and geriatric populations. Special conditions also occur, including renal failure, trauma, maxillofacial, dermatologic (e.g., burns), neurologic, psychiatric, cardiac, obstetric, neonatal, oncologic, ophthalmologic, dental, and other types of cases. No restrictions exist on the type of patients who might come to the emergency department or the dramas that can unfold there. Thus nurses who do not properly assess patients arriving for assistance have no excuses.

Organized Assessment Approach

Following an organized approach to assessment is very important, but most important is the idea that each nurse must develop and consistently use an approach that is meaningful to the individual. The first area of assessment should always be the cardiovascular and respiratory systems, including vital signs. A primary assessment of every patient for whom the emergency nurse has responsibility is mandatory, regardless of the patient's complaint. This survey takes only 30 seconds, and it includes airway, breathing, and circulation assessment. Vital signs are very significant indicators of current and future conditions. The body has a remarkable compensatory mechanism, and vital signs serve as indicators of how well that compensatory mechanism is functioning. Vital signs are "trended" (i.e., repeated overtime) and documented frequently in emergency settings so that they most accurately reflect the patient's status and effectively predict outcomes.

The general survey can be performed almost simultaneously with the primary survey, extending to areas such as level of consciousness, quality of speech, organization of thought, general appearance (e.g., dress, hygiene, skin color, facial expression, posture, motor activity while the patient sits or undresses, odors on skin or breath), and degree of distress. One very important aspect of assessment is the establishment of a therapeutic relationship. The nurse should provide privacy when talking with the patient, and he or she should utilize touch and verbal explanations to reassure the patient before performing any examination and procedure.

Assessment Priorities at the Time of Arrival

The triage nurse or EMS crew "delivers" patients to the treatment area to a primary nurse who is responsible for the care of that individual during the remainder of his or her stay in the emergency department. Included in the care that is expected of this primary nurse is the timely assessment of patients and the provision of written evidence of nursing assessments as the patients progress through the evaluation. However, this does not mean that nurses should perform complete physical assessments on every patient. Related pathophysiology should be explored and prior history, in addition to chief complaint and vital sign assessment, documented. For example, a patient who arrives with abdominal pain should be assessed for nausea, vomiting, diarrhea, and constipation. Additionally, appetite, weight loss, urinary problems, and skin turgor should be assessed. The abdomen should be examined for firmness, distension, point-tenderness, location and radiation of the pain. If possible, the patient should quantify the pain using the 1 to 10 pain scale (i.e., 10 being the worst pain, 1 being the least) and identify the type (e.g., burning, sharp, gnawing, cramping), onset, and duration of pain. Pulses in the lower extremities and swelling should also be assessed. History of congestive heart failure, bowel obstruction, flu, possible intake of spoiled food, ulcer disease, gastrointestinal bleeding, cirrhosis, bowel cancer, and other similar conditions should be assessed as well.

Another assessment priority pertains to trauma patients. A primary survey of the ABCDs (i.e., *a*irway, *b*reathing, *c*irculation, and *d*isability-neurologic status) must be assessed and documented at arrival as baseline data and should reflect consistency among all medical and nursing assessments. (If not, the nurse may someday be required to justify why the absence of breath sounds were noted during his or her primary assessment but were not conveyed to the physician.)

Also imperative is the assessment of the mechanism of injury (e.g., whether the patient was restrained or unrestrained via seatbelt, was ejected, was the driver or passenger, and the amount of vehicle damage—inside and outside). The EMS crew can be very helpful in this regard. This information can save time and lives by directing the clinical focus toward those internal structures and systems most vulnerable to specific types of injuries. Make note of any "field sticks" (i.e., intravenous [IV] devices started outside the hospital) at the time of arrival: needle gauges, location, fluid type, fluid amount (e.g., bag size, number, amount infused), and site condition (e.g., red, painful, swelling, draining, dressing intact). Policy may require that field sticks be changed more frequently than "hospital sticks"; therefore accurate documentation spares the patient from an increased risk of infection.

Some routine assessment parameters are considered standards of care, such as those used for head injury patients. A minimally acceptable assessment would include the mental status, level of consciousness, motor movement, posture, and pupillary status.

Assessment in the emergency department is designed to facilitate the recognition of life-threatening emergencies and collect enough data to establish priorities of care within a very busy setting. At all times, and for all patients, the emergency nurse is expected to elicit and communicate appropriate findings, including abnormalities, any worsening of symptoms, or changes in acuity level to the physician for further management. Documentation must reflect that this took place.

Monitoring

Many patients are placed on cardiac, blood pressure, and oxygen saturation monitors by primary nurses on arrival to the treatment area. This could be decided on the basis of clinical history alone or in combination with current complaints. When using a cardiac monitor, an initial strip should be timed and placed in the nursing record. If keeping the patient on a cardiac monitor remains necessary, then the nurse must document that monitoring was continued during periods when the patient was out of the emergency department (unless it is noted that the physician authorized otherwise). For example, the nurse would chart the following:

To CT scan with RN and respiratory therapist maintaining airway per Ambu bag and oxygen. Cardiac, oxygen saturation, and blood pressure monitoring maintained.

The standard of care is that vital signs are to be assessed every 4 hours at a minimum in the emergency department, and more often as the clinical condition warrants (e.g., every minute, if necessary).

The following case illustrates the importance of communicating assessment findings to the emergency department physician:

A 40-year-old female was transported to the emergency department by the EMS. She was complaining of a sudden, severe onset of right flank pain with nausea and vomiting that occurred while driving on the interstate from Florida to her home. At the time of the patient's arrival in the emergency department, the medics reported their belief that she might have a kidney stone, so a triage nurse assigned the patient to a noncritical bed. The receiving nurse insisted on talking directly with the patient and her family and immediately noted that the patient was pale, diaphoretic, and had a rapid pulse and low blood pressure. Her husband expressed that the patient's usual state of health was vigorous, and that her condition was very uncharacteristic. Within 10 minutes of her arrival, a physician was called to the bedside by the primary nurse. By the time the patient had been in the emergency department for 20 minutes, IV access had been established, a nasogastric (NG) tube and Foley catheter had been inserted, and she had been seen by a surgical resident. A computerized tomography (CT) of the patient's abdomen revealed an abnormality near the right kidney. The patient's condition deteriorated to the point that she required successful fluid resuscitation for shock and an emergent packed red blood cell transfusion for a critically low hemoglobin level. The diagnosis, made using angiography, was a ruptured right renal artery aneurysm. The patient's life was saved and liability was averted (anecdotal report, 1997).

Charting tips: The assessment of the RN and the involvement of the physician and other professional staff in the evaluation and plan of care were evident in the record, as were the time of the initiation of IV access, aseptic technique, needle gauge, blood flow, number of IV insertion attempts, NG insertion and verification of placement, and Foley catheter insertion using sterile technique.

PLANNING AND COLLABORATION

The ENA practice standard regarding planning states, "Emergency nurses shall formulate a comprehensive nursing care plan for the emergency department patient and collaborate in the formulation of the overall patient care plan" (ENA, 1995b).

Pace of the Emergency Department

Things happen quickly in the emergency department, but despite the variety and range of patient problems, a large body of knowledge thankfully exists that permits a reasonable number of tests and treatments. In this setting the goal is to stabilize a patient for the short term so that further diagnostic tests and management can be planned. Because of the need for rapid evaluation and treatment, nurses must exhibit a strong reliance on medical knowledge and protocol. The plan of care is often reflected in physician orders and in documented nursing assessments and interventions rather than in a formal written care plan. Therefore documentation by nurses of the times that orders were written and subsequently implemented and times that changes in patient status or pertinent clinical information were communicated to a physician together form a "tapestry" of care that reflects adherence to the standards of care as guidelines.

Preparedness

The key element of planning is preparedness. Emergency department nurses prepare for the unexpected; that is, the crises that will surely occur in this environment. Nurses should do this at the beginning of every shift by checking crash carts, defibrillators, endotracheal tube handles and lights, external pacemakers, pediatric emergency equipment, and suction equipment in every room. They should ensure that equipment and supplies are present and in working order so that patient care is not delayed. (This, too, should be documented for future reference.) Instances have occurred in which emergency department patients have aspirated and later died of adult respiratory distress syndrome because the suctioning apparatus did not work or nurses could not find the necessary equipment in the heat of the moment.

Safety

One standard of emergency nursing is that the emergency nurse should maintain a safe environment for coworkers, patients, himself or herself, and others in the department. This would include preventing hostile visitors from remaining at a patient's bedside or routinely anticipating the presence of weapons, then confiscating them from specific patient populations (e.g., those patients who might be homicidal or suicidal).

The following anecdotal case shows the importance of preparing for the care and safety of a fetus:

> A young woman who was 32-weeks pregnant was assaulted in a parking lot by a man trying to steal her car. She sustained severe head and abdominal injuries requiring admission to the intensive care unit (ICU). The patient remained in the emergency department for 6 hours while her assessment and consultations were completed. At no time was she placed on a fetal monitor. No consultation took place between emergency nurses and obstetric nurses, even though the facility had advanced capability for high-risk delivery and a neonatal ICU (NICU). Within 30 minutes of her arrival in the ICU, the fetus was noted to be in distress. (A fetal monitor was placed immediately by the ICU staff.) An emergency obstetrical team was activated and performed a cesarean-section. The infant has until at least age 21 to demonstrate developmental, physical, medical, or emotional problems that could be attributed to the emergency department nurses' failure to detect fetal distress in a foreseeable situation (anecdotal report, 1997).

Charting tips: The nurse's notes revealed a breach of standards; that is, a failure to provide a safe environment for the fetus in the emergency department and a failure to anticipate or plan for fetal monitoring and care per the applicable standard (i.e., the standard of care for obstetrical nurses). This fetus was clearly jeopardized. Had fetal monitoring been instituted in the emergency department, the time of placement should have been recorded, and monitor strips should have been placed in the record. The time of contact with labor and delivery nurses should be recorded in the emergency department nursing notes along with time of arrival for such assistance. If the ICU notes show that the infant was in distress from the time the fetal monitor was placed on arrival to the ICU, little, if any, defense exists for failing to obtain obstetric support in the emergency department.

IMPLEMENTATION

The ENA practice standard regarding implementation states, "Emergency nurses shall implement a plan of care based on assessment data, nursing diagnosis, and medical diagnosis" (ENA, 1995b).

Competency

The nurse should function independently within the parameters established for nursing practice in the emergency department, which may include life- or limb-saving measures. An emergency nurse must be able to perform and document nursing and medical treatments, includ-

ing times, according to accepted standards. One is not expected to know everything or be able to perform every procedure, but a competent nurse must be able to anticipate the need for special expertise as indicated by the clinical situation, and he or she must seek it and document all such efforts.

The advent of computerized charting has eliminated many concerns about handwriting. But competency issues will remain, as noted by the Joint Commission's requirements to maintain evidence of staff competency in key clinical areas, and by the increased numbers of lawsuits alleging that individual nurses failed to competently perform critical procedures according to existing standards. The following are examples of areas in which emergency nurses should routinely demonstrate competency, with relevant charting suggestions included:

• *Medication administration.* Nurses should always record the location of intramuscular (IM) injections. With irritants, such as IV Phenergan (promethazine), document the amount and type of the diluent. If breaking a glass vial is necessary, either note that a filtered needle was used or be certain that other nurses are prepared to testify that "usual practice" is to use filtered needles when extracting medication from glass vials.

Consider the following example:

> A 42-year-old woman was seen in the emergency department for pain caused by an ovarian cyst. An injection of Demerol (meperidine) was prescribed. The nurse giving the injection damaged the sciatic nerve with the needle, causing permanent injury and limiting the patient's active lifestyle. The hospital settled for $410,000 (Laska, 1997b).

Charting tips: Was the injection site recorded? Was a notation made in the record about patient response to medication, or a complaint about numbness, pain, or redness at the site? Was the physician notified? What was done about it? Was the discomfort improved at discharge?

• *IV access.* When initiating IV access, nurses should document that aseptic technique was used, a blood return was obtained, no swelling or redness was present at the site. The number of attempts at access by each nurse and the anatomic locations of failed attempts should be recorded.
• *Chest tubes.* The nurse should document the use of sterile technique, taping, placement verification, that lines are intact and functioning, and the use of the color and amount of output.
• *NG tube.* Placement and verification, including color and amount of output, should be documented.
• *Restraint use.* Documentation should include efforts to establish a rapport with the patient and instruct the patient on alternatives to restraints, and requests that the family remain at the bedside. Protection of patient privacy, the

provision of hygiene, diet, elimination opportunities, the release of restraints, and the condition of skin under the restraints should also be documented.

- *Lethal rhythm recognition and treatment.* Nurses need not record every nuance of the cardiac rhythms in the record. The standard of care for emergency nurses is to be able to recognize and be prepared to assist in the management of ventricular fibrillation, ventricular tachycardia with symptoms, pulseless electrical activity, asystole, and the bradydysrhythmias. Nurses must be careful not to overstep their responsibilities into the area of medical diagnosis when they should be describing and verifying diagnostic observations before placing them in the medical record; for example: "Atrial fibrillation with ventricular rate of 40 per Dr. P."
- *Splinting and Ace wraps.* Nurses should note the type of device, location, and circulatory status after splinting; for example: "No deformity or bruising, + swelling, + pain to touch at right ankle. Patient able to wiggle all toes right foot, to feel touch. Pulses palpable right foot."
- *Spinal immobilization.* Particularly with cervical collars, nurses should document the position (if present) when the patient arrives from the field, along with the baseline neurologic status of the patient. Furthermore, the nurse should do the following: document that the cervical collars was maintained when the patient left the emergency department for an x-ray or CT study; note the presence of the collar when the patient returns, along with the neurological status of the patient; and document the presence of the cervical collar and neurological status when the patient leaves the department for admission or for surgery. If the patient was combative for any reason, such as a head injury or intoxication, the nurse should note this in the record along with a description of the behavior; for example, "Ambulatory at scene, walked 2 miles to call EMS," or "Sat up in bed after removing cervical collar and stated, 'There is nothing wrong with me,'" or "Kicking and spitting at staff—4 police officers required to subdue patient."

A second example of failure to implement a safe plan of care based on the patient's diagnosis follows:

> A 33-year-old machine operator suffered multiple injuries in an auto accident. His cervical collar and head blocks were removed in the defendant emergency department. One doctor interpreted the x-rays as normal but ordered a consultation with a second doctor. The second doctor ordered the replacement of the collar and additional x-rays. These films showed moderate anterior subluxation to C6, consistent with locked facets at C6-C7. The patient was transferred to a regional medical center, where he was found to be quadriplegic at the time of arrival. The defendants claimed that the patient refused to allow them to keep the cervical collar in place, was intoxicated and abusive and difficult to manage, resulting in unreadable x-rays. The jury awarded $11.5 million, in-

cluding $500,000 for the patient's wife's claim of loss of consortium (Laska, 1997d).

- *IV conscious sedation.* The nurse should note the baseline vital signs, including pulse oximetry. Include the monitor strip.
- *ABGs.* Collecting the sample, understanding the results, and communicating them to the physician are essential for the nurse. Document that the Allen test was used to verify collateral arterial circulation before the arterial puncture, and that pressure was applied at the puncture site until bleeding was controlled.
- *Domestic violence and sexual abuse recognition and reporting.* The nurse should document signs of injury and ensure that the appropriate agencies are notified.
- *Knowledge of age-appropriate behavior from infancy through childhood.* The nurse should describe the playfulness, fussiness, and response of young children to stimuli. For example, for a 3½ month old not to arouse at all during an examination or for a 78-year-old to become hysterical at the prospect of returning home with a caregiver is abnormal.
- *Use of defibrillators, external pacemakers, transverse pacemakers.* The nurse should document when these devices are used in the emergency department.
- *Arterial and central lines.* The nurse should document the placement and verification. (Remember to chart that sterile technique was used.)
- *Endotracheal tube.* The nurse should document placement and verification.
- *Ventilator.* The nurse should document settings.

Flowsheets

The complexity of emergency department nursing responsibilities and the pace in the department necessitate the use of flowsheets for documentating the nursing process. One example is the use of a trauma flowsheet to manage trauma patient care and documentation (Figures 11-1, 11-2, and 11-3). Important information, such as the Glasgow coma scale, trauma score, and pupil measurement scale, are part of the record and should be readily available for reference, as are diagrams, which are useful in marking the patient's injuries or burns. Having a section for noting in detail the prehospital care as well as the arrival times of the trauma team and consultants, from specialties such as neurosurgery, orthopedics, and plastic surgery, as illustrated, is also helpful.

Another example is the frequent observation flowsheet (Figure 11-4), which provides check-off areas for standard documentation and helpful scoring information, such as pupil sizes and pediatric level of consciousness. Such forms allow the busy nurse to document information that would otherwise require many lines of narrative charting and could easily be omitted from the record in the rush to deliver

Text continued on p. 221

TRAUMA FLOWSHEET — Section 1 of 2

USE SPACE BELOW IF IDENTIFICATION
PLATE IS NOT AVAILABLE

NAME _____   ROOM NO. _____   IDENTIFICATION PLATE

TIME INJURED: _____   ALLERGIES: ☐ Unknown _____   AGE: _____

ARRIVAL TIME: _____   MEDICATIONS: ☐ Unknown _____   SEX: M   F

                                          LAST TETANUS: ☐ Unknown _____   LMP: _____

                                          PAST MEDICAL HISTORY: ☐ Unknown _____

                                          LAST MEAL/FLUIDS: _____

ARRIVED BY: ☐ Private vehicle   ☐ Ambulance
                    ☐ Ambulatory   ☐ Aeromedical   ☐ Transfer _____

PRE-HOSPITAL REPORT

MECHANISM OF INJURY:		IMMOBILIZATION:	O₂ THERAPY:	☐ MAST Applied

MECHANISM OF INJURY:
☐ MVC
☐ Restrained
☐ Air bag: Present   Y   N
            Deployed   Y   N
☐ Child seat
☐ Helmet

☐ Pedestrian
☐ Fall _____ ft.
☐ GSW
☐ Stab
☐ Burn
☐ Other_____

IMMOBILIZATION:
☐ C-Collar
☐ Back board

O_2 THERAPY:
☐ Non-rebreather mask
☐ BVM   ☐ Oral Airway
            ☐ Nasal Airway
☐ Intubated ☐ Oral
             ☐ Nasal
             ☐ RSI

☐ MAST Applied
Splints: ☐ R Leg   ☐ L Leg
         ☐ R Arm   ☐ L Arm
☐ IVF _____ cc
☐ PRBC _____ cc
☐ CPR _____ min

Estimated speed _____   ☐ Meds given: _____

ACTIVATION CRITERIA

☐ **TRAUMA CALL**

☐ Extrication time > 30 minutes.
☐ Ejection from a motor vehicle.
☐ Death in the same passenger compartment
☐ Fall of 20 feet or greater; or 2 x the height of the patient.
☐ GCS of 8 or less and/or unstable vital signs.
☐ Reported widened mediastinum/transected aorta.
☐ Full thickness burns 20% BSA or > with/without associated injury.
☐ Arrest: blunt mechanism, CPR > 5 minutes.
☐ Request of the EMS who have reason to suspect injury may involve threat of loss of life or limb.
☐ Other: _____

☐ **TRAUMA ALERT**

☐ Difficult airway (inability to obtain or intubate with O_2 saturation < 90%)
☐ Shock
☐ Known severe closed head injury, blunt chest or abdomen injury, or pelvic fracture with shock.
☐ Penetrating head, neck or torso injury with difficult airway or shock.
☐ Limb threatening ischemia or proximal amputation.
☐ Known spinal cord injury with paralysis.
☐ Multiple casualty incident.
☐ Pregnant patient (20+ weeks) with significant injury or shock.
☐ Arrest (penetrating mechanism)

TRAUMA TEAM RESPONSE				CONSULTANTS			
	Called	Arrived	Name	Service	Name	Called	Will See
1st Call							
2nd Call							
3rd Call							
Attending							
ED Attending							
Nurse R							
Nurse L							
RN Recorder							
Respiratory							
Radiology							
Phlebotomist							
Social Services							

TRAUMA FLOWSHEET

Figure 11-1 Trauma flowsheet.

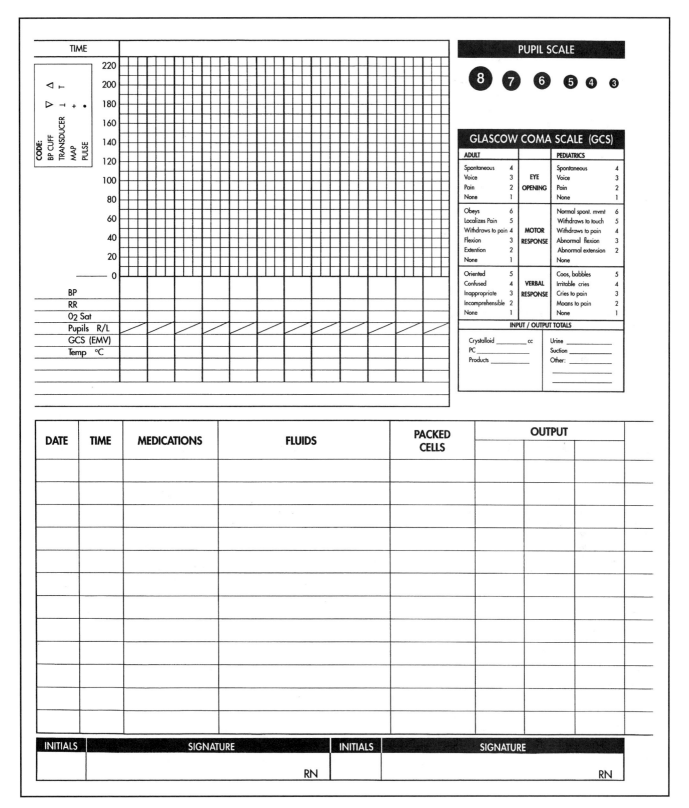

Figure 11-1, cont'd Trauma flowsheet. *Continued*

TRAUMA SCORE

SB/P	RR	GCS	
> 89	10-29	13-15	4
76-89	> 29	9-12	3
50-75	6-9	6-8	2
1-49	1-5	4-5	1
0	0	3	0
_____	_____	_____	_____

Admit to: _____ To O.R. from E.D. @ _____

Report called by: _____ to: _____

Expired in E.D.: _____ Pronounced by: _____ M.D.

   Time: _____ M.E. Notified: ☐ Y ☐ N ☐ N/A

Organ/Tissue Procedure Initiated by: _____

CLOTHING:
☐ Released to: _____
☐ To floor with patient
☐ Cut off ☐ ED ☐ PTA
☐ Given to Medical Examiner

   Family counseled at: _____

VALUABLES:
☐ No valuables found on admission to E.D.
☐ Valuables in E.D. Lock-Up
☐ Valuables released to: _____
☐ Valuables to hospital safe

NURSING DIAGNOSIS:

SOCIAL SERVICE NOTES: _____

NOTES

☐ See Addendum

INITIALS	SIGNATURE	INITIALS	SIGNATURE
	RN		RN

Figure 11-1, cont'd Trauma flowsheet.

PRIMARY SURVEY TIME: _____

AIRWAY WITH CERVICAL SPINE CONTROL

☐ Patent
☐ Artificial   ☐ Oral   ☐ BVM
             ☐ Nasal
             ☐ Intubated: ☐ Oral
                          ☐ Nasal
☐ Obstructed

INTERVENTIONS;

☐ Suction
☐ Oral/nasal airway   ☐ BVM
☐ Intubated oral/nasal # _____ Fr._____cm/_____
☐ Cricothyrotomy #_____Fr.
Cervical spine   ☐ Immobilized

Performed by: _____ Time: _____
Performed by: _____ Time: _____
Performed by: _____ Time: _____
Performed by: _____ Time: _____
Performed by: _____ Time: _____

BREATHING:

☐ Spontaneous/no distress
☐ Spontaneous/distressed   (<10 > 29)
☐ Absent
Chest expansion: ☐ Symmetrical   ☐ Asymmetrical
Trachea deviation: ☐ R   ☐ L

Breath Sounds: _____

Crepitus/subcutaneous air: _____

INTERVENTIONS:

☐ 100% O2 nonrebreather   ☐ BVM assisted
☐ Chest tube: R/L_____Fr.   ☐ Air   ☐ Blood _____ cc   Performed by: _____ Time: _____
☐ Chest tube: R/L_____Fr.   ☐ Air   ☐ Blood _____ cc   Performed by: _____ Time: _____

CIRCULATION:

Skin: ☐ Warm   ☐ Dry   ☐ Moist   ☐ Cool   ☐ Pink   ☐ Pale   ☐ Mottled
Pules present: Carotid R/L   Femoral /L   Radial R/L
Obvious bleeding: _____

INTERVENTIONS:

☐ Bleeding controlled by: _____
☐ IV access: Peripheral / Central _____ ga.   Site_____   Performed by: _____ Time: _____
☐ IV access: Peripheral / Central _____ ga.   Site_____   Performed by: _____ Time: _____
☐ IV access: Peripheral / Central _____ ga.   Site_____   Performed by: _____ Time: _____
☐ Pericardiocentesis results: _____   Performed by: _____ Time: _____
☐ CPR with ACLS protocol   ☐ See code sheet   Initiated by: _____ Time: _____
☐ Thorocotomy R L   ☐ Open massage   ☐ Internal defibrillator   Performed by: _____ Time: _____

DISABILITY:

☐ Awake   ☐ Responds to verbal   ☐ Responds to pain   ☐ Unresponsive

---

TEAM RECORDER: _____ **RN**

TEAM LEADER _____ **MD**

PRIMARY NURSE: _____ **RN**

KEY FOR ABBREVIATIONS

MVC	=	Motor Vehicle Crash	**MAST**	=	Military Anti Shock Trousers
GSW	=	Gun Shot Wound	**GCS**	=	Glasgow Coma Score
C-Collar	=	Cervical Collar	**BSA**	=	Body Substance Area
BVM	=	Bag-Valve-Mask device	**Fr**	=	French
RSI	=	Rapid Sequence Induction	**PTA**	=	Prior to Admission

Figure 11-1, cont'd   Trauma flowsheet.

DATE	MILITARY TIME	MICU	AMBULANCE	AIR	REFERRING M.D.

TRANSFERRING FACILITY	TYPENEX NUMBER	TRAUMA ALERT

☐ YES ☐ NO   MILITARY TIME:

BLOOD PRESSURE / PULSE / CARDIOVASCULAR

FAMILY NOTIFIED ☐ YES ☐ NO   PHONE #: _____ TIME:

CARDIOVASCULAR
INVASIVE LINES (IV, A-LINE, CVP)

TYPE	GAUGE

PHARMACOLOGIC
ALLERGIES:
CURRENT MEDS:

DRUGS	AMOUNT	ROUTE	TIME	INIT'S
1.				
2.				
3.				
4.				
5.				
6.				
7.				
8.				
9.				
10.				

BLOOD PRESSURE values: 200 190 180 170 160 150 140 130 120 110 100 90 80 70 60 50 40

PULSE values: 200 190 180 170 160 150 140 130 120 110 100 90 80 70 60 50 40 30 25 20 15 10 5 0

TIME

HI-FLOW TUBING/RAPID INFUSER YES ☐ NO ☐
PERIPHERAL PULSES:
EKG TIME: RHYTHM:
MAST: FIELD   TAA   TIME
INFLATED ☐ YES ☐ NO ☐ LEGS ONLY
ARREST ☐ YES ☐ NO   CPR ☐ YES ☐ NO
OPEN THORACOTOMY   TIME:

GASTROINTESTINAL
SALEM SUMP: SIZE   TIME:
DRAINAGE: COLOR   AMT.
ABDOMEN: SOFT ☐ FIRM ☐
          TENDER ☐ NON-TENDER ☐ UTO ☐
PERITONEAL LAVAGE: ☐ YES ☐ NO TIME:
AMT. INFUSED: AMT. DRAINED:
RECTAL EXAM: DR:
HEMETEST RESULTS: ☐ POS. ☐ NEG.

TEMP:
TIME:

GCS/TS
Pulse OX
RESP

| TETANUS TOX. | 0.5 ml | SQ | LOT # | |
| HYPER TET. | 250 u | IM | LOT # | |

COMMENTS:

LIVING WILL: YES ☐ NO ☐ UTO ☐ N/A ☐

X-RAYS	DONE	TIME	LAB	DONE	TIME	GENITOURINARY		
C-SPINE			Ua			FOLEY: SIZE:		TIME
SKULL			T&S			CYSTO YES NO		TIME
CHEST			T&X __ UNITS			HEMASTIX RESULTS		TIME
PELVIS			ADULT PKT			INTAKE	OUTPUT	
L SPINE			PEDI. PKT			CRYSTALLOID	URINE	
T SPINE			CK/MB			BLOOD	N/G	
OTHER:			DIC PROF.			COLLOID	CHEST TUBE	
			PREGNANCY			MEDS	R:	
			OTHER:			CT CONTRAST	L:	
						OTHER	OTHER	

NEUROLOGICAL
EXTREMITIES: PUPILS/REACT:
MAE YES ☐ NO ☐   O.D.   O.S.
ADM. W/CERVICAL IMMOB.   ☐ YES ☐ NO
CERVICAL PRECAUTION:

Drawn by:
Site:
TOTALS   TOTALS

CATSCAN	TIME
HEAD	
SPINE	
ABD	
PELVIS	

H I S T O R Y

RESPIRATORY
ADM. STATUS:
AMBU BAG   N ETT   O ETT   MASK   N/C
OXYGEN   L/MIN
BREATH SOUNDS: PRESENT   R   L
                CLEAR   R   L
                DIMINISHED R   L
ADVENTITIOUS SOUNDS:
TAA AIRWAY   MASK   N/C   N ETT   O ETT
ANESTHESIA INTUBATION: PULSE OX: CO₂:
VENTILATOR SETTING
CHEST TUBES: R#   L#
AUTO TRANSFUSION: YES ☐ NO ☐
O₂/FIO₂ CHANGES: TIME:
TRACH/CRIC: ☐ YES ☐ NO   TIME:

FINAL DISPOSITION
TO: TIME: EXPIRED ☐ YES ☐ NO
                                    TIME PRONOUNCED:

1. CONT. 2. BURN
3. FX DISLOC 4. ABR
5. LAC. 6. AVUL.
7. PUNCT. 8. GSW
9. CRUSH 10. AMP
11. HEMATOMA

CONSULTANTS

KEY
CERVICAL IMMOBILIZATION
P.C = PHILADELPHIA COLLAR
SN = STIFF NECK
NL = NECK LOCK
L.B. = LONE BOARD
↑ = BP TAKEN IN ERECT POSITION
HID = HEAD IMMOB. DEVICE

RN SIGNATURE	INT.'S	TRAUMA SURGEON SIGNATURE	INT.'S
PRIMARY RN			
SECONDARY RN			

PLACE PATIENT
I.D. LABEL AND TYPENEX #
HERE

COOPER HOSPITAL/
UNIVERSITY MEDICAL CENTER

SOUTHERN NEW JERSEY
REGIONAL TRAUMA CENTER

TRAUMA ADMITTING RECORD

Figure 11-2 Trauma admitting record. (Courtesy Cooper Hospital University Medical Center, Camden, NJ.)

NARRATIVE

TRAUMA SCORE FOR SOUTH JERSEY

		Value	Points
A.	Systolic Blood Pressure	>89	4
		76-89	3
		50-75	2
		1-49	1
		0	0
B.	Respiratory Rate	10-29	4
		>29	3
		6-9	2
		1-5	1
		0	0

C. Glasgow coma Scale

1. **Eye Opening**

Spontaneous	____ 4
To Voice	____ 3
To Pain	____ 2
None	____ 1

2. **Verbal response**

Oriented	____ 5
Confused	____ 4
Inappropriate words	____ 3
Incomprehensible words	____ 2
None	____ 1

3. **Motor response**

		Total GSC Points		Score
Obeys commands	____ 6			
Purposeful movement (pain)	____ 5	13-15	=	4
Withdraw (pain)	____ 4	9-12	=	3
Flexion (pain)	____ 3	6-8	=	2
Extension (pain)	____ 2	4-5	=	1
None	____ 1	3	=	0

TOTAL GCS POINTS
(1 + 2 + 3) _____

TRAUMA SCORE
(TOTAL POINTS = A + B + C) _____

VALUABLES

☐ TO SAFE   ☐ TO FAMILY   ☐ TO BEDSIDE

Figure 11-2, cont'd Trauma admitting record.

HARBOR-UCLA MEDICAL CENTER

TRIAGE

ARRIVED: DATE & TIME

MODE OF ARRIVAL
- ☐ Ambulatory
- ☐ Paramedic _____ SQUAD
- ☐ Ambulance
- ☐ Other _____

WHEREWITH
- ☐ Stretcher
- ☐ Wheelchair
- ☐ Restraints
- ☐ Other _____

FROM:
- ☐ Home
- ☐ Nursing Home
- ☐ Outside Hospital
- ☐ Other _____

CARE PRIOR TO ARRIVAL:
☐ NONE GIVEN

Chief Complaint/Mech. of Injury:

SKIN COLOR
- ☐ normal
- ☐ pale/ashen
- ☐ cyanotic
- ☐ flushed

MOISTURE
- ☐ normal
- ☐ dry
- ☐ moist
- ☐ profuse

SKIN TEMP.
- ☐ hot
- ☐ warm
- ☐ cool
- ☐ cold

PUPILS
- ☐ equal   ☐ responsive
- ☐ unequal   ☐ sluggish
- ☐ fixed   ☐ pin point
- ☐ dilated

MENTAL STATUS
- ☐ awake, oriented to time, place, name
- ☐ responds to loud verbal stimuli
- ☐ responds to painful stimuli
- ☐ non responsive to painful stimuli

Allergies:

Initial Assessment:
_____ Yrs./Old   ☐ F   ☐ M

Current Medication:

T   P   R   B/P   HT.   WT.

NURSING ACTIONS AT TRIAGE
- ☐ None   ☐ HCT _____
- ☐ Ice   ☐ Visidex _____
- ☐ Elevate   ☐ Dextrostix _____
- ☐ Splint   ☐ Cooling Measures
- ☐ Dressing   ☐ X-Rays _____
  - ☐ Wet   ☐ Other _____
  - ☐ Dry
  - ☐ Pressure
- ☐ Patient Teaching _____

LNMP   GR   P   AB   PRENATAL CARE

Significant Past Medical Problems:

Tetanus Status: **R.N. Signature:**

CLASSIFICATIONS AT TRIAGE
- ☐ Emergent
- ☐ Urgent
- ☐ Non-emergent

TRIAGE DISPOSITION
- ☐ AAC
- ☐ M.A.
- ☐ OB/GYN
- ☐ PEDS.
- ☐ Other _____

NURSING FLOW SHEET

Time	B/P	Pulse	Resp.	Temp.	Init.	Time	B/P	Pulse	Resp.	Temp.	Init.	Treatments and Diagnostics Procedures	Initial
												O₂ at Liters/min via	
												Hct	
												Visidex/Dextrostix	
												U.C.G.	
												Sed. Rate	
												Visual Acuity	
												OD OS	

Time	Medication or IV Solution	Dose/Amts.	Route/Site	Type/Gauge Needle	IV Rate	Amt. Infused & Time	Initial

A · Abrasion
B · Burn
C · C/O Pain
D · Draining Wound
E · Ecchymosis
F · Fracture
G · Possible FX
H · Hematoma
I · Foreign Body
L · Laceration
P · Penetrating Wound
R · Rash
S · Scar
X · Decubitus
+ · Pulse Present
− · Pulse Absent

INTAKE

		Initials	Signature/Classification	Initials	Signature/Classification
Parential					
Oral					
Other					
Time	Total				

OUTPUT

Foley		
Void		
Gastric		
Chest	R	
	L	
Emesis		
Time	Total	

Monitor (Not Applicable)

Time	Rhythm	Initials	Time	Rhythm	Initials

DEPARTMENT OF EMERGENCY NURSING INITIAL ASSESSMENT AND FLOW SHEET
COUNTY OF LOS ANGELES DEPARTMENT OF HEALTH SERVICES
HH107-76E358 (10/85)

Figure 11-3 Trauma flowsheet. (Courtesy Harbor-UCLA Medical Center, Torrance, Calif.)

DIAGNOSTICS							
	TIME		TIME		TIME		TIME
☐ **UA**		**X-RAY**		☐ ABG F₁0₂ _____		☐ GLUCOSE	
☐ VOID ☐ CATH.		☐ CHEST		☐ AMYLASE		☐ PT/PTT	
☐ CL CATCH		☐ ABD SERIES		☐ BUN		☐ GRAM SMEAR	
CULTURES SENT		☐ C-SPINE		☐ CREATININE		☐ BETA HCG	
☐ THROAT		☐ OTHER		☐ CBC		☐ TYPE/CROSS	
☐ G.C.				☐ HCO₃		# units	
☐ CSF		☐ EKG		☐ NA		☐ Rh TYPE & SCREEN	
☐ BLOOD				☐ K		☐ HOLD RED TOP TUBE	
☐ WOUND				☐ CL		☐ CARDIAC ENZYME	
☐ OTHER						☐ OTHER_____	

EMERGENCY NURSING NOTES

TIME		TIME	

☐ ADMITTED | Ward/Unit: | Date: | Time:

Transported Via: ☐ Stretcher ☐ Wheelchair ☐ Walk | Time:

☐ Family ☐ Friend | Notified: ☐ Yes ☐ No

Relationship:

Discharge Disposition: ☐ Home ☐ AMA

Report Given To:

☐ Referral: | Telephone:

Primary Nurse's Signature:

Discharge Teaching:

Figure 11-3, cont'd Trauma flowsheet.

USE SPACE BELOW IF IDENTIFICATION
PLATE IS NOT AVAILABLE

NAME _____   DATE _____

NUMBER _____   BED NO. _____   IDENTIFICATION PLATE

Condition on Arrival: T_____   P_____   R_____   B/P_____   Allergies: _____

Disoriented _____   Shock _____

Hemorrhaging _____   Unconscious _____   Admitting   A.M.

Alert _____   Apprehensive _____   Nurse: _____ Time: _____   P.M.

| Time | Skin | Pulse | Temp. | B/P | Resp. | Conscious Level | Pupils | | O₂ | Fluids In I.V. / P.O. | Output | | Nurses Notes (medications, procedures, observations, I.V. - time puncture mode and locations) |
							R	L			Urine	Drain-age	
											Total	Total	Total

Codes:

Skin
N - normal
M - mottled
B - cyanotic
J - jaundiced
P - pale
F - flushed
D - diaphoretic
C - cold

Conscious Level
1. Alert
2. Oriented (T-time; P-Place N-name; A-all)
3. Confused
4. Responds to verbal stimuli
5. Responds to pain
6. No Response
7. Decerebrate

Pupil Reaction
> greater than
< lesser than
= equal
R reactive
NR non-reactive
C constricted
D dilated

Cardiac monitor   (   )
Respirator   (   )
Hare Splint   (   )
Tetanus Taxoid _____
Hyper-Tet _____
Other _____
_____
_____
_____

Transferred to _____   Valuables: _____   Clothing: _____

Transferred at _____ a.m.   Hospital Safe _____   To Family _____

_____ p.m.   To family (name) _____   To Unit _____

Report given to _____ R.N.

Nurse's signature _____

EMERGENCY DEPARTMENT CRITICAL CARE RECORD

Figure 11-4 Critical care record.

NURSES NOTES

Time	Skin	Pulse	Temp.	B/P	Resp.	Conscious Level	Pupils R	Pupils L	O$_2$	Fluids In I.V. / P.O.	Output Urine	Output Drainage	(medications, procedures, observations, I.V. - time puncture mode and locations)
											Total	Total	

EMERGENCY DEPARTMENT CRITICAL CARE RECORD

Figure 11-4, cont'd Critical care record.

IVs must be assessed q 2 hours on adults and q 1 hour for children and critical drug infusions (pressors and vesicants). Use pumps on children 0-17 years old and adults weighing <60 kg. Change IV sites, tubing, and fluid bags q 72 hours and field sticks within 24 hours of initiation.

Addressograph

NURSING IV CARE RECORD

IV# _____ DATE AND TIME STARTED: _____

Enter times of assessment:															
Location _____ Gauge _____															
Site (± R/E/D) dressing: (± Dry, intact)															
Pump in use															
Comments:															

IV# _____ DATE AND TIME STARTED: _____

Enter times of assessment:															
Location _____ Gauge _____															
Site (± R/E/D) dressing: (± Dry, intact)															
Pump in use															
Comments:															

DATE: _____
RN INITIALS/SIGNATURE _____   RN INITIALS/SIGNATURE _____

Figure 11-5 Nursing IV care record.

emergency care. Likewise, the care of IV sites has become such a concern that a separate flowsheet with cues about the expected documentation of site checks and dressings is presented (Figure 11-5).

Nursing Responsibility for Patient and Family Teaching

According to the ENA practice standards on teaching, "Emergency nurses shall assist the patient and significant others to obtain knowledge about illness and injury prevention" (ENA, 1995b).

Nurses are expected to offer information to the patient and family in a way that is consistent with their ability to understand and to offer explanations about treatment before initiation whenever possible. The patient and family should be involved in therapeutic decision making as much as circumstances permit. The nurse should provide a written or verbal explanation of medications, treatments, self-care, referral, and prevention.

Discharge Instructions

The standard of care requires that instructions be given at the educational level of the patient or caregiver. Emergency nurses have available to them a variety of prepared materials for patient education and they are also expected to use their nursing judgment to prepare the patient or caregiver for discharge. Box 11-2 identifies essential elements that must be included in discharge instructions for emergency department patients.

A lack of documentation can seal the fate of the patient, who could suffer permanent damage or die as a result of an inability to recognize dangerous symptoms, and the nurse, who failed to note whether the patient could read or understand the information before leaving the care facility. For this reason, forms should generate duplicate copies; that is, one for the patient and one for the permanent record. If a patient must use crutches or perform dressing changes, the nurse must document whether the patient correctly performed a return demonstration after receiving instruction.

Charting tips: Do the nurse's notes state that the patient verbalized an understanding of the discharge instructions, or do they just get signed? Notes should reflect that the patient was referred to an orthopedist, family physician, ophthalmologist, cardiologist, surgeon, physical therapist, psychiatrist, or other healthcare provider, as indicated by the final diagnosis. The phone number should be written on the discharge instructions unless the nurse notes that the patient has the number.

The nurse should include written instructions at the time of discharge on what to do when symptoms worsen or recur (Figure 11-6). Reasonable care must also be taken to ensure the presence of and the instructions to caretakers for patients who might be unable to recognize warning signs after

---

> ### Box 11-2
>
> ### Essential Elements of Discharge Instructions
>
> - Provide the emergency facility's name, phone number, and the date.
> - Record the patient's name, medical record number, and signature (or the signature of the caregiver).
> - Witness the signature indicating understanding of the instructions.
> - Provide general instructions related to the chief complaint or discharge diagnosis, including symptoms indicating a need to return to the emergency department. For lacerations, nurses should include signs of infection and the dates and times the patient should return for wound checks and suture removal. Specify the frequency of dressing changes, and instruct the patient to keep dressings clean and dry. For broken bones and sprains, specify the intermittent application of ice or heat and how many days it is to be used. Also instruct the patient on proper use of ace bandages.
> - Individualize instructions related to specific injuries (e.g., head injury), postsedation precautions, and outpatient diagnostic tests.
> - Give the patient the names of medications prescribed in the emergency department with appropriate precautions, such as "no alcohol, driving, or operating equipment while taking _____." Patients may require drug teaching sheets.
> - Provide the name of the follow-up physician with the phone number and time for contact.
> - Specify the number of days the patient should take off from work and the date to return.
> - Provide a statement qualifying emergency department treatment as first aid care, requiring ongoing care by a physician, and the importance of reading and following all instructions provided.

---

discharge; for example, patients with head injuries, the elderly, or the debilitated. This could involve calling to make a report to a nursing home or personal care home, or locating a family member, in order to provide instructions. The reflection of such efforts in the medical record is essential. Joint Commission standards specify that a copy of the emergency services provided should be available to the practitioner or medical organization providing follow-up care when authorized by a patient or a legally authorized representative (JCAHO, 1996). This information helps to ensure the continuity of care.

Consider the following example:

A 35-year-old woman was injured during a jet ski race when she was struck by a competitor's jet ski. She was originally treated in the emergency department, then an orthopedic surgeon took over her care. She claimed that at the time of discharge, she was instructed to apply ice directly to the area for 24 hours a day for 10 days, and that she suffered frostbite to her skin as a result of these instructions, which required two surgical debridements and resulted in disfigurement of her leg and calf. The physicians

Head Injury

The first 24 hours after a head injury are the most important, although after effects may appear much later. It is important that a responsible person awakens the patient every 2 hours for the first 24 hours and watches for the following symptoms. If any of these occur, call your doctor or return to the emergency department.

1. Persistent headache, nausea or vomiting more than twice.
2. Weakness, numbness or paralysis of the arms or legs.
3. Blood or clear fluid from the ears or nose.
4. Blurred vision; unequal pupils (one larger than the other).
5. Convulsions.

No alcoholic beverages.
Take nothing stronger than aspirin or Tylenol for pain.

Eye Injuries

1. If your eye has been patched it is difficult to judge distance. Do not drive a vehicle or use hazardous equipment.
2. Do not rub your eyes.
3. Avoid bright lights and glaring sunshine. Wear sun glasses.
4. If your eye is patched it must be rechecked within 24 hours by your family doctor or an ophthalmologist. If you are unable to obtain an appointment in 24 hours, return to the emergency department.

X-RAY

The x-ray report which you have received is only a preliminary interpretation of the films. The radiologist will give your physician a complete report following his interpretation. You will be contacted by the Emergency Department if this differs from the preliminary report. You should contact your family doctor or the orthopod to whom you have been referred within 3 days if you are still having symptoms so that he/she may review the final report.

Abdominal Pain

1. Eat a bland diet for 24 hours. Avoid caffeine containing beverages such as coffee, tea, cola sodas, cocoa, chocolate and alcohol; fatty, greasy, spicy, highly seasoned foods; strongly flavored vegetables.
2. You should be rechecked by your doctor in 24 - 48 hours.
3. If the pain becomes worse, a fever or vomiting occurs, return to the emergency department.

Nose Bleed

After you leave the Emergency Department.

1. Keep your nose and head above the level of your heart. Sleep on your back with your upper body elevated on pillows.
2. Do not blow your nose.
3. Do not sneeze or cough.
4. Do not drink hot liquids.
5. Do not apply hot packs to your face.
6. Do not take any medication with aspirin in it.
7. Do not drink alcohol.
8. If nose starts to bleed again:
   a. Sit up.
   b. Pinch the lower one-half of the nose (not just the tip) between the thumb and index fingers.
   c. Pinch for 10 minutes continuously.
   d. If unable to stop bleeding, call your doctor or return to the emergency department.

Use of Crutches

1. Stand with injured foot off the ground. Place tips of crutches 18 inches apart and 6 inches in front of good foot.
2. Position hands on hand grips with tops of crutches against ribs. Keep elbows slightly bent and close to your body. Bear weight on your hands, not on underarms. Never lean on crutches with underarms.
3. Push down on hand grips, lift good leg, and swing forward through the crutches, placing weight back on good leg.
4. Wear sturdy, low-heeled shoes.

Allergic Reaction

1. Rest. Stay cool. Do not engage in activities which may cause your body to become overheated.
2. Apply ice to swollen areas.
3. If the rash gets progressively worse, call your doctor or return to the emergency department.
4. If you become SHORT OF BREATH, or develop TIGHTNESS IN THE THROAT OR CHEST PAIN, go to the emergency department immediately. If symptoms are severe call an ambulance for transport.

Figure 11-6 Emergency discharge instructions sheet. (Courtesy Mercy Community Hospital, Havertown, Penn.)

argued that she developed necrosis at the point of impact, not from the ice application. Furthermore, they stated that their instructions were to use ice only intermittently and to place it on the splint or dressing, not directly to the skin. The jury found in favor of the physicians (Laska, 1997g).

The discharge instructions and the emergency nurses' documentation about the patient's responses to them were undoubtedly an exhibit at this trial.

EVALUATION AND COMMUNICATION

According to the ENA practice standards regarding evaluation, "Emergency nurses shall evaluate and modify the plan of care based on observable responses by the patient and attainment of patient goals" (ENA, 1995b).

General Practice

The nurse must continuously evaluate the patient's care based on observable outcomes to determine the patient's progress toward outcomes and goals, and must document patient responses to treatment interventions and progress. Joint Commission standards (1996) state that the medical record of the patient receiving emergency, urgent, or immediate care should note "the conclusions at termination of treatment, including final disposition, condition at discharge, and instructions for follow-up care." When discharging a patient, the nurse should include a notation evaluating the patient's status at the time of leaving the emergency department. Likewise, when a patient is removed from a cardiac monitor, some notation should be made about the reason; for example, "Patient is pain-free with normal

ECG and normal cardiac enzymes. Cardiac source of pain ruled out by emergency department physician."

Evaluation Priorities

Pulse Oximetry and Vital Signs

The same standard applies to pulse oximetry as to cardiac monitoring: if the patient is sick enough to require a baseline reading, then another reading is indicated before discharge. Likewise, pulse, respirations, and blood pressure should be noted and documented at the time of discharge to prove that the patient's leaving was safe. If a concern exists about a fever developing, returning, or having been resolved during the course of care, then the temperature should be recorded at the time of discharge.

Medication Effects

Equally important is the ability of nurses to demonstrate that they were aware of possible side effects of medication such as nitroglycerin, dopamine, IV morphine, Versed (midazolam), Norcuron (Necuronium), Dilantin (phenytoin), diltiazem, and a host of medications that either drop or raise the blood pressure, respirations, and pulse. Documenting the vital signs (including cardiac strips) before, during, and after drug administration, the effect of the drug (e.g., reduced pain or fever, change in blood pressure, or cardiac rhythm), or adverse reaction to the drug (e.g., anaphylaxis) supports the nurse's contention that he or she was aware of the side effects and benefits of the drug and was monitoring the patient.

Intake and Output

When a patient is admitted to the hospital, the primary nurse is responsible for calculating and recording how much fluid was received in the emergency department and how much output occurred through urinary bladder, NG tube, chest tube, or other drainage system. This is particularly important for burn, bleeding, cardiac, renal, pediatric, diabetic, and head injury patients because too much (as well as too little) fluid can produce disastrous outcomes.

Evaluation of Resources and Coping

The emergency nurse must collaborate with the patient and family to elicit essential information with accuracy and timeliness. He or she should act as a liason by providing the treatment team with accurate and timely information regarding the patient's clinical condition. Furthermore, he or she should communicate verbally and in writing all information pertinent to patient care. If the emergency nurse discovers impediments to discharge in the process of providing care, he or she must communicate them to the physician or social worker so that arrangements can be made to accommodate the limitations at the time of discharge; these could include illiteracy, a lack of running water, homelessness, an unstable environment, a situation endangering a child, or an inability to purchase the prescribed medication. The worksheet in

Figure 11-7 is proposed to assist emergency nurses in evaluating and documenting resources or coping deficits that must be addressed before discharge.

In the following cases the failure to evaluate the patients before discharge resulted in two deaths and two lawsuits. In the third case, an astute nurse adhering to the standard of care saved a child's life.

> A woman was brought into the emergency department in respiratory distress. The defendant doctor gave her two prescriptions and released her within 30 minutes of her arrival. The following day, she again had difficulty breathing, which became worse after she took the medication prescribed by the defendant. She returned to the emergency department, where she died of bronchopneumonia. The jury returned a verdict of more than $1.8 million for the plaintiffs (Laska, 1997f).

Charting tips: What were the medications? Did she receive doses in the department? If so, what was her reaction? What did the nurses' notes say about this patient's condition at the time of discharge? Were vital signs and oxygenation status at the time of discharge evaluated? Did she have a fever? Was she short of breath?

> A 40-year-old woman arrived at the emergency department with a swollen tongue possibly because of an allergic reaction. She was treated with antiallergic medication, but the swelling did not subside. She died from "choking on her tongue" (i.e., an obstructed airway) 5 hours later. The plaintiff contended that an alternative airway (i.e., intubation) should have been established when the medication failed to work. The jury award was $356,866 (Laska, 1997c).

Charting tips: Where were the emergency department nurses while this patient's condition was deteriorating? Did the nurses' notes indicate that the nurses were aware of the increased distress or of a lack of improvement with the medication? Were repeated attempts to get the physician involved documented? Was the charge nurse notified of the problem and was the chain of command activated if the physician failed to respond to the nurses' concerns?

> A 4-year-old child with a history of recurrent, chronic otitis media was seen in the emergency department for a fever. Before discharge, he was treated with Tylenol (acetaminophen) and an antibiotic injection. Following department policy, the emergency nurse asked his parents to remain for 30 minutes after the injection to evaluate for a possible allergic reaction.
> After 15 minutes the father expressed his desire to leave. The nurse repeated her instructions to remain for 30 minutes. Twenty minutes after administration of the antibiotic, the child developed sudden, severe respiratory difficulty. He required emergent intubation and was successfully resuscitated after anaphylaxis. Had the nurse allowed the parents to leave with this child as requested, he would have arrested in his parents' car (anecdotal report, 1997).

Addressograph

EMERGENCY DEPARTMENT RESOURCES/COPING EVALUATION

ELDER/PHYSICALLY/MENTALLY CHALLENGED	**NSG Dx/PLAN**
• Does senior/adult display appropriate understanding of illness/injury?	☐ Knowledge deficit R/T: _____ _____ _____
• Does patient live alone? ☐ No 　☐ Yes: ☐ House ☐ Apartment ☐ Room ☐ Homeless	
• If elder couple, are there indicators that they are at risk? ☐ No 　☐ Yes: _____	☐ Social isolation
• Who would you call first if you needed help? _____ Any indication that patient is unable to meet/have problems with any of the following (check all that apply)?	☐ Self-care deficit ☐ Impaired home maintenance management
☐ Personal grooming/hygiene　☐ Nutritional needs 　☐ Support system　　　　　☐ Mobility issues 　☐ Housing/shelter　　　　　☐ Medical care/medications 　☐ Other needs/issues: _____	☐ Resources to contact for help: _____ _____ _____
• Is patient from an institution or personal care/nursing home? ☐ No 　☐ Yes:　Name/contact _____　Phone _____	☐ Social Services consulted ☐ ER MD aware
NEONATE/PEDIATRIC/ADOLESCENT	**NSG Dx/PLAN**
• Displays cognitive development appropriate for age? ☐ Yes 　☐ No: _____	☐ Knowledge deficit R/T: _____ _____ _____
• If injury, is someone other than the patient responsible? ☐ No ☐ Yes (If yes, this **must** be investigated.)	☐ Altered family processes
• If bicycle, automobile, or all-terrain vehicle (ATV) accident, were appropriate restraints/safety devices (e.g., helmet, pads) in use? ☐ No ☐ Yes	☐ Altered parenting ☐ Active/potential family violence
• Are there any verbal/nonverbal cues from patient or caregivers of physical/emotional/psychologic abuse? ☐ No 　☐ Yes: _____	☐ Social Services consulted ☐ ER MD aware

Figure 11-7 Emergency department resources/coping evaluation.

Charting tip: When a patient decides to leave against department policy, documenting statements made about leaving and obtaining appropriate signatures on an "against medical advice" (AMA) form is vital. This form must provide evidence that the patient was informed of and accepted the risks of leaving the emergency department before the completion of evaluation and treatment. Joint Commission standards (1996) require notation in the medical record when a patient leaves AMA. In these situations careful documentation of instructions provided to the patient is particularly important.

THE NURSE AS PATIENT ADVOCATE

The ENA practice standard regarding human worth states that "Emergency nurses shall provide care based on philosophic and ethical concepts, such as reverence for life and a respect for the inherent dignity, worth, autonomy, and

Addressograph

RELATIONSHIPS/BELIEFS/VALUES	NSG Dx/PLAN

RELATIONSHIPS/BELIEFS/VALUES

- Are you being hurt/frightened/hit by anyone at home or in your life?

  ☐ No ☐ Yes ☐ Spouse ☐ Boyfriend/girlfriend ☐ Unknown

  Have the police been notified? ☐ No ☐ Yes

- Does the patient have any religious/cultural/dietary needs that might influence evaluation or treatment? ☐ No
  ☐ Yes: _____

- Is there an identified language or hearing barrier that could affect the patient's understanding of discharge instructions? ☐ No
  ☐ Yes: _____

- Does the patient have Advanced Directives?

  ☐ No: Does the patient want more information? ☐ No ☐ Yes

  ☐ Yes: ☐ Medical power of attorney ☐ Living will ☐ Organ donor

NSG Dx/PLAN

☐ Fear/powerless

☐ Knowledge deficit R/T:

_____
_____
_____

☐ Impaired social interaction

☐ Spiritual distress

☐ Ineffective coping (circle one):
  Family
  Individual

☐ Chaplain notified

☐ Social Services consulted

☐ ER MD aware

BEHAVIORAL MEDICINE	NSG Dx/PLAN

BEHAVIORAL MEDICINE

Is the patient suicidal? ☐ No ☐ Yes   Homicidal? ☐ No ☐ Yes

Is there someone with the patient who is willing to be the applicant for a Mental Hygiene Petition? ☐ No ☐ Yes: _____
(Instruct this person to remain until the application is completed and notarized. Document the person's phone number before he or she leaves the ED.)

Does the patient have a behavioral health care provider: ☐ No
  ☐ Yes: _____ Phone: _____

NSG Dx/PLAN

☐ Ineffective patient coping

☐ Impaired thought process

☐ Potential for violence

☐ Social Services consulted

☐ ER MD aware

Figure 11-7, cont'd   Emergency department resources/coping evaluation.

individuality of each human being, and on a resolution to act dynamically in relation to people's beliefs'' (ENA, 1995).

The nurse must respect the dignity, confidentiality, and privacy of patients and obtain the appropriate consents for treatment. Patients should be informed of their legal rights as required and the medical records should reflect adherence to patient screening and transfer policies and regulations.

Nursing Role in the Transfer of Patients

Nursing management of patients in need of transfer to other facilities highlights the legal implications of the emergency nurse's responsibility for patient advocacy and for demonstrating respect for human worth as reflected in appropriate documentation.

COBRA Legislation

The Consolidated Omnibus Budget Reconciliation Act (COBRA) of 1985 requires that any hospital receiving Medicare funds evaluate all patients who come into the emergency department. This legislation was designed to stop the "dumping" of indigent patients for economic reasons. The law requires that hospital personnel stabilize a patient or manage the active labor of a pregnant woman before the patient can be transferred to another facility. The receiving facility must agree to accept the patient and have enough space and qualified personnel to care for them. The transferring hospital must provide the receiving hospital with medical records and transport the patient using qualified personnel and equipment, including life support, if indicated.

Physicians can be fined $50,000 for each COBRA violation. Joint Commission standards reiterate some components of COBRA legislation; in July 1987 the Joint Commission required all hospitals to begin keeping documentation validating compliance with the standards concerning transfer of patients. Thus the transfer of emergency department patients is a special concern with legal ramifications and documentation priorities.

Documentation Requirements

To support compliance with the standard requiring stabilization, documentation must include the following (Waxman, 1988):

- A copy of the sending hospital's treatment record
- Measures taken or treatment implemented at the sending facility
- A description of the patient's response to treatment
- The results of measures taken to prevent further deterioration in the patient's condition

Documentation responsibilities of emergency department personnel related to the transfer of patients are listed in Box 11-3. Figures 11-8, 11-9, and 11-10 are examples of transfer forms used to comply with these standards.

Consider the following anecdotal report in which a patient's treatment for sepsis was delayed for more than 13 hours because of improperly carrying out the transfer procedure:

A 24-year-old black male with known sickle cell disease arrived at an emergency department complaining of fever, chills, and pain progressively becoming worse over 12 hours. A catheter port had been placed 2 days before his arrival in the emergency department. His temperature was 102.3° F, and he had not been given an antibiotic. The patient refused to allow blood cultures to be taken or IV fluids to be administered after two unsuccessful attempts at accessing his port. His attending physician was paged within 15 minutes of the patient's arrival but did not answer for an hour. When he responded to the emergency department physician, his orders were that the patient be transferred to another hospital where, it was understood, he would arrange and manage further treatment. The record reflects the attending doctor's intention to admit the patient with sickle cell crisis, rule out sepsis.

No antibiotic was ordered. Five hours elapsed from the time of the decision to transfer until EMS arrived to transport the patient. The patient spent a total of 7 hours in the sending emergency department. During this time, his white blood cell count elevated 8 points above normal and

---

Box 11-3

Documentation Responsibilities for the Transfer of Patients

- Records should indicate that the hospital is following the law and examining all patients, regardless of financial status.
- A chart must be made for each patient who enters the emergency department, regardless of whether the patient is seen by the physician. The triage nurse should include vital signs, a brief history, and the triage classification. The physician should sign every chart.
- Charts should never be discarded or destroyed.
- The medical record should contain adequate information about the patient's status and the treatment provided.
- To justify the transfer, the physician must determine and document that the benefits of transfer outweigh the risks, and specify each benefit.
- The patient must consent to the transfer in writing.
- The transfer form should provide a guideline to ensure that complete information is documented and sent with the patient before the transfer occurs.

---

he had a hemoglobin level of 7.0. His fever rose to 104° F, his blood pressure dropped to 110/50 from 130/80, and his pulse rose to 150 beats per minute, all symptoms of impending septic shock. He was given Tylenol (acetaminophen), pain medication, oxygen, and oral fluids. No antibiotics or blood transfusions were initiated.

No forms were found bearing the patient's signature to support his refusal of IV fluids, although the chart showed that he resisted further attempts to access his catheter port after two unsuccessful attempts by staff. No documentation by the emergency department nurse was made to indicate that she provided a report about the patient to the receiving facility, or that she had determined where the patient was to go upon arrival (i.e., to the emergency department or nursing unit). And finally, no record was found to indicate that the patient had agreed to the transfer or that he had been informed of the need, risks, or benefits of transfer.

The patient's condition was classified as stable at the time of transfer by the sending emergency department. His attending physician did not see him for 23 hours after his arrival at the receiving hospital. IV fluids and antibiotics were ordered by phone, but they were not started until 5 hours after admission—13 hours after the patient's initial entry into the healthcare system and 25 hours after his symptoms began.

Laboratory test results the following day showed a white blood cell count 37 points above normal and a hemoglobin level unchanged from the previous emergency department result. The patient died of cardiac arrest 1½ days after admission (anecdotal report, 1997).

The sending emergency department could be held liable for negligence for not administering blood or antibiotics and could be accused of dumping—even though the transfer was requested by the patient's regular doctor. A COBRA violation could be reported. All emergency department

Saint John's Health System
Anderson, IN 46016

**This form should accompany all patients at time of transfer

REASON FOR TRANSFER: DIAGNOSIS_____

_____ HOSPITAL/PHYSICIAN RECOMMENDS   _____ SPECIALTY PROCEDURES   _____ OTHER

_____ PATIENT/FAMILY REQUEST   _____ SPECIALTY COVERAGE

Physician's Certificate of Transfer

All transfers have the inherent risks of traffic delays, accidents during transport, inclement weather, rough terrain or turbulence, and the limitations of equipment and personnel present in the vehicle. I hereby certify that, based on the information available to me at the time of transfer, the medical benefits reasonably expected from the provision of appropriate medical care at another medical facility outweigh the increased risk to the individual, and in the case of labor to the unborn child, from effecting the transfer.

This certification is based on the following:

BENEFITS OF TRANSFER: RISKS OF TRANSFER:

_____   _____

_____   _____

_____   _____

Physician's Signature_____ Date_____Time_____

Transfer to_____ by_____
         Receiving Facility   Conveyance (Type of Transport)

_____ spoke with _____who
      Transferring Physician   Receiving Physician
accepted the patient for transfer at_____.
                            (time)

Consent to Transfer

I hereby consent to transfer to another medical facility. I understand that it is the opinion of the physician responsible for my care that the benefits of transfer outweigh the risks of transfer. I have been informed of the risks and benefits upon which this transfer is being made. I have considered these risks and benefits and consent to transfer.

Signature of Patient or Responsible Person_____ ❏ Patient ❏ Relative ❏ Other

ON CALL PHYSICIAN DID NOT APPEAR

_____ "ON CALL" PHYSICIAN DID NOT APPEAR TO TREAT PATIENT IN E.R. AFTER BEING REQUESTED TO DO SO BY EITHER HOSPITAL PERSONNEL OR E.R. PHYSICIAN.

Physician Name:_____

Physician Address:_____

_____

| Pt. Registration #: |
| Pt. Name: |
| Date: |

WHITE-Original   YELLOW-Transfer Copy   PINK-Administration

678-3-1294   Emergency Medical Condition Transfer Form

B-C Note	C-Lab	D-X-Ray	E-Diag	F-Surgery	G-Therapy	H-Orders	I-Nurses	J-Misc.

Figure 11-8 Emergency medical division transfer form. (Courtesy St. John's Health System, Anderson, Ind.)

USE SPACE BELOW IF IDENTIFICATION PLATE IS NOT AVAILABLE

NAME _____   ROOM NO. _____

PHYSICIAN CERTIFICATION

THIS FORM MUST BE COMPLETED BY THE PHYSICIAN AND WITNESSED BY A HEALTH CARE PROFESSIONAL.

ALL APPLICABLE BOXES SHOULD BE CHECKED:

☐ It is in my/our best opinion that this individual (or legally responsible person acting on the individual's behalf) noted below is alert, oriented, and has the ability to understand his or her current situation.

☐ This individual is not competent to understand his or her situation, and despite reasonable efforts we have not been able to contact responsible family or friends. Documentation of these efforts is included on the patient's medical record.

☐ Patient's medical condition at transfer: ☐ Stable   ☐ Unstable

☐ I have explained to this individual (and/or the legally responsible person acting on the individual's behalf), if possible, the nature of his or her medical problem in clear language and the benefits and the risks of transfer.

THE NATURE OF THE MEDICAL PROBLEM IS: _____

THE REASON FOR TRANSFER IS: _____

THE RISKS OF TRANSFER INCLUDE: There will be temporary reduced accessibility to ancillary medical services, and the services of specific health care professionals, there is the risk of an unforeseeable motor vehicle or airplane crash, there is the risk of a delay caused by traffic, weather, or a mechanical breakdown. **THE FOLLOWING SPECIAL RISKS APPLY BECAUSE OF THE CONDITION OF THE PERSON TO BE TRANSPORTED: (If none, state none)** _____
_____
_____
_____

THE BENEFITS OF TRANSFER INCLUDE: _____

THE RISKS OF NOT BEING TRANSFERRED INCLUDE: _____

RECEIVING HOSPITAL: _____ **NAME OF ACCEPTING PHYSICIAN:** _____

☐ **BASED UPON THE INFORMATION AVAILABLE TO ME AT THE PRESENT TIME, THE MEDICAL BENEFITS REASONABLY EXPECTED FROM THE PROVISION OF APPROPRIATE MEDICAL TREATMENT AT THE RECEIVING HOSPITAL OUTWEIGH THE INCREASED RISKS FROM BEING TRANSFERRED AND TRANSFER IS ACCEPTABLE.**

☐ **TRANSFER IS INAPPROPRIATE.**

_____   _____   _____   _____
Physician's Signature   Date   Witness Signature   Date

PATIENT CONSENT AND REQUEST

MUST BE COMPLETED BY THE PATIENT OR OTHER RESPONSIBLE PARTY

I understand the conditions, risks, and benefits of transfer outlined above and certify that any questions or concerns that I may have had about transfer have been adequately addressed and with this in mind I (**check one**):

☐ **Consent and request to be transferred to:** _____

☐ **Refuse to be transferred at this time and accept the risk of the decision as noted.**

_____   _____   _____
Individual's Signature (or legally responsible party)   Date   Individual's Name (PRINTED)

Responsible party's relationship to patient: _____

WHITE COPY: Chart   YELLOW COPY: Receiving Facility   _____   _____
                                                                  Witness Signature   Date

CONSENT AND REQUEST FOR TRANSFER TO OUTSIDE FACILITY

Figure 11-9 Consent and request for transfer to outside facility. (Courtesy Charleston Area Medical Center.)

PATIENT TRANSFER CHECKLIST/WORKSHEET

To be completed on all patients transferred to another facility. All items must be completed before patient is cleared for the transfer.

1. ☐ Consent and Request for Transfer is complete and signed by the M.D. and the patient/or family.

2. ☐ Evidence of physician analysis of risks and benefits of transfer is evident on physician certification and progress notes.

3. ☐ Verification that receiving facility has necessary medical personnel, space, equipment, and have accepted the patient.

4. ☐ Nurses notes reflect mode of transport. (Ambulance, private vehicle, helicopter)

   Personnel required for the transport: RN _____

   Medic: _____

5. ☐ Nursing transfer note written and includes discharge vital signs and disposition of personal belongings.

6. ☐ Report called to receiving facility with documentation of who received the report:

   _____

7. ☐ Copy of patient's record including lab, x-rays, EKG, ABG and any other relevant tests.

_____

Signature of Nurse Completing Form

Date: _____ Time: _____

Review By: _____
                          Charge Nurse

Figure 11-10 Patient transfer checklist and worksheet. (Courtesy Charleston Area Medical Center.)

nursing documentation would be scrutinized in such a case. Whether the sending emergency department was vindicated or not, its personnel would have to participate in the legal process and their documentation would significantly impact their accountability.

Charting tips: *Always* document the time when calling to make a report to the receiving facility and include the name of the RN who took the call of the accepting facility. This will clarify whether the patient is being transferred to another emergency department or is to be directly admitted.

In either instance, it can be proven that nursing personnel at the receiving facility were notified about the patient before his or her arrival. Note every instance—both time and content—when an attending or emergency department physician is notified of changes in the patient's condition, as well as any requests for antibiotics or fluid resuscitation. In the event of EMS delays, record the time of any inquiries made to the EMS dispatcher about the expected time of arrival (ETA) of the transport crew, the reason for the delay, and notification of the charge nurse or physician of any delays. In the event of abnormal vital signs at the time of discharge, also chart the communication of this information to the physician.

Other Issues Concerning the Nurse's Duty to Act as a Patient Advocate

The opportunity to protect patient rights or uphold the dignity of vulnerable persons occurs every time someone arrives in the emergency department for care. The following six situations involve a failure to act as a patient advocate and illustrate the powerful impact emergency nurses have on human lives:

1. A judgmental attitude toward substance abuse and intoxicated patients leads to a missed diagnosis of diabetic ketoacidosis.

   An EMS crew brought in one of the emergency department "regulars," who was unresponsive. He had been incontinent of urine, was unkempt, and malodorous. At the time of arrival the patient's skin was pale, hot, and dry. His level of consciousness was assessed as lethargic, and his speech was slurred. The medics' assessment was "he's drunk again," so they did not start an IV or check his blood sugar at the scene. But the receiving nurse was unconvinced by the EMS crews' evaluation after looking at the patient. The patient had no odor of alcohol, and the alarming dryness of his skin, his slurred speech, and his history of insulin-dependent diabetes (elicited from the medics) prompted her to check his blood sugar at the bedside. The patient's blood sugar was too high to be read. The nurse immediately obtained physician assistance and started IV access. Serum glucose tests confirmed that his blood sugar value was over 900, and the patient was later admitted to the ICU on an insulin drip. His blood alcohol test result was negative (anecdotal report, 1997).

   Charting tips: Note the time and content of all assessments, blood sugar tests (e.g., Accuchecks), IV access, abnormal laboratory results, and communications with physicians. This demonstrates to expert reviewers that all possible efforts were made in a timely fashion in the event of patient disability or death.

2. Failure to activate the chain of command nearly results in the loss of a limb.

   A teenage boy was discharged without pedal pulses after a "four-wheeler" wreck. At the time he arrived at the

facility he had faint pulses in the affected foot. A fractured knee was the diagnosis. The nurses repeatedly documented that they were unable to verify circulation—even using an ultrasonic Doppler—over a 4-hour period. Although they informed the emergency physician early in the course of evaluation that they were having difficulty finding pedal pulses, the nurses did not document further communication with him about the boy's status, even though he developed severe pain distal to the injury, and exhibited decreased temperature and sensation in the foot. The physician discharged the patient and the nurse did not challenge this disposition. Instead, she documented that the patient had no detectable pulses in the affected foot at the time of discharge and that she had informed her charge nurse of this fact after the patient left. The charge nurse did not contact the patient or his family to return for further evaluation. A few hours later, his parents took him to a different facility, where emergency surgery was required to save his leg (anecdotal report, 1996).

   Charting tips: Making the observation that a patient has limb-threatening changes is not sufficient. Documentation must show that the physician was notified and, if he or she failed to take action, that the charge nurse, nursing supervisor, department director, and medical staff chief, if necessary, were all notified on the patient's behalf. Documentation must reflect the content and time that important clinical communication took place.

3. Failure to follow advance directives. If a patient arrests and is resuscitated in spite of a living will specifying that no resuscitation took place in the event of cardiac arrest, and the patient is left in a persistent vegetative state, who pays for this medical care? Can the family sue the hospital, physician, and nurses for disregarding the advanced directives? The answer is *yes*.

4. Failure to offer an autopsy or organ donation. This can promote suspicion in the family about the quality of care, prevent resolution of the grieving process, and result in legal action.

5. Failure to protect patient confidentiality, *even from family members (when the patient is an adult or mature minor)*. This can result in the illegal release of drug screening results or alcohol levels to the press, police, or the victims of a drunk driver, and it can impact the legal process to such a degree that a felony conviction could be denied. Emotional anguish results when the death of a patient is reported by the press before the family has been notified. Obviously such violations of confidentiality also breach the standard of respect for human worth and the responsibility of emergency nurses to act as patient advocates, and thus they form the basis for legal action.

6. Failure to ensure the safety of compromised or endangered patients after discharge. Documentation must reflect that the nurse made an effort to do each of the following:

   • Report dangerous situations to the proper authorities (e.g., Adult/child protective services, community homeless shelters, violence shelters, home health nurses, police departments, or social services).

- Provide transportation for and ensure the safety of compromised patients after discharge (e.g., blood alcohol levels above 100, inability to walk, slurred speech, or confusion). For example, giving an 85-year-old patient who arrived in her pajamas by EMS a bus ticket or even a free cab ride home is not acceptable emergency department nursing practice. Severely compromised patients should be discharged only to a responsible adult, if nurses have confirmed and documented that discharge is acceptable.
- Provide for the protection of life and limb when a reasonably prudent nurse would consider them endangered. Discharging a child into the care of an abusive parent is not acceptable, even when the custodial parent has been admitted after an accident; discharging a psychotic, hallucinating individual with or without stated suicidal or homicidal intent would be unacceptable as well. Nursing documentation must reflect activation of the chain of command as appropriate to safeguard the public and patient from harm. Nurses may have an additional duty to notify police or the intended victims of a homicidal patient, especially in the event of a patient's elopement from the emergency department.

SUMMARY

The emergency nurse has a vital responsibility to coordinate care of assigned patients from the time of arrival until departure and to anticipate problems after discharge. In spite of sometimes poorly planned efforts to reduce healthcare costs, emergency nurses face an increased responsibility as patient advocate to monitor the work of nonlicensed personnel and physician's assistants. The presence of physician supervision does not relieve nurses of this role.

Nurses are not always named as parties to lawsuits. Indeed, many lawyers want to avoid the perception of bullying nurses through direct litigation. The reader, however, should see that in the not so distant future, attorneys will recognize the impact that nurses have on patient outcomes through their responsibility to adhere to recognized standards of care and by their application of the nursing process, and they, as will the general public, will increasingly demand accountability from individual nurses.

Few nursing specialty areas experience the range of disastrous patient outcomes that result from the failure to follow established practice standards in the emergency department. Still fewer specialty areas enjoy the degree of freedom and independent judgment that is enjoyed by emergency nurses. However, with this freedom, as with other privileges, comes a price: responsibility. For emergency nurses that price is serving as patient advocates as established by law.

Nurses who fail to protect patients by acting as patient advocates further fail by preventing the impact of poor care on that patient's quality of life and survival, which impacts the family or significant others as well. Patient advocacy will increasingly become the focus of malpractice litigation against emergency nurses because attorneys and patients will discover both the duty of the nurse and the relationship of the nurse's failure in this duty to their health, and they will hold hospitals responsible through their emergency department. The authors hope that when that day comes, emergency nurses will be well prepared and their documentation, as well as their professional practice, will withstand scrutiny.

INTENSIVE CARE DOCUMENTATION
Ann Marie Santarelli-Kretovics, RN, BSN, MS

The American Association of Critical Care Nurses (AACN) states that critical care nursing involves the diagnosis and treatment of human responses to actual or potentially life-threatening illness (AACN, 1989). The scope of critical care nursing practice is defined by the interaction of the critical care nurse, the critically ill patient, and the environment that provides adequate resources for the provision of care.

Patients enter the critical care environment to receive intensive nursing care for a variety of health problems. The continuum of patient symptoms ranges from the patients that need frequent monitoring and require little intervention to the patient with multisystem failure requiring interventions to support the most basic of life functions. While the environment generally supports a nurse to patient ratio of 1:2 (depending on patient needs), one nurse may care for 3 patients and, occasionally, a patient may require the assistance of more that one nurse to survive. The support and treatment of these patients requires an environment in which information is readily available from a variety of sources and is organized in such a manner that decisions can be made quickly and accurately. Information is obtained through a balance of both human intervention and technologic assistance. Indeed, the critical care environment is highly technical by nature.

Documentation challenges in the critical care area relate to the intensity of nursing care, the performance of highly repetitive, technical tasks at frequent intervals, and complex patient problems. Timely, comprehensive, and meaningful documentation is a challenge for even the most competent and experienced bedside critical care nurse.

While most of the current documentation systems in the critical care setting consist of a manual medical record, the advantages of computerized, automated bedside records for this environment are well recognized. Computers that are interfaced with bedside equipment can provide continuous data flow. Interfaces also assist in the active treatment of patients because they require little physical intervention by the nurse. For example, investigators have developed a closed-loop system interfacing an infusion pump with the bedside monitor. The system automatically delivers the appropriate dose of vasoactive drugs in response to the blood pressure measurement. Both simple and complex calculations are completed in an instant. Laboratory test results and other ancillary information can be readily available at the bedside, negating the need for the nurse to seek out and find pertinent pieces of information on which to base further treatment decisions. Despite these advantages, computerized critical care information systems have not seen widespread acceptance, probably because of the cost of systems. (Such costs include both the hardware and the ongoing technical support required to maintain the system.)

The introduction of the microprocessor in the 1970s created an explosion of computer-driven bedside equipment lasting through the 1990s. This equipment has impacted the critical care environment and consequently the documentation of the care provided. State-of-the-art computerized patient monitoring systems and other lifesaving devices, such as external defibrillators, have the capacity to capture, record, and store the patient's vital signs and any significant events. Indeed, nurses frequently rely on these systems, particularly the bedside monitoring systems, to capture the vital signs as they become involved in the active treatment of highly unstable patients. In these cases the nurse will document retrospectively based on the information recorded and stored by the device. Nurses frequently use these printouts as an addendum to flowsheet charting. As a result, a review of nursing documentation may include a mix of manual and computerized records.

THE BEDSIDE FLOWSHEET

The flowsheet is the cornerstone of bedside critical care nursing documentation. A well-constructed, comprehensive flowsheet communicates and reflects the standard of care of the primary patient population served by the unit. The data should be organized so that assessments and routine interventions are predetermined and the nurse is cued to ensure that documentation is complete and addresses all essential areas of nursing intervention. Depending on the patient population that is served, the cues may vary; for example, the flowsheet of the cardiovascular intensive care unit (CVICU) may have very specific assessment parameters that cue the nurse to document the quality and amount of chest-tube drainage hourly, whereas the records of the coronary care unit (CCU) may not specify this parameter because patients with an acute myocardial infarction do not

routinely have chest tubes inserted. The actual process for designing a flowsheet is beyond the scope of this discussion; however, Box 11-4 lists information sources that could aid in flowsheet construction.

Flowsheet design can be as variable as the organizations that create them. Some organizations create forms that open out like a road map; for example, the flowsheet may be the size of four 8.5-inch × 11-inch pieces of paper that fold out to be 32 inches × 11 inches, but it may contain as many as eight sides. A landscape orientation presents information across the sheet so that all significant parameters can be viewed in light of the recorded interventions. Other organizations prefer to keep the pages in a portrait orientation (i.e., such as the format of this page). The pages may also be folded in to create a compact document. Regardless of the presentation of the form, information, such as vital signs, medication administration, laboratory data, and other ongoing assessment and intervention information, is generally placed conspicuously. Other more routine, or "scripted," information, such as nursing interventions or total body assessments, will be embedded more strategically in the form. The time column generally is blank, which allows the nurse to designate the frequency of vital signs or other significant events based on patient status. As a result, one form or a compilation of many forms may represent a 24-hour period of documentation. This timed charting is done as events unfold, as opposed to block charting, which is generally used in the narrative note as part of a description, or overall snapshot, of the patient's condition for a given time period.

The purpose of the flowsheet is to provide an ongoing, continuous record of the patient's status. This may be in increments ranging from a few minutes to once an hour. Nurses should remember, however, that the flowsheet is only a piece of the total picture of nursing process

---

Box 11-4

Information to Consider When Constructing a Critical Care Flowsheet

- Documentation standards of the American Nurses Association (ANA) and AACN
- Specific standards of care, as defined by specialty organizations and current literature
- Equipment considerations (e.g., calibration, alarm and alert settings, functional settings)
- Unit policy and procedures
- Pertinent patient safety issues (e.g., restraints, skin protocols, nutritional assessment)
- Clinical data (e.g., intake and output, vital signs, assessments, ABGs, medication and IV administration)
- Laboratory test results and other ancillary department information

documentation, to be used in conjunction with the progress notes and other essential pieces of documentation to completely describe the delivery of nursing services to the client. Documentation must include attention to all aspects of the nursing process: assessment, diagnosis, planning, intervention, and evaluation. Documentation of the patient's response, progress, or deterioration and the patient's achievement of outcomes is a necessary part of documentation as well. Figures 11-11 and 11-12 provide examples of critical care flowsheets.

DOCUMENTATION ISSUES IN CRITICAL CARE AREAS

Charting Passive Observations

When utilizing the flowsheet, the nurse must fill it out completely to provide comprehensive and accurate information regarding the patient's clinical status and active interventions. Although experienced critical care nurses are well versed in the use of flowsheet documentation, nurses should be aware of two common pitfalls in its use; casual charting and relying too heavily on the flowsheet.

Casual Charting

Casual charting is defined as the practice of casually (i.e., following the lead of the previous nurse) checking off certain parameters. For example, when going through the head-to-toe assessment prompts in the flowsheet, the night nurse may check the boxes in the same way as the evening nurse did in the previous shift. The nurse will then use the nurses' notes or hourly entries to chart the actual (specific) assessment information, which could obviously result in a discrepancy if the patient's condition has changed or inconsistencies occur in the actual level of care provided. Because the chart is a legal document, all areas must reflect the actual care given to the patient. A second type of casual charting occurs when the nurse ignores the preprinted assessment altogether and documents in the nurses notes "Assessment as previously noted."

Reliance on Flowsheets

Another error that nurses frequently make when using the flowsheet is that they tend to depend too heavily on the flowsheet to describe the entire course of care delivered. Thus the flowsheet essentially becomes the only tool used to document care. In addition to his or her observations, the nurse is required to evaluate and document the patient's response to the care provided. When relying too much on the flowsheet, the nurse may neglect to chart in the nurses notes the patient responses, with the documentation consisting only of treatments and assessments.

SOURCES OF LIABILITY

Vieira (1997) notes that in a review of one professional liability insurer's database, suits were identified that involved documentation issues (one issue being the insufficient or lack of documentation). She details the following case as an example of insufficient documentation:

A 56-year-old man was admitted to the surgical intensive care unit (SICU) following a pneumonectomy. The progress notes contained a nursing admission note to the unit. The flowsheets indicated a 5-day course of respiratory distress, extubation and reintubation, and a continuing course of changes in ventilatory rate, volume, and oxygen concentration. Although the flowsheets contained relevant subjective and objective data, no documentation was made in the progress notes by any nurses or physicians for 11 days to provide a rationale for the ventilatory management of the patient. The patient died, and the family successfully pursued a wrongful death action against the healthcare heathcare providers and the hospital (Vieira, 1997).

This section discusses common documentation issues affecting the defense of critical care nurses included in lawsuits. The sources of liability include the following:

- Omission of critical thinking
- Inadequate evaluation of patient status
- Missing or incomplete documentation of changes in patient condition before an arrest and resuscitation
- Documentation of physician notification regarding changes in a patient's condition

Omission of Critical Thinking

"Critical thinking forms the basis for quality documentation" (Chase, 1997). Critical thinking requires the use of nursing judgment in several areas, including initial judgments about patient's status, decisions about treatment options, and evaluations of the effectiveness of interventions.

If critical care nurses are expected to form judgments, then a failure to record those judgments could be seen as providing less than the standard of care (Chase, 1997). The recording of critical judgments requires that the nurse go beyond the flowsheet data, which documents only passive observations. The nursing progress notes will frequently be a recap of the information provided on the flowsheet, restated in narrative form. When documenting this way the nurse may omit important information about the patient's progress and miss the opportunity to demonstrate the impact of nurses' contributions to the patient's outcome. Consider the following nursing progress note:

Extubated at 2300. Vital signs stable. Respirations at 20/min. On 3 L/min nasal cannula. Mediastinal and leg dressings dry and

Text continued on p. 251

CARDIO-THORACIC INTENSIVE CARE RECORD

OPERATION _____

PAGE _____ POD# _____

DATE _____

IMPRINT/LABEL

	TIME	TEMP	HEART RATE	BLOOD PRESSURE	MEAN BP	CVP	LAP	R	PA SYS / DIAS	CO / CI	SVR / PVR	CARDIAC INFUSIONS				
A																
B																
C																
D																
E																
F																
G																
H																
I																
J																
K																
L																
M																
N																
O																
P																
Q																
R																
S																
T																
U																
V																
W																
X																
Y																
Z																

Figure 11-11 Critical care flowsheet. (Courtesy Cleveland Clinic, Cleveland, Ohio.)

MEDICATION SCHEDULE

MED

A _____ F _____

B _____ Pre-op Wt. _____

C _____ Present Wt. _____

D _____

E _____

INTAKE

	SIGNIFICANT EVENTS	MEDICATION DOSES AND ROUTES	BLOOD	COLLOID	A	B	C	D	E	F
A										
B										
C										
D										
E										
F										
G										
H										
I										
J										
K										
L										
M										
N										
O										
P										
Q										
R										
S										
T										
U										
V										
W										
X										
Y										
Z										

Figure 11-11, cont'd Critical care flowsheet. *Continued*

24 HOUR INTAKE								24 HOUR OUTPUT				
	PO TUBE	IV CRYST	BLOOD COLLOID	TPN			TOTAL	URINE	NG	CT		TOTAL
OR/PACU												
6A - 2P												
2P - 10P												
10P - 6A												
TOTAL												

		OUTPUT				LAB RESULT											
		URINE			CHEST TUBE		NEURO							Hgb /		BUN /	
		TOTAL	HOURLY	N.G.	TOTAL	HOURLY	PUPIL SIZE	COMA SCALE	K	Na	PT	PTT	GLUCOSE	Hct	SGOT	CR	WBC
A																	
B																	
C																	
D																	
E																	
F																	
G																	
H																	
I																	
J																	
K																	
L																	
M																	
N																	
O																	
P																	
Q																	
R																	
S																	
T																	
U																	
V																	
W																	
X																	
Y																	
Z																	

Figure 11-11, cont'd Critical care flowsheet. (Courtesy Cleveland Clinic, Cleveland, Ohio.)

NOTATION KEY
✓ INTACT / IN PLACE / COMPLETED   **U** - UPPER   **LO** - LOWER   **A** - ALL   **ON / OFF**
   ↑ - UP   ↓ - DOWN   **R** - RIGHT   **L** - LEFT   **S** - SUPINE   **P** - PRONE
* SEE NURSING PROGRESS REPORT   **SEE PER

Date _____

				7AM	8	9	10	11	12N
HYGIENE	Bath:	Self	Assist	Total						
	Mouth:	Self	Assist	Total						
	Back:	Self	Assist	Total						
	Peri Care	Self	Assist	Total						
ACTIVITY	Bedrest: Turn and Position	Self	Assist	Total						
	Chair:	Self	Assist	Total						
	Ambulatory:	Self	Assist	Total						
	Range of Motion:	Active	Passive							
	Sleep:									
NUTRITION	Feeding:	Self	Assist	Total						
	Force / Restrict Fluids		cc							
	Day:	Eve:		Night:						
	Calorie Count									
	Appetite / Diet Consumed (%)									
	Bowel Movement:	C – Continent		I – Incontinent						
TREATMENTS	Special Mattress / Bed:									
	Monitor / Telemetry Checks:	15 - 20 min.		30 min.						
	Hemodynamic Assessments (Swan, A-line, IABP, CVP) : 15 - 20 min. 30 min.									
	Infusion Pump Checks									
	Transducers: Zero and Calibrate									
	Cough and Deep Breathe:									
	Incentive Spirometry:									
	Suction:									
	Pulse Oximetry:									
	Trach Care:									
	Wound Assessment:									
	1.									
	2.									
	3.									
	Wound Care:									
	1.									
	2.									
	3.									
	Tube Care									
	1.									
	2.									
	3.									
	Pacemaker Checks:									
	PAS Stockings:									
	Pulse Checks:									
	Procedure Preparation (specify):									
	Hypothermia / Hyperthermia									
	Emotional Reassurance - Patient	Reassurance / coping								
	Emotional Reassurance - Family	Reassurance / coping								
SAFETY	Call Bell Within Reach									
	Side Rails									
	Restraints									
	Isolation									

Figure 11-11, cont'd   Critical care flowsheet.   *Continued*

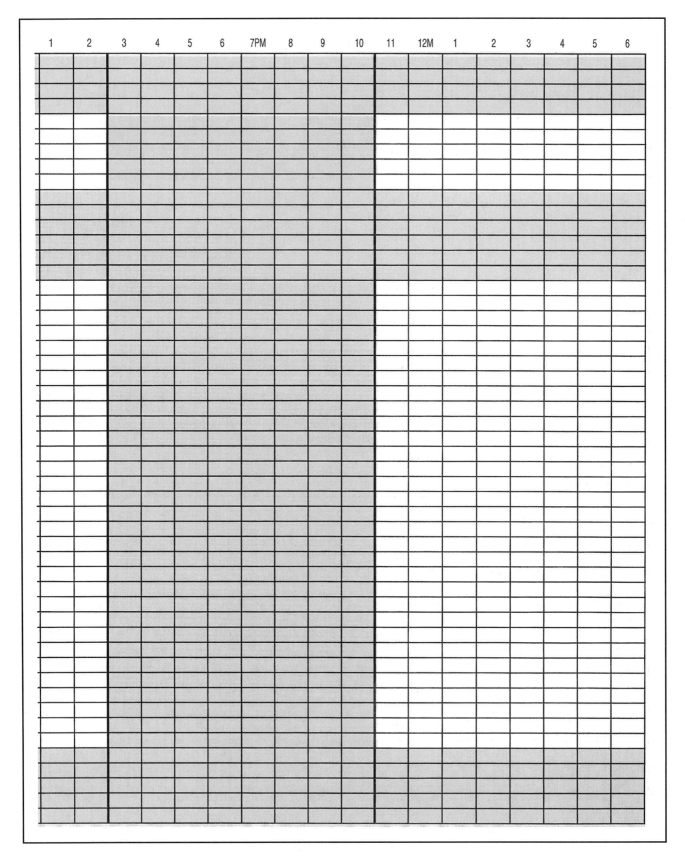

Figure 11-11, cont'd   Critical care flowsheet. (Courtesy Cleveland Clinic, Cleveland, Ohio.)

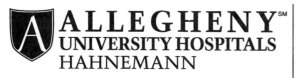

ALLEGHENY™
UNIVERSITY HOSPITALS
HAHNEMANN

PATIENT CARE FLOW SHEET

ADDRESSOGRAPH

DATE	ALLERGIES	TODAY'S WEIGHT				ET NT TUBE
RM#			LBS		KG	
	NONE	YESTERDAY'S WEIGHT				POSITION R / L
POST-OP DAY #	DIET		LBS		KG	TYPE ORAL NASAL
		ADMISSION PRE-OP WT.				INSERTION DATE
HOSPITAL DAY #	FLUID RESTRICTIONS		LBS		KG	LENGTH
		HT	BSA		CM	

EQUIPMENT CHECK
Circle the appropriate item and/or complete information in the boxes below.

PACEMAKER on/off	on / off	on / off	on / off
Mode			
Rate/MA			
CHEST TUBE Water Seal (cm)			
Suction on/off	on / off	on / off	on / off
CHEST TUBE Water Seal (cm)			
Suction on/off	on / off	on / off	on / off
CHEST TUBE Water Seal (cm)			
Suction on/off	on / off	on / off	on / off
Gastric Suction high/low	high / low	high / low	high / low
inter./cont.	inter. / cont.	inter. / cont.	inter. / cont.
Gastric Suction high/low	high / low	high / low	high / low
inter./cont.	inter. / cont.	inter. / cont.	inter. / cont.
Hypo/Hyper themia Blanket	on / off	on / off	on / off
Foley			
Traction type			
Weight (lbs)			

CHECK RECORD	INITIALS			DESCRIPTION OF SITE
	DAYS	EVES.	NIGHTS	
INVASIVE LINES / TUBES - Dressing Changes & Site Care Initials signify completion of dressing change				

ISOLATION TYPE ☐ NA

THERAPEUTIC BED ☐ NA ☐ OTHER (LIST) _____
  ☐ ZONEAIRE

FALL RISK ASSESSMENT ☐ NO RISK ☐ IMPAIRED MEMORY ☐ UNSTEADY GAIT
  ☐ HISTORY OF FALLS

SAFETY CHECK

ID Bracelet			
Allergy Bracelet			
O₂ Set Up			
Suction Set Up			
Airway			
Top Rail Up / Bottom Rail Up			
Monitor Calibration			
Bed in Low Pos.			
Monitor Alarms On			
Ventilator Alarms On			
Call Bell In Reach			

RESTRAINT EVALUATION ☐ NA ☐ HARM TO SELF / OTHERS
  APPLICATION TIME _____ / INITIALS _____

RESTRAINT TYPE: ☐ INVOLUNTARY (REQUIRES TIME LIMITED ORDER
  ☐ VOLUNTARY (REQUIRES INFORMED CONSENT)
  ☐ MEDICAL IMMOBILIZATION (REQUIRES UNIT PROTOCOL)

CHECK THOSE THAT ARE APPROPRIATE (CIRCLE APPROPRIATE EXTREMITY)
☐ WRISTS R / L ☐ ANKLE R / L MITTS R / L ☐ VEST
☐ OTHER

TRANSFER TO: _____ TIME: _____
TRANSFER TO: _____ TIME: _____

DAY SIGNATURES		**EVENING SIGNATURES**		**NIGHT SIGNATURES**	
INITIALS	SIGNATURE FULL NAME & TITLE	INITIALS	SIGNATURE FULL NAME & TITLE	INITIALS	SIGNATURE FULL NAME & TITLE

Figure 11-12 Critical care flowsheet. (Courtesy Allegheny University Health Care System, Philadelphia.)

Continued

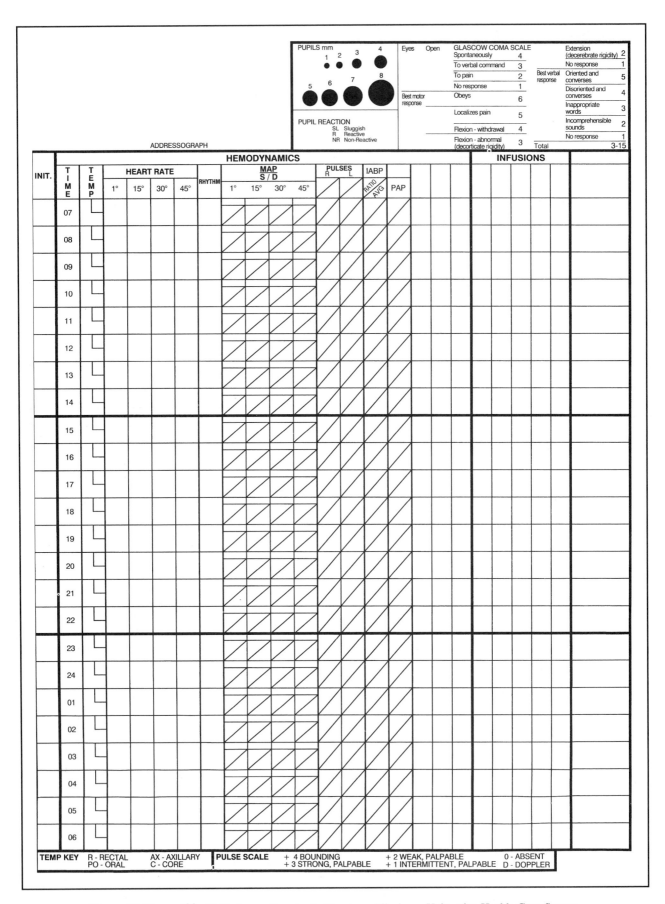

Figure 11-12, cont'd Critical care flowsheet. (Courtesy Allegheny University Health Care System, Philadelphia.)

LIMB MOVEMENT

5. Normal - Ability to move an entire extremity without assistance to a position and hold against gravity and resistance

3. Lift - ability to lift an entire extremity without assistance but cannot hold

1. No movement

4. Lift and Hold - Ability to move an entire extremity without assistance to a position but cannot sustain against resistance.

2. Move Laterally - ability to move entire extremity without assistance but cannot lift.

Allegheny University Hospitals, Hahnemann Division

ADDRESSOGRAPH

| | NEUROLOGICAL ASSESSMENT | | | | VENTILATION | | | LABORATORY DATA | | |

Figure 11-12, cont'd   Critical care flowsheet.   *Continued*

DRUG / CONCENTRATION

I	
II	
III	
IV	
V	

ADDRESSOGRAPH

TIME	CRYSTALLOIDS								M E D S	TPN	COLLOIDS			ALIMENTATION				TOTAL INPUT	TOTAL OUTPUT	BALANCE
														PO						
07																				
08																				
09																				
10																				
11																				
12																				
13																				
14																				
8 TOTAL																				
15																				
16																				
17																				
18																				
19																				
20																				
21																				
22																				
8 TOTAL																				
23																				
24																				
01																				
02																				
03																				
04																				
05																				
06																				
8 TOTAL																				
24 TOTAL																				

24° BALANCE

48° BALANCE

Figure 11-12, cont'd Critical care flowsheet. (Courtesy Allegheny University Health Care System, Philadelphia.)

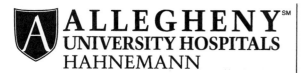

ALLEGHENY℠ UNIVERSITY HOSPITALS HAHNEMANN

PATIENT CARE FLOW SHEET

ADDRESSOGRAPH   ADDRESSOGRAPH

URINE			GI				DRAINS						PAIN MANAGEMENT						
TIME	CC'S		NG	RESIDUAL		STOOL						PD DRAIN	PD NET BAL	KEY	DOSE DELIVERED / INTERVENTION / LOCATION OF PAIN	PAIN SCALE	RESPONSE TIME	PAIN SCALE	PAIN KEY	
07																			PCA	
08																			E - EPIDURAL	
09																			IP INTRA-PLEURAL	
10																			IT-INTRA-THECAL	
11																			IM	
12																			IV - BOLUS	
13																			PO	
14																				
8 TOTAL																			INTERVENTION	
15																			M - MEDICATE	
16																			P - POSITION	
17																			R - RELAX	
18																			**OTHER SEE NOTE	
19																				
20																				
21																				
22																				
8 TOTAL																			PAIN SCALE	
23																			0 - 10	
24																			0 - NO PAIN	
01																			10 - WORST PAIN	
02																				
03																				
04																				
05																				
06																				
8 TOTAL																				
24 TOTAL																				

DOCUMENT ALL NARCOTICS IN THE LOCATION RELEVANT TO YOUR UNIT. (NARCOTICS CONTROL SHEET OR PYXIS SYSTEM).

Figure 11-12, cont'd Critical care flowsheet.   *Continued*

ADDRESSOGRAPH

		PROCEDURES												RESTRAINTS							
	HYGIENE	POSITION	ANTIEM THERAPY	RESP SUCTION	DESCRIPTION OF SECRETIONS	COUGH/DEEP BREATHE	INCENT SPIROM	PERCUSS. VIBRATION	TRACH CARE	ROM			ALTERNATIVES	APPLIED	DISCONTINUED	RELEASED Q2	CHECKED Q2	REASSESSES	NUTRITION/ FLUIDS	INITIALS
07																				
08																				
09																				
10																				
11																				
12																				
13																				
14																				
15																				
16																				
17																				
18																				
19																				
20																				
21																				
22																				
23		•																		
00																				
01																				
02																				
03																				
04																				
05																				
06																				

Figure 11-12, cont'd   Critical care flowsheet. (Courtesy Allegheny University Health Care System, Philadelphia.)

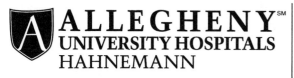

ALLEGHENY^{SM}
UNIVERSITY HOSPITALS
HAHNEMANN

PATIENT CARE FLOW SHEET

Patient Plan Of Care reviewed with patient and / or family

☐ Yes ☐ NA see exception note

ADDRESSOGRAPH

NURSING DIAGNOSIS	TARGET OUTCOME	TODAY'S GOAL: Patient will:	EVALUATION	If patient does not meet goals in Notes
☐ 1.Activity Intolerance	Tolerate Activity	_____	☐ Yes ☐ No	Initials _____
☐ 2.Ineff . Airway Clearance	Clear Airway	_____	☐ Yes ☐ No	Initials _____
☐ 3. Anxiety	Not Anxious	_____	☐ Yes ☐ No	Initials _____
☐ 4. High Risk for Aspiration	No Aspiration	_____	☐ Yes ☐ No	Initials _____
☐ 5. Ineffective Breathing Pattern	Effective Breathing Pattern	_____	☐ Yes ☐ No	Initials _____
☐ 6. Decreased Cardiac Output	Normal Cardiac Output	_____	☐ Yes ☐ No	Initials _____
☐ 7. Constipation	Normal Bowel Elim	_____	☐ Yes ☐ No	Initials _____
☐ 8. Diarrhea	Normal Bowel Elim	_____	☐ Yes ☐ No	Initials _____
☐ 9. Fear	No Fear	_____	☐ Yes ☐ No	Initials _____
☐ 10. Fluid Volume Alteration	Normal Fluid Volume	_____	☐ Yes ☐ No	Initials _____
☐ 11. Impaired Gas Exchange	Normal Gas Exchange	_____	☐ Yes ☐ No	Initials _____
☐ 12. Incontinence, Bowel	Continent	_____	☐ Yes ☐ No	Initials _____
☐ 13. Incontinence, Urine	Continent	_____	☐ Yes ☐ No	Initials _____
☐ 14. High Risk for Infection	No Infection	_____	☐ Yes ☐ No	Initials _____
☐ 15. High Risk for Injury	No Injury	_____	☐ Yes ☐ No	Initials _____
☐ 16. Alt Nutrition:	Well Nourished	_____	☐ Yes ☐ No	Initials _____
☐ 17. Pain	Comfort	_____	☐ Yes ☐ No	Initials _____
☐ 18. Self Care Deficit	Self Care Independence	_____	☐ Yes ☐ No	Initials _____
☐ 19. High Risk for Impaired skin Integ	Intact Skin	_____	☐ Yes ☐ No	Initials _____
☐ 20. Impaired Skin Integrity	Improved Skin Integrity	_____	☐ Yes ☐ No	Initials _____
☐ 21. Impaired Swallowing	Normal Swallowing	_____	☐ Yes ☐ No	Initials _____
☐ 22. Impaired Tissue Integrity	Normal Tissue Integrity	_____	☐ Yes ☐ No	Initials _____
☐ 23. Altered Tissue Perfusion	Adequate Tissue Perfusion	_____	☐ Yes ☐ No	Initials _____
☐ 24. Altered Urinary Elimination	Normal Urinary Elimination	_____	☐ Yes ☐ No	Initials _____
☐ 25. Ineffective Thermo Regulation	Normal Themo. Reg.	_____	☐ Yes ☐ No	Initials _____
☐ 26. _____	_____	_____	☐ Yes ☐ No	Initials _____
☐ 27. _____	_____	_____	☐ Yes ☐ No	Initials _____
☐ 28. _____	_____	_____	☐ Yes ☐ No	Initials _____

PATIENT FAMILY TEACHING

Instruction Key:	1 - Written Information, 2 - Discussion, 3- Demonstration, 4 - Audio / Video, 5 - Class / Group, 6 - Other
Readiness to Learn:	E - Eager to Learn, U - Seem Interested, A - Very Anxious, UC - Uncooperative, D - Denies need for education
Response Key:	VU - Verbalizes Understanding, RD - Return Demonstration, NR - Need Reinforcement, RT - Refuses Teaching
	SC - Significant Other Taught, *see exception note

Time	Readiness To Learn	Instruc Key	Teaching Outcomes	Response Key	Initials

Figure 11-12, cont'd Critical care flowsheet.   *Continued*

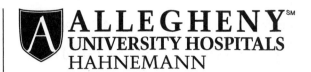

ALLEGHENY℠
UNIVERSITY HOSPITALS
HAHNEMANN

PATIENT CARE FLOW SHEET

KEY: ✓ = negative assessment   * = abnormal finding   → = no change from previous entry

ADDRESSOGRAPH

1. Place a " ✓ " in the box if the appropriate findings are the same as the parameters for each system. This constitutes a "negative assessment."

2. When the findings for any assessment differ from the parameters given or from the previous assessment, place a "*" in the box for that category. The "*" refers the reader to the "Notes" section and/or to the appropriate sections of the flow sheet. If additional space is needed, continue on Addendum Notes.

3. When there is no change in the assessment from a previous "*" entry, the current entry may be indicated with an " → ".

RESOURCE FOR ASSESSMENT: BATES, BARBARA; A GUIDE TO PHYSICAL EXAM, J.B. LIPPINCOTT, PHILA., 1992

☐ ADMISSION ASSESSMENT

Health Assessment	TIME												
A. Neurological: Alert and oriented to person, place and time Speech clear and understandable. Memory Intact. Behavior appropriate to situation. Pupils equal, reactive to light and accommodation Active range of motion (ROM) of all extremities, symmetrically equal strength. No paresthesia. Intact cough and gag reflexes.													
B. Cardiovascular: Regular apical pulse. Capillary refill <2 seconds. Palpable bilateral peripheral pulses. No peripheral edema. No calf tenderness.													
C. Pulmonary: Resting respirations 10-20 per minute, quiet and regular. Equal bilateral breath sounds. Vesicular breath sounds in all lungs fields. Bronchial breath sounds over major airways. No adventitious sounds. Clear sputum. Pink nailbeds and mucous membranes. Lungs clear.													
D. Gastrointestinal: Abdomen soft and non-distended. Active bowel sounds (5-24 per minute). No pain on palpation. Tolerates prescribed diet without nausea and vomiting. Bowel movements within own normal pattern and consistency.													
E. Genitourinary: No indwelling catheter in use. Able to urinate without pain. Undistended bladder after urination. Urine is clear, yellow to amber color.													
F. Surgical Dressing/Incision: Dressing dry and intact. No evidence of redness, increased temperature or tenderness in surrounding tissue. Sutures/staples/steri-strips intact. Sound edges well-approximated. No drainage present.													
G. Skin Integrity: Skin color within patient's norm. Skin warm, dry and intact. Moist mucous membranes.													
H. Psychological: Interacts and communicates in an appropriate manner with other persons (including family, significant others, health care personnel).													
I. Educational: Patient and/or significant others communicate understanding of patient's health status, plan of care and expected response.													
J.													

☐ ADMISSION
☐ REASSESSMENT

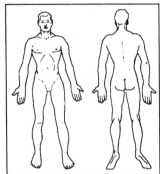

Instructions

(1) Circle areas of skin breakdown on diagram

(2) Assign a number to each area circled & describe in the spaces provide below

Site/number					
Stage					
Size (cm)					
Appearance					
Drainage					
Odor					
Cond. Surr. Skin					

If Necrotic tissue is present staging cannot be confirmed until wound is visible

Codes   Stage

Stage I   - Reddened Area
Stage II   - Blister / Skin Break
Stage III   - Skin break exposing subcutaneous tissue
Stage IV   - Skin break exposing muscle / bone

Appearance
P - Pink   S - Slough   E - Eschar
H - Hydrocolloid dressing intact

Odor
O - None   M - Mild
F - Foul

Drainage
S - Serosanguinous
P - Purulent   O - None

Condition of Surrounding Skin
I - Inflamed   M - Macerated
N - Intact / Normal

Braden Score	
Sensory	
Moisture	
Activity	
Mobility	
Nutrition	
Friction/Shear	
Total	

Figure 11-12, cont'd   Critical care flowsheet. (Courtesy Allegheny University Health Care System, Philadelphia.)

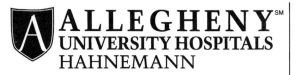

PATIENT CARE FLOW SHEET
NOTES

ADDRESSOGRAPH

TIME	

Figure 11-12, cont'd   Critical care flowsheet.   *Continued*

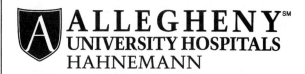

PATIENT CARE FLOW SHEET
NOTES

ADDRESSOGRAPH

TIME	

Figure 11-12, cont'd Critical care flowsheet. (Courtesy Allegheny University Health Care System, Philadelphia.)

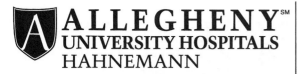

ALLEGHENY[SM]
UNIVERSITY HOSPITALS
HAHNEMANN

**PATIENT CARE FLOW SHEET
NOTES**

HEMODYNAMIC STRIPS

Figure 11-12, cont'd   Critical care flowsheet.   *Continued*

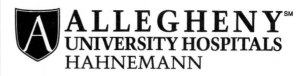

ALLEGHENY℠
UNIVERSITY HOSPITALS
HAHNEMANN

PATIENT CARE FLOW SHEET

HEMODYNAMIC STRIPS

Figure 11-12, cont'd Critical care flowsheet. (Courtesy Allegheny University Health Care System, Philadelphia.)

intact. Monitor shows NSR with occasional PVCs. Pacer off. Chest tubes draining dark red. Foley draining amber urine. NG in right nares to low suction. Report given to family and physician. Resting at intervals.

With the exception of the description of the drainage, this note gives no more information that could readily be found on the flowsheet record. This nurse cared for the patient for 8 hours and recorded hourly data on the flowsheet, then wrote this note, which fails to describe whether the patient is improving or deteriorating or what the nurse actually did to impact the patient's achievement of outcomes.

According to Chase (1997), a useful strategy in preparing a meaningful note is for the nurse to identify what patient problem or major issue was the focus of nursing care. In the previous example the nursing care of the patient focused on interventions to maintain a patent airway. Incentive spirometry was done once an hour, the patient was encouraged to frequently cough and breath deeply, and the nurse ensured that the prescribed aerosol treatments were provided. In addition, the nurse maintained the flow of oxygen-enriched air, did frequent respiratory assessments, and checked ABG values periodically. While all of these interventions and assessments could be pieced together by reviewing the flowsheet, what could not be captured is the actual evaluation of the effectiveness of these interventions. The nurse should use the nursing progress notes to document critical thinking, particularly in terms of describing the patient's response to interventions and making judgments about the patient's progress; for example:

Extubated and placed on NC at 3 L/min. Respirations are regular and easy at 20/min. Experienced mild anxiety immediately following extubation, which subsided with targeted encouragement. Sao_2 95%-100%. Providing periods of rest between C & DB and use of IS. Alert and oriented with clear speech. Aerosol treatments by RT. Patient taught to splint chest to cough. Is able to cough and expectorate sputum. Patient maintaining a patent airway with good gas exchange.

This note demonstrates a relationship between the patient problem, the interventions provided, and the patient's response, and it clearly states that the patient is breathing without difficulty and tolerating the removal of the ET tube. The note also describes nursing's unique contributions to the patient's outcome (being able to breathe unassisted).

Chase (1997) provides the following additional suggestions for improving documentation of critical thinking:

- Focus on major patient problems that require nursing care.
- Think in terms of patient problems that require nursing care.
- Report judgments about the data.
- Include patient responses to the nursing interventions.
- Document patient outcomes.
- Include a predictive thought for care (see following section for more information).

Inadequate Evaluation of Patient Status

Mayberry and Croke (1996) found that despite ongoing efforts to educate nurses in their professional responsibilities, the number of nurses named as defendants in malpractice actions has not decreased significantly over the last 10 to 15 years. In their review of 200 case summaries involving nurses in litigation, they identified several major categories of issues that formed the basis of the various lawsuits. One of these categories is the failure to document, including the failure to document a patient's progress and response to treatment.

In addition to ensuring that the individual nurse accurately documents all of the care provided, the practice of documenting nursing judgments provides an ongoing evaluation of the patient's progress or deterioration and helps to explain the rationale for any treatments or interventions that are initiated. Critical care nurses are frequently required to care for patients of whom they have no previous knowledge. Browsing through many pages of flowsheets is time-consuming, and expectations that the nurse could do this before caring for each patient are unrealistic. Verbal reports and summary sheets attempt to provide the nurse with an overview of the information necessary to assume care of patients with some sense of continuity. In addition to nurses formulating judgments when evaluating the patient's status, Chase (1997) also suggests that nurses anticipate the course of continued care, providing direction toward expected outcomes in the form of predictive thoughts documented in the nurse's notes. In this way the nurse communicates in a prescriptive manner about the link between the patient's current problems, any interventions found to be effective, and suggestions about the future direction of care to achieve the desired outcomes. Consider the progress note example discussed previously. The addition of a predictive thought gives direction to any future care and increases the continuity of care for the patient, as shown in the following:

Extubated and placed on NC at 3 L/min. Respirations are regular and easy at 20/min. Experienced mild anxiety immediately following extubation, which subsided with targeted encouragement. Sao_2 95%-100%. Providing periods of rest between C & DB and use of IS. Alert and oriented with clear speech. Aerosol treatments by RT. Patient taught to splint chest to cough. Is able to cough and expectorate sputum. Patient maintaining a patent airway with good gas exchange. **Suggest continuing with this plan of care and consider longer rest periods as breath sounds continue to improve.**

These strategies, which encourage nurses to go beyond the passive, "observation-based" documentation of the flowsheet, serve to communicate an ongoing assessment of overall patient status and provide valuable information regarding the patient's progress or deterioration. Nurses should use these documentation strategies to verify that ongoing monitoring of the patient's overall condition has occurred.

Documentation of Changes in Patient Condition: Arrest and Resuscitation

Documentation of arrest and resuscitation efforts presents a special challenge to the critical care nurse. While some arrest situations are anticipated from a recognition of the deteriorating condition of the patient, many are not. The nurse must be able to sort out the cause of the arrest in a matter of moments and proceed accordingly. Organizations may vary as to the amount of support provided to the nurse who is attempting to resuscitate a patient in arrest. In larger organizations, structured teams of nurses and physicians may respond, whereas in others, the nurse proceeds with support from the unit staff according to the standard written protocols. The challenge of documentation of these events is that it requires the nurse to attend to very specific details in very rapid succession in an extremely stressful situation, particularly if unanticipated.

Unanticipated arrest situations in the critical care area are generally heralded by an alarm. Every piece of equipment attached to the patient may have an alarm capability. Experienced nurses are able to distinguish which alarms require immediate investigation, such as the ventilator or heart monitor, and which do not. Sophisticated, state-of-the-art ECG monitoring systems provide different sounds for varying levels of alarm situations, helping the nurse to distinguish the presence of potentially lethal cardiac dysrhythmias by their sound.

Many critical care flowsheets may designate an area in the nursing interventions for the documentation of alarm status to cue the nurse, not only to document in regard to this very important issue, but also to ensure that all alarm parameters are set to the appropriate limits for that patient and the alarms are set to the "on" position. Even when the alarms are activated, a nurse must be present to respond to the signal. The following case illustrates the importance of the nurse finding someone to cover his or her responsibility if unavailable to respond to alarms:

A 41-year-old, unmarried woman from Texas was hospitalized for a severe abdominal infection. During surgery she became dependent on the ventilator. She was transferred to the SICU, where her ventilator tubing became disconnected. The SICU nurse allegedly abandoned the patient and left the unit without obtaining any one to cover for her. Furthermore, the off-site monitoring station was allegedly not staffed. The defendant resident was allegedly sitting across the hall from the unit when the ventilator, ECG, and central venous pressure (CVP) alarms went off. It was estimated that the alarms were on for at least 8 minutes before a response occurred. The patient ended up in a vegetative state resulting from total anoxic encephalopathy. She lived in this state for more than 4 years before she expired. The decedent's parents believed that the tubing and the ventilator were defective, and they settled with all manufacturers early in the discovery process for $52,000. The defendants claimed that adult respiratory distress syndrome

was the cause of death, and that the decedent would not have survived, regardless of their actions. The defendant hospital and doctor settled for a total of $190,000 plus a waiver of the decedent's medical bills of about $1 million (Laska, 1997e).

Most organizations provide a "code" sheet for the documentation of resuscitation efforts. Like the flowsheet, this record should cue the nurse to document important facts about the specific episode. Because arrest situations are associated with significant changes in the patient's condition and may be linked to unexpected poor outcomes, clear and accurate documentation of the events is essential. In fact, documentation of these events is so important that organizations will frequently designate in the policy and procedure who should assume the role of recorder. For example, when nurses from Emory University Hospital developed a CPR flowsheet, they constructed the form so that events would be documented in chronological order (Padilla, 1990). The end result is a clear summary of resuscitation events, eliminating the need to rewrite medications and other treatments and facilitating the evaluation of the resuscitation effort. Another organization used the actual Advanced Cardiac Life Support (ACLS) protocols to form the basis for their code documentation (Sander, 1989). Box 11-5 lists key items to document in the case of an arrest and resuscitation.

Documentation of the arrest and resuscitation efforts is made on the code sheet and cardiac rhythm strips. The flowsheet and the nurse's progress notes should reflect assessment data before and after the code. The code sheet, progress note, rhythm strips, and the flowsheet must reflect a consistent recording of timed events to accurately reflect the care provided. Evaluation consists of comparing the documented data with the current ACLS standard of care. Because this is such an important clinical issue, many organizations have a system whereby each arrest is evaluated in a formal manner and feedback is given to the providers regarding their performance and adherence to current standard of care. Indeed, the con-

---

Box 11-5

Key Items to Document on a Code Sheet

- Time and type of arrest (e.g., lack of pulse or breath)
- Initiation of CPR
- Rhythm initially and after medications, defibrillation and application of internal pacemaker
- Intubation, oxygen therapy, and ABGs
- Time and wattage of defibrillation; patient's response to defibrillation
- Medications and IVs (i.e., type, dosage and time, name of person administering)
- Pupillary reactions
- Members of the resuscitation team
- Patient outcome, including disposition

sequences of not providing the standard care in these instances can be devastating and costly, as related in the following example:

> The plaintiff, age 24, underwent open-heart surgery at the defendant hospital. She developed bilateral pleural effusions, tachycardia, and increasing cyanosis 2 days after surgery. On the fifth day after surgery, a physician's assistant performed a thoracentesis. The plaintiff developed a severe persistent cough, but she was not examined by a physician. Her heart rate decreased, resulting in cardiac arrest. An emergency code blue was called, and 15 minutes later the wrong medications were administered. The plaintiff vomited, aspirated, and was intubated. She was resuscitated, but she suffered paralysis from T6 down resulting in the loss of bowel and bladder control. The plaintiff alleged that the defendants were negligent in failing to properly monitor and treat her cardiopulmonary status, in failing to timely call the code, and in failing to properly respond to her arrest. The plaintiff maintained that she suffered paralysis from a prolonged lack of blood flow to her spine. The defendants contended that the plaintiff's paralysis was the result of a vascular abnormality in her spine, and they denied negligence. A $2 million verdict was returned against the hospital (Laska, October 1993).

Documentation of Changes in Patient Condition: Physician Notification

Patients in the critical care areas are frequently seen by several doctors in a 24-hour period. In large teaching hospitals, interns and residents attend to patients under the guidance of the staff physician. In organizations without a teaching program the attending physician generally consults one or more specialty physicians when the patient has complex medical problems. With many physicians caring for one patient, the nurse must coordinate and organize the implementation of prescribed treatments and ensure that information is communicated to the appropriate physician. Most routine information is communicated through the flowsheet, whereas other information is communicated through written reports or verbally during physician rounds. Ongoing information describing the patient's condition is relayed either in person (as the physician makes additional rounds) or by telephone. Each and every communication with the physician should be documented either in the progress notes or comments section of the flowsheet.

When significant changes occur in the patient's condition, a physician, preferably the one who admitted the patient, should be contacted immediately after the nurse completes the assessment. In large teaching hospitals the intern or resident may be contacted as the "on-call" physician. Whether a notification is made to the intern, resident, or attending physician, the nurse must docu-

ment the notification and note the response of the physician to the call. Failure to report important changes to a physician or allowing the patient's condition to deteriorate over time without insisting that the physician see the patient is below the standard of care. When working with residents or interns, the nurse may have to insist that the resident notify the attending doctor when the nurse judges that the patient is not responding to treatment by the intern or resident.

If the attending physician is not responsive after notification to a level that matches the severity of the patients condition, the nurse may need to reiterate his or her concerns to the physician. If the patient's condition continues to deteriorate, after repeated notification of the physician, the nurse must go to the next level in the chain of command, as defined by organizational policy and procedure. This may be a nursing supervisor (who provides "next-step" information) or perhaps the physician who serves as the director of the critical care unit. Nurses must document every attempt to obtain physician intervention. Mandell (1993) stresses that a delay or an omission in notifying the appropriate medical personnel can significantly increase the level of injury or otherwise bring harm to the patient, as the following case illustrates:

> The plaintiff's decedent underwent a successful cardiac angioplasty at the hospital. The surgeon's partner had agreed to be responsible for all postoperative care following surgery. At 2:00 PM the decedent complained of a terrible headache. At the same time, his blood pressure became abnormally elevated, and he was also experiencing nausea and vomiting. The decedent was suffering from a cerebral hemorrhage. The nurse contacted the doctor by phone to report the patient's condition. The doctor did not come in to see the patient and he did not request a consultation by another physician. Instead, he prescribed medicine for the headache and the blood pressure. Throughout the day the decedent's blood pressure remained abnormally elevated. The nurse continued to telephone the doctor, who did not come in to examine the patient or request a consultation by a neurologist or other physician. At 3:00 AM the decedent was comatose, having suffered a cerebral hemorrhage. Plaintiffs claimed the decedent's complaints of headaches and the abnormal elevation of blood pressure accompanied by nausea were evidence of cerebral hemorrhage, which mandated immediate personal attendance by a physician, discontinuing heparin administration, administration of Nipride (nitroprusside), and a CT scan. The failure of the defendant doctor to come to the hospital to attend to his patient or request another physician to do so constituted gross negligence. The nurse on duty had only one patient, the decedent. The plaintiff claimed the nurse should have recognized the severity of the patient's condition and followed the standard of care, which required that she report her concerns. She should have given a more accurate report to the physician. The physician argued that complaints of nausea and headache are common following angioplasty,

and that the patient had a history of migraine headaches and elevated blood pressure. The doctor appropriately ordered medication to lower the blood pressure. Furthermore, he was in contact with the hospital by phone and no personal appearance was needed. The hospital argued that the nurses appropriately reported the patient's condition to the doctor, and that nurses must defer to doctors' judgment. The case was settled for $300,000 (Laska, 1997a).

Mandell (1993) describes a nurse's failure to notify the physician of important information regarding the patient condition as an act of omission (in that the nurse is held accountable for what was not done). These "failure-to-act" suits often allege that the patient was harmed by a lapse in nurse-physician communication" (Mandell, 1993). These acts of omission may take several forms, including the failure of the nurse to provide the physician with all the relevant information; failure to inform the physician in a timely manner; or simply failing to summon the physician when indicated.

SUMMARY

When utilizing the strategies mentioned, the nurse provides clear, concise documentation of nursing care and reduces the likelihood of controversy that might arise over discrepancies in charting. Because carrying around the flowsheet to ensure that all entries are made accurately and timely is impractical, each nurse should develop a system to capture information that can then be documented later at regular intervals. Making entries as close as possible to the time of events is wise because it decreases the chance of error and eliminates charting based on "what you think happened when." The following list provides practical tips for the completion of documentation:

1. Use the flowsheet as intended and completely fill out all areas.
2. Link the activities to patient outcomes. Use narrative notes to link patient problems to interventions and outcomes. Make judgments about the patient's progress.
3. Ensure that the flowsheet and the progress notes are consistent.
4. Complete the code sheet as designated by the organization. Be familiar with current ACLS standards of care.
5. Document every communication with medical providers.

REFERENCES

AACCN: *Standards for nursing care of the critically ill,* Prentice Hall, Englewood NJ, 1989, The Association.

AHA: *Textbook of advanced cardiac life support,* Dallas, 1994, The Association.

Chase S: Charting critical thinking: nursing judgments and patient outcomes, *DCCN* 101(16):102, March/April 1997.

ENA: *Standards of emergency nursing practice,* ed 3, Park Ridge, Ill, 1995b, The Association.

JCAHO: *1997 accreditation manual for hospitals,* Oak Brook Terrace, Ill, 1996, The Commission.

Laska L, ed: Cardiopulmonary status not properly monitored after open heart surgery, *Medical Malpractice Verdicts, Settlements and Experts* p 5, October 1993.

Laska L, ed: Failure to diagnose cerebral hemorrhage after cardiac, *Medical Malpractice Verdicts, Settlements and Experts* p 54, March 1997a.

Laska L, ed: Injection for ovarian cyst hits sciatic nerve, *Medical Malpractice Verdicts, Settlements and Experts* p 15, June 1997b.

Laska L, ed: New York woman suffers allergic swelling of tongue, *Medical Malpractice Verdicts, Settlements and Experts* p 11, May 1997c.

Laska L, ed: South Carolina man develops quadriplegia after auto accident, *Medical Malpractice Verdicts, Settlements and Experts* p 14, June 1997d.

Laska L, ed: Texas woman becomes ventilator dependent after surgery, *Medical Malpractice Verdicts, Settlements and Experts* p 17, June 1997e.

Laska L, ed: Texas woman dies of pneumonia one day after cursory treatment and discharge from emergency room, *Medical Malpractice Verdicts, Settlements and Experts* p 14, April 1997f.

Laska L, ed: Woman claims she was told to apply ice directly to skin of injured area twenty-four hours a day for ten days, *Medical Malpractice Verdicts, Settlements and Experts* p 38, June 1997g.

Mandell M: What you don't say can hurt you, *Am J Nurs* 93(8):15, 1993.

Mayberry A, Croke E: Issues leading to malpractice show little change: a review of the literature, *J Legal Nurse Consult* 7(2):16, 1996.

Padilla M, Purcell J: Using a structured cardiopulmonary resuscitation flowsheet, *Focus Crit Care* 17:490, 1990.

Rea R et al: *Emergency nursing core curriculum,* ed 3, Philadelphia, 1987, WB Saunders.

Sander P, Holm RP, Powers J et al: CPR in a small hospital, *Am J Nurs* 89:812, August 1989.

Selfridge-Thomas J, Shea S: *Emergency nursing standards of care and quality improvement,* Philadelphia, 1994, WB Saunders.

Vieria A: Documenting in the patient record: the lawyer's view, *DCCN* 16: p 108, 1997.

Waxman J: Protecting emergency room patients, *Trial* p 58, July 1988.

ADDITIONAL READINGS

Alexander M: Two important lessons: caution with telephone triage and believing the caregiver, *J Emerg Nurs* p 149, April 1996.

AHA: *Textbook of pediatric advanced life support,* Dallas, 1994, The Association.

Bradley V: Innovative informatics—toward a common language: nursing uniform data set (ENUDS), *J Emerg Nurs* p 248, June 1995.

Bradley V, Heiser R: Using data to discover new patterns: a triage quality indicator, *J Emerg Nurs* p 435, October 1996.

Cahill J: *Nurses handbook of law & ethics,* Springhouse, Penn, 1992, Springhouse.

Campbell JE: *Basic trauma life support,* Englewood Cliffs, NJ, 1995, Brady.

Carpenito L: *Handbook of nursing diagnosis,* ed 7, Philadelphia, 1997, JB Lippincott.

Carpenito L: *Nursing diagnosis: application to clinical practice,* Philadelphia, 1995, JB Lippincott.

East T: Computers in critical care, *Crit Care Nurs Clin North Am* 7(2):203-217 May/June 1995.

ENA: *Emergency nursing pediatric course,* Park Ridge, Ill, 1993, The Association.

ENA: *Emergency Nurses Association position statements,* Park Ridge, Ill, 1995, The Association.

ENA: *Trauma nursing core course provider manual,* ed 4, Park Ridge, Ill, 1995, The Association.

Fischback FT: *Documenting care: communication, the nursing process, and documentation standards,* Philadelphia, 1991, FA Davis.

Frisch N: Challenges for the new year . . . use of syndromes in nursing, the need for careful review and assessment of the accuracy of nursing diagnoses found in patient records, and the necessity to add diagnoses when there is clearly a nursing need, *Nurs Diagn* p 3, January/March 1996.

George J, Quattrone M: Professional malpractice or simple negligence? *J Emerg Nurs* p 532, December 1993.

George J, Quattrone M: A matter of credibility, *J Emerg Nurs* p 69, February 1994a.

George J, Quattrone M: Blood alcohol tests in the emergency department, *J Emerg Nurs* p 232, June 1994b.

George J, Quattrone M: Erroneous reporting of sexually transmitted diseases, *J Emerg Nurs* p 148, April 1994c.

George J, Quattrone M, Goldstone M: Triage protocols, *J Emerg Nurs* p 65, February 1995.

George M, Quattrone M, Goldstone M: Risk management spotlight: increased risk potential of the ED triage nurse, *J Emerg Nurs* p 241, June 1996a.

George M, Quattrone M, and Goldstone M: Suicidal patients: what is the nursing duty to prevent a patient's self-inflicted injuries? *J Emerg Nurs* p 609, December 1996b.

George M, Quattrone M, and Goldstone M: Time standards from patient arrival to triage: spotlight on a potentially dangerous practice, *J Emerg Nurs* p 339, August 1996c.

George M, Quattrone M, Goldstone M: Persons brought to the emergency department by police: are they patients? *J Emerg Nurs* p 354, August 1997a.

George M, Quattrone M, Goldstone M: Slip and fall cases: beware, *J Emerg Nurs* p 633, December 1997b.

George M, Quattrone M, Goldstone M: The duty to document: what are the limits? *J Emerg Nurs* p 467, October 1997c.

Greenwood D: Nursing care plans: issues and solutions, *Nurs Manage* p 37, March 1996.

Groethe E: Documentation in critical care: a flowsheet format that communicates and saves time, *Focus on critical care* 18(3): p 241, April 1991.

Iyer P: *Nursing malpractice,* Tucson, Ariz, 1996, Lawyers and Judges Publishing.

Kidd P: Where did all the nurses go? The need to capture nursing, *J Emerg Nurs* p 191, June 1995.

Laska L, ed: California man suffers tibial fracture, *Medical Malpractice Verdicts and Settlements and Experts* p 12, May 1997.

Laska L, ed: New York man puts hand through glass: wound treated in emergency room, but no x-ray taken, *Medical Malpractice Verdicts Settlements and Experts* p 13, May 1997.

Laska L, ed: Texas woman treated in emergency room for laceration to knee, *Medical Malpractice Verdicts Settlements and Experts* p 14, June 1997.

Laska L, ed: Woman complaining of epigastric pain released from emergency room and dies hours later from arrhythmia, *Medical Malpractice Verdicts Settlements and Experts* p 13, December 1997.

Muhs S, Mooney F: Finally, an ICU flowsheet that makes sense, *RN,* 58(12):37, 1995.

Perry A, Potter G: *Clinical nursing skills and techniques,* St Louis, 1995, Mosby.

Pradat D, Tipton S: Trends in nursing liability: emerging professional roles and standards, *Defense Research Institute Modern Health Care Defense Issues* p 49, 1997.

Robinson D, Anderson M, Acheson P: Telephone advice: lessons learned and considerations for starting programs, *J Emerg Nurs* p 409, October 1996.

Rosenthal K: ICU-CCU flowsheet, *Critical Care Nurse* 8(12):58, 1992.

Rowe J: Emergency nursing assessment and notes, *J Emerg Nurs* p 138, April 1994.

Rowe J: Incorporating mechanism of injury into an emergency department's trauma triage protocol, *J Emerg Nurs* p 583, December 1996.

Simpson L, Lee-Jacobson L, Brennan C: Trauma nursing flowsheet, *J Emerg Nurs* p 239, June 1995.

Sullivan GH: Is your documentation all it should be? *RN* p 59, October 1996.

Warren J: NANDA news: from the President . . . the future of nursing diagnosis and nursing's language of practice, *Nurs Diagn* p 132, October-December 1996.

Zbilut J: More on critical thinking, clinical judgment, and documentation, *J Emerg Nurs* p 483, December 1995.

12

Perioperative Documentation

OPERATING ROOM DOCUMENTATION
Donna Cairone, RN, BS, BSN, CNOR, RNFA

The evolution of nursing documentation in the perioperative setting has been as dynamic as the technologic advances in this area. Nursing process, coupled with nursing diagnosis, has forged the way for a systematic, thought-provoking method of documentation that takes into account the patient's needs related to the preparation for surgery, the procedure itself, and the resultant recovery phase. The Joint Commission for the Accreditation of Healthcare Organizations (JCAHO) has addressed this advancement by mandating a multidisciplinary approach to the required functions of patient rights and organizational ethics, assessment of the patient, education, the continuum of care, care of the patient, surveillance and control of infection, and performance improvement. Further requirements include the documentation of nursing activity in the perioperative area, addressing target points such as patient and family education, preoperative assessment/baseline evaluation, nursing interventions and corresponding patient responses, and evaluation of the effect of the interventions as evidence of outcome of the nursing care delivered to patients and their significant others.

Today the perioperative environment is no longer defined simply as inpatient care. Complete, clear, and consistent documentation must occur in the hospital operating room (OR), surgical center setting, endoscopy suite, and doctor's office surgical suite. In addition to the legal implications of standardized care, documentation has become a tool for third-party insurance carriers to determine the acceptable type of care and its cost. Some hospitals have developed documentation tools that not only meet the care planning and medical information requirements, but may also be used for performance improvements, monitoring activities, and inventory control.

Finally, the pace of the perioperative environment requires that documentation be timely, precise, and concise. The forms used to collect all the required information must be user-friendly, consistent, and comprehensive. Checklists are often included, with significant space provided for interventions, nurse's notes, and important communications. Most importantly, the forms should have specific guidelines and instructions for use that facilitate clear documentation.

PREADMISSION DOCUMENTATION

In many institutions, preadmission testing and patient and family education for elective surgery usually occur within a week or two before surgery. The Joint Commission mandates the plan of care, and its documentation must be in the patient record before the procedure (JCAHO, 1996). The requirement to complete this documentation within this time span usually necessitates a highly specific system of documentation. Whether an organization decides to use separate forms to record the preoperative assessment and patient and family education needs, or a single multiple-page form to cover all stages of the perioperative process is a highly individualized decision that must meet the needs of the staff and the organizational systems in place. Evidence of the nursing process (i.e., assessment, diagnosis, planning, implementation, and evaluation) should be documented on the form. Emergent surgical patients must receive the same nursing assessments and interventions as those provided to elective surgical patients. When a lack of time prevents the fulfillment of the standard evaluations and documentation, the nurse should make notations about the emergent nature of the patient's surgery, nursing assessments completed, attempts made to contact or educate the family or significant others, any concerns voiced by the patient, and the nursing interventions made. Forms should be easily adapted to include all pertinent nursing diagnoses for emergent and nonemergent patients.

The preadmission process often begins with a patient interview designed to collect information pertinent to the patient's condition, the patient's knowledge of his or her condition, the patient's support systems, and plans for the recuperative period. Collection of samples for diagnostic and laboratory tests also begins at this time. The Joint Commission further mandates that the patient's history and physical information must be collected within 30 days prior to admission or the procedure and the preoperative diagnosis and diagnostic tests must be completed and recorded before the procedure (JCAHO, 1996). In elective surgical cases, organizations should allow information to be collected and stored in a secure and confidential place that will be available on the day of surgery. If surgery is to occur on the same day as the preadmission testing, the education and planning issues must be anticipated and addressed before the patient's arrival for the procedure. The establishment of an institutional care plan for preoperative patients may be valuable in this regard. Figure 12-1 illustrates this point.

PATIENT AND FAMILY PRE/POST SURGERY EDUCATION

With the increase in patient acuity and the shift to outpatient care, patient and family education should play a major role in restoring patients' health. Learning needs must be quickly assessed to meet the patient's educational requirements and recovery goals. The learning style of the individual or the significant other should be documented along with the results of the assessment. The patient or significant other should be able to identify the scheduled surgery and any pertinent preparations or instructions before the actual procedure. The patient's knowledge of his or her current and preoperative medications should be documented along with any possible food or drug interactions. The patient's expectations of the preoperative and postoperative periods should be discussed to prepare the patient for the level of care that will be needed, postoperative activities that are permitted, and the supplies or support persons that will be required. Finally, the signs and symptoms that require immediate contact with the physician (e.g., fever, vomiting, drainage, pain, and bleeding) should be reinforced with the patient. Figure 12-2 provides an example of a patient and family teaching record that serves as the account of the learning needs assessment, the teaching method used, the actual pertinent information to be conveyed, and the follow-up and evaluation. With staff time at a premium, such forms allow the nurse to evaluate the learner and document the key areas of teaching with a minimum of complexity. Charting space has also been provided on the back of the form to document in-depth discussions or concerns that will require follow-up before surgery. The content section of the form ensures the consistent communication of information that can be reinforced by interdisciplinary staff in the preadmission area. The interdisciplinary approach to patient care recommended by the Joint Commission can be seen in this form through the variety of information provided and the responsibilities of the various disciplines.

DOCUMENTING PERIOPERATIVE NURSING CARE

On the day of surgery the patient and family can experience great anticipation and stress. Patient anxiety, family demands, and other commitments make it imperative that the admitting nurse clarify that all necessary instructions have been followed. Preoperative checklists (Figure 12-3) are commonly used to ensure that the standard items are reviewed with each patient. These forms often include a list of individual items needed to facilitate a smooth surgical experience by eliminating or communicating potential problems. The list may include basics such as verifying of the identification band information, checking to ensure the patient has had nothing by mouth, ensuring that a signed consent is present, performing the surgical preparation, and arranging for the disposition of valuables brought to the hospital. This form should be specific to the institution and should serve as an easily accessible repository of pertinent information. When the preoperative checklist has been completed, the patient may then move to the surgical area for preoperative assessment by the perioperative nurse.

Once the eduation process has been completed, the next area of assessment should be the identification of the patient's physiologic and psychosocial baseline and the development of the nursing care plan based on the individual's nursing diagnoses. According to the Association of Operating Room Nurses (AORN), the primary recommended practice for the documentation of perioperative nursing care is that it "should reflect the patient's plan of care, including assessment, diagnosis, outcome identification, planning, implementation, and evaluation" (AORN, 1996). The nursing process must be evident from the time of admission to the time of discharge. Standard care plans using nursing diagnoses developed by the North American Nursing Diagnosis Association (NANDA) and the AORN standards of perioperative care are most often used for development of an institution's documentation forms.

OUTCOME STANDARDS AND NURSING DIAGNOSES

The AORN (1983) first published the *Patient Outcomes and Standards for Perioperative Care* in 1983. In 1991 they were renamed *Patient Outcomes: Standards of Perioperative Care* (1991). The shift to observable and measurable responses to perioperative nursing care made

Text continued on p. 263

BLESSING HOSPITAL
QUINCY, IL
INTRA-OPERATIVE RECORD

Emergency: ☐ Yes ☐ No

OR _____

Wound Classification 1 ☐ 3 ☐
2 ☐ 4 ☐

In room: _____ Blood # _____ EBL _____

OR Start: _____ Units Available _____ Units in OR _____

OR Complete: _____ Blood given: No. Units _____ Plasma _____ Other _____

Discharged to: PACU _____ Other _____ Medications/Irrigations _____

Report To: _____ _____

Operative Procedure: _____

_____

Pre-Op Diagnosis: _____

Post-Op Diagnosis: _____

Surgeon: _____ Assistant: _____

RN Circulator: _____ Scrub Personnel: _____

_____ _____ Observers: _____

Relief: _____ Relief: _____ X-Ray Personnel: _____

Anesthesia Method: ☐ General ☐ MAC ☐ Spinal ☐ Block ☐ Local-agents

Administered by: _____

Position: ☐ Supine ☐ Prone ☐ Jackknife ☐ Lateral ☐ Lithotomy ☐ Other: _____

Devices Used: ☐ Safety Strap ☐ Vac Pak ☐ Sandbag ☐ _____ Stirrups

☐ Headrest ☐ Mayfield H.H. ☐ Chest Rolls ☐ Pillow _____ Armboards Other: _____

Prep: ☐ Provoiodine Solution ☐ Provoiodine Scrub Shave: _____ Other: _____

ESU _____ Ground Site _____ Pad Area Shaved ☐ Yes ☐ No

Active Electrode: _____ Coag _____ Cut _____ Bipolar _____

Applied By: _____ Holder Used ☐ Yes ☐ No Pre-op ✔☐ Post-op ✔☐

Tourniquet: No. _____ Site: _____ Pressure: _____ Time↑ _____ Time↓ _____

Applied by: _____ Site: _____ Pressure: _____ Time↑ _____ Time↓ _____

Anti-embolism System: No.: _____ ☐ Thigh Hi ☐ Knee Hi Pressure _____ mmHG

Thermoregulation Unit No.: _____ Time: _____ Time: _____ Time: _____ Time: _____

☐ Esoph. ☐ Rectal ☐ Skin Temp: _____ Temp: _____ Temp: _____ Temp: _____

Urinary Cath. in place: ☐ Yes ☐ No Inserted in OR By: _____ Size: _____ Drainage: _____

Drains/Packs: Type and Site: _____

Specimens Hist: ☐ Yes X _____ ☐ No F.S. ☐ Yes ☐ No Cult ☐ Yes ☐ No Other _____

Counts Indicated: ☐ Not Indicated ☐ Initial Counts: _____ Final Counts: _____

Counts Correct: ☐ Yes ☐ No Sponge: ☐ Yes ☐ No Needle: ☐ Yes ☐ No Inst: ☐ Yes ☐ No ☐ NA

Action Taken: _____

Implants: (Sticker or Product No., Lot No., Sterilization Information) _____

_____

_____

_____

_____

Comments: _____

_____

_____

_____

Family Notified: _____

Figure 12-1 Intraoperative record. (Courtesy Blessing Hospital, Quincy, Ill.)

PERI-OPERATIVE NURSING DOCUMENTATION

Patient Identified: ☐ Verbally ☐ ID Band ☐ Family Member ☐ Operative Site

Permits Signed: ☐ OR ☐ Blood ☐ Anesthesia ☐ Sterilization ☐ Blood Refusal

Allergies: _____

Medical Condition: _____
_____

Lab Values: CBC_____ SMA_____ LYTS_____ EKG_____ CHEST_____ URINE_____

Previous Surgery: _____
_____

MOBILITY LIMITATIONS	**SKIN APPEARANCE**		**VISION**	**MENTAL/EMOTIONAL ASSESSMENT**	
	COLOR	CONDITION	_____	☐ Alert/Awake	☐ Crying
☐ None	☐ Normal	☐ Intact		☐ Drowsy	☐ Withdrawn
☐ Paralysis	☐ Flushed	☐ Rash	**HEARING**	☐ Cooperative	☐ Restless
☐ Arthritis	☐ Pale	☐ Diaphoretic	_____	☐ Responsive	☐ Resistive
☐ Prosthesis	☐ Cyanotic/Dusky	☐ Dry/Itchy		☐ Non-Responsive	☐ Combative
☐ Others: _____	☐ Jaundiced	☐ Mottled/Necrotic	☐ Dentures _____	☐ Apprehensive	☐ Others:_____
_____	☐ Bruise		☐ Caps		
	☐ Reddened Areas		Date:_____	Time:_____RN	

Patient Interview: ☐ Holding Areas ☐ Patient Room ☐ Chart Review ☐ OR Room   Date

PERI-OPERATIVE NURSING CARE PLAN

NSG. DIAG./OUTCOME STATEMENT	**NURSING INTERVENTIONS**	**EVALUATION/REASSESSMENT**
Potential increased anxiety related to peri-operative environment. Improved ability to cope with anxiety as evidenced by verbalization of anxiety and understanding of perioperative events.	1. Assess anxiety and understanding of perioperative events. 2. Explain perioperative events, according to developmental level. 3. Reorientation, support, and assurance during intra-operative phase of care.	☐ Expected outcome achieved.
Potential injury related to: 1. Perioperative environment 2. Anesthetized state 3. Positioning No injury sustained.	(All Intra operative Interventions) 1. Verify patient's indentity and operative site/procedures/surgeons. 2. Verify patient's allergies. 3. Implement safety devices. 4. Maintain proper body alignment, secure extremities 5. Maintain skin integrity. 6. Use appropriate prepping technique. 7. Suction equipment ready and available to anesthetist. 8. Protect integrity of tubes, catheters, etc. 9. Place dispersive electrode appropriately. 10. Have all equipment in proper working order. 11. Complete sponge, needle, and instrument counts. 12. Maintain Aseptic technique. 13. Transport to PACU with O$_2$.	☐ Expected outcome achieved.
Potential alteration of body temperature related to exposure and environment Maintain body temperature	1. Monitor temp 2. Hypo/Hyperthermia blanket 3. Avoid overexposure 4. Warm irrigation 5. Apply blankets pre and post op	☐ Expected outcome achieved

Figure 12-1, cont'd   Intraoperative record.

MERCY COMMUNITY HOSPITAL
Patient/Family Teaching Record
Pre/Post Surgery

Patient/Family Expected Outcomes By the end of Instruction, the Patient/Family will be able to:	Date	Responsible Discipline and Signature	Tchg. Meth.	Eval. F/U	Content Outline and Resources
DIAGNOSIS/PROBLEM					
Identify the surgery/procedure. **Review any special preparations needed prior to surgery/procedure**		Nursing			Information is specific to surgery/procedure to be done; should include approx. time involved for surgery/procedure, average length of time in hospital, SPU/SDA. Do not eat or drink anything after midnight of evening prior to surgery/procedure. Pre procedure: may need enemas, shave/prep, or special oral agents as prep.
MEDICATION					
State the names, action, dosages, frequency, side effects, possible food/drug interactions, specific precautions of pre-op medications		Nursing Pharmacy			Specific medication information will be available for the patient. List medications patient should take prior to admission per anesthesia (e.g.: Lanoxin, Theodur, etc.) Check with physician to determine continuation of prescribed meds. Post-op pain interventions will be provided, if indicated.

ADDRESSOGRAPH

Code: Teaching Methods - (Tchg. Meth.)	Evaluation/Follow-up - (F/U)
D: Discussion AV: Audiovisual H: Handout	1. Outcome achieved 2. Outcome unachieved 3. Reteach/Reinforce materials 4. Non-applicable

Figure 12-2 Patient and family teaching record. (Courtesy Mercy Health System, Havertown, Penn.)

MERCY COMMUNITY HOSPITAL   **PAGE 2 OF 2**   Pt. Name_____
PATIENT FAMILY TEACHING   Room #_____

Patient/Family Expected Outcomes By the end of Instruction, the Patient/Family will be able to:	*Date*	*Responsible Discipline and Signature*	*Tchg. Meth.*	*Eval. F/U*	*Content Outline and Resources*
TREATMENTS					
Explain the rationale for IV, post-op vital signs check, dressings, respiratory toileting, leg exercises.		Nursing Respiratory Therapy			IV is to assist in maintenance of fluid balance. Post-op vital signs check done to forestall problems and permit early intervention if needed. Dressings protect surgical site from trauma, contamination, and contain drainage. Respiratory toileting assists body in achieving optimal oxygenation. Leg exercises help with maintaining circulation and prevention of blood clot formation.
DISCHARGE PLANS					
Describe activity level and restrictions.		Nursing			Activity and restrictions will vary per procedure. <u>Physical Therapy</u> will teach exercises and/or use of assistive devices if indicated.
State symptoms to report to physician.		Nursing			Unusual bleeding, swelling pain, respiratory distress, fever.
State how and when to contact Emergency Medical System (EMS).		Nursing			Call "911" if symptoms become severe.
Identify available community resources.		Social Services			Refer to local pharmacy for supplies that may be needed; identify support groups in community; inform learner of local agencies specific to need. Assist with arrangement of referrals, if needed.

ADDRESSOGRAPH

Code: Teaching Methods (Tchg. Meth.) D: Discussion AV: Audiovisual H: Handout	**Evaluation/Follow-up (F/U)** 1. Outcome achieved 2. Outcome unachieved 3. Reteach/Reinforce materials 4. Non-applicable

Figure 12-2, cont'd Patient and family teaching record.

Pre-Operative Assessment:

Date: _____ Time: _____ **Allergies:** _____

Level of Consciousness: _____ Alert _____ Lethargic _____ Confused _____ Unconscious

Restraints in Place: _____ No _____ Yes Type: _____

Ability to Move Extremities: _____ No Difficulty _____ Other, Describe: _____
_____

Skin: _____ Intact _____ Other, Describe: _____
_____

IV Therapy: Site / Port-a-Cath: _____ Date Inserted: _____

Solution Infusing: Type / Amount: _____

Voided Last at: _____ AM / PM _____ Foley Catheter in Place and Functioning

Pre-Operative Checklist:

_____ Identification Bracelet on Patient	_____ Medication Kardex	_____ Blood Work Results in Chart
_____ Dentures Removed	_____ History & Physical	_____ Chest EKG Report in Chart
_____ Jewelry Removed / Secured	_____ Surgical Permit	_____ X-Ray Report in Chart
_____ Loose Teeth	_____ Blood Permit	_____ Urinalysis Report (notify Anesthesia
_____ Contact Lenses / Glasses Removed	_____ Breast Surgery Permit	if unable to get reports)
_____ Hairpins, Make-Up, Nailpolish is	_____ Medical Clearance	_____ Addressograph Plate
Removed / Sculptured Nails	(when ordered)	_____ All Chart Forms Stamped
_____ Prosthesis _____	_____ Anesthesia Permit	

_____ **NPO after** _____ **AM / PM**

_____ Patient Instructed Not to Get OOB Without Assistance _____ Verbalized Understanding

_____ Call Bell Within Reach. Patient Instructed on Use of Call System. _____ Verbalized Understanding

_____ Side Rails Up _____ Patient Verbalized Understanding of Patient Safety

Temp: _____ Pulse: _____ Resp: _____ B/P: _____
(1 Hour Before OR)

Pre-Op Med:

_____ Pre-Op Meds Given as Ordered: _____ Time:_____

_____ Pre-Op Meds Not Ordered

_____ Unable to Give Pre-Op Meds, "Please Notify Anesthesia if Unable to Give Pre-Med"

_____ Notified:_____

_____ Antibiotics Sent With Patient _____

_____
RN Signature

PEDS ONLY

Weight: _____ lbs. _____ kg

Loose Teeth: _____ No _____ Yes, Describe: _____

Last Fluid Intake: _____ AM / PM

Last Solid Food Intake: _____ AM / PM

If Child Has a Runny Nose, Cough, Fever, or Congestion, Notify Pediatric Resident or Anesthesia. Signs/Symptoms Present: _____

Physician Notified: _____

_____
RN Signature

Mercy
Health System
A Healthcare Ministry of the Sisters of Mercy

☐ MERCY FITZGERALD HOSPITAL
☐ MERCY HOSPITAL OF PHILADELPIA
☐ MERCY COMMUNITY HOSPITAL

PRE-OPERATIVE NURSES NOTES AND CHECKLIST

Figure 12-3 Preoperative nurses notes and checklist. (Courtesy Mercy Health System, Havertown, Penn.)

possible the creation of a template for evaluating the patient's responses to the specific nursing interventions. Table 12-1 lists the *Patient Outcomes: Standards of Perioperative Care* published by the AORN in 1997. The individual standards are easily cross-referenced to many nursing diagnoses, and the criterion listed provide concrete nursing actions with measurable parameters for evaluating patient status.

The practice of establishing standard care plans is quite common today in the OR environment. The use of the AORN standards and their measurable criteria should be evident in the care plans and the documentation of the implementation of these plans. The identification of nursing diagnoses that are universal to all surgical patients facilitates consistent documentation that focuses on areas of concern specific to a patient's condition and the planned procedure. Outcomes from these records should be measurable and useful for the evaluation of the quality of care for performance improvement.

PLAN OF CARE DOCUMENTS

All perioperative documentation tools must have an identification section that reflects the current available patient demographics, along with the correct date and time. This area often includes the patient's name, address, medical record number, social security number, age and date of birth, race, sex, religion, type of insurance, and attending physician's name. This information should always be verified to ensure the completeness and accurateness of the documentation. Other information that should be in this section includes a history of allergies, preoperative diagnosis, anticipated procedure, surgeon, method of anesthesia, and anesthesiologist and anesthetist. A log of surgical team members, including the identification of scrub, circulating, and relief nurses, should be kept along with times logged in and out. The patient's time of arrival in the operating suite, the mode of transportation, and accompanying safety devices are important points in establishing the patient's preoperative level of function. The history and physical, laboratory test results, and the availability of blood or special equipment should also be confirmed at this time. Verification of the patient's identification, the procedure to be performed, the side of the body to be operated on (if applicable), and the patient's consent should correlate with the scheduled surgery. The patient's level of consciousness must be recorded, particularly at times when consent is withheld, until the patient speaks to the operating surgeon. Correlation with heightened psychological states must be recorded here to present a clear picture of the patient's understanding and acceptance of the events to come. Legal proceedings are frequently initiated because of discrepancies between the signed consent and the patient's verbal communication at the time of surgery. A clear recording of the patient's mental status and any specific comments made

regarding consent can sway a jury's decision in a malpractice case.

Any physical, mental, or psychological limitations must be communicated between the preoperative nurses and the operating room nurses at this point. Problems in these areas should be addressed immediately through the nursing care plan. For example, nurses caring for a visually impaired individual should be prepared to give the patient verbal instructions as to what will be taking place around him or her. This information should be communicated early in the process, and communication should continue throughout the entire surgical stay, as applicable.

Patient anxiety is very understandable given fears about potential complications, the results of surgery, and the intimidating nature of the OR suite. The goal of decreasing anxiety can be accomplished by any number of basic nursing interventions. A documentation form using a checklist format with space provided for further evaluation comments is easy to use. This tool is particularly important for documenting reassessment at various times throughout the perioperative process. Ancillary staff members in this area may frequently make observations and identify problems. The RN has the responsibility of assessing and periodically reassessing the patient and recording such nursing interventions.

Preoperative physical assessment and observation should be documented in a review of systems format with ample space to record any nursing diagnoses made during the patient's evaluation and examination. The identification of nursing diagnoses universal to all surgical patients facilitates the creation of consistent documentation tools that focus on areas of specific concern, as shown in Figure 12-4. Because nursing assessment is the legal responsibility of the RN, space is also provided for the nurses' signatures next to the identified diagnoses. The presence of invasive devices, such as Foley catheters, IV lines, tracheostomies, prostheses, or sensory aids, should always be included in the assessment, as should the baseline vital signs.

SOURCES OF LIABILITY

This section discusses common sources of liability and suggestions for documentation. The liability issues discussed include skin assessment, patient positioning, and patient safety, including the use of assistive and electrical devices, counts (e.g., needles, sponges), medication administration, and implant insertion.

Skin assessment is a key area in the care of preoperative patients. Skin, as the barrier against the external stressors, protects the patient from trauma related to pressure or foreign objects, fluid and heat loss, and entry by infectious organisms. The skin should be assessed for evidence of wounds, pressure areas, growths, abnormal sensation, color, and poor circulation. This information will be critical when positioning the patient, preparing the skin, and applying assistive devices, such as tourniquets, electrocautery pads,

TABLE 12-1 Patient Outcomes: Standards of Perioperative Care

Standard 1.1 The patient is free from signs and symptoms of physical injury.

Criterion: The patient is free from any physical injury, including, but not limited to, skin breakdown or irritation, neuromuscular injury, and cardiopulmonary compromise.

Standard 1.2 The patient is free from signs and symptoms of injury caused by extraneous objects.

Criterion: The patient shows no signs or symptoms of injury caused by extraneous objects, including, but not limited to, skin breakdown, redness, skin blanching, and echymosis.

Standard 1.3 The patient is free from signs and symptoms of chemical injury.

Criterion: The patient shows no signs or symptoms of chemical injury, including, but not limited to, rash or blistering, allergic reaction, burn, and respiratory distress.

Standard 1.4 The patient is free from signs and symptoms of electrical injury.

Criterion: The patient shows no signs and symptoms of electrical injury. (Electrical injury may not be immediately apparent or observable and can occur from the skin surface to the deep muscle tissue.)

Standard 1.5 The patient is free from signs and symptoms of injury related to positioning.

Criterion: The patient returns to a preoperative functional status consistent with the surgical procedure. Postoperative evaluation includes cardiopulmonary, neuromuscular, and integumentary systems relative to positioning.

Standard 1.6 The patient is free from signs and symptoms of laser injury.

Criterion: The patient has no contact with the laser beam other than for the intended purpose and receives the minimum laser energy exposure to achieve the intended therapeutic value.

Standard 1.7 The patient is free from signs and symptoms of radiation injury.

Criterion: The patient has no signs or symptoms of radiation injury. Measures will be taken to avoid undue exposure to radiation.

Standard 1.8 The patient is free from signs and symptoms of injury related to transfer or transport.

Criterion: The patient has no signs or symptoms of injury related to transfer or transport. Evaluation includes neuromuscular and integumentary systems relative to transport.

Standard 1.9 The patient receives appropriate prescribed medication(s), administered safely, during the perioperative period.

Criterion: The patient receives correct medication in accurate doses. The patient has no signs or symptoms of untoward reaction, either systemic or local.

Standard 2.1 The patient is free from signs and symptoms of infection.

Criterion: The patient is free of signs and symptoms of infection throughout the stages of wound healing. The stages are as follows: immediate postoperative (inflammatory or defensive, 4-5 days); acute postoperative (fibroplastic or proliferative, 5-24 days); postoperative discharge/rehabilitation (maturation or remodeling, >24 days).

Standard 2.2 The patient has wound or tissue perfusion consistent with or improved from baseline levels established preoperatively.

Criterion: Wound or tissue perfusion is maintained or improved postoperatively. Tissue perfusion is assessed continually, including vital signs and observation of the skin color, capillary refill, turgor, temperature, and integrity.

Standard 2.3 The patient is at or returning to normothermia at the conclusion of the immediate postoperative period.

Criterion: Thermoregulation may be assessed and measured by rectal, esophageal, tympanic membrane, or other temperature monitoring devices.

Standard 2.4 The patient's fluid and electrolyte balance and acid-base balance is consistent with or improved from baseline levels established preoperatively.

Criterion: The patient's condition reflects the following: level of consciousness consistent with preoperative level or improved; elimination processes are consistent with operative procedure; fluid and electrolyte balance is consistent with or improved from preoperative status; acid-base balance is improved or consistent with preoperative status.

Standard 2.5 The patient's pulmonary function is consistent with or improved from baseline preoperative levels.

Criterion: Pulmonary status is consistent as verified by measuring arterial oxygen percent saturation, respiratory rate, skin color, and arterial oxygen pressure.

Standard 2.6 The patient's cardiac function is consistent with or improved from baseline levels established preoperatively.

Criterion: Status must be consistent or improved. Measurements should include, but are not limited to, blood pressure, heart rate, peripheral pulses, arterial pressure, and central venous pressure.

Standard 3.1 The patient demonstrates knowledge of the physiologic responses to the operation or other invasive procedure.

Criterion: The patient communicates the following: consent for the operation or invasive procedure; sequence of events during the perioperative period; outcome expectations in realistic terms; feelings about the operation or invasive procedure.

Standard 3.2 The patient demonstrates knowledge of the psychological responses to the operative or other invasive procedure.

Criterion: The patient communicates the following: consent for the operative or other invasive procedure; the sequence of events during the perioperative period; outcome expectations in realistic terms; feelings about the operative or other invasive experience.

TABLE 12-1   Patient Outcomes: Standards of Perioperative Care—cont'd

Standard 3.3 The patient demonstrates knowledge of nutritional requirements related to the operation or other invasive procedure.	*Criterion:* The patient communicates the following: outcome expectations in realistic terms; importance of NPO status not taking anything by mouth; need for IV hydration management; appropriate postoperative diet; appropriate actions to take for nausea, vomiting, and diarrhea.
Standard 3.4 The patient demonstrates knowledge of medication management.	*Criterion:* The patient communicates knowledge of medication used, outcome expectations, and appropriate actions for untoward reactions.
Standard 3.5 The patient demonstrates knowledge of pain management.	*Criterion:* The patient communicates the following: previous pain experience; outcome expectations; understanding of the plan for pain assessment and management; acknowledgement of pharmacologic and nonpharmacologic methods of pain management; the need to accurately report pain in a timely manner.
Standard 3.6 The patient participates in the rehabilitation process.	*Criterion:* The patient communicates the following: concerns; the date of the next planned visit, goals; sequence of perioperative events; and activities related to his or her care.
Standard 3.7 The patient demonstrates knowledge of wound healing.	*Criterion:* The patient communicates the sequence of wound healing, concerns, dressing care, and goals.
Standard 4.1 The patient participates in decisions affecting his or her perioperative care.	*Criterion:* Ensure the patient's involvement through informed consent, using family or surrogate decision-makers, advocating the patient's rights to self-determination affecting resuscitative measures, life-sustaining treatment, and end-of-life decisions.
Standard 4.2 The patient's care is consistent with the perioperative plan of care.	*Criterion:* The treatment and care received does not deviate from the perioperative plan.
Standard 4.3 The patient's right to privacy is maintained.	*Criterion:* Actions include, but are not limited to, providing mechanisms to protect privacy, securing patient records and belongings, entering appropriate and accurate information into records, and discussing or releasing information only in the context of care.
Standard 4.4 The patient is the recipient of competent and ethical care within legal standards of practice.	*Criterion:* Competent care providers meet the following criteria: they are cognizant of legal, institutional, professional, and regulatory standards; they have knowledge of ethical concepts and principles; they are informed about ethical decision-making processes; they maintain appropriate licensure or credentials; they participate in professional and continuing education activities.
Standard 4.5 The patient receives consistent and comparable levels of care from all caregivers, regardless of the setting.	*Criterion:* Care is delivered in a nondiscriminatory, nonjudgmental environment. Guidelines should include legal, institutional, professional, and regulatory standards.
Standard 5.1 The patient demonstrates and reports (as necessary) adequate pain control throughout the perioperative period.	*Criterion:* The patient demonstrates adequate pain management through cognitive responses, physiologic signs and symptoms, and nonverbal cues. These include using a pain severity index, changes in vital signs, and a decrease in expressed or apparent level of anxiety.
Standard 5.2 The patient's value system, life style, ethnicity, and culture are considered, respected, and incorporated (as appropriate) in the perioperative plan of care, which reflects the patient's level of function and ability during the perioperative period.	*Criterion:* The perioperative plan includes, but is not limited to, the client's cultural or ethnic practices, spiritual or religious beliefs, psychosocial barriers or support systems, physical and/or cognitive limitations, and language barriers.

Data from AORN: *Standards, recommended practices, and guidelines,* Denver, 1997, The Association.

restraint devices, casts, and dressings. The opportunity exists with almost every patient for injuries resulting from chemical burns caused by the prep solution, electrical burns caused by the cautery pad, or pressure wounds caused by the safety belt. A specific record of the types of prep solutions used and who used them, the location of the cautery pad and who placed it, and the safety belt position can be valuable when identifying the cause of injuries found later. Because most patients are immobilized for a period of time in the OR, the skin should always be reassessed at the end of each

Text continued on p. 270

IDENTIFICATION PROCEDURE:

PREOPERATIVE/HOLDING AREA:

_____ ARM BAND/SITE CHECKED   _____ ARM BAND/SITE CHECKED   _____ ARM BAND/SITE CHECKED

Patient Identified By: Patient Identified by: Patient Identified By:

_____   _____   _____

    SIGNATURE: NURSE   SIGNATURE:ANESTHESIA DEPT   SIGNATURE:ATTENDING SURGEON

PRE-OP ASSESSMENT

    Patient identification: verbal _____ armband _____ chart_____

    Verification of procedure: verbal _____ consent form _____ which side or extremity? _____

    Chart complete: lab tests_____ EKG_____ x-ray_____ history & physical _____ blood available _____

    Comments: _____

    Allergies: no_____ yes_____, list_____

    NPO after midnight: no_____ yes_____, comments_____

    Prostheses: no_____ yes_____, list_____

    Patient arrived in OR with: IV_____ NG tube_____ Foley_____ other_____, list_____

    Patient arrived via: stretcher_____ bed_____ side rails up_____ wheelchair_____ ambulatory_____

    Known infectious disease: no_____ yes_____, comments_____

Level of consciousness	**Skin condition**	**Psychological**	**Physical**
☐ alert	☐ cool	☐ calm/relaxed	☐ no limitations
☐ drowsy	☐ warm	☐ anxious	☐ language/ speech barrier
☐ disoriented	☐ dry	☐ upset/ crying	☐ hearing defect
☐ unresponsive	☐ flushed	☐ talkative	☐ vision impaired
	☐ diaphoretic	☐ withdrawn	☐ R.O.M. limited
	☐ excoriated		☐ paralysis
	☐ bruised		☐ cast/splint/traction

Nursing Diagnosis - Potential for Anxiety

    Plan _____ Give explanations clearly   _____ Listen to concerns: answer questions

        _____ Support and reassure   _____ Give comfort measures - warm blanket, pillow

    Goal - Decreased Anxiety

    Evaluation - decreased anxiety _____yes _____no   RN signature_____

    Comments:_____

INTRAOPERATIVE NURSING RECORD

PAGE 1 OF 3

MERCY COMMUNITY HOSPITAL

Figure 12-4 Intraoperative nursing record. (Courtesy Mercy Health System, Havertown, Penn.)

INTRA-OPERATIVE NURSING CARE

Nursing Diagnosis - Potential for Injury

Plan - A. Position safely

Type of position: ___ supine ___ prone ___ lateral ___ beach chair ___ lithotomy ___ jackknife

Positioning aids: ☐ arthroscopy leg holder   ☐ thermo mattress (setting_____)

        ☐ seat belt (where_____)   ☐ fracture table

        ☐ sandbag (where_____)   ☐ headrest

        ☐ rolled sheet (where_____)   ☐ stirrups

        ☐ vacupak   ☐ Wilson frame

        ☐ pillow (where_____)   ☐ hand table

        ☐ rt. armboard   ☐ unaffected leg support

        ☐ lt. armboard   ☐ other

Circulatory Supports: ___ TED's ___ Ace bandages ___ sequential stockings (setting _____)

B. Electro surgical unit safety: ___ ESU unit (number_____) ___ bipolar unit (number _____)

Grounding pad site_____ applied by _____ setting: coag ____ cut ____ tested ____

C. Tourniquet safety

tourniquet #_____ cuff site_____ applied by _____

time inflated _____ pressure _____ time deflated _____

D. Potential for Retained Foreign Body   Counts Performed by

☐ sponge count   correct ☐ yes, ☐ no   _____ / _____

☐ needles, sharp   correct ☐ yes, ☐ no   _____ / _____

☐ instrument   correct ☐ yes, ☐ no   _____ / _____

Goal - Patient will be at minimum risk for injury

Evaluation - Goal Achieved ____yes ____no   comments _____

R.N. signature_____

Nursing Diagnosis - Potential for Infection

Plan A. Maintain sterile technique, instruments, & supplies _____

B. Area shaved _____ by _____

C. Skin prep _____ by _____

_____ by _____

Goal - Patient will be at minimum risk for infection

Evaluation - All necessary precautions taken____yes, ____ no   comments _____

R.N. signature_____

Preoperative Diagnosis:_____

_____

Procedure:_____

_____

Postoperative Diagnosis:_____

_____

X- ray ____ yes, ____ no

Anesthesia: ____ General ____ MAC ____ Block (type_____) ____ Local ____ Spinal ____ Epidural

Anesthesiologist _____ Anesthetist_____

INTRAOPERATIVE NURSING RECORD

PAGE 2 OF 3

MERCY COMMUNITY HOSPITAL

Figure 12-4, cont'd Intraoperative nursing record. *Continued*

Times: Patient in OR at _____. Patient out at _____ Surgeon _____

Assistant _____ Other persons in the room _____

Scrub Nurses _____ in _____ out _____

_____ in _____ out _____

_____ in _____ out _____

Circulating Nurses _____ in _____ out _____

_____ in _____ out _____

_____ in _____ out _____

Medications ordered and given: _____

_____

_____

_____

_____

Irrigation Solution: _____

Physician's Signature _____

Vital Signs during Local Anesthesia:

Time																		
Blood Pressure																		
Pulse																		
Respirations																		
Pulse Oximeter																		

POST-OP ASSESSMENT

Implants: _____ yes, _____ no, _____ recorded on progress notes, other_____

Drains: **Packing:**   **Dressing:**   ☐ other

☐ penrose   ☐ chest tube   ☐ nasal   ☐ 4 x 4's   ☐ xeroform
☐ T-tube   ☐ Solcotrans   ☐ oral   ☐ nasal splint   ☐ adaptic
☐ sump   ☐ Hemovac   ☐ wound   ☐ band aids   ☐ brace
☐ Jackson Pratt   ☐ other _____   ☐ bias stockinette   ☐ webril
☐ urinary catheter _____   ☐ Ace bandage   ☐ splint
_____   ☐ foundation garment ☐ cast

Wound classification: _____ clean, _____ clean-contaminated, _____ contaminated, _____ infected

Skin condition: _____ good, _____ other, comments _____

Specimens: _____ yes, _____ no _____

_____

Cultures: _____ yes, _____ no _____

Patient discharged: _____ RR, _____ ICU. _____ room, _____ OP, report by _____

via : _____ RR stretcher, _____ bed, _____ side rails up, _____ wheelchair, _____ ambulatory

Date: _____ Signature of circulating nurse _____ Patient status _____

INTRAOPERATIVE NURSING RECORD

PAGE 3 OF 3
MERCY COMMUNITY HOSPITAL

Figure 12-4, cont'd   Intraoperative nursing record. (Courtesy Mercy Health System, Havertown, Penn.)

DATE	TIME	FOCUS	NURSING PROGRESS NOTES

NURSING PROGRESS NOTES

MERCY COMMUNITY HOSPITAL

Figure 12-4, cont'd Intraoperative nursing record.

procedure before transfer to the PACU. Abnormalities should be specifically documented by recording the size, shape, color, location, and nursing actions taken to protect the site. Injuries occurring while the patient is under anesthesia should be reported immediately to the surgeon and documented in the postoperative notes.

Once immobilized, the patient's potential for injury is greatly increased. According to the AORN standards, preventing injury from items such as surgical equipment, medications administered, positioning, and other extraneous objects is the responsibility of the nurse. These standards dictate many of the nursing interventions used to protect the patient. Once again, a checklist can help make the documentation of specific items and interventions timely and comprehensive. OR nurses involved in developing such a form may list the specific options used in the OR, thus tailoring the documentation tool to meet the specific needs of their patients.

Positioning of the patient varies according to the specific procedure and is based on what anatomy is to be exposed, maintaining patient comfort, and preventing injury related to pressure or restraint devices. Many positions are used in surgical procedures (e.g., supine, prone, lateral, beach chair, lithotomy, jackknife), and many more positional aids are used to prevent injury to the patient. The use of basic positional aids such as a seat belt, rolls, sandbags, pillows, armboards, or Vacupaks must be documented in the OR record to support the prevention of injury. The use of specialty tables, positioning frames, hyperthermia blankets, stirrups, and leg supports must also be documented as nursing interventions. Circulatory supports, such as antiemboli stockings, compression bandages, and sequential stockings, should also be included when documenting positioning equipment because stasis of blood flow is a direct result of immobilization.

The use of electrical equipment is quite common in the surgical setting. Bipolar cautery devices do not require grounding pads, and they must be designated by type on the OR record. Unipolar cautery devices do require the placement of an electrical grounding pad on the patient. Those individuals who have thick or dense hair at the grounding pad site should be shaved around the site to allow proper pad adhesion and prevent burns. The shave preparation should be documented along with the placement site and the individual who performed it. The settings for the cutting and coagulation functions of the instrument must be recorded, as should a notation of testing or verification performed by the surgeon or assistant. The laser and electrical equipment should always be recorded by a specific name and identification number. Printouts with the settings, number of shots, and other data should be attached to the OR patient record. Electrical burns caused by cautery devices may occur through the skin down into the muscle layer, and may be delayed in their appearance. The condition of the grounding pad site after the removal of the pad should be documented

in the skin reassessment. The following case highlights the importance of appropriate placement of the grounding pad:

> A California man sued his orthopedic surgeon and anesthesiologist after back surgery because of an electrocautery-device burn to his thigh. The patient maintained that he had a severe psoriasis condition at the site and the doctors had been negligent in placing the pad on the compromised skin. The physicians argued that assessment of the site and placement of the pad was not their duty. Although the decision was in favor of the physicians, a $20,000 verdict was awarded to the plaintiff from the defendant surgery center (Laska, 1997b).

One of the most frequent causes of OR liability is the loss of a sponge, needle, or instrument in the patient. The injuries incurred by a patient in such cases often yield a large financial settlement, as the following case illustrates:

> A 53-year-old woman was recently awarded $400,000 as a result of a sponge left in her abdomen during a hysterectomy. The sponge was not detected for 17 days despite "bowel dilatation suggesting obstruction or ileus." During the patient's subsequent surgery, a tooth was dislodged and the patient's blood volume became so low she suffered a cerebrovascular accident (Laska, 1997g).

The AORN recommends the practice of counting as a safeguard. However, institutional policy should dictate specifically what is to be counted. "Sponges should be counted on all procedures in which the likelihood exists that a sponge could be retained" (AORN, 1997). Furthermore, after an initial count, a count should be performed before the closure of a cavity within a cavity and at closure of the skin. Records of these counts may take two forms: a worksheet or a separate count record. Worksheets are usually specific to a type of instrument tray, and they can be included in the sterile tray during processing as an inventory of what should be included. This sheet is then handed from the scrub nurse to the circulating nurse for concurrent counting. Whether this work sheet is to be retained as part of the medical record or discarded at the end of the case should be the decision of the individual institution. The worksheet must be supported by strict guidelines for use. For example, data concerning instruments with multiple parts must be recorded to identify the number of pieces making the whole. Items used within or around an incision (e.g., towels or cautery scratch pads) should be recorded in a miscellaneous area.

The commonly used method of documenting counts uses a separate count record to be included in the OR patient record. Information should include the names of the counting nurses, activity of the counts, and the correctness of all counts. In the event of an incorrect count the corrective actions must be recorded in the permanent OR record for all required sponge, needle/sharp, and instrument counts. Policy may dictate the protocol for searches and any resulting x-ray procedures for missing items, but these must still be specifically reported to the surgeon and recorded as evidence of adherence to nursing policy. In negligence cases in which a surgical item is found to be inside a person's body, defending the nurses' level of practice without the documentation of concurrent, inclusive, and correct counts is impossible. The following complex case in California illustrates this point:

A patient who underwent gastroplasty for weight control experienced failure of the surgery. When she was evaluated, a sponge was detected in her abdomen. A second gastroplasty was performed, and the sponge was retrieved. The patient contended that the second surgery was only done to remove the sponge. "The defendant contended that the second surgery was a result of the original gastroplasty malfunctioning, not from the sponge." The physician settled for $25,000, and the hospital was found to be 75% liable for a total award of $100,000 (Laska, 1997e).

The administration of medications during surgery is often the shared responsibility of the anesthesiologist or anesthetist and the perioperative nurse. For patients managed by the anesthesiologist or anesthetist, the intake and output recordings are usually done by them with the assistance of the circulating nurse. The perioperative nurse is still responsible for recording any medications or fluids he or she has given. These medications may include IV sedation drugs, local anesthesia, antibiotics, hemostatic agents, and irrigation fluids. Medications must be documented in the record as ordered by the surgeon with the name, dose, time, and route of administration. The use of fluids to distend organs or flush cavities must be done appropriately and recorded by solution name and amount. The inappropriate use of large amounts of sterile fluid has been known to cause massive fluid shifts, which can be dangerous to the circulatory and neurologic systems and are therefore an area of liability that needs to be observed for and recorded carefully. The physician must sign this section just like any other doctor's order, and the RN must also sign the order to verify the administration of fluid. Fluid administration was a key factor in the following case:

A large settlement was awarded to a woman in Florida who underwent a myomectomy/endometrial ablation laser procedure. The surgeon used fluids under pressure to dilate the uterus. The patient experienced critical fluid overload, which caused her lungs to fill with fluid and precipitated a cardiac arrest. "The plaintiff alleged the defendant's nurses failed to properly monitor the intake and infusion fluids during the procedure; the hospital was therefore negligent for deviating from the prevailing professional standards of care." The woman received $175,000 from the hospital and an undisclosed amount from the surgeon and the anesthesiologist (Laska, 1997a).

The insertion of any type of implant during surgery requires specific, detailed documentation. Duplicate implant information is usually supplied as labels by the manufacturer. The labels should include the identification number of the implant, lot number, company, and sterility expiration date. The patient's name and demographics and an implant label are returned to the manufacturing company for registration. One label should be placed on the patient's perioperative record, and others may be kept by the surgeon or OR administration for record keeping, ordering, or performance improvement activities. Another label may be provided to the patient for his or her personal health records. In the event of an implant recall, the organization must have a process in place so that individuals who receive the items in question can be quickly identified.

At the conclusion of the procedure, postoperative assessment must be documented before the patient is transferred to the postanesthesia care unit (PACU). The type of procedure and the postoperative diagnosis must be recorded because they may differ from the preoperative procedure or diagnosis. Wound classification, as defined by the Center for Disease Control and Prevention (1998) should be recorded to assist the institution's infection control personnel. Wound classification is one of the predictors of risk for surgical wound infection. Surgeries can be classified as clean (I), clean-contaminated (II), contaminated (III), or infected (IV). The type of procedure, the time anesthesia was commenced, the time the incision was made, and the time the incision was closed also contribute to the use of a risk index that is used to proactively identify patients at risk of surgical wound infection. Any cultures obtained from the surgical site should be recorded by identity and disposition. Specimens obtained must be identified by anatomic site, labeled with the patient's demographics, and recorded in the OR record. The number and type of transfused blood products should be identified, and further documentation should be supplied in the progress notes or blood bank section of the medical record. The presence of drains, tubes, catheters, packing, and dressings must all be documented by site and type, as should the presence of any drainage. Reassessment of the skin should occur before leaving the OR. Particular attention must be paid to the mode of transportation and safety measures used when moving the patient. Finally, the unit to which the patient is transferred must appear on the record with the nurse's signature.

SURGERY-SPECIFIC DOCUMENTATION

Speciality areas in the OR often require highly specific equipment and procedures, which must be recorded. The following text describes items that should be included in surgery-specific documentation in addition to the general surgical items that have already been noted.

Neurosurgery

Neurosurgery frequently involves the use of cotton balls and cottonoid sponges, which may not be easily recorded on the standard sponge count sheet because of their variety. For specialized cases a microscope with microsurgical instruments, shunting material, nerve stimulators, intracranial pressure (ICP) monitoring devices, and stereotactic equipment may be used. The recording of the use of such equipment and the counts of instruments and microsurgical sutures must be meticulous. Documentation of all special monitoring devices (e.g., Swan-Ganz, CVP, or epidural catheters) must be included with the reported readings. The highly specific nature of neurosurgical procedures and technology may require individualized worksheets for monitoring and counts.

Cardiac, Thoracic, and Vascular Surgery

Cardiac, thoracic, and vascular surgery frequently use instruments with multiple parts, clamps, rubber shods, vessel loops, pledgets, gauze dissectors, catheters, and fine suture needles that may require additional meticulous counts. Required documentation also includes data regarding pressure monitoring devices with readings, irrigations, and solutions used, topical hemostatics used, amount of contrast dye administered, and type of graft material used. The use of anticoagulants may occur at the sterile field during surgery, and such use must be included in the medication administration record by the circulating nurse. The insertion of any type of graft must be documented, as previously mentioned. Cross-clamping of blood vessels to insert the graft should be timed and recorded as "clamp on time" and "clamp off time." Doppler devices are frequently used to provide evidence of peripheral pulses. The presence of the pulse at specific anatomical sites must be recorded with the date and time. The insertion of chest tubes, a check of the water seal, color, and amount of drainage, as noted, must be included on the patient record. Intake and output must be coordinated with anesthesia personnel and recorded before transfer to the PACU or surgical intensive care unit (SICU).

Gastrointestinal Endoscopic Procedures

Gastrointestinal (GI) endoscopic procedures are becoming quite common because of minimally invasive techniques that are more comfortable for the patient. If pictures are taken by video camera, a copy must accompany the medical record. Additional copies may be supplied to the physician and patient for his or her records.

Genitourinary Surgery

Genitourinary surgery utilizes many endoscopic procedures. The amount of nonhemolytic, isotonic, and nonelectrolytic irrigation solutions that are used can often reach thousands of milliliters. The appropriate type of solution must be verified by doctor's protocol or order, and the amount must be reported periodically during the process. The placement of stents and catheters must be recorded because the patient often leaves the OR with these items in place. In kidney transplant surgery the specifics of the donor-recipient match must be included in the chart for review before surgery.

Cesarean Section Births

Cesarean section births may be performed in the labor and delivery area, the OR, or a birthing center. Fetal heart tones should be monitored at the time of admission to the OR and notation should be made of contraction frequency, duration, and intensity. In the event of a prolonged surgical period before delivery of the baby, these parameters should be reassessed at an established interval. Institutional protocol should dictate the process for the identification of mother and child and the disposition of the placenta. This information is pertinent and should be included in the operative record.

Orthopedic Surgery

Orthopedic surgery often begins with the placement of a pneumatic tourniquet on the limb to decrease the amount of blood flow to the surgical site. This equipment should be checked before use, and padding should be placed between the patient's skin and the tourniquet. The surgical limb, the padding, and the tourniquet pressure setting must be documented in the patient record with the time that the tourniquet was inflated and deflated. The tourniquet must never be inflated longer than 2 hours to avoid damage to the limb; this may require that it be deflated before the end of a procedure. If this occurs, it should be clearly documented to avoid discrepancies in case the tourniquet must be reinflated to finish the case. Nerve damage can cause devastating and irreversible injuries, as the following case illustrates:

> Nerve damage was sustained by a Kentucky woman after arthroscopic surgery. Compression of the femoral nerve in her thigh caused permanent nerve damage, which left her with an unstable gait and an inability to run. The jury awarded the plaintiff a $330,000 verdict for negligence during the performance of her surgery (Laska, 1997f).

Any x-ray studies that are performed must be logged. Hardware inserted into the patient should be treated as an implant despite the absence of preprinted manufacturer's labels. Supply as much information as possible about the name, type, size, length, caliber, number, and manufacturer of the implant in the patient's record in the event of a product failure or recall. Glues used to secure prostheses should also be recorded, including information about the manufacturer, lot number, and expiration date. Because the law mandates that institutions report adverse events caused by medical devices, the OR should keep an additional log for all implantable devices used there. The use of local anesthetics, pulsed lavages, and intraarticular irrigations should be included in the section of the record used to document medication administration. Photos taken during arthroscopy procedures should also be included in the patient's records.

Conscious Sedation

In the fast-paced environment of ambulatory care, the development of conscious sedation has had a dramatic impact. This type of pain management allows patients to tolerate experiences that are normally unpleasant while maintaining a relaxed, cooperative state, stable vital signs, and enabling purposeful movement in the patient. The return to preoperative level of consciousness is quick and little residual effect occurs. These cases may require an additional registered nurse (RN) to preoperatively assess the patient, monitor the patient's vital signs, and administer medications. The Joint Commission dictates that continuous monitoring be documented at 5 to 15 minute intervals by personnel proficient in medication administration, airway evaluation, and emergency response measures (i.e., basic and advanced life support). Sedatives and other medications must be recorded in the chart with the dose, route of administration, time, and physiologic and psychological effects.

Local Anesthesia Procedures

Procedures performed with only local anesthetics should be monitored at the same intervals with the same level of professional competence as those procedures using conscious sedation. The preoperative assessment must be performed by an RN with particular attention paid to the arrangements made to transport the patient back home. Postoperative assessments should be complete and should include vital signs, level of consciousness, and comfort level of the patient. Postoperative instructions must be given and documented that they are understood (to the best of the patient's ability).

DOCUMENTATION OF PREOPERATIVE EMERGENCIES

Shock and Hemorrhage

Among the most common perioperative emergencies are shock and hemorrhage. Nursing interventions are based on assisting with temperature regulation and fluid replacement. The monitoring of intake and output by visual and laboratory analysis necessitates careful, rapid assessment. Transfusing warmed blood products while estimating blood loss helps restore fluid balance and normal temperature while the surgeon attempts to control the bleeding. Topical hemostatic agents will likely be used, and their use should be documented in the OR medication administration record. Situations that result in cardiac arrest should be documented, according to institutional policy, in standard code documents, the anesthesia record, or the nurse's progress note.

Malignant Hyperthermia

Malignant hyperthermia is a hypermetabolic state involving skeletal muscle. The administration of inhalation agents or neuromuscular blocking agents can precipitate leakage of myoglobulin into the bloodstream in specific individuals, causing a potentially fatal elevation in temperature. Treatment involves changing the anesthesia circuit to eliminate all remnants of the causative agents and administering IV dantrolene once every 10 minutes to counteract the metabolic chain reaction. The perioperative nurse's main responsibility is to reduce the body's rising temperature. A cooling blanket may be applied, cold packs may be placed on the large pulse points, cold, wet towels may be applied to the skin, or the patient may be packed in ice. Intravenous fluids and irrigants should be iced for core cooling. A nasogastric (NG) tube may be placed so that iced lavages can be performed. Time is critical to this type of emergency, and attention to medication administration times for documentation is crucial. Identifying the patient as "malignant hyperthermia susceptible" in the medical record is the surest way to prevent a repeat occurrence of this type of OR emergency in a patient.

Trauma

The arrival of a trauma patient in the OR causes a flurry of activity aimed at assessing and stabilizing the patient. Identification of the patient, notification of the family or significant others, previous medical conditions, and the existence of drug allergies are the most important information to be obtained and recorded. Medical evaluation may include x-ray studies, fluid aspirations, and laboratory studies, which may need to be done in the OR area. Trauma victims may need rapid induction of anesthesia, which often requires the bedside assistance of the circulating nurse. Once on the operating table, the extent of injuries may need to be further assessed, and surgery will begin. The nurse's recording of monitoring devices, intake and output, blood loss and administration, the insertion of implants, and the placement of drains is particularly important.

Forensics

The characteristics of crime victims admitted to the OR are similar to those of trauma patients. The nursing care of forensic patients, however, brings an added responsibility to collect and preserve evidence of the crime. Evidence may be physical or in the form of information given by the patient. Observations of evidence may include statements or actions of the patient or accompanying person, physical items that can be seen, quantified, or analyzed, or observations of unusual situations. Documentation must be specific, complete, accurate, and legible. Pertinent comments should be recorded in quotes. Wounds should be described with anatomic landmarks and specific characteristics. Physical items must be marked "forensic specimen" and should include the patient's name and identification number, the date and time collected, the specimen type, the site of collection, and the collector's name. Disposition of the specimen must also be recorded, including the name of the police personnel taking the specimens. The unexpected nature of these violent situations makes standardizing care plans difficult because of the various types of injuries sustained.

SUMMARY

Documentation in the fast-paced, varied environment of the perioperative area brings with it the responsibility to be accurate, concise, and complete and the corresponding accountability. The nursing process contributes insightful physical and psychosocial assessment, and the standards of care offer thoughtful, measurable interventions that facilitate positive patient outcomes. The regular reevaluation of the patient's condition and the nursing interventions performed provide evidence of the positive impact of the nursing process. The absence of appropriate documentation of the established standards of perioperative care indicates a lack of professional ability and a failure to uphold responsibilities for the nurse and the institution. A reduction in liability occurs when the communication of nursing interventions and patient responses is clear and reflects positive results. The documentation of this complex process can ultimately be the most important nursing intervention.

POSTANESTHESIA CARE
UNIT DOCUMENTATION

Jo Anne Kuc, RN, BSN

PACUs no longer restrict their scope to caring exclusively for postoperative patients. Today PACUs are specialized critical care units used for various complex sedation-related procedures, such as administering epidural blocks, elective cardioversion, electroconvulsive therapy, and post-angiogram procedures. While some PACUs focus on a specific patient population, such as pediatrics, others incorporate broad services, such as ambulatory care centers. Discussing all of the documentation protocols for all types of surgical procedures and patients is impossible. Instead, this chapter focuses on documentation of adult PACU patients. The reader is encouraged to seek out other reference sources for additional information.

The primary role of the PACU nurse is to ensure that patients emerge safely from anesthesia. Compliance with the nursing standard of care for PACU patients can only be validated by timely, factual, and accurate documentation. Regardless of the method of documentation used (e.g., narrative, subjective data, objective data, assessment, plan (SOAP), problems, interventions, and evaluation (PIE), or computerized documentation, defensive PACU documentation should convey a message that the patient was cared for by a knowledgeable nurse, who is properly educated in critical care and anesthesia and practices approved PACU standards of care.

THE POSTANESTHESIA CARE
UNIT FLOW CHART

The environment of the PACU can change at any given moment. For this reason the PACU flow chart must be easy to use and be conducive to rapid and systematic recording of a patient's status. Incorporating flowsheets (check charting) into parts of the PACU record allows patient assessments to be documented in a matter of minutes.

Although check charting saves time, this type of documentation should be utilized carefully and not be taken lightly. Check charting implies that the task or assessment was done in accordance with PACU standards of care. Therefore the accuracy of the assessment can be challenged during testimony if a nurse explains his or her check notation improperly or erroneously when describing an assessment technique.

As in all nursing units, the PACU nurse should document in accordance with the nursing process. In the PACU, check charting should never be an overall substitute for narrative charting. Narrative documentation should be used to describe actual or potential patient problems, the implementation of a plan of care, and the evaluation of the patient outcome. Good narrative charting also should reflect that the nurse prioritized the needs of his or her patient while they were recovering from anesthesia. One cannot overemphasize that good PACU documentation conveys the patient's status, nursing observations and interventions, and the patient's response to treatment. The standard components of PACU documentation, shown in Box 12-1, should contain the following broad categories:

- Identifying the patient information e.g., using an Addressograph (name plate)
- Type of anesthesia
- Date and time of arrival
- Surgical information (e.g., name of surgeon, title of operation, name of anesthesiologist, admitting nurse, preoperative vital signs, patient medical history, allergies)
- Skin assessment
- Ventilation assessment
- Circulatory assessment
- Neurologic assessment
- Tubes or drains

Box 12-1

Standard Components of Postanesthesia Care Unit Documentation

Demographic Data

- Patient Addressograph
- Type of anesthesia (e.g., general, local, spinal)
- Date
- Arrival time
- Surgeon
- Anesthesiologist/certified registered nurse anesthetist (CRNA)
- Title of operation
- Admitting PACU nurse
- Significant preoperative medical history
- Preoperative vital signs
- Allergies

Patient Assessment

- Skin temperature (e.g., warm, dry, turgor, moist)
- Skin color (e.g., normal, pale, mottled, jaundice, cyanotic)
- Ventilation (e.g., spontaneous, labored, regular rate and rhythm)
- Method of oxygen administration (e.g., nasal, cannula, mask)
- Type of assisted ventilation (e.g., endotracheal tube, T-piece, percentage of Fio_2, ventilator rate and volume)
- Breath sounds (e.g., bilateral assessment, describing auscultation findings)
- Apical pulse (e.g., regular, irregular); if a cardiac monitor is used, note the type of rhythm
- Radial and femoral pulses, noting quality
- Drainage tubes (e.g., nasogastric, Foley, gastrostomy, Hemovac, Constavac, Jackson Pratt, chest)
- Invasive lines (i.e., subclavian, jugular, central venous pressure, arterial line, pulmonary artery catheter); note location of area and condition of site
- Level of consciousness (e.g., alert; lethargic; oriented to time, place, and name; obeys commands; responds to verbal stimuli; responds to pain purposefully; responds to pain nonpurposefully; no response to pain)
- Neurologic assessment (e.g., movement of upper and lower extremities, sensation in extremities, pupils)

- Vital sign grid recording blood pressure, pulse, respirations, temperature, and pulse oximetry

Fluid Balance

- Type of intravenous solution, noting amount of volume upon arrival, time begun, amount of solution remaining at the time of discharge; for blood products, note blood bank number and blood type
- Total PACU intake, (including parenteral and piggyback port medications, and blood products)
- Total PACU output (e.g., urine, suction, emesis, chest tube)

Anesthesia

- Orders given by anesthesiologist
- Anesthesiologist's signature authorizing discharge of patient from PACU

PACU Diagostic Studies

- Time and results of laboratory tests
- Time and results of x-ray studies
- Verification that physician was notified of results

PACU Narrative

- Time of notation
- Medications given
- Narrative PACU nurses notes

Post Anesthesia Recovery Score

- Done at time of patient arrival and every 30 minutes until time of discharge

Discharge Information

- Name of receiving nurse and time report was given
- Time and date patient was discharged from the PACU
- Signature of PACU discharge nurse

- IVs, monitoring devices, and infusion record
- Level of consciousness
- Vital sign graph
- Intake and output
- Diagnostic tests section
- Narrative notes
- PACU/Aldrete scoring system (optional)
- Discharge information
- Name of PACU nurse

Figure 12-5 is an example of a PACU record used in same day surgery.

Though not required, most PACU flow charts incorporate a postanesthesia scoring system as part of the patient care assessment. Several scoring systems are available, the most widely used being the Aldrete system. The Aldrete format is easy to use, and it incorporates objective and retrievable data on the patient's movement, respiration, circulation, consciousness, and skin color. If a PACU form does not use a scoring system, the narrative nurse's notes must reflect that the patient is stable, responsive, and free from complications and has adequately recovered from the major effects of anesthesia before discharge.

PATIENT ASSESSMENT

When the patient arrives in the PACU, the PACU nurse is given the name and age of the patient, the surgery or

FIRST STAGE RECOVERY

Date: _____ Time: _____ Side Rails up: _____ ☐ Call Bell in Reach

Admitting RN _____

Allergies _____ History _____

Type Anesthesia: ☐ General   ☐ Spinal   ☐ Regional   ☐ Local   ☐ Monitor Anesthesia Care

Anesthesiologist: _____ Surgeon _____

OR Intake: _____ IV count: _____ Total Intake: _____ Total Output: _____

Pain   O – 10 (O=none – 10=worst)

N/V   = Yes   O=No   * indicates see Nurses Notes

Vital Signs	TIME:							POST ANESTHESIA RECOVERY SCORE TIME:		
	temp:									
	Heart Rate:							Able to move 4 extremities voluntarily or on command = 2 Able to move 2 extremities ITY: voluntarily or on command = 1 ACTIV- Able to move 0 extremities voluntarily or on command		
	Cardiac Rhythm:									
	BP:									
	Respirations:							Able to deep breathe & adequate exchange = 2 RESPIRATION Dyspneic or Limited Breathing = 1 Apneic = 0		
	Breath Sounds:									
	O2 Sat:									
	O2 delivered							BP +/– 20% Pre-op Systolic Level = 2 BP +/– 20-50% Pre-op Systolic Level = 1 CIRCULATION BP +/– 50% Pre-op Systolic Level = 0 Children under 10 Apical pulse		
	Pain: (see above)									
	N/V Present:							Awake, coherent = 2 Arousable on calling = 1 CONSCIOUSNESS Not responding = 0		
	Dressing									
	IV site							Normal skin color = 2 Pale, dusky, blotchy, jaundiced, other = 1 COLOR Cyanotic = 0		
	Other:									
	Distal pulse site									
	mobility							Preop BP: Pulse: TOTAL:		
	capilliary refill									
	sensation							IV fluids / Meds		
	color									
	ext. temperature									
	Initials:									

NURSE'S NOTE

Figure 12-5   Same day procedures unit, first-stage recovery. (Courtesy Robert Wood Johnson University Hospital, New Brunswick, NJ.)

procedure performed, the name of surgeon, any significant medical history (e.g., allergies, anesthetic agents, other medications administered), the amount of intraoperative IV fluids and blood products administered, intake and output, any intraoperative problems, estimated blood loss, and any potential postanesthetic problems. In addition, the standard of care requires that the PACU nurse review the anesthesia record, admission history and physical, preadmission records, and preoperative check-list, which can contain important patient information impacting the recovery of the patient and the care rendered in the PACU.

Within minutes after the patient's arrival the PACU nurse should perform a rapid and systematic assessment of the respiratory, cardiovascular, neurologic, gastrointestinal, and genitourinary status of the patient. The initial priorities in PACU assessment are airway, circulation, and level of consciousness. Additional critical priorities include renal assessment and the status of the patient's recovery from spinal anesthesia.

Airway

One of the greatest risks of general anesthesia is respiratory compromise. Intravenous and inhalation anesthetic agents, muscle relaxants, narcotics, pain, and even surgery itself can compromise ventilation and perfusion. Muscle relaxants, patient anatomy, or improper patient positioning can cause the tongue to fall back and partially occlude the airway. Fluid overload or poor cardiac function can cause pulmonary edema. Bronchospasm can cause neurogenic pulmonary edema. Volume deficits from blood loss, shock, or third spacing can cause hypotension and poor perfusion. Third spacing is a shift of extracellular fluid from the plasma compartment to interstitial or transcellular spaces.

Documentation of the respiratory system status focuses on measures that were undertaken to prevent complications and promote optimal ventilation and perfusion. Complete assessment of the respiratory system involves more than counting and recording the respiratory rate once every 10 minutes; it should include a description of the quality and depth of respirations. Documentation should include a description of breath sounds (e.g., clear, rales, rhonchi), equal chest expansion, the presence of abnormalities such as intercostal retractions, abdominal or irregular breathing, or abnormal sounds such as stridor. The nurse should note the type of oxygen delivery system (e.g., nasal cannula, mask), the percentage of oxygen being administered, the pulse oximetry readings, and the presence and type of an artificial airway.

The use of a jaw thrust or head tilt to relieve simple airway obstruction should be recorded in the PACU record. Respiration rates below 10 per minute require notification of the anesthesia service and will likely require the administration of naloxone (Narcan). Appropriate and timely interventions should be undertaken and noted if naloxone is ineffective.

The following case underscores the consequences of substandard respiratory monitoring and assessment:

The patient (FC) was admitted to the PACU following a cholecystectomy. Extubation occurred in the OR, and the patient was transported to the PACU. Upon arrival the anesthesiologist informed the PACU nurse that the patient had received intraoperative narcotics and that the nurse should "watch his respirations." Oxygen was applied at 2 L/per minute, as was the standard protocol. The receiving PACU nurse admitted the patient, then asked a second nurse to watch the patient while she left the PACU. During testimony the primary nurse admitted that she did not receive a verbal response from the second nurse acknowledging that she would watch her patient. When the primary nurse returned to the PACU, she noted that the patient's respiration rate was 8 per minute. The anesthesiologist returned to the PACU and inquired about the patient's condition. He received assurances that the patient was stable. When he assessed the patient himself, the anesthesiologist observed that the patient had stopped breathing. The patient became bradycardic and eventually went into cardiac arrest. A heart rate was reestablished 20 minutes later; however, the patient remained comatose for over a year until the time of his death. The Superior Court found the anesthesiologist negligent for failing to ensure that his patient was stable before leaving the PACU. The Superior Court also found the PACU nurse negligent for the following actions: failing to ascertain the type of intraoperative drugs that were administered to the patient, leaving a patient without verifying that the patient would be adequately cared for, and failing to recognize that the patient had stopped breathing (Tammelleo, 1991).

Circulation

Vital Signs

The initial vital signs should be recorded and verbally communicated to the anesthesiologist at the time of the patient's arrival at the PACU. The PACU nurse then compares these vital signs with the preoperative and intraoperative values. Because the status of PACU patients can change very rapidly, the authors recommend that vital signs of stable PACU patients be recorded a minimum of once every 10 minutes for the first hour. More frequent recording of vital signs is warranted when the patient is unstable.

Pulses

Only radial and pedal pulses are routinely assessed and recorded; however, specific surgical procedures may require that the nurse record other pulses as well. (For example, rotator cuff surgery requires that the nurse assess the radial pulses, and femoral bypass surgery requires that the nurse assess the popliteal, posterior tibial, and pedal pulses.) Pulse quality should be described as normal, bounding, thready, palpable but obliterated with palpation, or absent. Palpable pulses can be graded using a +1 to +4 system. Doppler pulses should be described as "audible by Doppler" without a +1 to +4 grading format.

Color and Temperature

The nurse should describe the color of the patient's skin such as normal, pale, flushed, mottled, jaundice, or cyanotic. Areas of mottling or cyanosis should be noted. Certain surgical procedures require assessment of the capillary refill time. Capillary refill should be assessed and recorded in seconds and compared with the unaffected extremity. (Normal capillary refill is 3 seconds.)

Hypothermia is common in the PACU. A patient is considered hypothermic if the body temperature is below 96° F. Fortunately, various rewarming devices are currently available. The PACU record should reflect the type of rewarming device used, the length of use, and frequent recording of the patient's temperature. Before discharge from the PACU, the patient's temperature should be nearly normal.

Electrocardiogram Monitoring

When bedside electrocardiogram (ECG) monitoring is implemented, the PACU record should reflect the baseline cardiac rhythm and rate. A 6-second rhythm strip is mounted and maintained as a permanent part of the PACU record. Additional strips are warranted if and when new dysrhythmias occur and also before discharge.

Level of Consciousness

Emergence from anesthesia is directly related to the anesthetic agents administered and the individual's rate of metabolism and drug excretion. Documentation of the neurologic status should describe the patient's level of consciousness, degree of alertness, orientation, and his or her ability to follow simple commands or respond to tactile stimuli.

The PACU nurse may encounter patients with prolonged somnolence or emergence anxiety. More neurologically depressed patients may respond only to pain. In this case the nurse should record the patient's response to a sternal rub or fingernail pressure. Abnormal posturing, such as decorticate or decerebrate posturing, should be recorded and reported. The nurse should also note and record the presence of abnormal breathing, such as periods of apnea or Cheyne-Stokes respirations, which can indicate cerebral damage or injury to the pons and medullary centers of the brain. Finally, the PACU record should contain a pupillary assessment noting pupil size, equality, and reaction to light.

Surgery on an extremity, major blood vessels, or nerves requires documentation of the following:

- Movement of the extremity (e.g., movement of toes, dorsiflexion and eversion of feet)

- Movement of the fingers and the ability to touch each finger to the thumb
- Presence or absence of numbness, tingling, or decreased sensation
- Standard circulatory assessment as previously discussed

The following anecdotal report shows why a neurovascular assessment is important:

> A 68-year-old patient underwent a radical prostatectomy. His past medical history was significant: a femoral-femoral bypass surgery complicated by thrombosis of the graft and also deep vein thrombosis just 3 years prior. His vital signs were stable throughout the entire PACU stay. However, the PACU nurse neglected to perform a neurovascular assessment of the lower extremities. The patient was transferred to a general surgical unit. Not until the patient complained of severe right leg pain did the nurse assess his lower extremities. By this time, the patient had developed compartment syndrome, which eventually resulted in an amputation below the knee. During the trial the surgeon testified that the extent of compromise was such that it must have occurred shortly after surgery. Both the PACU nurse and the receiving surgical nurse were negligent in failing to perform a neurovascular assessment of a patient at high risk for neurovascular compromise (anecdotal report).

Renal Assessment

In addition to assessing and documenting the status of patient's airway, circulation, and level of consciousness, documentation of renal assessment and recovery from spinal anesthesia is critical. The renal assessment centers on fluid loss and hydration. At the time of arrival in the PACU the anesthesiologist should provide the nurse with the intraoperative intake and output, estimated blood loss, and the amount of fluids administered intraoperatively. The PACU nurse should record the type and location of all IV lines, the type and amount of IV solutions, and the rate of infusion. The descriptions of all drains, irrigations, catheters, tubes, and suction devices should also be recorded. Accurate documentation of intake and output is obtained by emptying all drainage devices at the time of arrival in the PACU and immediately before discharge. Assessment of all drainage devices should be performed frequently throughout the PACU stay and abnormalities should be recorded on the PACU flow chart.

RECOVERY FROM SPINAL ANESTHESIA

Spinal anesthesia (i.e., subarachnoid anesthesia or intrathecal anesthesia) induces sympathetic, sensory, and motor blockades. The nurse should note any adverse effects of spinal anesthesia, such as hypotension, bradycardia, urinary retention, nausea, vomiting, or postdural spinal headache. Knowledge of the type of anesthetic used during spinal anesthesia will serve as an indicator as to when motor function will return. Motor ability generally returns before sensory function.

Documentation should center on frequent assessment of motor and sensory function and the time bilateral toe or foot movement returns. Patients should not be discharged from the PACU until they can move their toes.

SURGERY-SPECIFIC DOCUMENTATION

The following serves as a guide for documentation specific to certain surgeries.

Vascular Surgery

Numerous vascular procedures are used for peripheral and major vessel disease, including coronary artery bypass surgery, carotid endarterectomy, abdominal aortic aneurysm repair, femoral-femoral bypass surgery and femoral-popliteal bypass surgery. The type of vascular procedure used, the risk factors, and the patient's status determine the type of preoperative invasive lines to be placed. Invasive monitoring devices include, but are not limited to, arterial lines, pulmonary artery catheters, or CVP catheters. Following is a sample nursing entry in the documentation of an invasive line:

Right radial arterial line and right chest PA catheter intact with no site redness, dressing intact, lines flushed and patent and connected to HDM, good wave form. Right hand warm with 3 sec. capillary refill. PA: 23/11 M: 12.

When the anesthesiologist inserts an epidural catheter to augment pain control, documentation of epidural analgesia should be performed, as outlined in this chapter.

Monitoring graft patency should be a priority in the PACU. Peripheral pulses and circulation should be assessed and documented every 15 minutes. Maintaining blood pressure within the normal limits is crucial. Prolonged hypotension can cause graft thrombosis (Lewis, Collier, 1992). Prolonged hypertension can cause a leakage of blood or a rupture of the suture line (Maldonado, 1996). Documentation should reflect appropriate administration of volume expanders, vasopressor agents, or antihypertensive medications.

Special notation of the patient's underlying cardiac rhythm is important. Ventricular dysrhythmia can occur in individuals with underlying heart disease, or it may be the result of hypoxia, hypothermia, or electrolyte imbalance. Nursing documentation should reflect that the nurse assessed the patient for the underlying cause of the complication. For example, notations of preexisting heart disease should be recorded, as should oximetry readings, the percentage of supplemental oxygen, the patient's temperature, and the warming methods used, the results of laboratory tests, and the medications given to correct abnormalities.

Patients with prosthetic vascular grafts are also at risk for infection. The PACU documentation should reflect the administration of broad-spectrum antibiotics (if ordered), the monitoring of the patient's temperature, and white blood cell-count results. If the patient has an NG tube, documentation should include the type of tube, patency, color and amount of drainage, and amount of suction.

Blood loss or prolonged aortic clamping can compromise renal perfusion. The patient may also have a Foley catheter. Hourly urine output should be recorded, and the surgeon should be notified of any drop in urine output below 30 ml per hour. Prolonged aortic cross-clamping can also cause motor or sensory compromise in the lower extremities. The PACU record should include an assessment once every 15 minutes of the following: color of extremities; femoral, popliteal, and pedal pulses; temperature of the extremities; capillary refill; movement; and sensation.

Following vascular surgery of the neck, such as carotid endarterectomy, documentation should include a description of the patient's voice, his or her ability to pronounce the letter "E," the symmetry of the patient's smile, and facial symmetry when the patient sticks out his or her tongue. Careful attention paid to potential problems and the documentation of prompt interventions facilitate a successful recovery.

Thoracic Surgery

Thoracic surgical procedures include, but are not limited to, bronchoscopy, mediastinoscopy, lung biopsy, lobectomy, thoractomy, and pneumonectomy. In addition to the basic respiratory assessment, the PACU nurse should be alert for, record, and promptly report any major cardiovascular and pulmonary complications that occur following thoracic surgery, including hypotension, low output syndrome, cardiac dysrhythmias, myocardial ischemia, myocardial infarction, pulmonary emboli, pulmonary torsion, pulmonary hemorrhage, chest tube leakage, and pleural drainage problems.

Specialized documentation should include the following:

- Bed position
- Assessment of breath sounds (e.g., wheezing, friction rub)
- Appearance of the chest anatomy (noting the presence or absence of asymmetry)
- Use of accessory muscles
- Presence and location (mediastinal or pleural) of drains and tubes
- Use of chest tube suction
- Palpation of the chest to assess for crepitus

Orthopedic Surgery

The PACU nurse should describe the surgical site (if visible), the status of the surgical dressing, and the location and type of drainage devices (e.g., Jackson Pratt, Hemovac). Assessment of patients who have undergone orthopedic surgery involving an extremity should also include a neurovascular assessment of the extremity. Any abnormalities should be recorded and promptly reported to the surgeon. Notations should also be made concerning casts, Ace wraps, complete circulatory assessment of the digits, capillary refill, and motor and sensory assessment. Following is an example of documentation after surgery for carpal tunnel syndrome:

Right hand and wrist gauze dressing dry and intact. Right arm elevated on two bath blankets. Right radial pulse palpable through dressing. Right fingers warm, color normal, with 3 sec. capillary refill present. Able to move all fingers well. States sensation normal to right hand and fingers. Denies numbness or tingling.

Examination of the patient's circulatory, motor, and sensory status should be recorded periodically throughout the PACU stay. The application of ice, slings, splints, or traction should be noted. Bleeding on casts or dressings should be circled and noted in the PACU record along with the time. The maintenance of an extremity in a particular alignment or specialized movement, such as a log roll, should be recorded.

In surgeries involving the spine, such as laminectomy, diskectomy, foraminotomy, and spinal fusion, specific documentation should include proper body alignment, log rolling, the maintenance of the patient in a flat position, the inspection of the surgical site and drains, and a neurovascular assessment of the extremities; for example:

Received awake and responsive. Log rolled to right side using three assistants. Lumbar dressing dry and intact. Legs and feet warm; moves toes and feet well. Demonstrates normal bilateral dorsiflexion and plantar flexion. Denies numbness, tingling, or decreased sensation. Pedal pulses 3+ bilaterally, feet warm with 3-sec. capillary refill bilaterally.

Even with the use of appropriate padding, patients undergoing prolonged surgical procedures are at risk for compartment syndrome, which can first become evident in the PACU. Compartment syndrome can involve any extremity. Complaints of unusual numbness of or pain in a nonsurgical extremity requires a complete neurovascular assessment, prompt notification of the orthopedic surgeon, and documentation.

Urological Surgery: Transurethral Resection of the Prostate

Transurethral resection of the prostate (TURP) is indicated when conservative therapies cease to be effective. Because of the blood supply in the area of the prostate, postoperative bleeding is common. Various solutions are used for continuous bladder irrigation (CBI), and the rate of infusion is fairly rapid.

In an effort to reduce significant surgical bleeding, the urologist may apply Foley catheter traction before the patient leaves the operating room. If Foley catheter traction is present, it should be noted in the PACU record. Similarly, if the PACU nurse assists the urologist in applying Foley catheter traction, the nurse should record the time of the procedure and name of urologist who did it. Additionally, if the Foley catheter is manually irrigated, the time of the irrigation and the amount and type of irrigating solution should be recorded.

Documentation focuses on describing the presence or absence of clots and any complaints of bladder spasms by the patient. Surgery on the prostate causes a breakdown of systemic urokinase, which normally breaks down clots and stimulates bleeding (Wilson, 1997). Documentation should therefore reflect the nurse's close monitoring of bleeding and the color of blood in the urine (e.g., light pink, dark red).

To control profuse urinary bleeding, the administration of aminocaproic acid may be necessary. The nurse should note the time of administration, the dosage of aminocaproic acid, and the patient's response. The nurse should be alert for and record any adverse reactions to aminocaproic acid, such as hypotension, bradycardia, or cardiac dysrhythmias, which can occur from inadvertent rapid administration of aminocaproic acid.

Patients undergoing TURP are also susceptible to hyponatremia caused by systemic absorption of irrigation fluid. The nurse should be alert for, record, and report the following warning signs associated with hyponatremia: an abrupt increase in blood pressure, confusion, bradycardia or a dramatic drop in heart rate below baseline levels. Uncorrected hyponatremia can cause seizures and lethal dysrhythmias. If treatment of dilutional hyponatremia is ordered, the nurse should record the administration time and dosage of diuretics and hypertonic saline.

Finally, strict intake and output is mandatory. This is accomplished by subtracting the total Foley catheter output from the amount of irrigant infused. (A standard CBI bag contains 3000 ml of solution.) The number obtained is the urine output, which should be a positive number. If the calculation is a negative number, the urologist must be notified.

Neurosurgery

Several types of neurosurgical procedures exist, including craniotomy, ventriculoperitoneal shunt, hematoma evacuation, arteriovenous malformation, and evacuation of brain tumors. Additionally, the PACU nurse may encounter multiple trauma victims with closed head injuries. The potential for significant cardiorespiratory and neurologic deterioration exists in the immediate postoperative period for neurosurgical patients. Documentation should focus on a comprehensive neurologic assessment. It is imperative that the nurse compare the PACU neurologic assessment with the preoperative status of the patient. Failure to emerge from anesthesia might indicate increased intracranial pressure or bleeding. A patient who is awake who suddenly becomes unresponsive may have developed underlying obstructive hydrocephalus or brain stem compression.

Other abnormalities that should prompt documentation and physician notification include the following:

- Slow, bounding pulse
- Widening pulse pressure
- Irregular breathing
- Apnea

These symptoms are all indicative of increased intracranial pressure. Apnea is particularly worrisome because it may represent a temporary or permanent impairment of the respiratory center.

The nurse should record a sensorimotor assessment, such as the following:

- Evaluating the symmetry of a patient's smile or ability to stick out his or her tongue
- Grasping strength of the hand
- Symmetrical movement of the extremities
- Dorsiflexion and plantar flexion of the feet and sensation of the extremities

Complicated brain surgery may cause increased cerebral edema, requiring postoperative ventilatory assistance. If an ICP monitor has been inserted, the PACU record should reflect periodic recording of the ICP pressure.

Swallowing difficulties should be noted because it might be a sign of stretching or manipulation of cranial nerves IX, X and XII and a heightened risk for aspiration, pneumonia, or hypoxia (Brash, Cullen, Stoelting, 1992). Systemic hypertension requires immediate treatment to prevent cerebral edema and hematoma formation. The PACU record should reflect the dosage of and time of administration of all medications used to prevent or reduce increased ICP, such as nitroprusside, steroids, diuretics, osmotic agents, or antihypertensive drugs.

Gastrointestinal Surgery: Laparoscopic Cholecystectomy

Laparoscopic-assisted laser cholecystectomy (LLC) is the most popular surgical technique for cholecystectomies. Injuries associated with LLC include intraabdominal bleeding caused by unexpected vascular injury, bladder injury, and trocar injury to the intestines. Though symptoms caused by associated complications might not manifest themselves in the PACU, documentation should still reflect close monitoring for these potential complications.

The PACU nurse should be alert for, record, and report any of the following symptoms of potential complications:

- Increasing abdominal girth
- Unusually severe abdominal pain
- Pallor
- Tachycardia
- Hypotension
- Diaphoresis
- Drop in urine output if a Foley catheter is in place

The PACU record should contain the details of IV antibiotic administrations, which are commonly given postoperatively to prevent infection.

Obstetrical Surgery: Caesarean Section

During the initial hours following a caesarean-section birth, the patient is at high risk for increased vaginal bleeding. At the time of arrival in the PACU, an IV with Pitocin, used to facilitate uterine contraction, will be hanging. The PACU nurse should palpate the fundus and describe its texture (e.g., firmness, boggy) and position. The fundus normally should be below the umbilicus.

Increased vaginal bleeding can be the result of uterine atony, which requires fundal massage and immediate notification of the obstetrician. The nurse should carefully record the following:

- Time of each fundal massage
- Estimated amount and color of blood expressed during the massage
- Presence or absense of and the size of clots
- Number of perineal pads used and frequency of changes

A blood loss of 500 ml is considered a hemorrhage and warrants immediate notification of the obstetrician.

After a caesarean section the patient will also have a Foley catheter placed. The color and amount of urinary output should be recorded at the time of arrival and assessed throughout the PACU stay. The presence of blood can be benign or indicative of a more serious complication, such as a bladder perforation. The presence of blood in the urine merits documentation and prompt notification of the obstetrician.

DOCUMENTATION OF COMMON POSTANESTHESIA PROBLEMS

Complications can occur following any surgical procedure. Anesthetic agents, underlying health problems or age of the patient, and emergency surgeries are a few of the factors that can heighten the incidence of postoperative complications. The PACU nurse must be constantly aware of potential complications associated with specific surgeries, must recognize, record, and report changes in the patient's condition, and must promptly intervene before detrimental effects occur. The following text describes a few of the specialized complications that can arise in the PACU.

Hypotension

Hypotension can be caused by fluid loss, decreased cardiac output, myocardial dysfunction, or decreased vascular resistance resulting from sepsis or medications. Identification of a potential cause is crucial to implementing the appropriate treatment. The PACU documentation should reflect optimal patient oxygenation at all times. When the patient is hypovolemic, nursing documentation should provide details of blood volume expansion using IV fluids, volume expanders, or blood products, and monitoring of hemoglobin and hematocrit levels. If the cause of the hypotension is myocardial dysfunction, nursing documentation should include the use of medications to stimulate myocardial contractility, such as the administration of digoxin, atropine, dopamine, or dobutamine.

In situations involving hypotension caused by decreased peripheral vascular resistance, documentation should include the use of measures such as volume expanders or vasopressor drugs (e.g., ephedrine, dopamine, Neo-Synephrine).

Laryngospasm

Laryngospasm can occur abruptly without warning and is a dire respiratory emergency. Careful nursing assessment and prompt intervention can prevent lethal complications. The depth of anesthesia can be directly related to laryngospasm; therefore extubation should be performed while the patient is in a deep plane of anesthesia or while the patient is awake (Murray-Calderon, Connelly, 1997). Patients who are extubated while in a light plane of anesthesia are more susceptible to laryngospasm.

Nursing documentation should include the following:

- Level of consciousnsess (e.g., fully awake, restless, confused, somnolent)
- Presence of noisy breath sounds (e.g., crowing, stridor)
- Use of intercostal muscles for breathing
- Pulse oximetry
- Skin color
- Vital signs

Documentation should reflect prompt notification of the anesthesiologist or CRNA, time called and response time.

The nurse should record the time and techniques used to treat laryngospasm, their effectiveness and the patient's response. Such interventions include the following:

- Jaw thrust to open the airway
- Suctioning to clear the airway
- Positive pressure using 100% oxygen via bag-mask

ventilation while maintaining the head and neck in a hyperextended position to break the bronchospasm (contraindicated in cervical spine surgery)
- Use of racemic epinephrine
- Use of succinylcholine chloride for muscle relaxation

Laryngospasm can evolve into noncardiogenic pulmonary edema. If noncardiogenic pulmonary edema occurs, treatment and nursing documentation should be similar to that of patients with cardiogenic pulmonary edema. The following documentation example concerns a patient who underwent a dilatation and curettage and then developed a laryngospasm, which evolved into noncardiogenic pulmonary edema. Vital signs were closely monitored and recorded on a separate graph:

1500	Received responsive, nodding to questions. Moves all extremities to command. Chest expansion symmetrical, lungs clear bilaterally. HOB @ 30. O_2 3 L/NC. Pulse oximeter: 92%. IV patent. No drainage on peripad. Denies pain.
1510	Sudden drop in pulse oximeter to 88% without change in color, respiratory rate, or respiratory quality. Denies shortness of breath or dyspnea. Breath sounds remain clear and equal bilaterally. Aerosol mask applied at 50%. Dr. Borden paged stat.
1511	Return call by Dr. Borden. States he is coming immediately. Placed on ECG monitor. NSR.
1512	O_2 saturation rapidly dropping into mid-60s. Respiratory rate unchanged. Inspiratory stridor audible. O_2 saturation verified by another pulse oximetry unit and remains in mid-60s. Patient placed on Ambu bag with 100% oxygen in conjunction with own respiration in effort to break possible bronchospasm. Pulse oximetry rising to 70% with Ambu bag.
1513	Dr. Borden at bedside and took over use of Ambu bag. Bilateral breath sounds audible with rales $\frac{1}{3}$ ↑ posteriorly. Less stridor audible. Pulse oximeter 84%. Stat chest x-ray ordered.
1515	Stat chest x-ray done. Remains awake and nodding to questions. 16 F Foley catheter inserted with 200 ml urine returned. 4 mg morphine sulfate given IV. 40 mg Lasix (furosemide) given IV. Pulse oximetry 88%.
1523	Respirations easy and regular without stridor. Chest x-ray viewed by Dr. Borden. Placed on 50% aerosol mask with pulse oximetry at 90%. Diuresing well.

Once the initial crisis is over, nursing documentation centers on the description of supportive care and assessment for secondary complications. The PACU nurse should document the general appearance of the patient, vital signs, percentage of supplemental oxygen, pulse oximetry values, time of administration and type of diuretic agent used, time taken and results of arterial blood gas (ABG) tests and chest x-ray studies, and the patient's response to treatment.

Adult Respiratory Distress Syndrome

Patients suffering from multiple trauma, sepsis, aspiration, or multiorgan failure, and those patients who received multiple intraoperative blood transfusions are susceptible to adult respiratory distress syndrome (ARDS) in the PACU. It has been shown that individuals who develop ARDS do so within the first 24 hours after surgery (Jones, Hoffman, and Delgado, 1994). In addition to recording a general assessment of the patient, nursing documentation should reflect actions performed to maximize oxygen delivery. These include the following:

- Pulse oximetry readings
- Sedation
- Endotracheal (ET) intubation and ventilator support with positive end-expiratory pressure (PEEP)

Standard documentation of the nursing care of ventilator patients should include the following:

- Type of ventilator
- Percentage of oxygen
- Tidal volume (TV)
- Ventilator rate (assist control or spontaneous intermittent mechanical ventilation [SIMV])

Document PEEP or pressure support (PS) as shown in the following:

Oral ET connected to Bear I; TV 1000, Fio_2 50%, SIMV 10, PEEP +5; PS +5.

The PACU nurse should also observe for and document complications resulting from the use of PEEP. Overly distended alveoli can cause a tension pneumothorax. If this occurs, the nurse should note the presence of tachypnea, increased dyspnea, decreased or absent breath sounds, tachycardia, bradycardia, or mediastinal shift. The anesthesiologist and surgeon should be immediately notified, and the time of the notification, as well as the information that was shared with the physicians, should be documented.

Decreased cardiac output can also occur from PEEP, and it is caused by decreased venous return. A drop in blood pressure should alert the PACU nurse to the potential for compromised cardiac output and perfusion. Documentation of pulmonary artery readings and cardiac output is critical. The nurse should note all communication with the appro-

priate healthcare providers regarding abnormal readings and the prompt initiation of inotropic agents, if ordered.

The following two cases emphasize the critical role PACU nurses play in caring for and monitoring patients at high risk for pulmonary complications:

A 62-year-old woman underwent an uncomplicated colon resection. She developed hypotension in the PACU and was treated with full resuscitation. Volume overload occurred, resulting in pulmonary edema. A pulmonologist was called in for treatment, and her condition began to improve. However, her condition changed, and she developed respiratory distress, which was not reported to the physician. She developed ARDS the following day and died. The plaintiffs contended that the PACU nurses were negligent in their monitoring of her intake and output status, which resulted in pulmonary edema. The plaintiffs also contended that the PACU nurses failed to appraise the doctors of a change in the patient's condition. The jury returned a $301,228 verdict for the plaintiff (Laska, 1997c).

The patient, a 43-year-old woman, underwent emergency surgery for a ruptured ectopic pregnancy. While emerging from general anesthesia, the patient vomited and aspirated. As a result, the anesthesiologist left the patient intubated for pulmonary hygiene and ventilation purposes. The nurse in the PACU connected the patient to 100% oxygen through the ventilator. However, the ventilator hose was disconnected, and the patient received room air at 21% oxygen, resulting in anoxic encephalopathy, from which the patient never recovered. The decedent remained comatose for 4 years and died. She was survived by her two children, ages 7 and 14. The case settled for $1.1 million (Laska, 1997d).

Postoperative Fever

The PACU nurse might occasionally encounter postoperative fevers. Evidence of shivering, chills, weakness, hypotension, tachycardia, tachypnea, or rash should be recorded. A fever with associated rash formation could indicate a drug-induced fever. Postoperative fever can also result from bacterial, fungal, or viral infections. Hemolytic hyperthermia can occur during or after blood transfusions or surgical stress.

The most life-threatening form of fever is malignant hyperthermia (MH). Because fever is a late sign of MH, nursing documentation should concentrate on the recognition and reporting of early signs of this syndrome, as described in the following list:

- Tachycardia
- Dysrhythmias
- Diaphoresis
- Muscle rigidity
- Cyanosis
- Unstable blood pressure
- Dilated pupils

Notation should be made of the following laboratory test results, which are indicative of MH:

- Arterial and venous acidosis
- Hypercarbia
- Hypoxemia
- Elevated creatinine phosphokinase levels
- Hyperkalemia
- Myoglobinuria

When MH is suspected, frequent recording of the patient's temperature is warranted, because the patient's temperature can rise rapidly—as much as 1° C every 5 minutes (Enright, Hill, 1989). The PACU record should also reflect the implementation of ventilatory support, the use and temperature setting of an ice mattress, and the administration of dantrolene (2.5 mg/kg IV). Additionally, all other supportive measures, such as treatment of cardiac dysrhythmias, acidosis, electrolyte imbalance, and hypoxia, and the patient's status should be clearly noted in the PACU record.

Anaphylaxis

All anesthetic agents can potentially cause anaphylaxis. Anaphylactic reactions can also occur because of incompatible blood given during transfusions, the administration of antibiotics or other medications, or latex sensitivity. If anaphylaxis occurs in the OR, surgery will be terminated as quickly as possible and the patient will be immediately transported to the PACU for further interventional care. The PACU nurse should note the use of all nonlatex equipment in cases involving latex allergy. The removal of any latex invasive devices, such as catheters and ET tubes, and the reinsertion of nonlatex devices should also be noted.

Except for the special precautions in latex allergy, the treatment of anaphylaxis remains the same. The PACU record should reflect basic patient monitoring, particularly airway evaluation, as previously mentioned. Hypotension is caused by vasodilation; therefore the administration of volume expanders should be clearly noted, as should the use of other medications for the treatment of anaphylaxis, such as epinephrine, antihistamines, catecholamines (epinephrine, norepinephrine, or isoproterenol), corticosteroids. aminophylline, albuterol, or sodium bicarbonate.

MISCELLANEOUS POSTANESTHESIA CARE UNIT PROCEDURES

Extubation

Patients are frequently extubated in the PACU. It is imperative that the PACU record contains appropriate information to support that a patient is ready for extubation. Accepted documentation criteria includes the following:

- Patient fully awake and able to follow commands

- Ability of the patient to sustain a head lift
- Minimal tidal volume of 5 ml/kg
- Forced vital capacity of 15 ml/kg
- Oxygen saturation higher than 90%, with Fio_2 less than 40% or negative inspiratory force more than −20 cm of water.

Following extubation, documentation should be done in accordance with the basic respiratory assessment, as previously outlined.

Premature extubation can have lethal consequences, as shown in the following case:

A woman underwent elective outpatient endoscopic surgery. The anesthesiologist administered a depolarizing muscle relaxant before ET intubation and during the surgery; however, the amount of the drug was not documented. The surgical procedure was uneventful and lasted 25 minutes. The patient was transported to the PACU with the ET tube in place. She exhibited signs indicating that the muscle relaxant had not been sufficiently reversed: She was unable to open her eyes on command; sustain a head lift for 5 seconds; she was tachycardic and tachypneic; and she required 100% oxygen to maintain adequate oxygen saturations. Despite the fact that she did not meet the criteria for extubation, the anesthesiologist extubated her, and she sustained a cardiopulmonary arrest 5 minutes later. The anesthesiologist was in charge of the "code blue" proceedings but did not follow ACLS protocols. Resuscitative medications were not administered in a timely manner. The patient was not reintubated appropriately. She was not defibrillated, and her ABG samples were not drawn until 18 minutes into the emergency. Although a heart rhythm was established 54 minutes later, the patient later died as a result of hypoxic encephalopathy. The case was presented to a medical review panel in Indiana, which found no negligence on the part of the anesthesiologist. Subsequently, a panel doctor changed his opinion at the time of deposition and testified that the anesthesiologist's care failed to conform to the standard of care. A maximum settlement amount of $750,000 was awarded (Court Summaries and Trial Reports, 1998).

This case makes it clear that the chronology of events was based on the PACU chart. Precise documentation of times is essential, but timely intervention is even more critical.

Electroconvulsive Therapy

Because muscle relaxants and sedatives are administered before electroconvulsive therapy (ECT), the PACU is a logical site for this outpatient procedure. The PACU nurse should verify completion of the standard preoperative check list and that the patient has had nothing by mouth before beginning the ECT procedure. The PACU record should reflect the nurse's close monitoring of vital signs, the use of continuous bedside ECG monitoring, pulse oximetry readings, and all protective measures in place to prevent injury.

Although the anesthesiologist is responsible for recording all aspects of anesthesia care, the PACU record should reflect the following:

- Administration of preoxygenation (administration of 100% oxygen to saturate red blood cells) before the shock therapy
- Dosage and time of administration of all medications given by the anesthesiologist and the PACU nurse
- Presence or absence of ectopy; number of shocks and shock strength
- Length and description of seizure
- Ventilation support during the procedure
- Patient's response
- Ventilation following the seizure

Following the patient's return to consciousness, ECT documentation is the same as for other PACU patients.

Nerve Blocks and Blood Patches

Various types of nerve blocks are performed in the PACU, including, but not limited to, subarachnoid, epidural, brachial plexus, intercostal, and stellate ganglion. Some of these procedures are performed preoperatively for postoperative pain control, whereas others are done on an outpatient basis for chronic pain management.

After standard patient preparation and appropriate presurgical work-up, the PACU nurse should ensure that the IV line is secure and functioning. Baseline vital signs, the cardiac rhythm via bedside ECG monitoring, the percentage of oxygen via nasal cannula or other oxygen delivery system, and pulse oximetry readings should all be recorded. The nurse should then assist with patient positioning.

After the procedure the PACU record should reflect the following:

- Vital signs
- Pulse oximetry readings
- Level of site of injection
- Condition of the site
- Any abnormalities (e.g., accidental intravascular or subarachnoid puncture)
- Hypotension
- Numbness
- Tingling
- Pain

When caring for outpatients, the level of pain relief should be recorded in those individuals who undergo nerve block for chronic pain relief. In addition, the PACU record should reflect all patient education and care instructions for the procedure.

When caring for postsurgical patients who have had volumetric epidural pumps connected following surgery, nurses are advised to use a specialized epidural flow chart that allows for the documentation of the following details:

- Vital signs
- Motor assessment
- Recording of a sensory level
- Level of sedation
- Pain scale
- Condition of the epidural site
- Verification of the epidural catheter position
- Dosage and rate of infusion of the epidural medications
- Bolus doses
- Adverse side effects

A patient may occasionally develop a postdural spinal headache, which occurs because of cerebrospinal fluid leakage at the puncture site. If conservative treatment fails to provide relief, the anesthesiologist may perform a blood patch. Generally 10 to 20 ml of blood is removed from the patient's peripheral vein and injected directly into the epidural space at the level of the spinal puncture. Relief of the headache should be almost instantaneous. In addition to the standard documentation listed above, documentation for a blood patch procedure should include the following:

- Name of the anesthesiologist
- Amount of blood drawn
- Amount of blood injected
- Epidural level
- Symptomology
- Response of the patient

Postprocedure assessment is the same for any PACU patient; however, because no sedation is required, patients may be discharged when their condition becomes stable.

The following two anecdotal cases involved direct patient injury caused by nursing negligence:

The patient (LV), in the first case was a 73-year-old lady suffering from chronic back pain. Her physician advised her to come to the hospital for a trial administration of an epidural infusion of bupivacaine and fentanyl. If LV achieved a good pain relief from the infusion, she was to return later for an implantable epidural catheter. After LV arrived in the PACU for the epidural trial, the epidural catheter was inserted without incident followed by a 2-hour infusion of bupivacaine and fentanyl. When LV received successful pain relief, the epidural infusion and catheter were discontinued and the nurse prepared her for discharge. Although she was stable, LV informed the PACU nurse of numbness and decreased sensation to her right leg. The PACU nurse, who was inexperienced in the care and management of patients receiving epidural analgesia, instructed LV to ambulate. While trying to do so, LV fell, fracturing her femur. The PACU nurse admitted during testimony, that she had never taken care of an epidural patient or received any formal instruction. In addition, the hospital did not have a policy about the care of epidural patients. Analysis of this case led to the conclusion that the PACU nurse was negligent for the following:

- Being unfamiliar with the care and management of patients receiving epidural analgesia
- Failing to perform a neurologic assessment
- Failing to inform the anesthesiologist about the patient's residual right leg numbness
- Allowing a neurologically compromised patient to ambulate
- Preparing an unstable patient for discharge
- Failing to ensure patient safety (anecdotal report)

In the second case the anesthesiologist inserted an epidural catheter preoperatively in MM, a 32-year-old patient, for postoperative pain control. The patient's hemicolectomy was done under general anesthesia. At the conclusion of surgery, the anesthesiologist injected the epidural catheter with bupivacaine. At the time of arrival in the PACU, the patient was stable, responsive, and pain free. Her PACU orders included a standard bupivacaine and fentanyl epidural infusion using a volumetric pump set at 7 ml per hour. After approximately 20 minutes the patient began to complain of severe abdominal pain. The epidural infusion was not yet available from the pharmacy. The PACU nurse notified the anesthesiologist and received orders for 6 ml of 1.5% Marcaine (bupivacaine) to be injected through the epidural catheter. After the PACU nurse injected the catheter with the medication, the patient underwent respiratory arrest. During the resuscitation the epidural catheter was aspirated and blood was obtained. The epidural catheter presumably migrated into a blood vessel during transport of the patient from the OR to the PACU. Instead of an epidural injection of Marcaine, the medication was given intravascularly. The PACU nurse notes failed to include the following information:

- Condition of the epidural site and dressing at the time of arrival in PACU
- Motor ability and sensory level of the patient
- Aspiration of the epidural catheter before the epidural injection of Marcaine (anecdotal report)

Radioactive Implants

Patients who enter the PACU with radioactive substances should be placed in an isolation room. The PACU nurse should obtain a pocket dosimeter from the OR nurse and record the initial dosimeter reading before entering the isolation room. The PACU nurse should clip the pocket dosimeter at his or her waist area while caring for the radiation patient. In addition to the PACU record, hospital policy may require documentation on a "personnel exposure monitoring data" form so that the amount of radiation received by all individuals who come in contact with the patient can be accurately recorded. Such information should include the following:

- Name of the PACU nurse
- Date

- Patient location
- Initial dosimeter reading when PACU care was initiated
- Time the patient leaves the PACU
- Final dosimeter reading and the total amount of exposure received by the PACU nurse

DISCHARGE ASSESSMENT

The PACU record should contain the necessary criteria to support the fact that the patient is stable to be discharged from the post anesthesia unit. In general, the patient should demonstrate the following:

- Patent airway
- Adequate TV
- Respiratory rate
- Oxygen saturation levels
- Stable vital signs and heart rhythm
- Alertness and ability of the patient to summon help from the nursing staff
- Tolerable level of pain
- Adequate return of patient's motor and sensory function
- Normal or near-normal body temperature

The PACU nurse should provide the receiving nurse with a full report and record the time of the report, the receiving nurse's name, and the time the patient left the PACU.

SUMMARY

The vulnerability of patients emerging from anesthesia underscores the unique role of the post anesthesia care unit. Higher acuity patients, expanding medical technology, advances in medical and nursing research, and hospital restructuring place additional challenges on the PACU nurse. Patients rarely remember the PACU nurse or the care rendered there; yet the PACU is a high-risk environment. Adverse outcomes do occur, but they can be minimized with astute patient monitoring, prompt reporting of abnormalities, and defensive documentation.

Today, more than ever, nurses are required to adhere to and improve on standards of nursing care. The American Society of Post Anesthesia Nurses (ASPAN) has created standards of care for post anesthesia care. The American Society of Anesthesiologists (ASA) has also developed standards of practice for post anesthesia care. The American Society of Pain Management Nurses will soon join in adapting formal standards of practice in acute and chronic pain management. Nurses interested in PACU nursing are encouraged to become familiar with these standards because the care they provide will be judged by them.

REFERENCES

AORN: Recommended practices for documentation of perioperative nursing care, *AORN J* pp 1145, 1148, 1150, June 1996.

AORN: Patient outcomes and standards of perioperative care, Denver, 1991, The Association.

AORN: *Standards, recommended practices, and guidelines,* Denver, 1997, The Association.

AORN: Patient outcomes and standards for perioperative care, Denver, 1983, The Association.

Brash PG, Cullen BF, Stoelting RK: *Clinical anesthesia,* ed 2, Philadelphia, 1992, JB Lippincott.

Center for Disease Control and Prevention: Draft guidelines for prevention of surgical site infections, 1998, Federal Register, 192: pp 167-183.

Court summaries and trial reports, *The Indiana Lawyer,* Section A p 14A, February 19, 1998.

Enright T, Hill M: Treatment of fever, *Focus Crit Care* 16:96, 1989.

JCAHO: *1997 Comprehensive accreditation manual for hospitals,* Oakbrook Terrace, Ill, 1998, The Commission.

Jones MA, Hoffman LA, Delgado E: ARDS revisited, *Nursing* 12:34, 1994.

Laska L, ed: A Florida woman's circulatory system becomes overloaded with fluid during myomectomy, *Medical Malpractice Verdicts, Settlements and Experts* p 19, July 1997a.

Laska L, ed: California man suffers bovie burn on thigh during orthopaedic surgery, *Medical Malpractice Verdicts, Settlements and Experts* p 41, April 1997b.

Laska L, ed: California woman dies of ARDS one day after colon surgery, *Medical Malpractice Verdicts, Settlements and Experts* p 19, May 1997c.

Laska L, ed: Faulty ventilator hose thwarts emergency tracheotomy: *Medical Malpractice Verdicts, Settlements and Experts* p 19, April 1997d.

Laska L, ed: Foreign object left after gastroplasty, *Medical Malpractice, Verdicts, Settlements and Experts* p 46, November 1997e.

Laska L, ed: Kentucky woman suffers nerve damage following arthroscopic knee surgery, *Medical Malpractice Verdicts, Settlements and Experts* p 41, April 1997f.

Laska L, ed: Sponge left in Virginia woman's abdomen during hysterectomy, *Medical Malpractice Verdicts, Settlements and Experts* p 53, May 1997g.

Lewis S, Collier I: *Medical surgical nursing: assessment and management of clinical problems,* ed 3, St Louis, 1992, Mosby.

Maldonado K: Care of patients after aortic aneurysm repair, *J Post Anesth Nurs* 11(1):29, 1996.

Murray-Calderon P, Connelly MA: Laryngospasm and noncardiogenic pulmonary edema, *J Perianesth Nurs* 12(2):89, 1997.

Tammelleo AD, ed: Recovery room nurse fails to monitor patient, *Regan Rep Nurs Law* 32(2):4, 1991.

Wilson M: Care of the patient undergoing transurethral resection of the prostate, *J Perianesth Nurs* 12(5):341, 1997.

SUGGESTED READINGS

Brazell NE: The significance and application of informed consent, *AORN J* 65(2): p 377, February 1997.

Christensen B: Hemodynamic monitoring: what it tells you and what it doesn't, *J Post Anesth Nurs* 7(5):338, 1992.

Fetzer-Fowler SJ: Caring for the ambulatory surgical patient who has a pacemaker, part II: intraoperative hazards and postoperative care, *J Post Anesth Nurs* 8(3):174, 1993.

Kuc J: Liability issues related to epidural analgesia, *J Legal Nurse Consult* 89(2):7, 1997.

Kuc J: Managing of acute myocardial infarction in the post anesthesia care unit, *J Post Anesth Nurs* 5(6):1, 1990.

McShane FJ: Epidural narcotics: mechanism of action and nursing implications, *J Post Anesth Nurs* 7(3):155, 1992.

Muro GA, Easter CR: Critical forensics for perioperative nurses, *AORN J* 60(4):585, 1994.

Murphy JM: Astute assessment by a perioperative nurse in the expanded role saves patient from malignant hyperthermia, *AORN J* 66(1):146, 1997.

Palmerini J: Developing a comprehensive perioperative nursing documentation form, *AORN J* 63(1):239, 1996.

Pape T: Legal and ethical considerations of informed consent, *AORN J* 65(6):1122, 1997.

Pasero CL, McCaffery M: Avoiding opioid-induced respiratory depression, *Am J Nurs* p 25, April 1994.

Pritchard V, Eckard JM: Standards of nursing care in the post anesthesia care unit, *J Post Anesth Nurs* 5(3):163, 1990.

Proposed recommended practices for sponge, sharp, and instrument counts, *AORN J* 61(2):404, 1995.

Recommended practices for managing the patient receiving conscious sedation/analgesia, *AORN J* 65(1):129, 1997.

Rothrock JC: *Perioperative nursing care planning,* ed 2, St Louis, 1996, Mosby.

Salzback R: Presurgical testing improves patient care, *AORN J* 61(1): 210, 1995.

Stein RH: The importance of communication between the anesthesiologist and the post anesthesia care unit nurses, *J Post Anesth Nurs* 6(4):279, 1991.

Tammelleo AD: Court holds "charting by exception" policy negligent, *Regan Rep Nurs Law* (12) p 1, May 1994.

13

Psychiatric and Home Care Documentation

PSYCHIATRIC DOCUMENTATION

Rosie Oldham, RN, BS

Pamela Meyer-Tulledge, RN, BSN, MA

The material contained in this chapter is specific to psychiatric documentation and is not meant to be all-inclusive. This chapter focuses specifically on critical documentation issues that commonly result in legal problems for psychiatric nurses.

The staff of every psychiatric institution must contend with numerous regulatory agencies in their community and meet their standards. Each institution has its own unique characteristics and problems. Some common deviations from accepted practice do occur in most settings in which nursing care is provided, and some pitfalls specific to each clinical area do exist. The intent of this section is to highlight common documentation issues in psychiatric nursing.

FAILURE TO PREVENT HARM TO SELF OR OTHERS

This section addresses situations in which patients may be injured. Nursing documentation is an important factor in the defense of nurses involved in this type of incident.

Suicidal or Violent Behavior

The nursing process dictates that the nurse must appropriately assess suicidal or violent patients. The nurse should diagnose, plan, and implement interventions to reduce the risk and evaluate the effectiveness of these interventions. The documentation should reflect this process.

Assessment

The psychiatric nurse must be able to assess the patient for signs of suicidal and/or violent behavior. Because patients are often unable to communicate their own perceptions of danger, the nurse must assess and document any hints of impending suicidal or violent behavior. Indicators include the following:

- Agitation
- Intense emotional affect
- Delusions
- Threatening hallucinations
- Any previous history of suicidal or violent behavior

Exhaustive search does not yield inappropriate results or extreme changes in affect: agitation, anger, or increasing anxiety (Chou, Kaas, and Richie, 1996).

The nursing assessment should be based on risk factors for the nursing diagnosis of risk for violence, as shown in Box 13-1. Initiating an involuntary commitment when a patient is evaluated as posing a risk to himself or herself or others is common practice. Nursing documentation may be used to justify this type of commitment. The specific behavior exhibited by the patient, the interventions used or refused by the patient, and the evaluation of the patient's responses should all be documented. In the following case the assessments of the healthcare team were significant factors in a patient's claim that he was unjustly committed to a psychiatric facility:

Box 13-1

Risk Factors for Violence

- Substance abuse or withdrawal
- Toxic reaction to medication
- Explosive, impulsive, or immature personality
- Paranoia
- Panic, manic, or rage state
- Antisocial characteristics
- Response to a catastrophic event
- Development crisis
- Significant change in lifestyle
- Actual or potential loss of significant other
- Loneliness
- Lack of support systems
- Dysfunctional communication patterns
- Feelings of alienation
- Physical, sexual, or psychological abuse
- Manipulative behavior
- Perceived threat to self-esteem
- Suicidal behavior
- Social isolation
- Effects of organic brain syndrome
- Temporal lobe epilepsy

From Taptich B, Iyer B, Bernocchi-Losey D: *Nursing diagnosis and care planning,* ed 2, Philadelphia, 1994, WB Saunders.

The plaintiff was a 25-year-old man who worked as a medical records clerk. He was involuntarily committed to the defendant's psychiatric hospital. He was released 34 days later after a court hearing. The plaintiff claimed that the applicable laws required that he be mentally ill to be committed and that the defendants had no evidence of mental illness to justify his commitment. The defendant contended that the plaintiff refused to cooperate with testing and evaluations; the hospital could therefore only look at the plaintiff's actions in making a determination about his mental state. The defendants claimed that the plaintiff exhibited signs of mental illness. A defense verdict was reached (Laska, 1998b).

The observations of the nurses and doctors, as documented in the medial record, were likely used to justify this patient's commitment.

Many legal cases involve nursing actions that contribute to a patient's self injury. The nurse may encounter legal difficulties when a patient is not assessed for risk factors of suicidal or violent behavior, or when the documentation does not reflect that this assessment was completed. In the following case the nurses did not properly assess a suicidal patient:

A 33-year-old male was committed to a state psychiatric hospital for severe depression accompanied by suicidal

thoughts. He had made several previous attempts at suicide. The man was allowed to go out on the hospital grounds on the first day accompanied by staff. The next day he was allowed to go out alone.

When the man returned from his first trip alone, he became extremely agitated and was crying, shaking, and telling the staff that he wanted to kill himself, but that he could not do it. The nurse notified the psychiatrist, and medication was ordered. The man later woke up in an extremely agitated state and was again talking of suicide. He was then medicated for a second time. Despite these two episodes, the nursing staff did not seek a physician's evaluation of the man.

The following day the man asked to go outside. He was told by a nurse that because of the difficulties he had experienced the previous day, he was not to go out. The man responded that he was feeling better, and the nurse then permitted him to go out alone. The man went outside and climbed up a ladder attached to a two-story smoke stack. He jumped off the ladder, falling to the ground below, and sustained multiple injuries.

The man alleged that the nursing staff was negligent in failing to call in a physician after he returned from his first trip outside. The defendants did not dispute that the man was in severe distress, was severely agitated, shaking, and crying, and had specifically advised the nurses that he wanted to kill himself. The man alleged additional negligence on the part of the nurses in permitting him to go outside the next day given the extreme reaction he had exhibited the day before. The case settled before trial for $125,000 (*Tort claims act—$125,000 recovery,* 1996).

Planning and Implementation

After assessing the patient's risk for suicide, the nurse should plan, implement, and document interventions to reduce the risk of injury. These interventions typically include removal of dangerous objects and careful monitoring of the patient. The diligent observation of a suicidal patient has been an issue in a number of cases, including the following one:

A 15-year-old boy was admitted to a locked psychiatric adolescent unit for attempting suicide at home by ingesting antidepressant medication and cough syrup. He was evaluated as a suicide risk and self-harm precautions were initiated. The precautions included visual checks of the patient (at 15-minute intervals) and the bathroom, which he was not permitted to use alone. A Beck Depression Inventory test was also conducted. The teen was permitted to wear his clothes and belt. On the day after admission the teen committed suicide by hanging himself in the bathroom.

The plaintiff alleged that three breaches of the standard of care occurred. First, the 15-minute check was not performed, and the teen was unsupervised for a period of almost 45 minutes. Second, the bathroom door was inexplicably unlocked, allowing the teen to make use of it in his suicide. Finally, the teen should not have been permitted to keep his belt. The plaintiff also alleged that the staff had not reviewed the results of the test, which would have clearly shown the teen to be depressed and suicidal. A settlement was reached for $485,000 (Laska, 1997e).

Hospital policies are based on knowledge of the risks of suicide and the appropriate interventions, as defined by usual and customary nursing practice. Questions raised by this case include the following:

- Why was the patient allowed to have a belt in light of his potential for suicide?
- Why was the bathroom door unlocked?
- Why was the patient not monitored according to physician's order?

In the event of a lawsuit, nurses will be evaluated on whether the incident could have been foreseen and whether they followed hospital policies. When deviations from the policies occur, the nurse may be asked to justify them. A suicide that occurs in a hospital is a sentinel event. As such, its occurrence necessitates an internal investigation and is to be reported to the Joint Commission.

Another area of potential liability involves episodes in which a patient harms others. If a patient injures someone, the documentation may be scrutinized to determine what steps the nurse took to prevent the incident. Consider the following case:

> A woman in Maine visited her son, who was in a psychiatric care facility. The visit took place inside one of the locked units. When she arrived in her son's room, the mother noticed a young woman putting her clothes into her son's dresser drawer. Not wanting to upset the woman or her son, the mother notified the nurses, who responded, "Oh, my goodness! Is that where she is? We've been looking for her." Later, when the mother was ready to leave, the same young woman approached her and began to beat and choke her. The son's mother sustained severe bruises, chipped teeth, and emotional distress.
>
> The young woman was under orders to be constantly observed by the staff members because of recent episodes of physically violent behavior. According to the hospital policies and guidelines, constant observation meant that a staff member should always be able to see the patient and should never be more than six steps away. However, because of the statute of limitations, the psychiatric facility was not held liable (Tammelleo, 1991).

The attending nurse had a responsibility to keep the patient under constant (literally) observation according to the physician's orders. The nurse had adequate knowledge of the young woman's history of violence. However, the patient obviously was not monitored under constant observation. If the nurse had kept the patient under constant observation as ordered, she could have prevented this incident. However, no warning may be given that a patient is suicidal or violent. When a patient attempts to or does commit suicide or exhibits violence toward others, the facility and healthcare providers can be held accountable. The plaintiff's attorneys will ask the jury to determine whether the nurse was aware of the patient's suicidal or violent intentions and whether the nurse acted reasonably given that information. If the psychiatric nurse suspects that a patient is at risk, accurate documentation is imperative.

Documenting Suicidal or Violent Behavior

A type of charting note that is hard to refute in court is a direct quote, coupled with documentation of the nurse's follow-up action. The initial note should state that the physician was notified, what safety precautions were ordered, and what time the precautions were initiated. Describe in concrete terms that conduct that posed a threat to the patient or others. Use direct quotes when necessary, such as "I plan to kill myself." In doing so, the nurse can avoid charges of false imprisonment and provide justification for involuntary commitment.

Carefully document all precautions taken against suicide when a patient expresses suicidal thoughts, if a change in behavior is noted, or the patient acts out against himself or herself in some manner (Northrop, Kelly 1987). Most psychiatric facilities use a seclusion record for a patient who is at risk to harm himself or others (Figure 13-1). The nurse should document on this form that the patient was monitored on a constant, one-to-one basis every 15 or 30 minutes, depending on the physician's order.

The nurse should document the following recommended information concerning a suicidal patient (Calfee, 1996):

1. Direct patient quotes about suicidal or violent thoughts, intentions, plans, and motives
2. Direct quotes from family and visitors who express concern about the patient's intentions
3. Data gathered regarding the patient's risk factors, such as a history of suicide attempts or violent episodes, the patient's ability to carry out the plan, possible reasons for suicide or harm to others, substance abuse, or previous psychiatric diagnosis
4. Actions taken in accordance with facility policy to remove items the patient could use to harm self or others
5. That the physician was notified if the patient verbalizes a specific plan or makes an attempt to harm himself or herself
6. The patient's whereabouts on the seclusion record (suicidal or violent), if ordered
7. That the patient was instructed about the precautions ordered and the reasons for the implementation of the precautions
8. That the patient was monitored according to the physician's order

When a patient threatens to harm another person, the healthcare professional may be obligated to breach confidentiality. The precedent established by the Tarasoff ruling requires nurses to notify a physician and warn any intended victims that the patient may be threatening to harm.

DANVILLE STATE HOSPITAL
Danville, Pa.

SECLUSION RECORD

DSH 207/10-90

Date: _____		Date: _____		Date: _____	
7:00 A.M. - 3:00 P.M.	**Code No., Initials**	**3:15 P.M. - 11:00 P.M.**	**Code No., Initials**	**11:00 P.M. - 7:00 A.M.**	**Code No., Initials**
7:00		3:15		11:15	
7:15		3:30		11:30	
7:30		3:45		11:45	
7:45		4:00		12:00	
8:00		4:15		12:15	
8:15		4:30		12:30	
8:30		4:45		12:45	
8:45		5:00		1:00	
9:00		5:15		1:15	
9:15		5:30		1:30	
9:30		5:45		1:45	
9:45		6:00		2:00	
10:00		6:15		2:15	
10:15		6:30		2:30	
10:30		6:45		2:45	
10:45		7:00		3:00	
11:00		7:15		3:15	
11:15		7:30		3:30	
11:30		7:45		3:45	
11:45		8:00		4:00	
12:00		8:15		4:15	
12:15		8:30		4:30	
12:30		8:45		4:45	
12:45		9:00		5:00	
1:00		9:15		5:15	
1:15		9:30		5:30	
1:30		9:45		5:45	
1:45		10:00		6:00	
2:00		10:15		6:15	
2:15		10:30		6:30	
2:30		10:45		6:45	
2:45		11:00		7:00	
3:00					

Code - Behaviors

1. Beating or kicking door
2. Yelling or screaming
3. Cursing
4. Crying
5. Laughing
6. Talking
7. Mumbling Incoherently
8. Standing
9. Walking or Pacing
10. Lying on Bed or Mattress
11. Sitting
12. Quiet
13. Sleeping
14. Requesting Release from Seclusion Room
15. Harmful to self
16. Threatening Staff or Assaultive to Staff
17. Disrobing
18. Crawling on floor
19. Non-communicative
20. Destructive to clothing/furniture
21. Destructive to room
22. Urinating/defecating on floor
23. Other: Please Note in Record of Patient

Code - Treatment

A. Meal Served
B. Other Nourishment served-Amount Accepted
C. Bath/Shower
D. Toilet
E. Visit by Physician
F. Verbal Intervention
G. Released from Seclusion
H. Medications
I. Refused Medications
J. Refused bathing/toileting
K. Resistive to care-bathing/toileting

Figure 13-1 Seclusion record. (Courtesy Danville State Hospital, Danville, Penn.)

In the Tarasoff case an Indian patient told his psychiatrist he was planning to murder his former girlfriend (Ms. Tarasoff). At the request of the psychiatrist, the police briefly detained the patient, then let him go because he appeared rational. Two months later the patient killed the young woman. The jury held the therapist liable for failing to warn the victim, stating that concern for the patient's right to confidentiality was less important than the need to protect the public.

If a patient threatens to harm himself, herself, or others, the nurse must act quickly—especially if the nurse does not know the patient. If the patient kills himself, herself, or someone else, and documentation exists to show that the nurse was aware of the patient's intentions, the nurse can be sued (Oliver, 1986).

When threats are brought to the nurse's attention, the intended victim should be warned and this action should be documented in the medical record. The nurse should also document that members of the healthcare team were advised of the threats. On the other hand the patient may say that he or she wants to hurt someone, but the nurse cannot learn the identity of the intended victim. In this situation, documenting the patient's exact words and the fact that the intended victim's name could not be determined is best.

Contraband

To provide clear direction to the nurse, psychiatric agencies have developed policies and procedures that specifically identify items that can cause harm to patients. No facility is completely safe from all items; however, efforts must be made to keep units as safe as possible. *Contraband* is a term used to describe any item considered to be a safety hazard or potentially dangerous to the integrity of the patients. At the time of admission, each patient's belongings should be thoroughly checked for contraband. The nurse should remove all potentially dangerous items and document each item on a contraband list form. The contraband should then be placed in a secured area and returned to the patient at the time of discharge. Certain hygiene items should be kept in a locked area from which the patient can either check them out or use them while being monitored by staff. The nurse should document in the clinical record that the patient's belongings were checked, the contraband list form (if used by the facility) was completed, and all contraband items were removed. Box 13-2 lists examples of contraband items.

The nurse is expected to assess the risk of harm and take necessary precautions to reduce this hazard. In the following case, the potential for the patient's injury to himself related to a dangerous item was ignored:

A 46-year-old California man committed suicide with dandruff shampoo and after-shave lotion on the fourth day after his admission to a psychiatric unit of an acute-care

---

Box 13-2

Examples of Contraband Items

- Razors
- Metal cans
- Sharp implements
- Glass containers or bottles
- Belts
- Flammable liquids, aerosol containers
- Medications, topical agents, mouthwash
- Drugs, alcohol
- Knives, guns, weapons
- Electrical devices
- Make-up, toiletries

---

facility. At that time, his orders were to be checked every 30-minutes. After his family brought in shampoo and after-shave lotion, he consumed them, resulting in a severe metabolic disorder from which he never recovered. The man's family claimed that the staff failed to make an adequate assessment of his suicidal potential, that he should have been checked more frequently, that he should not have been allowed to use dandruff shampoo and after-shave lotion without supervision, and that he displayed classic signs of suicide potential on the morning of the incident. The jury found both the physician and hospital negligent (Laska, 1993a).

REFUSAL OF TREATMENT

A recognition has developed of the need to respect and protect psychiatric patients' right to refuse treatment, which is protected by standards of practice and law when the patient is competent. Whether the patient understands the consequences of the decision to refuse treatment is an important consideration.

The following four generally accepted state interests override the patient's right to refuse treatment (Rouse, 1988):

1. Preservation of life
2. Prevention of suicide
3. Maintenance of the ethical integrity of the medical profession
4. Protection of innocent third parties

In a nonemergency situation the nurse must document the patient's refusal of treatment and the time the physician was notified. If required by state guidelines, the physician is usually responsible for documenting that the patient was informed of the alternative services available and the consequences of refusal of treatment. If the nurse believes that the refused treatment must be given to prevent serious harm to the patient or others, the nurse should document a factual and objective description of the signs and symptoms supporting this judgment, including information on whether the patient met the following criteria (Payson, Jakacki, 1985):

1. Competent to refuse treatment
2. Oriented to time, place, and person
3. Rational or nonrational in thought processes and judgment
4. Possibly dangerous to self or others, including making verbal or physical threats
5. Experiencing a rapid deterioration in condition

The nurse should also record the patient's response to treatment and document that the physician and nursing supervisor were notified about the situation. Courts usually support the right of healthcare professionals to take action when a patient poses a danger to himself, herself, or others and refuses necessary treatment.

Discharge Against Medical Advice

Releasing a mental health patient when it is reasonably foreseeable that the patient will harm himself, herself, or a third party is another area in which potential liability occurs. All patients who have voluntarily signed themselves into a psychiatric facility have the right to terminate their stay with or without the consent of the attending physician. The following are the only exceptions to this:

- Patients on "legal holds" (72-hour detentions, all legal certifications, and court commitments)
- Patients on conservatorships or with legal guardians
- Minor patients
- Patients with suicidal or homicidal ideations or intent

When a patient requests to leave the hospital against medical advice (AMA), the nurse's actions must be in accordance with the agency's policies and procedures. The patient should complete an AMA questionnaire (if it is used in the facility) before discharge so that the psychiatric nurse can assess the patient's mental status and his or her satisfaction with their hospitalization (Figure 13-2). An AMA statement that defines the patient's responsibility when leaving the hospital AMA must also be signed by the patient (Figure 13-3).

Documenting AMA Procedures

The most important information that the nurse can document in the clinical record at the time of a routine or AMA discharge is that an accurate assessment of the patient's current mental status was performed. Nurses will frequently document that the patient denied suicidal or homicidal behavior at the time of discharge. More extensive documentation must take place. Not only should the nurse document any verbalized threats or acts of violence that occurred during the course of hospitalization, but he or she should also document any direct statements made by the patient at

the time of discharge concerning his or her desire to harm himself, herself, or others. Furthermore, the nurse should document the patient's statements including intentions, plans, and motives. Doing this will protect the nurse if an injury that results in a lawsuit should occur in the future. In a court of law, retrospectively defining the patient's state of mind at the time of discharge without thorough documentation and direct quotes is difficult.

In the following case the patient was discharged from a hospital despite the patient's history of violent behavior, resulting in liability caused by the death of a third party:

A patient had been committed to state mental hospitals on 11 prior occasions. He had a history of aggressive, hostile behavior. He had been previously convicted for numerous crimes, including voluntary manslaughter (as a consequence of his beating a man's head against the sidewalk until the man died).

The man was again admitted for being dangerous to others. Two months later he was discharged because he was responding well to medication and was not perceived to be a threat or danger to others. However, it was indicated that the patient should be supervised after his release from the hospital. Documentation included the fact that his history and identified stressors could cause a crisis of violence in the community.

The patient was discharged, and 2 months later, he hit a man with a fence post, killing him. The plaintiff (the decedent's representative) sued the state for releasing the patient from the hospital when they knew (or should have known) that he was violent or dangerous to others. The commission found this breach of duty to be the proximate cause of the decedent's death because it was reasonably foreseeable that, if released, the patient would harm someone. The plaintiff was awarded $100,000 (*Psychiatrist's release from hospital of patient to stand trial*, 1996).

Documenting in the clinical record that the man's history and identified stressors might cause a crisis of violence and dangerousness in the community and then discharging him in disregard of this assessment is grossly negligent. The hospital had a duty to exercise reasonable care for the protection of third parties from injury by this patient. Consider the following case:

A 38-year-old man was voluntarily admitted to a psychiatric facility with a history of suicidal ideations. He was given lithium and placed on a 24-hour suicide watch. After 5 days he voluntarily discharged himself. Within 12 to 18 hours after discharge he hung himself. His minor children claimed that the decedent was never correctly treated for his suicidal ideations and that he was given drugs for manic depression instead of depression. The defendants denied any negligence, contending that they could not legally hold him after he had asked to be voluntarily discharged. The jury returned a $75,000 verdict for each of the two children (Laska, 1997c).

Charter Behavioral Health System
Of _____
Facility Name

AMA QUESTIONNAIRE

PATIENT NAME: _____ UNIT: _____ DATE: _____

DATE OF ADMISSION: _____ DATE OF REQUEST FOR D/C: _____

TIME OF ADMISSION: _____ TIME OF REQUEST FOR D/C: _____

What was your initial impression of the hospital? _____
_____

Did you expect to participate in the <u>Adult Services Treatment Program</u>? _____

How long did you expect to stay in the hospital? _____

How did your expectations match with your experience in the hospital? _____
_____

What did you hope to gain from your treatment program? _____
_____

How long did you expect it to take to resolve your issues and meet your therapy goals? _____
_____

What are your reasons for requesting discharge? _____
_____
_____

Please describe your level of satisfaction in the following areas:

PHYSICIAN: _____

NURSING STAFF: _____

COUNSELORS: _____

INTAKE: _____

FAMILY THERAPISTS: _____

Please indicate those staff member who offered assistance to you.
_____
_____

What do you think should have happened to assist you that has not occurred at this time? _____
_____
_____

What recommendations do you have that will assist Charter Behavioral Health System of AZ in improving the overall care of its patients? _____
_____
_____
_____

THANK YOU FOR YOUR RESPONSE.

(Do not maintain as part of record.)

Figure 13-2 AMA questionnaire. (Courtesy Charter Behavioral Health System, Chandler, Ariz.)

REQUEST FOR DISCHARGE BY VOLUNTARY PATIENT OR REPRESENTATIVE

REASON FOR REQUEST _____   PATIENT INFORMATION

_____   _____

_____   _____

To: _____   _____
                        Physician

Through: Physician or Registered Nurse

    I hereby request discharge from CHARTER HOSPITAL. I understand and agree that if I am discharged against the advice of my attending physician, I release the doctor, the hospital, and hospital staff from responsibility for any ill effects, loss or injury which may result from my early discharge.

_____ _____ , 19 __   _____ _____ , 19 __
Signature of Patient   Witness

                             Time   Title   Time

[Request may be made by someone other than Patient]

I hereby request the discharge of _____ . I understand and agree that if patient is discharged
                                        Patient
against the advice of the attending physician, I relieve the doctor, the hospital, and hospital staff from any responsibility for any ill effects, loss or injury which may result from early discharge.

_____ _____ , 19 __   _____ _____ , 19 __
Name of Person   Witness

_____   _____
Relationship   Time   Title   Time

If this request is made by someone other than the patient or the patient's legal guardian, the patient must show agreement by signing above before being discharged.

I withdraw my request for discharge.

_____ _____ , 19 __   _____ _____ , 19 __
Signature of patient   Witness

_____   _____
Signature if other than patient   Time   Title   Time

☐ **Discharge is recommended.**

☐ **Discharge is not recommended** for the following reason(s): _____

_____

_____

_____

☐ **Discharge Against Medical Advice (AMA)** _____

☐ **Involuntary hospitalization** _____

                                                 _____ , 19 __
CHARTER STAFF ACKNOWLEDGEMENT   Attending Physician

For AMA discharge

The undersigned recognizes that the requested discharge is against the advice and judgment of the staff and physicians of CHARTER HOSPITAL and that the staff and physicians believe this patient could benefit from continued treatment. Leaving the hospital is **NOT** in the best interest of the patient. I, the undersigned, do hereby fully and completely release the physicians, the hospital, and all hospital staff from responsibility for any ill effects, loss, or injury which may result resulting from the patient's early discharge.

_____ _____ , 19 __   Address of Witness _____
Patient Signature

_____ _____ , 19 __   _____
Parent or Guardian, if Applicable

_____ _____ , 19 __
Witness (Responsible Friend or Relative, if available)

CHART

Figure 13-3   Request for discharge by voluntary patient. (Courtesy Charter Behavioral Health System, Chandler, Ariz.)

When the patient requests to leave AMA, the nursing staff must adhere to the following steps:

1. Assess the patient's legal and mental status.
2. Notify the patient's attending physician and advise him or her of the following:
   - Patient's request for discharge
   - Patient's reason (as stated by the patient)
   - Assessment of the patient's current mental and physical condition
   - Any other information pertinent to the request

If the physician gives an order to discharge the patient AMA, process the order according to the agency's policies and procedures, as shown in the following steps:

1. Instruct the patient to read, complete, and sign the AMA statement and AMA questionnaire form.
2. Clearly document the entire incident in a discharge summary in the patient's clinical record.
3. Complete all discharge procedures.
4. Notify the admissions office, nursing supervisor, and administrator.
5. Complete an incident report.

Elopement

During hospitalization, elopement is always a risk, particularly if the patient has a history of runaway behavior. Healthcare facilities provide a treatment structure that can exert a continuous stressful force, and the urge to leave is often strong. A patient who leaves the hospital without staff permission is said to have eloped. Risks are involved when a patient elopes, including a physical risk to the patient and a legal risk to the hospital.

If a patient is missing, the nurse should attempt to locate the patient within the facility; then he or she should notify the supervisor, physician, and police, if indicated, documenting these actions when completed. When a patient is missing, the consequences may be serious, depending on the condition of the escapee. The police are usually notified if the patient is at risk for harming himself, herself, or others or has left the facility with medical devices in place, such as a heparin lock. The consequences of leaving AMA can be particularly severe when the patient is confused. Lawsuits are commonly initiated when a patient is injured or dies of exposure after leaving undetected. Serious injury or death that occurs after elopement from a hospital is a sentinel event, according to the Joint Commission. This requires the organization to make a thorough investigation of the events surrounding the elopment (see Chapter 6 for more information).

The following two cases demonstrate the potential legal consequences that can occur when a patient elopes:

A 36-year-old man who was being treated for schizophrenia at a mental health center was given a ½-hour grounds pass. However, he did not return, and he was found later that night—dead as a result of alcohol intoxication. The plaintiff alleged that the defendant was negligent in issuing the pass that allowed the man to escape. The jury returned a verdict for $459,130 (Laska, 1997d).

A 43-year-old Korean anesthesiologist was admitted to a psychiatric clinic with a history of depression, having recently attempted suicide by hanging himself in his bathroom. The man was diagnosed with major affective disorder, was depressed, had a high anxiety level with agitation, guilty and pessimistic ruminations, and suicidal ideation. The physician did not admit him to a locked unit, but instead assigned the man to an open unit where patients had various dining and ground privileges. His roommate reportedly saw him at 5:00 PM on the day of admission, and that was the last time he was ever seen. The nurse did not learn of his disappearance until she returned from dinner at 8:00 PM. The nurse called the supervisor, and a search of all units and rooms was conducted. A search was subsequently undertaken by the police, including the use of search dogs and helicopters, which did not reveal any trace of the man. The man disappeared from the clinic within 6 hours after his admission and was never found.

After an Order of the Court declaring the man to be dead in accordance with New Jersey, his widow brought suit against the psychiatric clinic. The jury found that the nurse had been negligent in her deviation from accepted nursing standards. The jury found the clinic to be negligent in that other members of its nursing staff also deviated from accepted nursing standards (Tammelleo, September, 1996). This case was appealed and retried in 1997, with a second jury also providing a verdict of negligence.

Nurses must adhere to the agency's high-risk policies and procedures. Nursing standards of practice dictate that the nurse must assist in maintaining a safe environment and must ensure resolution of any safety problems that occur during the shift.

Many psychiatric healthcare agencies have instituted an elopement precaution flowsheet to better monitor the whereabouts of the patient. Staff members are required to monitor the location of the patient once every 15 or 30 minutes, depending on the physician order. Adhering to the agency's high-risk policies is demonstrated by the completion of this required documentation. Progress notes should indicate the reason for such precautions, that the patient was informed of these precautions, and that an assessment of the patient's mental status was performed. If a patient does elope, accurate documentation is essential. Many lawsuits can be averted if the facility staff prevents elopement and takes prompt action to locate the patient when it does occur. Key documentation points related to elopement are shown in Box 13-3.

MEDICAL MANAGEMENT OF THE PSYCHIATRIC PATIENT

A nurse can be held liable if a medical condition is overlooked or neglected during a patient's psychiatric stay. The psychiatric nurse is often primarily focused on the

---

Box 13-3

Procedures for Managing and Documenting an Elopement

- Document that the patient had been adequately monitored, as demonstrated by the completion of the elopment precaution flowsheet.
- Document the time and location where the patient was last seen.
- Document the patient's mental and physical status at the time of the disappearance.
- Document that a room-to-room search was completed.
- Notify the physician.
- Notify family members who might know the patient's whereabouts.
- Notify the police if the patient is potentially harmful to himself, herself, or others. Follow the agency's policy for notifying the police, and document accordingly in the clinical record.
- Follow hospital policy for notifying the nursing supervisor and administrator.
- Complete an incident report.

---

patient's mental status, and the patient's medical status becomes secondary. Psychiatric patients often have medical problems that require assessment and intervention. Psychiatric treatment should not interfere with medical management. Symptoms of medical conditions should be clearly documented at the time of admission and throughout hospitalization. The nursing assessment should include both past and current psychiatric and medical issues.

Nursing Physical Assessment

The medial assessment is an integral part of the assessment portion of the nursing process; it includes skillful collection of subjective and objective data during the admission process.

Proficiency in performing the physical assessment increases the nurse's ability to make effective decisions in diagnosing, planning, implementing, and evaluating the patient's nursing care. Pertinent information from the past should be correlated to actual or potential medical problems of the patient.

The physical assessment should be completed on a nursing assessment form, as dictated by the agency, within the first 24 hours of admission. The problem list should also include any identified medical problems discovered at the time of admission. The nursing care plan includes any medical problems and appropriate interventions for each problem. The nursing progress notes must reflect that these interventions were implemented and should include the patient's response to these interventions.

The nurse should notify the physician at the time of admission or at any time during the patient's hospitalization if a patient is experiencing symptoms of a medical condition. The nurse should also document that the physician was notified. (Doing so can only protect the nurse from any future repercussions.)

Documenting Medical Findings

When documenting medical findings, consider the following steps:

1. Document the problem and symptoms clearly. Use direct quotes for clarity.
2. Document the date and time.
3. Notify the attending physician.
4. Document all appropriate interventions.
5. Initiate any medical progress, flowsheets, as dictated by agency's policies and procedures, and document their use.
6. Document the patient's response to interventions.
7. Document follow-up and any further recommendations.

The nurse must be able to perform an accurate physical assessment and evaluation. The psychiatric nurse must be skilled in determining whether the patient's complaints and symptoms are medical or psychiatric in nature. The following two cases demonstrate the importance of a proper medical assessment:

A 42-year-old woman was admitted to a psychiatric facility. The woman was recently divorced, and she was admitted for depression and anxiety. The woman was compliant and passive during the admission process. She had no history of suicide or violence.

Several days after her admission, the woman became belligerent and thought she heard doctors outside her door plotting to get rid of her. She refused to eat because she believed the food was poisoned. Her daughter denied that the patient had any previous similar behavior. The nurse did not review the woman's chart, but she did notify the physician about the patient's behavior. The woman was placed in seclusion for safety and medicated according to the physician orders.

Laboratory studies had been completed several times during the course of her hospitalization. The following day, her clinical record was reviewed, and it was discovered that the laboratory studies had revealed a BUN level of 56, which accounted for the increasing confusion and belligerence (anecdotal report).

A 62-year-old man who was hospitalized had a history of insulin-dependent diabetes mellitus for over 30 years. A standing order was in place authorizing the nursing staff to draw blood for the purposes of monitoring his blood sugar.

The daughter requested on more than one occasion that her father's insulin level be checked because his behavior indicated to her that something was wrong with his blood-sugar level. The nurses failed to monitor the man's blood sugar, and the man died.

The daughter maintained that her concerns about the nurses' failure to monitor her father's blood sugar were reported to the nurses several times. The daughter claimed that the nurses failed to act upon her requests. The court found that the daughter could not be overlooked in view of her claim that she recognized a blood-sugar problem. Her recognition of the problem was based on her personal observation of her father and his diabetic condition over the course of many years. The nurses' failure to monitor the man's blood sugar resulted in a suit against the nurses and the hospital that employed them (Tammelleo, 1995).

The nurses deviated from the usual and accepted standards of nursing care by failing to monitor the patient's blood sugar. In this case the nurses had clear knowledge of the patient's history of diabetes. The medical management of this patient was neglected by the nursing personnel. Nurses should listen to reasonable requests from family members who, in many cases, may be familiar with symptoms exhibited by patients.

Although this incident occurred in a medical unit, the psychiatric nurse should be advised to pay close attention. Psychiatric agencies frequently admit patients with medical problems, such as diabetes. The psychiatric nurse must be knowledgeable in both medical and psychiatric case management.

Chemical Withdrawal

Drug abuse involves the use of drugs for purposes other than legitimate medical reasons. The clinical manifestations may vary from one drug to another, but the underlying principles of nursing management are essentially the same.

Psychiatric facilities commonly provide treatment for patients with substance abuse problems. The standard of care, as determined by the clinical agency, requires the patient to receive individual pharmacologic treatment during the health maintenance, withdrawal, and recovery process. The nurse should use his or her knowledge of the signs and symptoms of substance abuse, withdrawal, and medication to guide the nursing process. Medical problems commonly coexist with the addiction disorder. The nurse should use this knowledge when monitoring the patient's care.

Many agencies use a chemical withdrawal assessment flowsheet to monitor the patient's symptoms during the withdrawal process. The flowsheet identifies medical symptoms associated with detoxification and allows the nurse to grade the severity of physical symptoms on a scale from 0 to 4. A section is often present on this flowsheet to document the patient's vital signs and medications. The chemical withdrawal assessment flowsheet should be completed once every 4 hours or as ordered until it is discontinued by the physician.

The following documentation tips relate to charting signs and symptoms of chemical withdrawal:

1. Document vital signs according to agency policy.

2. Contact the physician or administer medication as needed according to the agency's policies and procedures, for a blood pressure over 140/90, a pulse over 100 beats per minute, a temperature over 99.0° F, and a chemical withdrawal assessment score of 3 or above.

3. Document the results of the chemical withdrawal assessment flowsheet in the clinical record.

4. Chart all signs and symptoms of detoxification.

5. Document all medications administered and the patient's response. Librium (chlordiazepoxide) is frequently given in decreasing doses because of its sedating and anticonvulsant effect during detoxification.

6. Chart all details when the physician is notified that the patient is not responding to the current medical regimen, including any changes in orders.

7. Note the patient's sleep patterns and nutritional patterns.

8. Document any abnormal laboratory findings. Notify the physician of the abnormal results, and document that this was done.

Failure to adequately monitor a patient during withdrawal can result in a life-threatening situation, as shown in the following case.

A 36-year-old Native-American woman was admitted to a psychiatric facility for chemical dependency. She had an extensive history of alcohol abuse. The physician ordered Librium (chlordiazepoxide) on a regular schedule and as needed. The nursing staff initiated a chemical withdrawal assessment flowsheet and administered Librium according to the physician's orders. On the night in question the woman began to experience acute withdrawal symptoms, which progressed into the delirium tremors. The woman was placed in four-point restraints and transferred to the medical-surgical unit. The medical-surgical nurses kept the woman in the four-point restraints for 2 days without any range of motion to the extremities. The woman sustained severe contractures.

When the woman's clinical record was reviewed, it was noted that the nurse on the psychiatric floor had neglected to assess the woman because the chemical withdrawal assessment had not been completed every 4 hours. However, the chart reflected that the vital signs had been completed every 4 hours, and they indicated that the woman was in acute withdrawal. The nurses administered the regularly scheduled doses of Librium but no additional Librium had been given even though it was needed (anecdotal report).

This case presents compelling evidence that the nurses deviated from the accepted standards of nursing care by failing to adequately monitor the patient. The nurses made two errors in nursing judgment: (1) The nurses on the psychiatric floor did not properly monitor the woman's medical complications associated with the detoxification phase of her treatment, and (2) the medical-surgical nurses neglected to provide the necessary nursing care for a patient in restraints. It was later discovered that the medical-surgical nurses were not familiar with the hospital's protocol for the use of restraints.

Extrapyramidal Side Effects

Among the legal and ethical issues confronting nurses dealing with mentally ill patients are the use of neuroleptic medications and the management of their side effects. Standards of practice require that the nurse use professional judgment when administering prescribed treatments and medications. The nurse is responsible for knowing about neuroleptic medications, side effects, and toxic symptoms.

Extrapyramidal side effects (EPS) are common in patients receiving neuroleptic medications. These side effects are often overlooked and improperly assessed. They can be extremely uncomfortable and frightening to the patient. The nurse must be proactive in identifying and managing such side effects. The psychiatric nurse can be held liable if the patient is not assessed and monitored properly. Life-threatening medical complications can arise if the patient experiencing EPS is not treated in a quick, safe manner.

Documenting EPS

The Abnormal Involuntary Movement Scale (AIMS) is a common tool in psychiatric facilities. The AIMS test is a form used for recognizing acute EPS that lists all extrapyramidal side effects. The nurse should assess the patient once every shift and check off whether extrapyramidal side effects are present or absent. Some AIMS tests use a scale from 1 to 4. The nurse can then grade the severity of the symptoms. The patient's pulse and blood pressure should also be recorded on the AIMS form. The AIMS test may be kept with the medication administration record, and it becomes a part of the patient's legal record.

The nurse should document in the clinical record the results of the AIMS test and any antiparkinsonian drugs administered to counteract EPS. The accepted standard of nursing practice involves rapid administration of antiparkinsonian medications to quickly decrease symptoms.

If the patient does not respond to the medication, notify the physician. Document the patient's symptoms, response to the antiparkinsonian agents, and that the physician was notified (Figure 13-4).

Abnormal Laboratory Values

The psychiatric nurse should be constantly monitoring blood levels in patients who are receiving psychiatric medications. Blood levels should be frequently drawn to determine whether the medication is in a low, therapeutic, or toxic range and whether the dosage should be adjusted.

Laboratory test results often arrive when the physician is not present. Laboratory personnel commonly ask for and document the name of the nurse who was notified of an important abnormal laboratory test value. The psychiatric nurse must evaluate laboratory test results for toxic drug levels and notify the physician of these abnormalities. Document in the clinical record that the physician was notified and include any changes in orders.

In the following case a critically abnormal blood-test value went unnoticed, which led to permanent hospitalization of the patient in a psychiatric hospital:

> A 38-year-old woman with chronic manic-depressive disorder was a resident of an adult congregate living facility. She had been dependent on lithium for several years, and at one point she became groggy and sleepy, had slurred speech, and was mumbling. The plaintiff claimed that these were signs of lithium overdose. The lithium level drawn at the local mental health center was 3.5 (the maximum recommended level is 1.5). The plaintiff continued to receive lithium and went into a coma. She was left with permanent physical problems and an exacerbation in mental disability. She was confined to a state hospital. A $1,650,000 settlement was reached with the mental health facility contributing $750,000 and the adult group living facility providing $900,000 (Laska, 1993b).

The nursing staff was negligent in monitoring this woman's lithium level, which is considered a standard practice in psychiatric facilities. The nursing personnel should have been monitoring her lithium level, withheld her lithium, and ensured that the physician received this information.

Infection

Hospitalization increases a patient's contact with others who might have infections. Psychiatric patients are vulnerable to infections as a result of their decreased ability and desire to care for themselves. The nursing staff should be alert, should assess patients for infection, and should provide appropriate treatment. Nursing standards of practice dictate that the nurse should utilize appropriate nursing measures for infection control as exhibited by documentation on infection control reports and in daily nursing practice.

Many psychiatric facilities recognize the potential for infection and have therefore instituted an infection progress flowsheet (Figure 13-5). The flowsheet provides for accurate monitoring of the patient's symptoms and should be completed daily by the nurse. The nurse should document the type of infection, temperature, pain, swelling, inflammation, and exudate. A section for comments should be available to document any unusual findings or abnormal laboratory reports. The nurse may also be involved in completing an infection control report and notifying the appropriate departments. Figure 13-6 lists important data to be documented when an infection occurs.

Documenting an Infection

The nurse should document the following:

- Signs and symptoms
- That an infection control report was completed and an

Text continued on p. 304

Charter Behavioral Health Systems

AIMS EXAMINATION PROCEDURE

Patient Identification

DATE: _____

Prior to assessment, observe patient unobtrusively at rest (i.e.: in dayroom). Prior to assessment, ask whether there is anything in his / her mouth (i.e.: candy, gum) and if there is, ask them to remove it. *Note if Patient has False Teeth.*

0 = None 1 - Minimal 2 = Mild 3 = Moderate 4 = Severe	0	1	2	3	4
EXTREMITY MOVEMENTS — Ask patient to stand. (Observe in profile, observe all body areas facing patient). Have patient walk a few paces, turn and walk back. (Observe hand and gait.) Ask patient to extend both arms outstretched in front with palms down (observe trunk, legs and mouth). Have patient sit on chair with hands on knees, legs, slightly apart and feet flat on floor (look at entire body for movements). Ask patient to sit with hands unsupported (observe hands and other body areas.) Flex and extend patient's left and right arms (one at a time).					
Upper (arms, wrist, hands, fingers) include abortic movements (i.e.: rapid, objectively purposeless, irregular, spontaneous), athetoid movements (i.e.: slow, irregular, complex serpentine). Do not include tremor (i.e.: repetitive, regular rhythmic).					
Lower (legs, knees, ankles, toes) e.g.: lateral knee movement, foot tapping, heel dropping, foot squirming, inversion and eversion of foot.					
Trunk Movement (neck, shoulders, hips) e.g.: rocking, shrugging, twisting, squirming, pelvic gyration.					
0 = None 1 - Minimal 2 = Mild 3 = Moderate 4 = Severe	0	1	2	3	4
FACIAL AND ORAL MOVEMENTS — Ask patient to open mouth (observe tongue at rest within mouth). Do this twice. Ask patient to protrude tongue (observe abnormalities of tongue movement). Do this twice. Ask patient to tap thumb with each finger as rapidly as possible for 10 - 15 seconds separately with right hand, then with left hand (observe facial and leg movement).					
Muscles of Facial Expression, e.g.: movements of forehead, eyebrow, blinking, grimacing.					
Lips and Prioral Area, e.g.: puckering, smacking, sucking.					
Jaw, e.g.: biting, clenching, chewing, mouth opening lateral movement.					
Tongue (rate only increase in movement both in and out of mouth, not ability to sustain movement).					
0 = None 1 - Minimal 2 = Mild 3 = Moderate 4 = Severe	0	1	2	3	4
GLOBAL JUDGEMENTS — Severity of abnormal movements.					
Incapacitation due to abnormal movements.					
0 = None, Normal 1 = Aware, No Distress 2 = Aware, Mild Distress 3 = Aware, Moderate Distress 4 = Aware, Severe Distress	0	1	2	3	4
Patient's awareness of abnormal movements (rate only patient's report).					

Does the result of the AIMS require physician review? ☐ No ☐ Yes If Yes: Physician Signature:_____ Date/Time:_____

If yes, is there any further action required by R.N.? _____

_____

_____

Signature:_____ Date / Time: _____

ANY SCORE OF 1 OR MORE ON ANY ONE ITEM REQUIRES A PHYSICIAN REVIEW.

Figure 13-4 Abnormal involuntary movement scale. (Courtesy Charter Behavioral Health System, Chandler, Ariz.)

Charter Behavioral Health System

Of _____
  Facility Name

S.O.C. AND TREATMENT PLAN

TITLE: INFECTION TRANSMISSION, POTENTIAL FOR

Often associated with any infectious or contagious disease/condition

ADDRESSOGRAPH

Initiation: _____ R.N.

Date: _____

Renewal: _____ R.N.

Date: _____

Codes: V/D = Verbalizes/Demonstrates
  θ = Absence of

Type of infection: _____

I. GOALS:

Long term - patient will be free of the infectious disease process.

Short term - patient will demonstrate understanding of relationship between proper hygiene and infection; patient will understand and demonstrate methods to prevent the spread of infection.

II. PRESENTING S & S:

0. None
1. Elevated TPR
2. Swelling/redness/warmth of site
3. Purulent drainage/productive cough
4. Rash
5. Foul odor of site
6. Abnormal lab results
7. C/O burning/itching/pain
8. Fatigue/malaise
9. Diarrhea/vomiting
10. _____
11. _____

II.

DATE											
AM											
Code											
Initial											
PM											
Code											
Initial											
NOC											
Code											
Initial											

III. NURSING INTERVENTIONS:

1. Reassess potential for infection transmission
2. Cooling comfort measures (eg. tepid bath, sitz bath)
3. Encourage fluids
4. Observe and monitor for relief/exacerbation of symptoms
5. Administer antibiotics/apply topical antibiotics per M.D.
6. Diet per M.D./nsg discretion
7. Clean site and apply dressing per M.D./nsg discretion
8. Transport pt for E.R. evaluation per M.D.
9. Precautions/isolation per M.D./hospital polilcy
10. _____
11. _____

III.

DATE											
Time											
Code											
Initial											
Time											
Code											
Initial											
Time											
Code											
Initial											
Time											
Code											
Initial											
Time											
Code											
Initial											

IV. DAILY OBSERVATION OF PROGRESS OF INFECTION:

Date								
Temperature								
Swelling								
Inflammation								
Exudate								

Figure 13-5 Infection transmission flowsheet. (Courtesy Charter Behavioral Health System, Chandler, Ariz.)

Continued

V. PATIENT TEACHING
(specific to infection):

ITEM TAUGHT

	Method/Outcome-Initial	Date												Comments
1. Infection/Disease	A-1 KT	/	/	/	/	/	/	/	/	/	/			
2. Preventative Measures														
3. Medications														
4. _____														
5. _____														
6. _____														

Teaching Method:
A - verbal
B - demonstration
C - written material
D - audio/visual

Patient/Family Outcome:
1) able to state full knowledge
2) able to state some knowledge
3) unable to state knowledge
4) able to demonstrate full skill
5) able to demonstrate some skill
6) unable to show skill

VI. RESOLUTION:
1. Normal TPR
2. Lab results within normal limits
3. No signs/symptoms of infection

Resolution: _____ R.N.

Date: _____

INITIAL	RN SIGNATURE	INITIAL	RN SIGNATURE

NURSING STADARDS OF CARE/REASSESSMENT
FOR INFECTION TRANSMISSION, POTENTIAL

Figure 13-5, cont'd   Infection transmission flowsheet. (Courtesy Charter Behavioral Health System, Chandler, Ariz.)

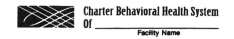

Charter Behavioral Health System
Of _____
Facility Name

REPORT OF PATIENT WITH
SUSPECTED INFECTION

_____
PATIENT ID

Patient Name _____ Room _____ Age _____ Sex _____

Date of Admission _____ Med. Record # _____ Attending M.D. _____

Indication(s) for RX _____

Site of suspected infection _____ Date of Culture _____

Antibiotic Name/Dosage _____ None ____ Start date _____

    Ordering M.D. _____ Admitted with infection? ☐ Yes ☐ No

CHECK ALL THAT APPLY

☐ A. CONTINUOUS OR INTERMITTENT FEVER OF 100.4 ON ANY 2 CONSECUTIVE DAYS.

☐ B. WBC OF OVER 12,000.

☐ C. UPPER RESPIRATORY OR OTHER BODY AREA WITH SUGGESTED EVIDENCE OF INFECTION OR INFILTRATE.

☐ D. USE OF ANTIBIOTIC FOR MORE THAN 72 HOURS.

☐ E. REDNESS, SWELLING OR PRURULENT DRAINAGE FROM SITE. CULTURE MAY BE NEGATIVE.

☐ F. PULOMARY RALES, DULLNESS TO PERCUSSION.

☐ G. ANY ABNORMAL BODY DISCHARGE, INCLUDING 3 OR MORE STOOLS/DAY FOR 2 DAYS.

☐ H. ORAL LESIONS, VISICLES, CORYZA OR OTTIS MEDIA.

☐ I. ADMISSION URINE WITH 10 OR MORE WBC AND MODERATE NUMBER OF BACTERIA.

☐ J. PHYSICIAN'S DIAGNOSIS OF INFECTION.

☐ K. OTHER: _____

Reporting Nurse _____ Date _____ M.D. notified ☐ Yes ☐ No

Culture Result _____ Sensitive to Antibiotic ☐ Yes ☐ No

If culture negative, was RX D/Cd? ☐ Yes ☐ No   Continued use documented ☐ Yes ☐ No

Response to therapy documented by M.D.? ☐ Yes ☐ No   By Nurse? ☐ Yes ☐ No

Adverse Reaction ☐ Yes ☐ No (If yes, specify) _____

Reported to Public Health ☐ Yes ☐ No   Committee Review Date: _____

Recommendation/Comments _____

_____

Nosocomial ☐ Yes ☐ No   Final Synopsis/Resolution (Include lab slips) _____

_____

_____   _____
INFECTION CONTROL NURSE   COMMITTEE CHAIRPERSON

WHITE — CHART   YELLOW — MAR BOOK

Figure 13-6 Report for patient with suspected infection. (Courtesy Charter Behavioral Health System, Chandler, Ariz.)

infection progress flowsheet (if used in the facility) was initiated

- Medications ordered for the infection and the patient's response
- Vital signs
- Any adverse effects, and that the physician was notified of these
- Subjective statements from the patient
- Results of cultures and abnormal laboratory findings

SUMMARY

This chapter presents some of the critical issues that influence psychiatric nursing documentation. Psychiatric nurses often encounter difficulties in meeting the regulatory agency's requirements for documentation and patient care. With a knowledge of common liability problems, the nurse can sharpen his or her charting skills that are specific to these issues.

Nurses must keep in mind that patients have ethical and legal rights, and that these rights can be easily violated. Nursing practice must be guided by the policies and procedures set forth by their agency and by the standards of psychiatric nursing practice. Effective documentation is essential to minimize the risks of liability.

HOME CARE DOCUMENTATION

Donna Ambler Peters, RN, PhD, FAAN

Home care is the fastest growing sector in health care today, and it can be expected to continue to grow until at least 2030, when the aged population will peak at 64.3 million people age 65 and older (Woerner, Donnelly, Edwards, 1993). Several other factors contribute to this exceptional growth rate, including the following: (1) improved medical technology, which has increased life expectancy and moved the care of sicker patients into the home; (2) patients' preference to have care provided in their own homes; and (3) demands from reimbursement sources that healthcare providers reduce costs while expanding patient access to services in a wide variety of settings. As a result, home health agencies are under significant pressure to provide efficient, high-quality, cost-effective care to a growing number of clients.

The single biggest problem when providing this type of care is the excessive time nurses spend documenting. Overall, documentation accounts for as much as 50% of home care nursing time (Braunstein, 1993). A survey of nine different agencies across the country was done by the Community Health Accreditation Program (CHAP) through their "In Search of Excellence in Home Care Project." The findings revealed that 44.3% of the staff responding either agreed (23.1%) or strongly agreed (21.2%) that they spend more time completing paperwork than they do giving care. Only 68.7% felt that the paperwork they had to do was manageable. The administrators and supervisors in these same agencies agreed with their staff. Of the managers responding, 45.6% either agreed (32.4%) or strongly agreed (13.2%) that employees in patient-care positions in their agencies were spending more time on paperwork than on patient care.

This chapter describes the changing documentation needs in home care. Furthermore, it discusses the requirements for documentation as identified by professional and regulatory standards, the scope of care, and fiscal and legal imperatives. Finally, it discusses moving to electronic documentation as a way to manage some of the documentation problems that home care presents.

CHANGING DOCUMENTATION NEEDS

The purpose of documentation in home care traditionally has been to establish both a need for services and a legal record, and to refresh a clinician's memory about what was done for the client. Documentation was done manually usually in narrative form, listing fragmented tasks. However, handwriting can sometimes be illegible, gaps can occur in the recording of the services provided, and the same data can be entered in several places on the chart by various disciplines. Definitions of terms and abbreviations are often not standardized, leaving them open to individual interpretation and misinterpretation.

However, because of the pressure to become more efficient in providing services and the escalation in the accountability to consumers and payers of home care, documentation in home care has become a decision-making and informational tool—not just a diary for documenting patient events. Therefore charting must not only contain an accurate reflection of nursing interventions, but also provide for the effective tracking of all elements in the provision of care and the analysis of outcomes. The reason for this imperative is the nature of home care and the home care industry, as discussed in the following points:

1. Care takes place in the patient's home and therefore is not witnessed by anyone except those rendering the care, the patient, and perhaps the patient's family. For others to observe what takes place is almost impossible; therefore the only way to know what has occurred is to read about it in the chart.
2. The chart is the foundation of evidenced-based care and the agency's quality management program; the

justification for reimbursement to the agency from Medicare, Medicaid, and managed care organizations; and the basis of legal protection. Today an agency must be able to track interventions and analyze results to continue to improve the level of care. Furthermore, without proper documentation regarding the seriousness of a patient's condition, patient and family expectations, the nursing interventions, the patient's reactions to the interventions, and the results of the interventions, an agency has no recourse against reimbursement denials that lead to financial losses. The agency and care provider may also have little recourse against legal suits.

3. Because the chart is the only way to identify the care rendered in the home, incomplete or inaccurate charting may distort the overall picture of the problems that were addressed, the interventions used, and the patient's response. The need for a comprehensive picture includes preventive care as well as any skilled treatments that are rendered.

4. Comprehensive charting is required for accurate communication and continuity of care. The home care team consists of nurses, therapists, aides, social workers, nutritionists, and physicians. These people are seldom present in the home at the same time. Other service agencies, particularly social service agencies, such as Meals on Wheels or other adult care services, provide home care. The need for communication and continuity of care continues to become more important as the home care industry expands and the delivery of services becomes more fragmented. For example, the use of per diem nurses and the rotation of staff for weekend and holiday coverage are recent trends that increase the number of nurses caring for a patient. Nurses, not physicians, are the case managers; therefore the nurse is the one responsible for coordinating the patient's care. Thus the nurse's documented word becomes the pivotal factor in maintaining continuity of care and provides evidence of the communication of significant clinical information to the physician.

INFLUENCES ON HOME CARE DOCUMENTATION

Documentation related to the clinical care of the patient at home is affected by professional and regulatory standards, the scope of care, patient input, the chosen data sets used, fiscal requirements, and legal imperatives.

Professional and Regulatory Standards

Professional standards define professional competency and, as such, are one way that the quality of nursing practice can be measured. In 1986, the American Nurses' Association (ANA) developed standards specifically for home health nursing based on the nursing process (ANA, 1986). There are also two major accrediting bodies that have published standards relevant to a home health agency's operation: the CHAP (1993) and the Joint Commission for the Accreditation of Healthcare Organizations. These regulatory organizations have similarly addressed specific requirements for documentation. For example, CHAP standards, which were last revised in 1993, require that the clinical record contains the following:

- Reason for service
- Referral source
- Diagnosis and prognosis
- Patient and family data base, including physical, psychosocial, and environmental data
- Contact person in case of emergency or death
- Client problems, plan of treatment, and both short-term and long-term goals
- Safety measures
- Functional limitations
- Physician's name
- Dietary, treatment, and activity orders
- Medication profile
- Evaluation of individual patient outcomes
- Appropriate, current, and signed medical orders
- Consent and authorization forms
- Documentation of interdisciplinary conferences and their outcomes
- Advance directives
- Copies of summaries sent to physician
- Timely clinical notes signed by the individual providing the services

In addition, federal government regulations also influence home care documentation. The Health Care Financing Administration (HCFA), which is responsible for the Medicare Program, is expected to mandate the collection of the Outcome and Assessment Information Set (OASIS) by the end of 1998. OASIS is a data collection tool made up of 89 questions—79 aimed at patient assessment of health and functional status, and 10 related to patient demographics. Box 13-4 provides an example of an OASIS-B question. These OASIS questions will have to be answered regarding all adult patients in home care (Medicare and non-Medicare), except for maternal-child health patients. Measurements will be made at the start of care, after a hospitalization, every 57 to 62 days during agency service, and at the time of discharge. Because OASIS is not a comprehensive assessment instrument, the OASIS questions must be integrated exactly as written into an agency's existing assessment form with duplicate questions removed. OASIS provides a way to collect the same data from all patients so that outcomes can be measured and compared within and across agencies over time.

Box 13-4

MO560 Cognitive Functioning

Patient's current level of alertness, orientation, comprehension, concentration, and immediate memory for simple commands.

0   Alert/oriented, able to focus and shift attention, comprehends and recalls task directions independently

1   Requires prompting (cueing, repetition, reminders) only under stressful or unfamiliar conditions

2   Requires assistance and some direction in specific situations (e.g., on all tasks involving shifting of attention), or consistently requires low-stimulus environment due to distractibility

3   Requires considerable assistance in routine situations; is not alert and oriented or is unable to shift attention and recall directions more than half the time

4   Totally dependent due to disturbances such as constant disorientation, coma, persistent vegetative state, or delirium

---

From Center for Health Services and Policy Research Center, Denver, 1997.

Scope of Care

Professional standards also dictate the scope of required documentation by requiring that a comprehensive plan of care be developed in consultation with the patient and all care providers, and include the following (CHAP, 1993):

- Types of services, supplies, and equipment needed
- Frequency of visits
- Prognosis
- Rehabilitation potential
- Functional limitations
- Mental status
- Activities permitted
- Nutritional requirements
- Medications and treatments
- Procedures to be performed, including amount, frequency, and duration
- Safety measures
- Discharge or referral instructions
- Other items, such as precautions and contraindications

Domains of the Care Plan

In order to be comprehensive, the patient care plan, which is the result of the team input from a case conference, as depicted in Figure 13-7, must include more than just the physiological problems of the patient. These are the most objective, simplest problems to observe, describe, and treat, and the easiest for which to obtain reimbursement. How-

ever, several other areas impact the patient and must be considered to ensure the quality of interventions and outcomes for physical problems. Important aspects to be addressed include the environment, the caregiver, the patient and family attitudes, and the resources needed and available, including patient strengths.

Environment

Documentation of the environment in which care is provided is required to ensure both the quality of care and safety. For example, when an elderly person is using a walker or wheelchair for the first time, knowing whether the toilet facilities are on the same floor as the bedroom is important. If not, a ground-floor room, such as a dining room, can be temporarily converted into a bedroom, and a bedside commode can be used. In this way all basic necessities are on the same floor. Physical adaptations may be required; for example, the width of doorways may not accommodate a wheelchair, or ramps may be needed for stairs leading to entrances. The nurse should document the plans for adaptations and then facilitate their implementation as possible. Safety measures should also be taken, such as removing throw rugs. Other items that should be noted include the following:

- Directions to the home, including the entrance to be used by the nurse
- Pets in the home, including type, number, and where they are housed (e.g., inside the home, in a fenced-in backyard)
- Environmental characteristics, including size of the residence, an assessment of cleanliness and safety, the availability of food, and hazards (e.g., clutter, lack of utilities)

Caregiver

Much of the actual patient care rendered may be done by significant others who may or may not live in the same household. These people may themselves be limited by age, physical disabilities, or time restrictions (e.g., employment). Because patient care may depend on the caregiver's abilities, documentation describing the characteristics of the primary caregiver is required. Notations could include the following:

- Name, address, and telephone number of the primary contact person with whom to arrange care
- Name, address, and telephone number of the primary caregiver (if different from above)
- Name, relationship, address, and telephone number of the nearest responsible relative with whom to make arrangements for cases of emergency
- Caregiver characteristics, including schedule of availability, degree of willingness, emotional stamina, physical ability, and level of understanding or knowledge

Community Nursing Service MULTIDISCIPLINARY CASE CONFERENCE

Signatures present at MDCC:

_____
_____
_____
_____
_____

Client _____
Medical Record Number _____
MDCC Date _____
Recertification Date _____
Start of Care Date _____
Previous Discharges _____
Funding _____
Team/Specialty _____
Case Manager _____
Physician _____
Supervisor _____

Diagnosis _____

SKILLED NURSE
Provider: _____ Visit Frequency: _____
Qualifying Skill: _____
Progress toward goals: _____

New or Continuing Concerns: _____

Treatment Plan: _____

Expected Outcome: _____
_____ Expected Discharge Date: _____

PHYSICAL THERAPY
Provider: _____ Visit Frequency: _____
Qualifying Skill: _____
Progress toward goals: _____

New or Continuing Concerns: _____

Treatment Plan: _____

Expected Outcome: _____
_____ Expected Discharge Date: _____

HOME HEALTH AIDE
Provider: _____ Visit Frequency: _____
Progress toward goals: _____

New or Continuing Concerns: _____

Treatment Plan: _____

Expected Outcome: _____
_____ Expected Discharge Date: _____

MEDICAL SOCIAL WORK
Provider: _____ Visit Frequency: _____
Progres towardgoals: _____

New or continuing Concerns: _____

Treatment Plan: _____

Expected Outcome: _____
_____ Expected Discharge Date: _____

Continued

Figure 13-7 Case conference documentation form. (Courtesy Service and Hospice Community Nursing, Salt Lake City.)

NUTRITION
Provider: _____ Visit Frequency: _____
Progress toward goals: _____

New or Continuing Concerns: _____

Treatment Plan: _____

Expected Outcome: _____
_____ Expected Discharge Date: _____

OCCUPATIONAL THERAPY
Provider: _____ Visit Frequency: _____
Progress toward goals: _____

New or Continuing Concerns: _____

Treatment Plan: _____

Expected Outcome: _____
_____ Expected Discharge Date: _____

SPEECH THERAPY
Provider: _____ Visit Frequency: _____
Progress toward goals: _____

New or Continuing Concerns: _____

Treatment Plan: _____

Expected Outcome: _____
_____ Expected Discharge Date: _____

PHARMACY Provider: _____ Visit Frequency: _____
Progress toward goals: _____

New or Continuing Concerns: _____

Treatment Plan: _____

Expected Outcome: _____
_____ Expected Discharge Date: _____

HOME MEDICAL EQUIPMENT
New or Continuing Concerns: _____

Treatment Plan: _____

Expected Outcome: _____
_____ Expected Discharge Date: _____

SPIRITUAL NEEDS
Provider: _____ Visit Frequency: _____
New or Continuing Concerns: _____

Treatment Plan: _____

Expected Outcome: _____
_____ Expected Discharge Date: _____

PATIENT CARE COORDINATOR _____ signatures present at MDCC
INTAKE _____ signatures present at MDCC
BILLING REPRESENTATIVE _____ signatures present at MDCC
OTHER _____ signatures present at MDCC

TYPE OF CONFERENCE: INITIAL DISCHARGE RECERTIFICATION INTERIM PHONE

Figure 13-7, cont'd Case conference documentation form. (Courtesy Service and Hospice Community Nursing, Salt Lake City.)

Patient and Family Attitudes

The attitudes of the patient, family, and other volunteers assisting in care may affect both the ability of the patient to cope with the situation and his or her motivation to improve. When establishing outcomes, for example, realistic outcomes must be considered in the context of the effort that the patient is willing or able to put forth. The nurse's role is to inform the patient of the pros and cons of the choices available and to support the patient in his or her efforts, regardless of the choice that is made. Documenting the emotional state and attitude of the patient, as well as that of others involved, is important, including the following (Eggland, 1993):

- The degree to which the patient's condition has altered the work schedule, employment, or educational activities of the patient, caregiver, and other family members
- Any family interactions that have changed as a result of the patient's condition, treatment, or care
- Ability of the patient and other family members to adjust to the demands of patient care, and how these demands have changed their lives, even if only temporarily

Patient Strengths and Resources

Successful home care depends on building on existing patient strengths and possibly using additional outside resources, including service and product resources. Using these building blocks is essential; therefore notations in the chart need to include patient strengths, such as the following:

- Support system, including health habits (e.g., exercise, diet)
- Names, addresses, and number of friends and neighbors who can help out if necessary
- Coping behaviors
- Financial status and needs

Notations about patient resources include the following:

- Name, address, and telephone number of the physician and pharmacy
- Name and telephone number of contact person for other special services, such as Meals on Wheels
- Name and telephone number of the patient's medical equipment supplier
- Supplies and equipment needed for care (e.g., ostomy supplies, hospital bed, wheelchair)

Physiological Care

Documentation of physiological care resembles that of other clinical settings and should include appropriate risk screenings for areas such as nutrition and infections. The following list indicates other key information that should be included (Eggland, 1993):

- Vital signs
- Chief complaints of the patient, including related signs and symptoms
- Description of the patient's condition, changes in the patient's condition, additional complaints, and potential complications related to the diagnosis and identified needs
- Treatment, medications, nursing interventions, and expected outcomes
- Patient education, including verbal and written instructions and demonstrations given to the patient and family
- Return demonstrations and verbalization of understanding of the instructions by the patient and family
- Patient outcomes, the response of the patient to treatments, and the reaction of the family

Addressing these areas is consistent with the holistic view of patients maintained by home health nurses. Furthermore, community health nurses define their unit of care as the entire family, not just the patient.

OMAHA CLASSIFICATION SYSTEM

One comprehensive framework for organizing the information in home care is the Omaha Classification System (OCS), which was originally developed by the staff and management of the Visiting Nurse Association of Omaha. It was originally developed by practicing community health nurses for use in community health. The system is composed of three parts, which have been described by Martin and Scheet (1992): (1) the Problem Classification Scheme, (2) the Rating Scale for Outcomes, and (3) the Intervention Scheme.

The Problem Classification Scheme is an orderly, nonexhaustive, mutually exclusive list of nursing diagnoses used by community health practitioners for data collection and problem identification. These diagnoses are organized within the four domains that represent the broad areas of community health practice: environment, psychosocial, physiological, and health behaviors. Each problem is modified with the words "Health Promotion," "Potential," or "Deficit/Impairment/Actual" and is referenced as an individual or family problem. Actual problems are described by signs and symptoms. For example, one problem listed in the physiological domain is: "Consciousness: Impairment"; the signs and symptoms include lethargic, stuporous, unresponsive, and comatose.

The Rating Scale for Outcomes is a five-point Likert Scale that measures patient progress within three concepts: knowledge, behavior, and status. This scale is used with each of the nursing diagnoses in the Problem Scheme to evaluate patient progress at regular time intervals, such as at the time of admission, at the midpoint of treatment, and at the time of discharge. For example, when evaluating

"Consciousness: Impairment" on a scale of 1 to 5 for knowledge, level 1 would be selected when the family cannot recognize change in status and level 5 would be selected when the family understands the current symptoms and anticipates future changes.

The Intervention Scheme is a taxonomy of categories and targets to be used with any diagnosis within the Problem Scheme, and it is helpful in developing plans for successive visits. It is organized into three levels of abstraction. The first level consists of four broad areas that describe community health nursing actions: (1) health teaching, guidance, and counseling; (2) treatments and procedures; (3) case management; and (4) surveillance. The second level consists of targets and objects of nursing actions that serve to further describe interventions (e.g., cardiac care, caretaking, and parenting skills). The third level of the scheme consists of client-specific information that is generated by the nurse or healthcare professional.

Community Health Intensity Rating Scale

One piece missing from the OCS is the determination of nursing intensity (i.e., the amount of resources that will be consumed). This intensity can be determined through the use of the Community Health Intensity Rating Scale (CHIRS), which is a comprehensive assessment form composed of 15 parameters that fully describe the scope of home care services (Peters, 1988). These parameters fall within the same four main domains as the Omaha Problem Scheme: environmental, including the patient's place of residence; psychosocial, including social issues or problems; physiological (i.e., body systems); and health behaviors, which identifies preventative areas and maintains a positive focus by identifying areas of patient strength (e.g., nutrition habits, exercise, screening tests). The parameters in each domain are listed in Table 13-1.

Each parameter contains a number of descriptors that reflect the scope of that particular parameter. For example, the descriptors in the nutrition parameter are prescribed diet, appetite, dietary intake, nutrition support system status, ability to shop for food, ability to prepare meals, and weight. Under each descriptor are several assessment items, each carrying an intensity from 0 to 4. The items under nutritional support system status are as follows: no nutritional support status (0); functional nutritional support system (2); self-care nutritional support system (2); new nutritional support system (3); and problems with the nutritional support system (4). The highest weight for each parameter is chosen as the parameter score. The total of all the parameter scores is the intensity score for the patient at the time of the assessment, and it can range from 0 to 60.

CHIRS scores which incorporate both physiological and nonphysiological patient needs have been found to significantly explain variation in nursing resource consumption in three different studies of home health and public health populations (Peters, 1988; Hays, 1992; Hays, 1995). At the University of Nebraska Medical Center College of Nursing, CHIRS has been used to provide a structure for community health patient assessments. Using the scores generated by CHIRS, students assess whether there were changes in patient intensity between the rating done at the beginning of the semester and at the end of the semester, facilitating a discussion of the impact of care on patient status. A companion tool, the School Health Intensity Rating Scale (SHIRS), is currently being developed for use in school health nursing (Burt CJ, Beetem MN, Iverson C et al, 1996).

Patient Input

Nursing care has always been patient focused. However, because the issues in home health care are subjective quality-of-life issues, the inclusion of the patient as a partner in the care is necessary. Furthermore, because care is being rendered in the patient's home, the patient's preferences must be honored because he or she is the decision-maker concerning the daily routine; that is, the patient decides when to get up, what to eat, and how and when to bathe. Eliciting and documenting patient preferences are important to communicating them to others, such as therapists and aides, who are providing care and to ensuring the best chance for successful outcomes. To achieve the desired outcomes, a contracting process must be maintained with the patient throughout the nursing process. What this means is that the nurse must document what the patient wants and what he or she is willing to commit to doing. When accountability is assigned for each intervention in the care plan, one of the team members responsible for some of the interventions may be the patient or the family.

The most important part of the contracting process is listening to the patient. The concept of listening is simple, but listening is not always easy. Most people do not listen with the intent to understand; instead, they listen with the intent to reply, so that during a conversation they are either speaking or preparing to speak. When nurses think they already understand the client's needs, they cause ineffective exchanges of information, misinterpretation, and ineffective care plans. For example, a home care nurse was visiting a retired professor who had surgery for cancer and subsequent reconstructive surgery, including a skin graft to his face. The nurse was there to provide wound care because of delayed healing, including infections. The recovery period had not been easy for the patient, but he remained in good spirits. The nurse assumed that his expected outcome was a healed wound, but when she asked him, she found out that he wanted explanations about what the doctor was telling him and what was happening. This expectation resulted in a different care plan—a teaching-oriented care process—from the original one that focused simply on demonstrating how to change dressings and care for the wound.

TABLE 13-1 Community Health Construct

Environmental Domain	
Finances	Available financial resources, including employment status, of an individual or family; reflects the adequacy and availability of income with regard to financial obligations
Housing safety and health	Condition of patient's home/neighborhood, including availability of necessary facilities and transportation to those facilities
Psychosocial Domain	
Community networking	Individual's family knowledge and use of community resources/services
Family system	Interpersonal relationships within the household (primary unit) and/or with relatives, friends, and significant others outside the household, such as church members, social group members, and fellow employees (This parameter does not reflect the family's ability to render skilled care unless that ability is marred due to interpersonal problems.)
Emotional/mental response	Mental status and expression of feelings, including sexual concerns, spiritual beliefs, depression, anxiety, and behavioral outcomes that arise from an individual's/family's perception of self as it relates to a change in health status
Individual growth and development	Early-adult life development of cognitive, physical, and social tasks, including ability to speak, read, and write
Physiological Domain	
Sensory function	The body function concerned with the use of senses, including vision, hearing, taste, touch, smell, proprioception, and an individual's perception of pain
Respiratory/circulatory function	The body function concerned with the transfer of gases to meet ventilatory needs and the supply of blood to body tissues by way of the cardiovascular system
Neuromusculoskeletal function	The body function concerned with integration and direction of body regulatory processes related to gross and fine-motor movements, including level of consciousness, speech patterns, muscle strength, coordination, skeletal integrity, and degree of physical independence/mobility
Reproductive function	The body function concerned with menstruation, family planning, fertility, pregnancy, lactation, and impediments to sexual activity; includes sexual organs and secondary sexual characteristics such as breasts
Digestion/elimination	The ability to ingest food and fluids, utilize nutrients, and excrete waste products from the body
Structural integrity	The character and intactness of the body's protective mechanisms, including skin and/or the immunological system
Health Behaviors Domain	
Nutrition	An individual's/family's selection, preparation, and consumption of nutrients, including significant cultural and health factors
Personal habits	An individual's/family's management of personal health-related activities; includes sleep activity patterns, personal hygiene, and avoidance of harmful materials; addresses patient/family habits or preferences, not ability to do ADLs
Health management	An individual's/family's management of their own health status, including their perception of health and their motivation to strive for an optimal level of wellness as demonstrated by regular participation in recommended health screenings/examinations appropriate for age and physical condition; participation in technical procedures; and adherence to prescribed therapeutic plans

ADLs, Activities of daily living.
Modified from Peters D: Examples of existing quality assurance programs in home health care: a hospital based agency. In Meisenheimer CG, ed: *Quality assurance for home health care,* p 255, 1989, Aspen Publishers.

One way to encourage nurses to ask questions is to provide space on the documentation forms for the patient's expected outcome by parameter, by nursing diagnosis, or by patient problem. The outcomes must meet the patient's expectations, not the nurse's perceptions of the patient's expectations.

Chart Information (Data Sets)

A number of forms (Box 13-5) are used in home care to document the nursing process. During the assessment phase, data are collected about the patient's needs through dialogue with the patient. In the diagnosis phase the patient's major problems and strengths are identified and discussed with the

---

Box 13-5

Forms for Documentation

The usual forms used to document home care include the following:

- Patient assessment
- Referral source information/intake form
- Discipline-specific (e.g., nurse, therapist, aide, social worker) care plans
- Physician's plan of treatment
- Medication sheet
- Clinical progress notes (narrative, flowsheet, or both)
- Miscellaneous (e.g., conference notes, verbal order forms, telephone calls)
- Discharge summary
- Reports to third-party payers

---

patient and caregiver. During the planning step, outcome measures that are mutually agreed upon need to be established with set time frames. Available resources that will assist in meeting the desired outcomes should be explored. A plan must be developed and responsibilities must be divided and assigned to all persons involved (e.g., patient, nurse, family, aide). During the implementation phase, the nurse must coach, support, encourage, assist, educate, and reward success. The evaluation step includes comparing and documenting measurements or results with the established expected outcomes (benchmarks) and adjusting time frames, future outcomes, or the plan of action accordingly.

The content of these forms is determined by the information that is important for a particular client. For example, with the mandate of OASIS, chart forms are being revised to include the OASIS data set in the assessment, clinical notes, and discharge forms. Figure 13-8 provides an example of a cardiorespiratory and genitourinary assessment that includes the OASIS data set. Furthermore, with the proliferation of managed care, many short assessment forms are being developed to focus on the specific problem being addressed.

Finally, with the increasing use of electronic documentation, agencies need to evaluate the clinical data set for their agency. For data to be useful, they must be relevant, current, consistent, accessible, accurate, timely, and comprehensive (Peters, 1997).

One of the implications of this requirement is the use of consistent language for all clinical care using either agency language or one of the recognized nursing languages. These include NANDA (North American Nursing Diagnosis Association), NIC (Nursing Intervention Classification), NOC (Nursing Outcome Classification), or Home Health Care Classification System. The language needs to address the full scope of agency services. The challenge is to determine the level of the language to be

used. For example, is "take vital signs" a sufficient intervention or should each vital sign (e.g., blood pressure, temperature, pulse, respirations) be listed as a separate intervention? Or should even more specificity be used, such as "take blood pressure in the left arm, with patient in sitting position"?

Defining an agency data set also means using the same choices each time a similar question is asked. For example, in examining the choices for quality of pulse, practitioners would choose from the same list of choices (e.g., bounding, thready, regular, irregular, weak) instead of creating their own response. The agency personnel must reach a consensus about what those choices will be.

Fiscal Requirements

Fiscal requirements also influence the type of information to be included on the chart forms. Documentation must demonstrate adherence to the protocol of insurers if the agency is to be reimbursed for services. Insurers vary in their requirements for information. Some demand that agencies use the insurer's forms, whereas others permit the agency to send in the information on its own forms. Some insurers want a copy of the entire clinical record, whereas others only ask for periodic reports. Furthermore, some insurers want the assurance of a designated clinical pathway. The current trend is for "paperless" billing using electronic claims processing. However, this does not eliminate the need for preparing and sending patient records or reports as requested by the insurer.

In home care, as in other aspects of the healthcare system, the physician is usually identified as the gatekeeper to payment, which means that the physician must order the services of the other healthcare professionals to ensure that the services rendered were necessary so that the agency will receive payment. When these services must be performed by a professional, they are frequently referred to as "skilled care." Payment is rarely available for long-term care, chronic care, health maintenance, health promotion, or personal care (Gould, Rech, 1989), although this may change with some of the new payment methodologies under managed care.

MEDICARE FORMS 485 AND 486

The most frequent insurer for home health care is Medicare. Medicare requires a Medicare certification and plan of treatment form that was developed by the HCFA: forms 485 and 486. Form 485 is the Plan of Treatment, which must be signed by the physician. Form 486 is the Medical Update and Patient Information form, which is used to provide Medicare with supplemental information. Until recently, these forms had to be submitted with all bills to Medicare in order to justify payment. In an effort to reduce paperwork, however, Medicare no longer routinely requires these

9. **CARDIORESPIRATORY:** Temperature _____ Respirations _____

BLOOD PRESSURE: Lying _____ Sitting _____ Standing _____

PULSE: Apical rate _____ Radial rate _____ Rhythm _____ Quality _____

CARDIOVASCULAR:

_____ Palpitations	_____ Dyspnea on exertion	_____ BP problems	_____ Murmurs
_____ Claudication	_____ Paroxysmal nocturnal dyspnea	_____ Chest pain	_____ Edema
_____ Fatigues easily	_____ Orthopnea (# of pillows _____)	_____ Cardiac problems	_____ Cyanosis
_____ Pacemaker _____		(specify)_____	_____ Varicosities
(Date of last battery change)		_____ Other (specify) _____	

COMMENTS:

RESPIRATORY:

History of: _____ Asthma _____ Bronchitis _____ Pneumonia _____ Other (specify)

_____ TB _____ Pleurisy _____ Emphysema _____

Present Condition:

_____ Cough (describe) _____ _____ Sputum (character and amount) _____

_____ Breath sounds (describe) _____ _____ Other (specify) _____

(M0490) When is the patient dyspneic or noticeably **Short of Breath?**

☐ 0 - Never, patient is not short of breath
☐ 1 - When walking more than 20 feet, climbing stairs
☐ 2 - With moderate exertion (e.g., while dressing, using commode or bedpan, walking distances less than 20 feet)
☐ 3 - With minimal exertion (e.g., while eating, talking, or performing other ADLs) or with agitation
☐ 4 - At rest (during day or night)

(M0500) **Respiratory Treatments** utilized at home: **(Mark all that apply.)**

☐ 1 - Oxygen (intermittent or continuous)
☐ 2 - Ventilator (continually or at night)
☐ 3 - Continuous positive airway pressure
☐ 4 - None of the above

COMMENTS:

10. **GENITOURINARY TRACT:**

_____ Frequency	_____ Nocturia	_____ Dysmenorrhea	_____ Gravida/Para
_____ Pain	_____ Urgency	_____ Lesions	_____ Date last Pap test
_____ Hematuria	_____ Prostate disorder	_____ Hx hysterectomy	_____ Contraception
_____ Vaginal discharge/bleeding	_____ Other (specify) _____		

(M0510) Has the patient been treated for a **Urinary Tract Infection** in the past 14 days?

☐ 0 - No
☐ 1 - Yes
☐ NA - Patient on prophylactic treatment
☐ UK - Unknown

(M0530) **When** does Urinary Incontinence occur?

☐ 0 - Timed-voiding defers incontinence
☐ 1 - During the night only
☐ 2 - During the day and night

(M0520) Urinary Incontinence or Urinary Catheter Presence:

☐ 0 - No incontinence or catheter (includes anuria or ostomy for urinary drainage) [**If No, go to Section 11 - Gastrointestinal Tract**]
☐ 1 - Patient is incontinent
☐ 2 - Patient requires a urinary catheter (i.e., external, indwelling, intermittent, suprapubic) [**Go to Section 11 - Gastrointestinal Tract**]

COMMENTS: (e.g., appliances & care, bladder programs, catheter type, frequency of irrigation & change)

Figure 13-8 Start of care assessment. (Courtesy Center for Health Services and Policy Research, Denver.)

submissions. However, form 485 must be completed, signed by the physician, and retained in the patient's files. Form 486 is only necessary if Medicare requests a medical review of the case. This decrease in external control means that agencies must ensure that patient documentation demonstrates medical necessity, home-bound status, and skilled care (NAHC, 1993).

When completing form 485, several key criteria must be met to meet Medicare specifications. The medical diagnosis must use the International Classification of Diseases terminology. The primary diagnosis listed on form 485 should be the main reason the patient is receiving home health care services, although it is not always the primary diagnosis listed on the referral. Other diagnoses should then be listed in order of importance. The treatment orders should be listed by discipline, and they must be clear and specific to the medical diagnosis, indicating both frequency and duration; for example:

- A skilled nurse must visit three times per week for 3 weeks, then once per week for 2 weeks.
- Vital signs must be checked every visit.
- Colostomy care must be taught.
- A 4-gram sodium, low-fiber diet must be taught.

Orders for medications must include size of the dose, frequency, method of administration, and an indication that the orders are new or changed to determine the patient's need for education or review. A need exists for goals, rehabilitation potential, a discharge plan specific to the medical diagnosis, and a summary of the clinical status of the patient (Monica, 1988).

Tips for Reimbursement Documentation

Several key factors also exist regarding documenting for reimbursement (Box 13-6). The nurse must document evidence that the patient is in need of skilled care. The initial assessment should be documented in the data base, and clinical progress notes should then be written for each visit. Four key factors should be considered: documentation of direct skilled care; documentation of patient instruction; documentation of skilled observation; and evaluation and documentation of the patient's home-bound status (Monica, 1988).

LEGAL CONSIDERATIONS

Litigation in home care has rarely occurred, so little case law exists that is directly related to malpractice issues involving nurses in home care. However, several factors could lead to a possible explosion of lawsuits, including the increased use of advanced technology and discharging patients from hospitals who are sicker and more unstable (Warner, Albert, 1997). The following are the three main categories of risks in home care (Brueckner, Pace, 1989):

Box 13-6
Documentation for Dollars

Direct Skilled Care

These are specific tasks, such as catheter changes, wound care, treatments, and injections. Charting must be specific, including the length and complexity of the treatment.

Patient Instruction

Instructions should be broken down to a specific drug, diet, treatment, or exercise. Instructions should continue until the nurse can document that the patient, family, or both demonstrate the ability to perform the activity independently or that they verbalize understanding of the instructions (e.g., instructions about medication side effects).

Charting should use descriptive terms, such as the color of the exudate or sputum and the severity of pain (perhaps using a pain-rating scale of 0 to 10).

Home-Bound Status Evaluation

Home-bound status is required for Medicare reimbursement. The reason that the patient is home-bound must be documented at the time of admission and at least once weekly thereafter. Functional limitations must be described clearly and stated in measurable terms. The nurse must be careful to support the statements of other disciplines about the status of the patient. For example, the nurse should not write that the patient is ambulating without difficulty while the physical therapist is providing gait-training services to the patient. The nurse's statement could disqualify the therapy services from payment.

---

1. Home care services are provided in an uncontrolled environment.
2. Services are generally provided such that only long-distance supervision is in place.
3. Positive outcomes for services depend on the compliance of patient and family.

In essence the autonomy of patients and their ability to direct and control their own care is far greater in home care than for any other sector of the healthcare delivery system. Thus it is important that home care personnel be certain that patient expectations are realistic in regard to the type of services that can be delivered at home. Common areas of vulnerability for the agency nurse include impaired communication, lack of continuity of services, ineffective patient education, and supervision of other staff (Warner, Albert, 1997).

Impaired Communication Among All Professionals Responsible for Care

The importance of recording information communicated to a physician about a change in condition is illustrated in the following case:

A 400-pound, 42-year-old woman underwent surgery to repair a hernia and remove her right ovary. The patient showed signs of pulmonary embolism, which she reported. The surgeon prescribed Coumadin (warfarin). The patient died at home of a pulmonary embolism 15 days after surgery. The plaintiff claimed that the defendant home care nurse did not report two episodes of shortness of breath to the defendant surgeon. The surgeon also claimed that he was not told of the two episodes. This case resulted in a defense verdict (Laska, January 1998a).

Documentation of conversations with physicians can provide legal protection for the nurse. Therefore the nurse must note every attempt to reach a physician, the time and content of any messages left, the facts conveyed in all conversations, and any efforts to communicate with others about a given situation, including with whom the conversation occurred and what was said (Sullivan, 1994).

Lack of Continuity of Services

The difficulty in providing reasonable nursing care with a variety of nursing personnel is illustrated in the following case:

A 72-year-old male, who was an insulin-dependent diabetic, had long-standing peripheral vascular disease and diabetic neuropathy that resulted in a left leg amputation below the knee several years earlier. Just before the referral for home care services, the patient sustained an injury to his right leg that developed into small ulcerations. The patient was referred to home care for daily wet-to-dry saline dressings for 2 weeks. The orders also specified that the nurses should monitor the status of the lesions.

In the 18 days that the patient received care, daily visits were made on 15 days. No documentation was made to explain why two of the three visits had been missed. Six different nurses provided care during this time. Some wound measurements were made, but the majority of the nurses simply described the amount of drainage and whether they believed that the wounds were healing. Because of the number of different nurses involved in the case and the failure to quantify wound measurements, the nurses were unable to see the deterioration of the patient's condition. On the nineteenth day of his care, he was admitted to the hospital, where he underwent surgical debridement of the lesions, IV antibiotics, and invasive diagnostics. He ultimately had to have his right leg amputated.

The patient brought suit against the home care agency, stating that the lack of continuity of care was the proximate cause of his injury. Treatment appeared to be ineffective, as evidenced by the development of peripheral edema, increased drainage, and necrotic tissue at the base of the lesions. No documentation was made to indicate that any of this was communicated to the podiatrist in charge of the patient's care. Furthermore, the final entry by the last nurse to see the patient at home differed significantly in terms of wound dimensions, necrosis, and drainage from that of

the physician who admitted the patient to the hospital. The conflicting information and inadequate documentation in the home care record placed the agency in the poorest legal position possible (Warner, Albert, 1997).

Ineffective Education of the Patient or Family Regarding Proper Care

The importance of documenting patient education is illustrated by the following case:

A 42-year-old Texas woman with juvenile-onset diabetes underwent treatment by a home care and home infusion company for a series of infections. These companies provided services and medications for daily treatment of self-administered IV solutions of antibiotics in the patient's home. She claimed that the defendants (the service providers) failed to properly instruct her on how to mix antibiotics with saline solution, resulting in inadequate dosages for the ongoing infections. As a result, the plaintiff had to have her lower leg and right foot amputated. The defendants argued unsuccessfully that the plaintiff had been properly instructed and monitored, but that she had been negligent in failing to follow the treatment course provided. The verdict was for $4.1 million, including $2 million in punitive damages (Laska, 1997b).

Documentation is essential in such cases. The nurse should address the actual interventions, the methods used to teach the patient, the patient's response to the teaching, the adverse effects that might occur if the procedure is performed incorrectly, when return demonstrations were performed by the patient, and the patient's lack of compliance (if any), including the patient's reactions and responses to these issues. Documented evidence of information given regarding what to do in the event of an equipment malfunction, including who to notify and what initial measures to take, can also provide a good defense against possible litigation. Equally important (as previously mentioned) is documenting any and all communication with the physician and other healthcare providers.

Supervision of Other Staff Members

The registered nurse often is responsible for supervising home care aides. After providing (and documenting) orientation to the policies of the agency, the agency nurses become responsible for long-distance supervision of the aides. Periodic on-site observations enable nurses to monitor the quality of care. Accidents, injuries, and complications may result in allegations of inadequate supervision and instruction of the aides. Sources of liability may include the following: burns from cigarettes or hot water; medication errors; adverse drug reactions; patient's refusal of treatment; patient complaints; unexpected changes in the patient's condition; falls from the bed, chair, or a hoyer lift; development of decubitus ulcers; sexual assault or abuse by the aide; malfunction or improper use of equipment; and theft (Abbott, 1996). Specific instructions provided to the aide should be documented in the medical record. The medical record should clearly support the supervisory nature of the registered nurse's visits to the home.

Adequate documentation serves to protect the home care nurse from liability. A good example of this is the following case:

A 3-month-old Minnesota baby received all his well-child care from his family practice physicians. The county nursing service had been involved in the mother's prenatal care and made follow-up home visits after the child was born. The child was brought to the county clinic with complaints of a cough and fever at age 2½ months. Over the next 9 days he was seen intermittently by his family physician and the county nurses. The physician's records differed dramatically from the poor condition reflected in the nursing service records. The child was ultimately admitted to the hospital, where he was observed to be obtunded, posturing, and hypertonic. He was diagnosed with *Haemophilus influenzae* meningitis and died despite aggressive treatment. The mother claimed that the defendant doctor negligently failed to diagnose and treat the child's pneumonia, resulting in sepsis and ultimately meningitis. The settlement was for $100,000. The comprehensive documentation on the nursing records kept them from being named as defendants in the suit (Laska, 1997a).

DOCUMENTATION MANAGEMENT

Home healthcare workers have unique problems in accessing the clinical record. The record is needed by many different persons, including the nurse, therapists, the supervisor, quality-management staff, and billing personnel. Some of these people are in the office, where the chart is located, and some are in the home (at different times) with the patient, where the care is rendered. Therefore information must often be recorded on more than one form at different locations, a time-consuming process that can create inconsistencies that affect reimbursement and cause problems in getting the properly recorded information to the right place in a timely manner.

The main challenge in home health care is documenting the care accurately, completely, consistently, clearly, quickly, and concisely. This dilemma is handled in various ways by different agencies. Some agencies have the nurse take part of the chart to the home and then return it to the main office or satellite office. However, problems arise if a change in schedule occurs after the nurse leaves the office. The nurse may then need to visit without any written information about the patient. Another approach is to use NCR paper to make multiple copies of all recorded information. However, illegible copies can be a drawback with this approach. Some agencies use a daily sheet so that the nurse can document each visit on a separate sheet. This alternative sometimes results in misplaced sheets and lost

information. In addition, the history of the patient is often unavailable when the visit is made. Other agencies keep the patient's record in his or her home. Still others use dictating equipment so that the nurse can dictate the visit while in the home or immediately afterward. The dictation is transcribed at the agency and put into the chart later. Nurses tend to be most comfortable taking brief notes in the home and writing them in the record later to conform to all the required standards. Later, however, is sometimes late in the day or even later in the week, creating the possibility for inaccuracies or incompleteness.

Other challenges to compiling a complete patient record include reminding the therapists (who are often under contract or work part time and therefore are not in the office very often) to document on the chart in a timely fashion. Ensuring that a verbal order from the physician is documented in the record can also be time-consuming. The nurse must call the doctor from the patient's home or from the agency's office and must complete a verbal order form, which is then sent to the physician to be signed. The nurse must follow-up to ensure that the verbal order form is returned in a timely manner and is placed in the records.

Computerized Patient Records

Computerized patient records offer solutions to many of these problems. Some home care nurses document using lap-top computers or other data-entry devices, which may also be used to update the patient's clinical record. When computer patient records are fully integrated, the record is accessible at many different locations simultaneously—by the nurse and the therapist, at the billing office, in the patient's home, in the physician's office, and at the hospital. This accessibility provides stronger links, leading to better continuity of care. The record can be retrieved by phone wherever or whenever needed, giving the nurse access to the patient's history and plan of care regardless of scheduling changes. The nurse can document care as it is delivered, improving both the accuracy and completeness of the record. The computer can also take information that has been entered only once and reformat it for various administrative, billing, and clinical purposes, including generating Medicare forms 485 and 486. The electronic patient record makes it easier to read notes and find information (Braunstein, 1993). Computerized patient records can potentially reduce documentation time, which many agencies report to be a problem. They also help create a much-needed data base in home care that can assist in the further development of protocols for treating specific outcomes and the use of critical pathways, as described in Chapter 3.

Electronic records are not without problems, however. Lap-top computers can be lost or stolen, and patients have been known to complain about nurses entering data into a computer instead of being attentive to their needs. However, most of these issues can be overcome through the proper implementation of computerized mobile systems. Conversion to mobile documentation transforms the entire documentation system within an agency and affects every agency employee. Examples of agency processes that need to be redefined include the business infrastructure, patient-clinician interactions, and clinician work habits (Peters, 1997a). The business infrastructure will be changed by computerization because staff will no longer need to come into the office every day. Thus the agency has to decide how it is going to support staff offsite: How will they be informed about changes or have a chance to discuss cases with their peers? Patient-clinician interaction changes with the introduction of an electronic device that some perceive to be a barrier. Experience seems to indicate, however, that this is more a measure of staff discomfort than a patient issue. An effort must be made to maintain ongoing staff training for both computer skills and the use of software programs. Changes in clinician work habits seem to create the most trouble. As previously stated, many staff members are in the habit of finishing paperwork at the end of the day. However, the effectiveness of computerized systems is maximized by using them in real time (i.e., during the visit). Changing the way daily work is completed requires ongoing support and encouragment, but when successful, it improves the accuracy and comprehensibility of information recorded in the patient's records.

SUMMARY

This chapter describes and reviews the changing documentation needs of home care nursing. Home care documentation is influenced by the following: professional, regulatory, and accreditation standards; the definition of the scope of care; patient attitudes, strengths, resources, and needs; the data sets and language used; requirements of third-party payers; and legal imperatives.

The nature of home care creates unique challenges to documentation. Documentation is time consuming, not only because similar information must be recorded in several places, but also because of the need for several healthcare providers to have chart accessibility in different locations at the same time. One way that this is being addressed is through electronic mobile documentation, and this chapter investigates the reasons why agencies should consider converting to such systems.

REFERENCES

Abbott K: Home care and nursing risk management, *J Nurs Law* 3(3):41, 1996.

ANA: *Standards of home health care nursing,* Kansas City, Mo, 1986, The Association.

Braunstein M: The electronic patient records solution, *Caring* 12(7):30, 1993.

Brueckner G, Pace D: Implementing an effective home care risk management program, *Perspect Healthc Risk Manage* p 25, Fall 1989.

Burt CJ, Beetem MN, Iverson C et al: Preliminary development of the school health intensity rating scale, *J Sch Health* 66(8):286, 1996.

Calfee B: Documenting suicide risk, *Nursing* 26(7):17, 1996.

CHAP: *Standards of excellence for home care organizations,* #21-2327, New York, 1993, National League for Health Care and CHAP.

Chou K, Kaas M, Richie M: Assaultive behavior in geriatric patients, *Journal of Gerontological Nursing,* p 31, November 1996.

Eggland ET: *Nursing documentation resource guide,* Gaithersburg, Md, 1993, Aspen.

Gould EJ, Rech PL: Documentation. In Meisenheimer CG, ed: *Quality assurance for home health care,* Rockville, Md, 1989, Aspen.

Hays BJ: Nursing care requirements and resource consumption in home health care, *Nurs Res* 41(3):1138, 1992.

Hays BJ: Nursing intensity as a predictor of resource consumption in public health nursing, *Nurs Res* 44:106, 1995.

Laska L, ed: Suicide committed with dandruff shampoo and after-shave lotion, *Medical Malpractice Verdicts, Settlements and Experts* p 48, March 1993a.

Laska L, ed: Woman taking lithium for manic depressive disorder goes into coma due to toxic levels, *Medical Malpractice Verdicts, Settlements and Experts* p 48, March 1993b.

Laska L, ed: Death of 3-month-old boy in Minnesota, *Medical Malpractice Verdicts, Settlements and Experts* p 40, July 1997a.

Laska L, ed: Diabetic Texas woman treated for infections by self-administered infusions of IV antibiotics at home, *Medical Malpractice Verdicts, Settlements and Experts* p 29, February 1997b.

Laska L, ed: Nevada man commits suicide after voluntary discharge from psychiatric hospital, *Medical Malpractice Verdicts, Settlements and Experts* p 47, May 1997c.

Laska L, ed: Schizophrenia patient goes AWOL and dies from alcohol poisoning, *Medical Malpractice Verdicts, Settlements and Experts* p 47, May 1997d.

Laska L, ed: Teen suicidal risk not monitored at hospital psych ward—hangs himself with belt, *Medical Malpractice Verdicts, Settlements and Experts* p 41, September 1997e.

Laska L, ed: Failure to timely diagnose and treat pulmonary embolism blamed for obese woman's death—Ohio defense verdict, *Medical Malpractice Verdicts, Settlements and Experts* p 13, January 1998a.

Laska L, ed: Medical record clerk committed to psychiatric ward after threatening to kill five coworkers, *Medical Malpractice Verdicts, Settlements and Experts* p 20, January 1998b.

Martin KS, Sheet NJ: *The Omaha system: a pocket system: a pocket guide for community health nursing,* Philadelphia, 1992, WB Saunders.

Monica ED: Documentation. In Harris MD, ed: *Home health administration,* Owings Mills, Md, 1988, Rynd Communications.

NAHC: NAHC achieves major paperwork reduction victory, *Homecare News* p 18, May 1993, The Association.

Northrop C, Kelly M: *Legal issues in nursing,* St Louis, 1987, Mosby.

Oliver R: Legal risks when the patient has emotional problems, *RN* p 51, December 1986.

Payson A, Jakacki M: Out of control, *Am J Nurs* p 1335, 1985.

Peters DA: The development of a community health intensity rating scale, *Nursing Research* 37(4):202.

Peters D: Examples of existing quality assurance programs in home health care: a hospital based agency. In Meisenheimer CG, ed: *Quality assurance for home health care,* Rockville, Md, 1989, Aspen.

Peters DA: Mobile computing: pencil to pentium, *The Remington Report* 5(2):43, 1997a.

Peters DA: The details are in the data, *Computertalk* 5(2):43, 1997b.

Peters DA: Quality documentation: quality care, *Caring* 7(10):3034, 1998.

Psychiatrist's release from hospital of patient to stand trial created liability for death of third party killed by patient, despite recommendation of continued supervision, *Medical Malpractice by Specialty* 4(12):14, 1996.

Rouse F: Living wills in the long term care facility, *J Long Term Care Adm* p 14, Summer 1988.

Simmons D: *A classification scheme for client problems in community health nursing,* DHHS No HRA 80-16, Washington, DC, 1980, US. Department of Health and Human Services, Health Resources Administration, Bureau of Health Professions, Division of Nursing.

Sullivan GH: Home care: more autonomy, more legal risks, *RN* p 63, May 1994.

Tammelleo A: "Constant observation" means "constant observation," *Regan Report Nurs Law* 31(10):4, 1991.

Tammelleo A: Nurses fail to monitor blood sugar despite family pleas, *Regan Report Nurs Law* 36(3):2, 1995.

Tammelleo A: Psych patient disappears—death presumed, *Regan Report Nurs Law* 37(4):1, 1996.

Tort claims act—$125,000 recovery, *Malpractice by Specialty* p 32, 1996.

Taptich B, Iyer B, Bornocchi-Losey D: *Nursing diagnosis and care planning,* ed 2, Philadelphia, 1994, WB Saunders.

Warner I, Albert R: Avoiding legal land mines in home health care nursing, *Home Health Care Manage Pract* 9(6):8, 1997.

Woerner L, Donnelly D, Edwards P: Challenges facing the home health care industry, *Nursing Dynamics* p 5, May 1993.

SUGGESTED READINGS

Eggland E: Charting smarter: using new mechanisms to organize your paperwork, *Nursing* 25(9):34, 1995.

Fiesta J: Psychiatric liability, Part I. *Nursing Management* p 10, July 1998.

Fiesta J: Psychiatric liability, Part 2. *Nursing Management* p 18, August 1998.

Fiesta J: Psychiatric liability, Part 3, *Nursing Management* p 16, September 1998.

Laska L, ed: Failure to properly treat suicidal patient-death, *Medical Malpractice Verdicts, Settlements and Experts* p 46, May 1997.

Laska L, ed: Utah man attempts suicide by overdose of medication, *Medical Malpractice Verdicts, Settlements and Experts* p 47, May 1997.

Laska L, ed: Woman hangs self in psychiatric facility after learning of impending arrest upon discharge, *Medical Malpractice Verdicts, Settlements and Experts* p 4, July 1997.

Lawrence K: *Home health care: forms, checklists and guidelines,* ed 2, Rockville, Md, 1998, Aspen.

Marrelli TM: *Handbook of home health standards and documentation guidelines for reimbursement,* St Louis, 1998, Mosby.

Martin KS, Sheet NJ: *The Omaha system,* Philadelphia, 1991, WB Saunders.

McCabe v Tucson Psychiatric Institute: wrongful death, *The Trial Reporter* p 3, January 1997.

Menenberg S: Standards of care in documentation of psychiatric nursing care, *Clin Nurse Spec* 9(3):140, 1995.

Nelson J: The influence of environmental factors in incidents of disruptive behavior, *J Gerontol Nurs* p 19, May 1995.

Peters DA, McKeon T: *Transforming home care: quality, cost, and data mangement,* Gaithersburg, Md, 1998, Aspen.

Psychiatrists not liable for patients violent conduct following voluntary in-patient psychiatric treatment, *Medical Liability Reporter* p 159, June/July 1997.

14

Long-Term Care Documentation

Rita Cavallaro, RN, C, LNHA, MS, Joyce R. Newman, RN, C, CLNC, C-GN, Patricia Iyer, RN, MSN, CNA

The basic principles of documentation in long-term care are the same as the universal principles of nursing documentation discussed earlier in this text: professional responsibility and accountability. Progress notes are still the primary means of communication between nurses and other members of the healthcare team. Documentation must clearly communicate the nurse's decision-making process, assessments, diagnoses, planning, and evaluations, including the patient's response to nursing interventions. Nursing documentation also addresses patient and family education, discharge planning, and psychological and psychosocial factors. The clinical record is the key to reimbursement and serves as an important legal document. Documentation is used for evaluating and planning services and for quality improvement activities, and it is also an important part of the survey, certification, and licensure activities of external reviewers. Documentation must therefore be complete, objective, consistent, and accurate.

THE NURSING HOME RESIDENT

Long-term care residents who require nursing home care take up residency in the nursing home so that they can live where skilled nursing care is available. The length of time a resident may live in one or more facility can vary depending on the acuity, disability, chronicity, and multiplicity of his or her condition. Living arrangements, geography, and the strength of support networks in the resident's family and community also have an impact on the length of the resident's stay in long-term care facilities. Nurses in the long-term care setting promote functional independence and self-determination, and they assist residents in achieving the highest attainable level of mental, physical, and psychosocial well-being in a homelike environment. The healthcare providers are effectively guests in the residents' home (albeit an institutional home), which requires that they

exhibit a diligent respect for the resident's individual rights, preferences, and needs. Long-term care often requires long, hard work to bring about incremental improvements in the rehabilitation, restoration, preservation, or adaptation of functional skills. Furthermore, long-term care includes continuing to provide quality care to residents over a long time period despite their progressively deteriorating conditions. Nursing personnel often become the confidants of the resident or family members. The nursing home environment, contrary to that of the acute care setting, seeks to preserve normal lifestyles and minimize extraordinary problems, which establishes a significantly different focus for nursing documentation.

Demographic Factors

Most residents in long-term care facilities are 75 years and older. In fact, the median age of nursing home residents is 81 years. Residents of nursing homes are typically elderly, white, widowed females. The level of acuity of hospital patients and the rapid discharge from the acute care setting is reflected in the elevated acuity of these elderly residents when they are admitted into long-term care facilities. If today's medical-surgical units look like yesterday's intensive care units, then yesterday's medical-surgical units are today's long-term care units, with one exception: Long-term care patients are often of an advanced age and, as a result, may suffer from chronic health problems that make them more vulnerable to acute conditions. Long-term residents are coming to facilities in worse health than ever before.

As the society of the United States ages, the reality is that, although many elderly people are indeed living longer, they experience more disabilities in their later years. This is especially true for women. Men die at a younger age than women, skipping the intermediate stages of disability or spending less time in those stages (Markides, 1989). Before placement in a nursing home, most nursing home residents have already received a significant amount of home care provided by family members, friends, or community agencies. The complex functional problems of these individuals lead to complex medical conditions and increased social burdens for their caregivers.

Clinical Needs of Residents

One fourth of nursing home residents are dependent in all six activities of daily living (ADLs) (i.e., feeding, dressing, bathing, toileting, continence, and mobility), and 93% need assistance in at least one ADL (Matteson, McConnell, 1988). Cognitive impairment affects more than one half of nursing home residents. As the number of cognitively impaired residents increases in the nursing home population, so, too, does the incidence of behavioral problems that are often the most burdensome aspect of providing care.

Nursing homes provide a protective, safe environment that enhances the competence of the residents and provides opportunities for meaningful social interaction. Long-term care professionals can provide close monitoring and effective treatment of chronic and acute conditions while paying attention to health promotion and therapeutic goals. Long-term care currently focuses on resident strengths and minimizes excessive disabilities (Matteson, McConnell, 1988).

FREQUENCY OF DOCUMENTATION

The frequency of long-term care documentation often differs from that of acute care. Each state's Department of Health may dictate the frequency of charting; for example, the following New Jersey regulations regarding nurses' notes are typical of long-term care requirements.

Medicaid patients shall have daily summaries for the first 5 days after admission, written by staff of each shift and at the end of 5 days the records shall be updated once per week for the next 4 weeks. Then summaries shall be written once every 30 days for the next 60 days following admission. Thereafter, documentation shall be a minimum of every 3 months or when there is a change in the clinical status of the patient requiring provision of nursing services in accordance with N.J.A.C. 10:63-1.3. All clinical records shall be updated at intervals based on the seriousness of each patient's condition in accordance with the standards of professional practice. A comprehensive assessment shall be completed a minimum of once every 12 months. Thereafter, summaries shall be written once every 90 days (*New Jersey Register,* 1990).

Some facilities may use worksheets to keep track of the dates when completing summaries (Figure 14-1). The influence regulatory agencies have on nursing practice and documentation in the long-term care setting cannot be overstated. The nursing home industry has become one of the most regulated industries in this country. Much of the documentation in long-term care is based on both federal and state regulations. If nurses' notes were intended for information purposes only, nurses would probably make fewer notations, but they would likely be more informative and useful (Matteson, McConnell, 1988). The interdisciplinary comprehensive assessment and care plan is the primary focus of the Federal and State OBRA survey.

All of these factors have generated a change in the content of nursing documentation and in the tools used to document long-term care nursing. Several factors, including informed consumers, regulatory agencies, third-party payers, and the evolution of gerontologic and long-term care nursing, have influenced the documentation of interventions, the outcomes of residents, and the responses of residents to nursing care significantly.

DEVELOPMENT OF THE MINIMUM DATA SET AND RESIDENT ASSESSMENT PROTOCOLS

As early as 1959 a Senate subcommittee focused on the delivery of quality care and its variations from one long-term care facility to another and from one state to another. The Health Care Financing Administration (HCFA) proposed several reforms in the 1970s.

In the early 1980s the U.S. Congress called for a study of existing regulations and asked for recommendations that would help long-term care facilities in providing satisfactory care for their residents. The HCFA contracted with the Institute of Medicine of the National Academy of Sciences to conduct this study (AHCA, 1990). Congress incorporated many of their recommendations into the Omnibus Budget Reconciliation Act (OBRA) of 1987, commonly referred to as OBRA '87. This legislation has had the most sweeping effect in recent history on long-term care documentation, and perhaps on long-term care nursing services in general. OBRA '87 has been recognized as a significant legislation for long-term care reform in Medicare and Medicaid. Most of the provisions became effective on October 1, 1990.

Since then, the intention of HCFA has been to continue with ongoing evaluation and refinement of the Resident Assessment Instrument (RAI). The goal is to include the most current changes in clinical practice and assessment methodologies and accommodate the changing needs of nursing home populations (HCFA, 1995).

OBRA '87 includes provisions requiring that states adopt regulations that mandate a specified minimum number of registered and licensed nursing staff. This provision effectively eliminated the regulatory distinction between skilled-care and intermediate-care facilities. The law also expands requirements for quality assessment, adds to residents' rights, and requires additional training for certified nursing assistants.

The nursing home reform law (OBRA '87) provides a regulatory framework for ensuring good clinical practice

RESIDENT _Jane Doe_ ADM DATE _9-10-94_ MDS DATE _9-25-94_

NURSES' NOTES

1. Daily summaries for the first five (5) days after admission written by staff of each shift

   _9-10_   _9-11_   _9-12_   _9-13_   _9-14_

2. At the end of five days, weekly summaries for the next four weeks (which completes one month)

   _9-17_   _9-24_   _9-31_   _10-7_

3. Then summaries will be written once every 30 days for the next 60 days (which brings you up to the third month and the first quarter)

   _10-30_   _11-30_

4. Thereafter, documentation is a minimum of every 3 months (or quarterly) on the quarterly nursing summary sheet and QR FORM.

   _12-25-94_   _3-25-95_   _6-25-95_

All clinical records shall be updated when there is a change in the resident's clinical status, and based upon the seriousness of the resident's condition in accordance with the standards of professional practice. A comprehensive assessment (MDS) shall be completed a minimum of once every 12 months and summaries (PLUS MDS QUARTERLY REVIEWS) every 90 days. (As residents are discharged and readmitted these schedules of charting can and should be dove-tailed to coincide with the established MDS & QUARTERLY charting as long as a new MDS is not necessary and not result in unnecessary duplicate charting.)

These documentation regulations were published August 20, 1990 in the Long Term Care Manual Chapter 10:63-1.14. for facilities receiving Medicaid funds. Standards that are applied to Medicaid/Medicare patients are usually expected to apply to all residents as a minimum standard of care in a facility receiving these funds.

REP '91

Figure 14-1 Worksheet used to identify dates for completing the summaries. (Developed by Rita Cavallaro.)

by recognizing the importance of comprehensive assessment as the foundation for planning and delivering care to nursing home residents. The RAI is simply a new standardized way to do what clinicians have always done (i.e., assessing, planning, and providing individualized care). The HCFA's efforts in developing the RAI and associated policies have always been directed toward the question "What is the right thing to do in terms of good clinical practice, and for all nursing home residents?" (HCFA, 1995).

RESIDENT ASSESSMENT INSTRUMENTS

The HCFA used an interdisciplinary process to develop the RAI. The tool was created by experts in the care of nursing home residents (representing many professional disciplines), the nursing home residents, the nursing home industry, and consumer groups. The project team worked together with expert clinicians, consultants, a national advisory board, and hundreds of reviewers from nursing homes across the country. More than 50 draft versions of the minimum data set (MDS) were refined and reviewed. The development of the RAI involved several major tasks, such as determining what areas of a person's health status and functioning should be assessed in the MDS and how to organize the elements within a workable conceptual framework (AHCA, 1990). The purpose of the RAI is to help the nursing home staff assess the resident's capability, needs, and strengths. These assessment findings are addressed when the facility's interdisciplinary team meets to develop an individualized care plan for each resident.

The following information is from the *Federal Register* (1997):

This final rule establishes a resident assessment instrument for use by long-term care facilities participating in Medicare and Medicaid programs when conducting a periodic assessment of a resident's functional capacity. The resident assessment instrument (RAI) consists of a minimum data set (MDS) of elements, common definitions, and coding categories needed to perform a comprehensive assessment of a long-term care facility resident. (Figure 14-2 is the first page of this tool.) A State may choose to use the Federally established resident assessment instrument or an alternate instrument that has been designed by the State and approved by us. These regulations establish guidelines for use of the data set and designation of the assessment instrument.

The resident assessment instrument is intended to produce comprehensive, accurate, standardized, reproducible assessment of each long-term care facility resident's functional capacity.

State computerization requirements are effective [as of] June 1998. Facilities must enter information from the resident assessment into a computer, in accordance with HCFA-specified formats. At least monthly, the facility must transmit electronically the information contained in each resident assessment to the State.

The government, through the actions of the HCFA, was seeking a way to mandate a minimum standard of care that all citizens would be assured of receiving should they enter a long-term nursing care facility. To provide the minimum standard of care throughout the country, they determined that an MDS must be collected in a standardized way by all facilities seeking reimbursement from the government. In 1995 this was accomplished when the RAI included the MDS, version 2.0. Not only is there a coordinated approach to multidisciplinary care in long-term care, but there is also a fully integrated interdisciplinary approach to assessment and care planning. This emphasis is directly reflected in the documentation practices now being used in long-term care.

The interdisciplinary approach must take precedence over documentation practiced in the acute care setting that is strictly nursing-oriented.

Geriatric problems and care have long been understood to be part of a complex system that require therapies and services involving all professional disciplines. The needs of the diverse, complex geriatric population cannot be met by only one discipline (Matteson, McConnell, 1988).

USE OF MINIMUM DATA SETS AND RESIDENT ASSESSMENT PROTOCOLS IN LONG-TERM CARE FACILITIES

The RAI is composed of three parts: the MDS, resident assessment protocols (RAPs), and the Utilization Guidelines.

Minimum Data Set

At the time of admission, the professional registered nurse (RN) begins to assess and collect information, and within 24 to 48 hours he or she will institute an interim or initial care plan in accordance with the standards of practice and the facility's policies and procedures. The assessment should incorporate information needed to complete the appropriate MDS, and the care plan should accurately reflect the resident's characteristics, strengths, and needs. The social worker, recreational therapist, and dietitian all must complete their assessments of the resident, usually within 7 days of the time of admission.

The law states that the MDS must be completed according to the following criteria:

Within 14 days of admission; promptly after a significant change in the resident's physical or mental condition; and in no case less often than once every 12 months. The nursing facility must examine each resident no less than once every 3 months, and as appropriate, revise the resident's assessment to ensure the continued accuracy of the assessment. The results of the resident's assessment are used to develop, review, and revise the comprehensive care plan. Each assessment must be conducted or coordinated with participation of other health professionals and an RN, who must sign and certify the completion of the assessment. Each individual who completes a portion of the assessment must sign it to certify the accuracy of that part. Individuals who willfully and knowingly certify (or cause another individual to certify) a material and false statement in a resident assessment are subject to civil or criminal penalties (i.e., financial penalties) (*Federal Register,* 1989, 1991a, 1991b).

In addition, the RAIs and care plans must be kept in the resident's clinical record for a period of 15 months. The requirements for resident assessment found in the HCFA standards are applicable to all residents of Medicare (Title 18) skilled nursing facilities or Medicaid (Title 19) nursing facilities.

MINIMUM DATA SET (MDS) — VERSION 2.0
FOR NURSING HOME RESIDENT ASSESSMENT AND CARE SCREENING

BACKGROUND (FACE SHEET) INFORMATION AT ADMISSION

SECTION AB. DEMOGRAPHIC INFORMATION

1.	DATE OF ENTRY	Date the stay began. Note — Does not include readmission if record was closed at time of temporary discharge to hospital, etc. In such cases, use prior admission date
		☐☐ — ☐☐ — ☐☐☐☐
		Month Day Year

| 2. | ADMITTED FROM (AT ENTRY) | 1. Private home/apt. with no home health services
2. Private home/apt. with home health services
3. Board and care/assisted living/group home
4. Nursing home
5. Acute care hospital
6. Psychiatric hospital, MR/DD facility
7. Rehabilitation hospital
8. Other |

| 3. | LIVED ALONE (PRIOR TO ENTRY) | 0. No
1. Yes
2. In other facility |

| 4. | ZIP CODE OF PRIOR PRIMARY RESIDENCE | ☐☐☐☐☐ |

5.	RESIDENTIAL HISTORY 5 YEARS PRIOR TO ENTRY	(Check all settings resident lived in during 5 years prior to date of entry given in item AB1 above)
		Prior stay at this nursing home — a.
		Stay in other nursing home — b.
		Other residential facility — board and care home, assisted living, group home — c.
		MH/psychiatric setting — d.
		MR/DD setting — e.
		NONE OF ABOVE — f.

| 6. | LIFETIME OCCUPATION(S) (Put "/" between two occupations) | ☐☐☐☐☐☐☐☐☐☐☐☐☐☐☐ |

| 7. | EDUCATION (Highest Level Completed) | 1. No schooling 5. Technical or trade school
2. 8th grade/less 6. Some college
3. 9-11 grades 7. Bachelor's degree
4. High school 8. Graduate degree |

| 8. | LANGUAGE | (Code for correct response)
a. Primary language
0. English 1. Spanish 2. French 3. Other |
| | | b. If other, specify ☐☐☐☐☐☐☐☐ |

| 9. | MENTAL HEALTH HISTORY | Does resident's RECORD indicate any history of mental retardation, mental illness, or developmental disability problem?
0. No 1. Yes |

0.	CONDITIONS RELATED TO MR/DD STATUS	(Check all conditions that are related to MR/DD status that were manifested before age 22, and are likely to continue indefinitely)
		Not applicable — no MR/DD (Skip to AB11) — a.
		MR/DD with organic condition
		Down's syndrome — b.
		Autism — c.
		Epilepsy — d.
		Other organic condition related to MR/DD — e.
		MR/DD with no organic condition — f.

| 1. | DATE BACK-GROUND INFORMATION COMPLETED | ☐☐ — ☐☐ — ☐☐☐☐ |
| | | Month Day Year |

SECTION AC. CUSTOMARY ROUTINE

| 1. | CUSTOMARY ROUTINE | (Check all that apply. If all information UNKNOWN, check last box only.) |
| | (In year prior to DATE OF ENTRY to this nursing home, or year last in community if now being admitted from another nursing home) | CYCLE OF DAILY EVENTS |

| | | a. |
Stays up late at night (e.g., after 9 pm)
Naps regularly during day (at least 1 hour)	b.
Goes out 1+ days a week	c.
Stays busy with hobbies, reading, or fixed daily routine	d.
Spends most of time alone or watching TV	e.
Moves independently indoors (with appliances, if used)	f.
Use of tobacco products at least daily	g.
NONE OF ABOVE	h.

EATING PATTERNS
Distinct food preferences	i.
Eats between meals all or most days	j.
Use of alcoholic beverage(s) at least weekly	k.
NONE OF ABOVE	l.

ADL PATTERNS
In bedclothes much of day	m.
Wakens to toilet all or most nights	n.
Has irregular bowel movement pattern	o.
Showers for bathing	p.
Bathing in PM	q.
NONE OF ABOVE	r.

INVOLVEMENT PATTERNS
Daily contact with relatives/close friends	s.
Usually attends church, temple, synagogue (etc.)	t.
Finds strength in faith	u.
Daily animal companion/presence	v.
Involved in group activities	w.
NONE OF ABOVE	x.
UNKNOWN — Resident/family unable to provide information	y.

END

SECTION AD. FACE SHEET SIGNATURES

SIGNATURES OF PERSONS COMPLETING FACE SHEET:

a. Signature of RN Assessment Coordinator			Date
b. Signatures	Title	Sections	Date
c.			Date
d.			Date
e.			Date
f.			Date
g.			Date

☐ = When box blank, must enter number or letter

☐ a. = When letter in box, check if condition applies

Figure 14-2 The minimum data set face sheet. (Developed by HCFA.)

A "facility" may include a distinct part of an institution but does not include an institution for mental diseases. The "facility" for Medicare and Medicaid purposes (including eligibility, coverage, certification, and payment) is always the entity which participates in the program, whether that entity is composed of all of or a distinct part of a large institution (*Federal Register,* 1989).

Common practice is to complete MDS and RAPs for all Medicare and Medicaid residents. The MDS is a collection of several pages (including the face sheet) of resident information (see Figure 14-2). It contains approximately 500 items with information regarding demographic, physical, mental, and psychosocial function. The time frame for assessment of the resident's status is 7 days unless otherwise noted. However, the assessment reference date should be individualized within the limits of the regulations to most accurately reflect the resident's condition (e.g., over the past 7 days, over the past 14 days). One way to implement a standardized method of assessment is to calculate the fourteenth day after admission for a Medicaid resident (or fifth and fourteenth day after admission for the Medicare resident), then enter this date as the assessment reference date, which is the designated endpoint of the assessment. In this way, every member of the healthcare team is operating within the same frame of reference. This also gives new residents some adjustment time in the facility and provides the staff with enough time—within the limits of the regulated schedule for completion—to assess the resident in a variety of situations and across all shifts.

The nurse may conduct the entire assessment alone, but the intent of OBRA '87 is that staff from the various disciplines involved in the resident's care should participate in the comprehensive assessment process to enhance the interdisciplinary care planning process. Certain sections of the MDS clearly should be completed by other disciplines. For example, Section F (Psychosocial Well-Being) may be completed by the social worker; Section N (Activity Pursuit Patterns) may be completed by the recreational therapist; and Section K (Oral/Nutritional Status) may be completed by the dietitian.

Facility policies and procedures must clearly stipulate which discipline is responsible for completing each section. If any member of the team may not be available to complete the assessment in a timely manner, then that individual or discipline should not be included in the policies and procedures. Nurses provide care for the resident 24-hours-a-day, 7-days-a-week, and virtually nothing is included on the MDS that the nurse cannot assess or answer. Therefore, because the completion date of the assessment and the nurse's coordination of the resident assessment are regulated by law, the nurse could have to complete the assessment rather than leave the MDS incomplete. For the facility to receive Medicare and Medicaid funding, the MDS must be completed within the time limits established and defined in the *Long-term care facilities resident assessment instrument (RAI) user's manual,* version 2.0 (HCFA, 1995). The

nurse (assessment) coordinator, who may be the charge nurse, supervisor, or a MDS coordinator hired specifically for this job, must sign and date the MDS; this signing signifies both the completion of the assessment and the accuracy of every section not signed by another professional.

Federal regulations require that the RAI assessment must be conducted or coordinated with the appropriate participation of health professionals. While some aspects of the assessment process are dictated by regulations, facilities have great flexibility in determining how to integrate the RAI into their own day-to-day operations. The RN coordinator must also sign the RAP summary form to signify completion of the RAI (HCFA, 1995). Every item on the assessment must be answered; if not, then the assessment is not considered to be complete. A comprehensive care plan cannot be developed without a comprehensive assessment.

The resident, the family, and nurses' aides all play an integral role in the comprehensive assessment and care planning process. Communication between licensed nursing personnel and nursing assistants is critical because the nursing assistants directly provide the care to residents. Communication between shifts is of the highest importance as well. The assessment must reflect the resident's status over all shifts. Nurses must understand the importance of documenting and communicating the resident's response to care and interventions on all shifts in a descriptive way (for example, describing the resident's cognitive patterns, ability to perform ADLs, mood, and behavior). The MDS provides a framework for documentation, including indicators and descriptors that facilitate a standardized assessment.

Triggers

Built into these indicators are items referred to as triggered conditions. Triggers are specific MDS responses indicating the presence of clinical factors that may or may not represent a problem or needs that should be included in the care plan. When using the HCFA forms, one must use the trigger legend to identify the triggered items (Figure 14-3). Healthcare professionals may very well be required to assess an item or group of related items to determine whether the resident has a particular need, strength, or problem that should be considered for possible care planning decisions. Although any single MDS item does not necessarily have to show up on the care plan as a problem, the team must consider it in their care planning process. Furthermore, they must document their decision to proceed or not proceed with the care plan, the reason for that decision, and the location of the information that supports that reason. Care should be taken when deciding not to proceed with care planning when the issue is imperative to the health of the individual.

Following are the four types of triggers:

- Factors suggesting a potential problem that warrants

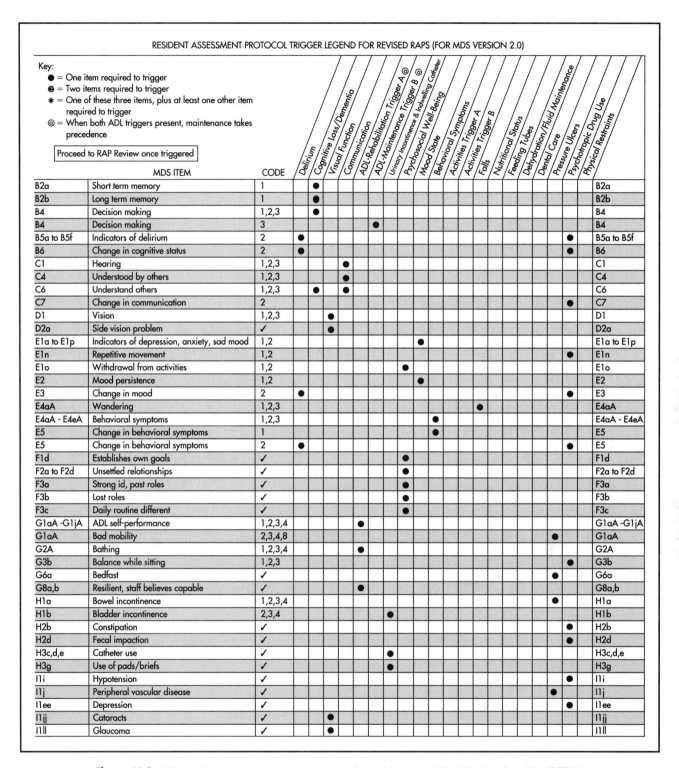

Figure 14-3 The resident assessment protocol trigger legend for revised RAPS. (Developed by HCFA.)

Continued

additional assessment and consideration of a care plan intervention

• Broad screening triggers that assist staff in identifying problems that are hard to diagnose

• Factors that are aimed at the prevention of problems

• Factors that are aimed at identifying candidates with rehabilitation potential

Triggers on items may affect the majority of nursing home residents or have the greatest impact on their daily

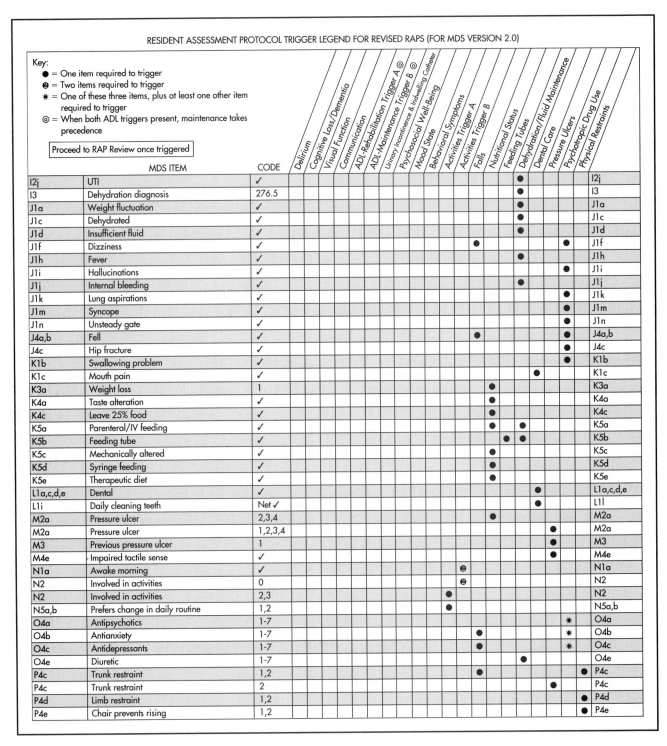

RESIDENT ASSESSMENT PROTOCOL TRIGGER LEGEND FOR REVISED RAPS (FOR MDS VERSION 2.0)

Key:
- ● = One item required to trigger
- ❷ = Two items required to trigger
- ✳ = One of these three items, plus at least one other item required to trigger
- ◉ = When both ADL triggers present, maintenance takes precedence

Proceed to RAP Review once triggered

MDS ITEM		CODE	Delirium	Cognitive Loss/Dementia	Visual Function	Communication	ADL-Rehabilitation	ADL-Maintenance Trigger A ◉	ADL-Maintenance Trigger B ◉	Urinary Incontinence & Indwelling Catheter	Psychosocial Well-Being	Mood State	Behavioral Symptoms	Activities Trigger A	Activities Trigger B	Falls	Nutritional Status	Feeding Tubes	Dehydration/Fluid Maintenance	Dental Care	Pressure Ulcers	Psychotropic Drug Use	Physical Restraints	
I2j	UTI	✓																	●					I2j
I3	Dehydration diagnosis	276.5																	●					I3
J1a	Weight fluctuation	✓																	●					J1a
J1c	Dehydrated	✓																	●					J1c
J1d	Insufficient fluid	✓																	●					J1d
J1f	Dizziness	✓														●						●		J1f
J1h	Fever	✓																	●					J1h
J1i	Hallucinations	✓																				●		J1i
J1j	Internal bleeding	✓																	●					J1j
J1k	Lung aspirations	✓																					●	J1k
J1m	Syncope	✓																					●	J1m
J1n	Unsteady gate	✓																					●	J1n
J4a,b	Fell	✓														●							●	J4a,b
J4c	Hip fracture	✓																					●	J4c
K1b	Swallowing problem	✓																					●	K1b
K1c	Mouth pain	✓																		●				K1c
K3a	Weight loss	1															●							K3a
K4a	Taste alteration	✓															●							K4a
K4c	Leave 25% food	✓															●							K4c
K5a	Parenteral/IV feeding	✓															●	●						K5a
K5b	Feeding tube	✓																●	●					K5b
K5c	Mechanically altered	✓															●							K5c
K5d	Syringe feeding	✓															●							K5d
K5e	Therapeutic diet	✓															●							K5e
L1a,c,d,e	Dental	✓																		●				L1a,c,d,e
L1i	Daily cleaning teeth	Net ✓																		●				L1l
M2a	Pressure ulcer	2,3,4															●							M2a
M2a	Pressure ulcer	1,2,3,4																			●			M2a
M3	Previous pressure ulcer	1																			●			M3
M4e	Impaired tactile sense	✓																			●			M4e
N1a	Awake morning	✓												❷										N1a
N2	Involved in activities	0												❷										N2
N2	Involved in activities	2,3									●													N2
N5a,b	Prefers change in daily routine	1,2									●													N5a,b
O4a	Antipsychotics	1-7																				✳		O4a
O4b	Antianxiety	1-7										●										✳		O4b
O4c	Antidepressants	1-7										●										✳		O4c
O4e	Diuretic	1-7																	●					O4e
P4c	Trunk restraint	1,2										●											●	P4c
P4c	Trunk restraint	2																			●			P4c
P4d	Limb restraint	1,2																					●	P4d
P4e	Chair prevents rising	1,2																					●	P4e

Figure 14-3, cont'd The resident assessment protocol trigger legend for revised RAPS. (Developed by HCFA.)

quality of life or care. Many items that are not triggered are still important to the care of nursing home residents, and these should not be dismissed. It is also necessary to note that the MDS, because it is a *minimum* data set, does not always address all aspects of care for every resident.

Additional assessments, documentation, and care planning must be done as required by the individual's needs, problems, concerns, and circumstances.

Nurses (or other healthcare professionals, when appropriate) should compare the completed MDS with the trigger legend. Once the MDS triggered items are identified from the MDS sections and marked on the trigger legend, the nurse should "walk up" the columns to find the problem areas that correlate to the triggered items. The problem areas should then be checked off on the RAP Summary Sheet.

Resident Assessment Protocols

Resident assessment protocols are problem-oriented frameworks used for additional assessment and problem identification, and they form the final link to decisions about care planning. The RAPs in the HCFA's RAI cover 90% to 95% of the areas that are addressed in a typical nursing home resident's care plan. The HCFA's manual contains the RAPs.

The main part of each RAP is the Guideline section (Figure 14-4). For clarification, the Utilization Guidelines are the HCFA regulatory names for instructions on how the RAI must be used, such as the definition of "Significant Change" found in the *Long-term care facilities resident assessment instrument (RAI) user's manual,* version 2.0 (HCFA, 1995). The guidelines facilitate additional assessment of relevant resident factors and provide a framework for the clinical decision-making process that is used to develop a care plan. The Guidelines section of each triggered RAP should be used to determine whether a problem exists, to identify relevant causal factors, and to develop an individualized care plan appropriate to the needs of the resident.

This system is designed so that the healthcare professionals refer to the RAPs for the following information: clinical, assessment, care planning, and intervention. The assessor must document summary information that will assist the interdisciplinary team in determining whether a problem or need exists, and if so, the type of care plan that should be developed. The assessor who completes each RAP should summarize the following information:

- Complications and risk factors, including the presence of causal factors that may be identified by the guidelines
- Need for referrals to appropriate healthcare professionals
- Reasons for deciding whether to proceed with care plans for triggered problems

If the triggered RAP is not a problem for the resident, the documentation should include the clinical factors from the RAP review process that support the decision. This documentation can be made anywhere in the clinical record, including the progress notes, flowsheets, care plans, or on the RAP Summary Sheet itself. It is important to remember that if a resident problem exists but does not trigger an RAP, the interdisciplinary team must address it in the care plan.

Resident Assessment Protocol Summary Sheet

If the problems are really triggered, they should be checked off on the RAP Summary Sheet, which is referred to as completing the RAPs. Whereas the Trigger Legend is a worksheet that does not have to be kept in every resident's clinical record, the RAP Summary Sheet must be included (Figure 14-5). On the RAP Summary Sheet is a column entitled "Location of Information." The nurse should indicate in this column where the supporting documentation can be found. The column entitled "Care Planning Decision" is filled in last by the staff member who completed that section of the MDS and the appropriate RAP. The assessor is making a clinical judgment to determine whether the MDS and RAP information indicates that this area should be included in the care plan for this resident. The RAPs provide the problem-identification link between assessment and development of care plan goals. Furthermore, RAPs include definitions of triggered conditions and structured frameworks for organizing assessment information (AHCA, 1990).

The RAP Summary form must be completed and signed by the nurse coordinator within 14 days of admission. In so doing, the facility has reached closure of the comprehensive assessment process, as required by law.

THE INTERDISCIPLINARY CARE PLANNING PROCESS

The process of care planning involves examining the resident as a whole and building on the measured characteristics of the individual resident using the standardized MDS items and definitions. Care planning is a process with several steps that may occur at the same time or in sequence. The RAI process should be completed as the basis for care plan decision making (HCFA, 1995). Within 7 days of the completion of the assessment a comprehensive care plan must be developed that includes measurable goals and timetables for meeting a resident's medical, nursing, mental, and psychosocial needs as identified in the comprehensive assessment. The care plan must describe the following:

(i) The services that are to be furnished to attain or maintain the resident's highest practicable physical, mental, and psychosocial well-being
(ii) Any services that would otherwise be required but are not provided due to the resident's exercise of rights, including the right to refuse treatment

The law also states that this care plan must be developed by an interdisciplinary team that includes the attending physician, a registered nurse with responsibility for the resident, and other appropriate staff in disciplines as determined by the resident's needs; and to the extent practicable, the participation of the resident, the resident's family, or the resident's legal representative (*Federal Register,* 1989, 1991b, 1992).

PHYSICAL RESTRAINTS RAP KEY (For MDS Version 2.0)

TRIGGER — REVISION	GUIDELINES

Review for efficacy, side effects and alternatives if one or more of the following:

- Use of trunk restraint [a]
  [P4c = 1,2]
- Use of limb restraint
  [P4d = 1,2]
- Use of chair that prevents rising
  [P4e = 1,2]

Review factors and complications associated with restraint use:

- **Behavioral Symptoms:** Repetitive physical movements **[E1n]**; Any behavioral symptoms **[E4]**; Part of behavior management program **[P1be, P2; from record]**
- **Risk of Falls:** Dizziness **[J1f]**; Falls **[J4a, J4b]**; Antianxiety **[O4b]**; Antidepressant **[O4c]**

- **Conditions and Treatments:** Catheter **[H3c,d]**; Hip fracture **[J4c, I1m]**; Unstable/acute condition **[J5a,b]**; Parenteral/IV and/or feeding tube **[K5a,b]**; Wound care/treatment **[M5f,g,h,i]**; IV meds **[P1ac]**; Respirator/Oxygen **[P1ag, P1al]**

- **ADL Self performance [G1]**

- **Confounding problems to be considered:**
  — Delirium **[B5]**
  — Cognitive loss/dementia **[B2, B4]**
  — Impaired communication **[C4, C6]**
  — Sad/anxious mood **[E1, E2]**
  — Resistance to treatment/meds/nourishment **[E4e]**
  — Unmet psychosocial needs **[F1, F2, F3]**
  — Psychotropic drug side effects **[see record, J1e,f,h,i,m,n]**

- **Other factors to be considered:**
  Resident's response to restraint(s); use of alternatives to restraints; resident/family/staff philosophy, values, wishes, attitudes about restraints **[record, observation, discussion]**

[a] Note: Code 2 also triggers on the Pressure Ulcer RAP. Both codes trigger on the Falls RAP

Figure 14-4 Physical restraints RAP key. (Developed by HCFA.)

After the completion of the MDS assessment on day 14, the interdisciplinary care plan must be developed and completed by day 21. If the assessment was completed on day 10, the care plan should be done by day 17. No regulation dictates how this interdisciplinary care planning is to be carried out with all the required disciplines. Interdisciplinary care planning can be done with verbal and written communication—as long as it is documented and the care plan actually shows the input of all appropriate disciplines. The standard of practice that has evolved, however, is a regularly scheduled interdisciplinary care-planning meeting or conference, which ensures a collegial process. Staff from all the responsible disciplines have the opportunity at this time to discuss their findings and make the final care planning decisions, and decisions made independently before the conference may be changed. If this happens, the RAP Summary Sheet should not be amended; however, the decision-making process should be documented. The RAP guidelines are not meant to be prescriptive or to replace the clinical judgment of the staff as long as evidence of underlying rationale for the care plan exists. Should the team decide that additions should be made to the care plan that were not identified through the MDS and RAP system, these items should not be added to the RAP

- Unmet psychosocial needs (e.g., social isolation, disruption of familiar routines, anger with family members)
- Sad or anxious mood
- Resistance to treatment, medication, nourishment
- Psychotropic drug side effects (e.g., motor agitation, confusion, gait disturbance)
- If a behavior management program is in place, does it adequately address the causes of the resident's particular problem behaviors?

Other Factors to be Considered.

Resident's Response to Restraints

In evaluating restraint use, it is important to review the resident's reaction to restraints (e.g., positive and negative, such as passivity, anger, increased agitation, withdrawal, pleas for release, calls for help, constant attempts to untie/release self). This will help determine whether presumed benefits are outweighed by negative side effects.

Review MDS items on other potential negative effects of restraint use, such as declines in functional self-performance, body control, skin condition, mood and cognition, since restraints have been in use.

Alternatives to Restraints

Many interventions may be as effective or even more effective than restraints in managing a resident's needs, safety risks, and problems. To be effective the intervention must address the underlying problem.

- Review resident's record and confer with staff to determine whether alternatives to restraints have been tried.
- If alternatives to restraints have been tried, what were they?
- How long were the alternatives tried?
- What was the resident's response to the alternatives at the time?
- If the alternative(s) attempted were ineffective, what else was attempted?
- How recently were alternatives other than restraints attempted?

Philosophy and Attitudes

In reconsidering the use of restraints for a resident, consider the philosophy, values, attitudes, and wishes of the resident regarding restraint use, as well as those of his family/significant others, and caregivers. Consider the impact of restraints on facility environment and morale.

- Is there consensus or differences among affected parties in choosing between resident independence and freedom in favor of presumed safety?

Figure 14-4, cont'd   Physical restraints RAP key.

Summary Sheet either. Only those items actually triggered by the MDS are to be checked off and commented on in the RAP Summary Sheet.

Care Plans

Care plans (Figure 14-6) should provide individualized guides to comprehensive, resident-oriented care. The health-care team's success in writing care plans is often influenced by the tool they use. Every care plan should do the following:

1. State the problem, need, strength, and nursing diagnosis simply and understandably.

2. Include measurable goals and resident outcomes.
3. Provide reasonable time frames within which those goals are to be achieved.
4. Identify specific interventions that the staff will implement to assist the resident in achieving those goals.

The design of the form can do the following:

1. Help or hinder the team in accomplishing its required documentation.
2. Enhance interdisciplinary contributions, communication, and multilevel implementation of the plan of care.

Resident's Name:		Medical Record No.:	

1. Check if RAP is triggered.
2. For each triggered RAP, use the RAP guidelines to identify areas needing further assessment. Document relevant assessment information regarding the resident's status.
   - Describe:
     — Nature of the condition (may include presence or lack of objective data and subjective complaints).
     — Complications and risk factors that affect your decision to proceed to care planning.
     — Factors that must be considered in developing individualized care plan interventions.
     — Need for referrals/further evaluation by appropriate health professionals.
   - Documentation should support your decision-making regarding whether to proceed with a care plan for a triggered RAP and the type(s) of care plan interventions that are appropriate for a particular resident.
   - Documentation may appear anywhere in the clinical record (e.g., progress notes, consults, flowsheets, etc.).
3. Indicate under the <u>Location of RAP Assessment Documentation</u> column where information related to the RAP assessment can be found.
4. For each triggered RAP, indicate whether a new care plan, care plan revision, or continuation of current care plan is necessary to address the problem(s) identified in your assessment. The Care Planning Decision column must be completed within 7 days of completing the RAI (MDS and RAPs).

A. RAP PROBLEM AREA	(a) Check if triggered	Location and Date of RAP Assessment Documentation	(b) Care Planning Decision — check if addressed in care plan
1. DELIRIUM	☐		☐
2. COGNITIVE LOSS	☐		☐
3. VISUAL FUNCTION	☐		☐
4. COMMUNICATION	☐		☐
5. ADL FUNCTIONAL/ REHABILITATION POTENTIAL	☐		☐
6. URINARY INCONTINENCE AND INDWELLING CATHETER	☐		☐
7. PSYCHOSOCIAL WELL-BEING	☐		☐
8. MOOD STATE	☐		☐
9. BEHAVIORAL SYMPTOMS	☐		☐
10. ACTIVITIES	☐		☐
11. FALLS	☐		☐
12. NUTRITIONAL STATUS	☐		☐
13. FEEDING TUBES	☐		☐
14. DEHYDRATION/FLUID MAINTENANCE	☐		☐
15. DENTAL CARE	☐		☐
16. PRESSURE ULCERS	☐		☐
17. PSYCHOTROPIC DRUG USE	☐		☐
18. PHYSICAL RESTRAINTS	☐		☐

B. _____   2. ☐☐ — ☐☐ — ☐☐☐☐
1. Signature of RN Coordinator for RAP Assessment Process   Month   Day   Year

_____   4. ☐☐ — ☐☐ — ☐☐☐☐
3. Signature of Person Completing Care Planning Decision   Month   Day   Year

Figure 14-5   RAP Summary Sheet. (Developed by HCFA.)

3. Serve as the hub of team documentation.
4. Reduce extraneous and redundant documentation.

Nurses can demonstrate their understanding of the nursing diagnosis by translating that diagnosis into the universal language of the MDS.

It is extremely helpful for the wording of the nursing diagnosis to use phrases such as "related to," "as evidenced by," or "as manifested by." Such wordings define the problem area and nursing diagnosis within the context of the resident and clearly state the condition so that other professionals and paraprofessionals understand it. The target

dates provide an expected reasonable time frame for achievement of the goal, and the review dates for the evaluation demonstrate the annual and quarterly assessment and care planning process in one centralized, easily accessible location. The evaluation may be a statement as simple as "Progress being made," "Goal not met," or "Goal met." But a better practice is to expand on the descriptive documentation; for example:

- "Progress being made. Resident increased ambulation from 10 to 20 feet with assist of two."

RED BANK CONVALESCENT CENTER, INC.
RESIDENT CARE PLAN

RAP Problem Areas:
 1. Delirium
 2. Cognitive Loss
 3. Vision
 4. Communication
 5. ADL/Rehab
 6. Incontinence/
    Catheters

 7. Psychosocial
 8. Mood State
 9. Behavior
10. Activities
11. Falls
12. Nutritional
    Status

13. Feeding Tubes
14. Dehydration/Fluid
    Maintenance
15. Dental Care
16. Pressure Ulcers
17. Psychotropics
18. Phys. Restraints

DATE STARTED (month,day,year)		PROBLEM/NEED/STRENGTH	GOALS Include patient outcome and target date of attainment.	TARGET DATE (month,day,year)		
10/20/93	#					
	1	ADL DEFICIT IN EATING	RESIDENT WILL GAIN 5 lbs IN 3 MONTHS	1	20	94
		RELATED TO:				
		NEUROMUSCULAR IMPAIRMENT	RESIDENT WILL CONSUME 75-100% ALL MEALS	4	20	94
		MANIFESTED BY:	WITHOUT ASSISTANCE OF STAFF			
		TREMORS OF Ⓡ HAND				
		WT. LOSS 5 lbs.				

Figure 14-6 Resident care plan. (From Red Bank Convalescent Center, Red Bank, NJ.)

Continued

RESIDENT _Jane Doe_

DIAGNOSIS _Parkinsonism_

DOCTOR _xyz_

STAFF INTERVENTIONS Include frequency, duration, and focus	RESPONSIBLE DISCIPLINES	REVIEW DATE (month,day,year)			EVALUATION Include date and initials
1- OT EVAL FOR ASSISTIVE DEVICES	NSG, OT	1	20	94	GOAL MET - SEE NEW GOAL, CONTINUE PLAN
2- PROVIDE ASSISTANCE AND TRAINING with UTENSILS and PLATE GUARD	OT				with MINIMAL STAFF Assist to PROMOTE FULL INDEPENDENCE
3- PROVIDE ASSISTANCE with meals when necessary	NSG				
4- MONITOR r RECORD MEAL INTAKE	N, D, OT				
5- RECORD WEEKLY WTS fo/mo then MONTHLY WTS	N, D				
6- PROVIDE ROM r LARGE MUSCLE EXERCISE	N, Act, OT				
7- PROVIDE SUPPORTIVE COUNSELING r PROMOTE INDEPEN	N, SS				

Figure 14-6, cont'd   Resident care plan. (From Red Bank Convalescent Center, Red Bank, NJ.)

```
                    TEAM CARE PLANNING SIGNATURES
_____

DATE    1/20/94                        DATE_____
RN  Mary White, Rn                     RN_____
SW  Pat Black, MSW                     SW_____
ACT June Brown, CRT                    ACT_____
DIET Eileen Gray, RD                   DIET_____
CNA  Anne Smith, CNA                   CNA_____
     Jane Doe                          _____
     Cathy Doe, daughter               _____
     Pam Evans, OT                     _____


DATE_____    DATE_____

RN_____    RN_____

SW_____    SW_____

ACT_____    ACT_____

DIET_____    DIET_____

CNA_____    CNA_____

_____    _____

_____    _____

_____    _____


OTHER_____    OTHER_____
_____    _____
_____    _____
_____    _____
_____    _____
_____    _____
```

Figure 14-6, cont'd Resident care plan.

- "Goal not met. Resident unable to ambulate 10 feet. See new goal."
- "Goal resolved. Resident ambulates 20 feet without assist."

Once new target dates have been entered, the periodic (quarterly) review and revision requirement is complete.

The Quarterly Review: The Federal Format and Process

Staff members must systematically monitor the resident's status between annual assessments. The quarterly review focuses assessment on a particular subset of MDS items to help the staff to detect gradual changes in resident status.

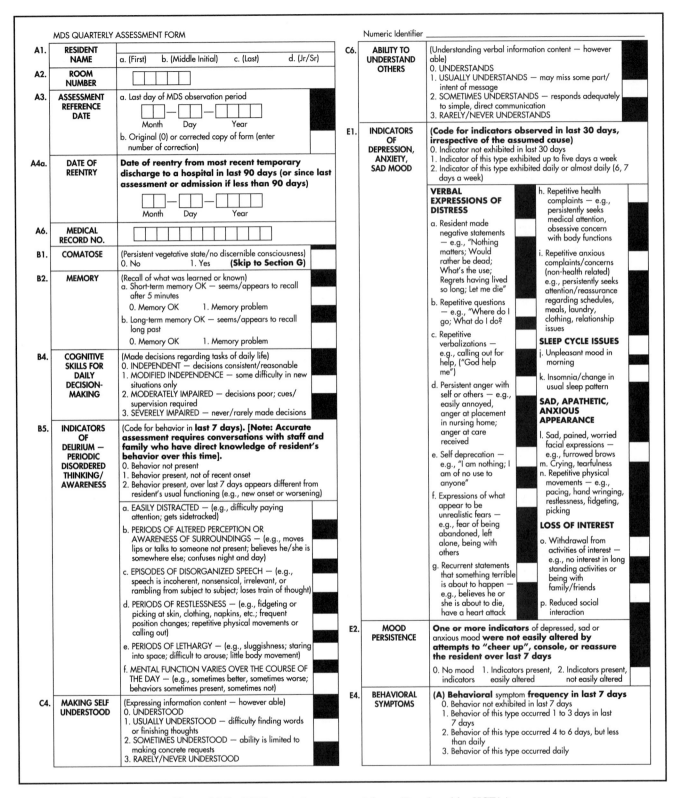

Figure 14-7   MDS quarterly assessment form. (Developed by HCFA.)

This subset has been defined by the HCFA as a minimum quarterly assessment. This core of critical indicators helps the staff track the resident's decline or improvement. The quarterly review also provides a source of information for determining whether the care plan should be revised. A facility is not obliged to use the HCFA quarterly review form as long as the core items in the form it uses are exactly the same (Figure 14-7). An identifiable summary

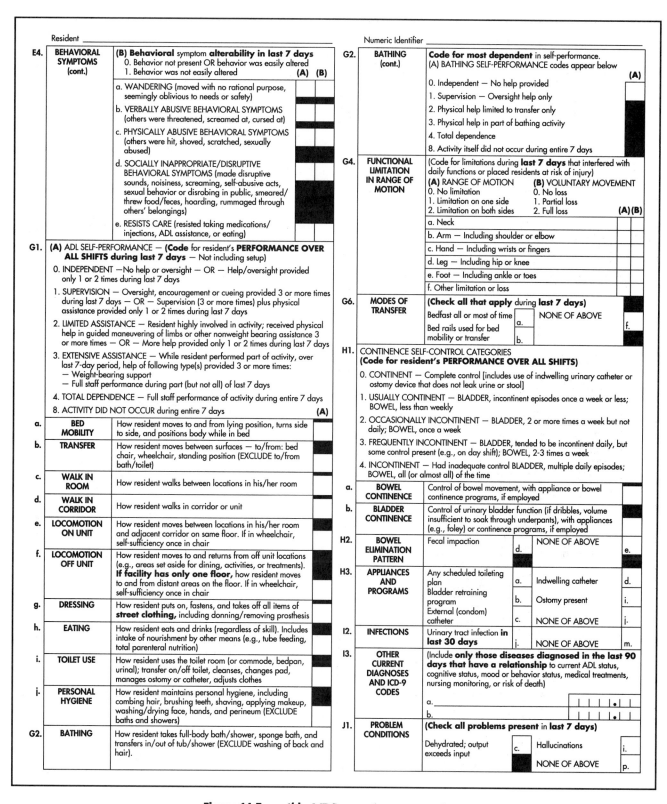

Figure 14-7, cont'd MDS quarterly assessment form. *Continued*

of the resident's status must be documented. Sometimes nurses prefer to include narrative notes in what is purely a codified review (Figure 14-8). In any event, the resident and the plan of care must be reviewed at least once every

90 days and revised as necessary based on the resident's needs. When using a good care plan tool, the care plan does not have to be rewritten each time, but instead it can demonstrate the continuity of care and progression of the

Resident _____ Numeric Identifier _____

J2.	**PAIN SYMPTOMS**	(Code the **highest level of pain** present in the **last 7 days**) a. **FREQUENCY** with which resident complains or shows evidence of pain 0. No pain **(skip to J4)** 1. Pain less than daily 2. Pain daily	b. **INTENSITY** of pain 1. Mild pain 2. Moderate pain 3. Times when pain is horrible or excruciating

J4.	**ACCIDENTS**	**(Check all that apply)**	Hip fracture in **last 180 days** — c.
		Fell in **past 30 days** — a.	Other fracture in **last 180 days** — d.
		Fell in **past 31-180 days** — b.	NONE OF ABOVE — e.

J5.	**STABILITY OF CONDITIONS**	Conditions/diseases make resident's cognitive, ADL, mood or behavior status unstable — (fluctuating, precarious, or deteriorating)	a.
		Resident experiencing an acute episode or a flare-up of a recurrent or chronic problem	b.
		End-stage disease, 6 or fewer months to live	c.
		NONE OF ABOVE	d.

K3.	**WEIGHT CHANGE**	a. **Weight loss** — 5% or more in **last 30 days**; or 10% or more in **last 180 days** 0. No 1. Yes
		b. **Weight gain** — 5% or more in **last 30 days**; or 10% or more in **last 180 days** 0. No 1. Yes

K5.	**NUTRITIONAL APPROACHES**	Feeding tube	b.
		On a planned weight change program	h.
		NONE OF ABOVE	l.

M1.	**ULCERS** **(Due to any cause)**	(Record the number of ulcers at each ulcer stage — regardless of cause. If none present at a stage, record "0" (zero). Code all that apply during **last 7 days**. Code 9 = 9 or more.) **[Requires full body exam.]**	**Number at stage**
		a. Stage 1. A persistent area of skin redness (without a break in the skin) that does not disappear when pressure is relieved	
		b. Stage 2. A partial thickness loss of skin layers that presents clinically as an abrasion, blister, or shallow crater	
		c. Stage 3. A full thickness of skin is lost, exposing the subcutaneous tissues — presents as a deep crater with or without undermining adjacent tissue	
		d. Stage 4. A full thickness of skin and subcutaneous tissue is lost, exposing muscle or bone	

M2.	**TYPE OF ULCER**	(For each type of ulcer **code for the highest stage in the last 7 days** using scale in item M1 — i.e., 0 = none; stages 1,2,3,4) a. Pressure ulcer — any lesion caused by pressure resulting in damage of underlying tissue b. Stasis ulcer — open lesion caused by poor circulation in the lower extremities

N1.	**TIME AWAKE**	**(Check appropriate time periods over last 7 days)** Resident awake all or most of the time (i.e., naps no more than one hour per time period) in the:	
		Morning — a.	Evening — c.
		Afternoon — b.	NONE OF ABOVE — d.

(If resident is comatose, skip to Section O)

N2.	**AVERAGE TIME INVOLVED IN ACTIVITIES**	**(When awake and not receiving treatments or ADL care)** 0. Most — more than 2/3 of time 2. Little — less than 1/3 of time 1. Some — from 1/3 to 2/3 of time 3. None

O1.	**NUMBER OF MEDICATIONS**	**(Record the number of different** medications used in the **last 7 days**; enter "0" if none used)

O4.	**DAYS RECEIVED THE FOLLOWING MEDICATION**	**(Record the number of DAYS** during **last 7 days**; enter "0" if not used. Note — enter "1" for long-acting meds used less than weekly) a. Antipsychotic b. Antianxiety d. Hypnotic c. Antidepressant e. Diuretic

P4.	**DEVICES AND RESTRAINTS**	Use the following codes for **last 7 days:** 0. Not used 1. Used less than daily 2. Used daily Bed rails a. — Full bed rails on all open sides of bed b. — Other types of side rails used (e.g., half rail, one side) c. Trunk restraint d. Limb restraint e. Chair prevents rising

Q2.	**OVERALL CHANGE IN CARE NEEDS**	Resident's overall level of self sufficiency has changed significantly as compared to status of **90 days ago** (or since last assessment if less than 90 days)
		0. No change 1. Improved — 2. Deteriorated —
		                           receives fewer receives more
		                           supports, needs support
		                           less restrictive
		                           level of care

R2. **SIGNATURES OF PERSONS COMPLETING THE ASSESSMENT:**

a. Signature of RN Assessment Coordinator (sign on above line)

b. Date RN Assessment Coordinator signed as complete   ☐☐ — ☐☐ — ☐☐☐☐
                                                        Month   Day   Year

	Title	Sections	Date
c. Other Signatures			
d.			Date
e.			Date
f.			Date
g.			Date

Figure 14-7, cont'd   MDS quarterly assessment form. (Developed by HCFA.)

resident's status. Each resident's clinical record will have at a minimum one face sheet (Figure 14-9), two MDS forms, and three quarterly review forms from the time of admission.

SIGNIFICANT CHANGES IN CONDITION

If a significant change in the resident's status is identified, either through the quarterly review process or at any other time, a complete MDS should be documented and the care

Patient's Name:_____

Room:_____ Date:

NURSING SUMMARY AND EVALUATION

1. General Appearance and Vitals: T_____ P_____R_____B/P_____

   _____

2. Cognitive and Communication Patterns_____

   _____

3. Physical Function, ADL, Potential_____

   _____

   _____

4. Continence_____

   _____

5. Mood and Behavior_____

   _____

6. Nutrition, Appetite, Weight_____

   _____

7. Restorative Nursing and Progress (treatments, dressings, PT, OT, B&B training, etc)

   _____

   _____

8. Socialization and Activities_____

   _____

9. Disease/Diagnosis Status_____

   _____

   Rep 91ᵉ

Figure 14-8 Narrative summary. (Developed by Rita Cavallaro.)

SECTION A. IDENTIFICATION AND BACKGROUND INFORMATION

1.	**RESIDENT NAME**	a. (First) b. (Middle Initial) c. (Last) d. (Jr/Sr)
2.	**ROOM NUMBER**	☐☐☐☐☐
3.	**ASSESSMENT REFERENCE DATE**	a. Last day of MDS observation period ☐☐ — ☐☐ — ☐☐☐☐ Month Day Year b. Original (0) or corrected copy of form (enter number of correction)
4a.	**DATE OF REENTRY**	**Date of reentry from most recent temporary discharge to a hospital in last 90 days (or since last assessment or admission if less than 90 days)** ☐☐ — ☐☐ — ☐☐☐☐ Month Day Year
5.	**MARITAL STATUS**	1. Never married 3. Widowed 5. Divorced 2. Married 4. Separated
6.	**MEDICAL RECORD NO.**	☐☐☐☐☐☐☐☐☐☐☐
7.	**CURRENT PAYMENT SOURCES FOR N.H. STAY**	(Billing Office to indicate; **check all that apply in last 30 days**)

7. payment			
Medicaid per diem	a.	VA per diem	f.
Medicare per diem	b.	Self or family pays for full per diem	g.
Medicare ancillary part A	c.	Medicaid resident liability or Medicare co-payment	h.
Medicare ancillary part B	d.	Private insurance per diem (including co-payment)	i.
CHAMPUS per diem	e.	Other per diem	j.

8.	**REASONS FOR ASSESSMENT** [Note — If this is a discharge or reentry assessment, only a limited subset of MDS items need be completed]	a. Primary reason for assessment 1. Admission assessment (required by day 14) 2. Annual assessment 3. Significant change in status assessment 4. Significant correction of prior full assessment 5. Quarterly review assessment 6. Discharged — return not anticipated 7. Discharged — return anticipated 8. Discharged prior to completing initial assessment 9. Reentry 10. Significant correction of prior quarterly assessment 0. NONE OF ABOVE b. **Codes for assessments required for Medicare PPS or the State** 1. Medicare 5 day assessment 2. Medicare 30 day assessment 3. Medicare 60 day assessment 4. Medicare 90 day assessment 5. Medicare readmission/return assessment 6. Other state required assessment 7. Medicare 14 day assessment 8. Other Medicare required assessment
9.	**RESPONSIBILITY/ LEGAL GUARDIAN**	(Check all that apply)

9.			
Legal guardian	a.	Durable power attorney/ financial	d.
Other legal oversight	b.	Family member responsible	e.
Durable power of attorney/health care	c.	Patient responsible for self	f.
		NONE OF ABOVE	g.

10.	**ADVANCED DIRECTIVES**	(For those items with supporting **documentation** in the medical record, **check all that apply**)

10.			
Living will	a.	Feeding restrictions	f.
Do not resuscitate	b.	Medication restrictions	g.
Do not hospitalize	c.	Other treatment restrictions	h.
Organ donation	d.	NONE OF ABOVE	i.
Autopsy request	e.		

SECTION B. COGNITIVE PATTERNS

1.	**COMATOSE**	(Persistent vegetative state/no discernible consciousness) 0. No 1. Yes **(If yes, skip to Section G)**
2.	**MEMORY**	(Recall of what was learned or known) a. Short-term memory OK — seems/appears to recall after 5 minutes 0. Memory OK 1. Memory problem b. Long-term memory OK — seems/appears to recall long past 0. Memory OK 1. Memory problem

3.	**MEMORY/ RECALL ABILITY**	(**Check all** that resident was **normally able to recall during last 7 days**)

3.			
Current season	a.	That he/she is in a nursing home	d.
Location of own room	b.	NONE OF ABOVE are recalled	e.
Staff names/faces	c.		

4.	**COGNITIVE SKILLS FOR DAILY DECISION-MAKING**	(Made decisions regarding tasks of daily life) 0. INDEPENDENT — decisions consistent/reasonable 1. MODIFIED INDEPENDENCE — some difficulty in new situations only 2. MODERATELY IMPAIRED — decisions poor; cues/ supervision required 3. SEVERELY IMPAIRED — never/rarely made decisions
5.	**INDICATORS OF DELIRIUM— PERIODIC DISORDERED THINKING/ AWARENESS**	(Code for behavior in the **last 7 days**.) [Note: Accurate assessment requires conversations with staff and family who have direct knowledge of resident's behavior over this time.] 0. Behavior not present 1. Behavior present, not of recent onset 2. Behavior present, over last 7 days appears different from resident's usual functioning (e.g., new onset or worsening) a. EASILY DISTRACTED — (e.g., difficulty paying attention; gets sidetracked) b. PERIODS OF ALTERED PERCEPTION OR AWARENESS OF SURROUNDINGS — (e.g., moves lips or talks to someone not present; believes he/she is somewhere else; confuses night and day) c. EPISODES OF DISORGANIZED SPEECH — (e.g., speech is incoherent, nonsensical, irrelevant, or rambling from subject to subject; loses train of thought) d. PERIODS OF RESTLESSNESS — (e.g., fidgeting or picking at skin, clothing, napkins, etc.; frequent position changes; repetitive physical movements or calling out) e. PERIODS OF LETHARGY — (e.g., sluggishness; staring into space; difficult to arouse; little body movement) f. MENTAL FUNCTION VARIES OVER THE COURSE OF THE DAY — (e.g., sometimes better, sometimes worse; behaviors sometimes present, sometimes not)
6.	**CHANGE IN COGNITIVE STATUS**	Resident's cognitive status, skills, or abilities have changed as compared to status of **90 days ago** (or since last assessment if less than 90 days) 0. No change 1. Improved 2. Deteriorated

SECTION C. COMMUNICATION/HEARING PATTERNS

1.	**HEARING**	(With hearing appliance, is used) 0. HEARS ADEQUATELY — normal talk, TV, phone 1. MINIMAL DIFFICULTY when not in quiet setting 2. HEARS IN SPECIAL SITUATIONS ONLY — speaker has to adjust tonal quality and speak distinctly 3. HIGHLY IMPAIRED/absence of useful hearing
2.	**COMMUNICATION DEVICES/ TECHNIQUES**	(**Check all that apply** during last 7 days)

2.	
Hearing aid, present and used	a.
Hearing aid, present and not used regularly	b.
Other receptive comm. techniques used (e.g., lip reading)	c.
NONE OF ABOVE	d.

3.	**MODES OF EXPRESSION**	(**Check all used** by resident to make needs known)

3.			
Speech	a.	Signs/gestures/sounds	d.
Writing messages to express or clarify needs	b.	Communication board	e.
		Other	f.
American sign language or Braille	c.	NONE OF ABOVE	g.

4.	**MAKING SELF UNDERSTOOD**	(Expressing information content — however able) 0. UNDERSTOOD 1. USUALLY UNDERSTOOD — difficulty finding words or finishing thoughts 2. SOMETIMES UNDERSTOOD — ability is limited to making concrete requests 3. RARELY/NEVER UNDERSTOOD
5.	**SPEECH CLARITY**	(Code for speech in the **last 7 days**) 0. CLEAR SPEECH — distinct, intelligible words 1. UNCLEAR SPEECH — slurred, mumbled words 2. NO SPEECH — absence of spoken words
6.	**ABILITY TO UNDERSTAND OTHERS**	(Understand verbal information content — however able) 0. UNDERSTANDS 1. USUALLY UNDERSTANDS — may miss some part/intent of message 2. SOMETIMES UNDERSTANDS — responds adequately to simple, direct communication 3. RARELY/NEVER UNDERSTANDS
7.	**CHANGE IN COMMUNICATION/ HEARING**	Resident's ability to express, understand, or hear information has changed as compared to status of **90 days ago** (or since last assessment if less than 90 days) 0. No change 1. Improved 2. Deteriorated

Figure 14-9 First page of the minimum data set, version 2.0, for nursing home resident assessment and care screening, full assessment form. (Developed by HCFA.)

plan should be revised. According to the HCFA "Final Rule" (dated June 1998), a "Significant Change" has been further defined and clarified as "a decline or improvement in a resident's status that will not normally resolve itself without intervention by staff or by implementing standard disease-related clinical interventions, that has an impact on more than one area of the resident's health status and requires interdisciplinary review or revision of the care plan." Before the completion of the MDS, the onset of a suspected significant change should be documented in the progress notes. All interventions and the resident's responses to these interventions must be carefully documented. If the care providers believe that the change in clinical status is not major or permanent, then substantial reasons for the decision not to complete a new MDS assessment must be documented as well. If there is not sufficient evidence to prove response to treatment by the fourteenth day after the onset of a change, then a full MDS for significant change must be completed. Significant change can be anything positive or negative, such as the following: the resident's recovery of his or her ability to walk or use his or her hands to grasp small items; the loss of his or her ability to perform two or more ADLs; a serious complication; improved behavior, mood, or functional status such that the existing care plan no longer matches the current needs of the resident.

SUMMARY OF THE INTERDISCIPLINARY RESIDENT ASSESSMENT AND CARE PLANNING PROCESS

The following list summarizes the interdisciplinary resident assessment and care planning process:

- At the time of admission, discipline-specific assessments and the initial care plans should be done; the nursing assessment and care plan must be finished within 24 to 48 hours, and those other disciplines must be completed within 7 days. Furthermore, nurses should follow Medicare/Medicaid requirements for charting.
- The MDS must be completed no later than 14 calendar days after admission for Medicaid residents. The nurse coordinator is responsible for the timely completion of the MDS.
- The Interdisciplinary Resident Care Plan (IDCP) must be finished within 7 days of the completion of the MDS. The IDCP conference must be scheduled between days 14 and 21.
- Amendments can be made to the MDS within 21 days after admission, but only in the following specific circumstances:

  1. Information necessary to complete the MDS is not available by the fourteenth day but becomes available within 21 days.

  2. Continued observation of and interaction with the resident provides a different clinical picture than the initial impression of the resident's cognitive patterns, potential for self-care improvement or rehabilitation, psychosocial well-being, mood and behavior patterns, activity pursuit patterns, and oral-nutritional status.
  3. Factual information error is caused by incorrect copying of things such as resident numbers, address, social security number, or ICD-9 codes.

- Ongoing progress notes should be made as the resident's status and events warrant.

Quarterly Reviews and Summaries of Resident Status and Resident Care Plan

Quarterly reviews and summaries of the resident's status and care plan must be date-specific to the completion date of the MDS. A quarterly review must be done once every 90 to 92 days. Scheduling completion of the quarterly review as close as possible to the date of completion of the MDS using the 90 to 92 day rule to standardize the process is advisable. The IDCP conference should be scheduled within the following week. If appropriate, making summary entries after the team has met, discussed reassessment, and reviewed the care plan is also advisable. Care cannot be planned without first providing an appropriate assessment. The annual MDS must be completed no later than once every 365 days.

If an MDS was completed for a significant change 1 month after the initial MDS was finalized, then the schedule for reassessment should be based on the completion of the second MDS. The date of the annual MDS, however, should be keyed to the date of the last MDS.

A BRIEF REVIEW OF THE SURVEY PROCESS AS IT RELATES TO DOCUMENTATION AND MDS

The OBRA survey process is oriented to the resident's outcome. The resident is the primary source of information regarding demonstrable quality of care, quality of life, and resident rights. The resident, the MDS, and the care plan are all an important part of assessment and care planning. If any one of these areas is not addressed, the facility will be cited for a deficiency, which can be costly for the facility in terms of monetary fines, closure to new admissions, or loss of certification for participating in Medicare and Medicaid. The surveyors should select a random sampling of residents to serve as subjects. They should then carefully review each item of the MDS (and quarterly reviews) for each one of these residents, developing the picture of the resident that the data has captured. Next the surveyors should proceed to the care plans to determine whether they match the assessments, and then they should observe the residents to determine whether their status matches that of the assessments and care plans. Finally the surveyors should observe the actual delivery of care.

COMPUTERIZATION OF THE RESIDENT ASSESSMENT INSTRUMENTS

As of June 1998 all Medicare- and Medicaid-certified nursing homes were required to electronically submit all subsequent MDS assessment, discharge, reentry records, and background information to the state database using the timing requirements found in the *Long-term care facilities resident assessment instrument (RAI) user's manual,* version 2.0. The state is required to submit the information in their database to the HCFA on a monthly basis. The state compares this information with the HCFA specifications to determine whether the sequence of assessment types is correct. For example, after a comprehensive assessment has been submitted, the state should expect to receive three quarterly review assessments, approximately 90 to 92 days apart, followed by an annual comprehensive assessment, no later than 365 days from the date of the last comprehensive assessment. With OBRA in mind, one can presume that the computerized format will make available data that will affect reimbursement to long-term care facilities.

One benefit of computerization is the reduction in documentation time. Resident assessments that can take 1 hour to complete manually can be performed in less time with computer assistance. Updates for quarterly reviews and care plan development can also be completed in less time than the manual method. Unfortunately many computer systems are being developed that are not necessarily designed for nursing. Although the RAI is a universal tool, the care planning piece can vary in design, content, and multidisciplinary assumptions. When the nurse's thoughts do not match the logic of the computer, nurses may decide the computer is correct and allow the computer to influence their decision-making process. In addition, depending on the type of process that is implemented, computerization may decrease the collegial dialogue necessary for the development of nursing knowledge (Vlasses, 1993). This problem can be overcome by entering the data while the healthcare team confers rather than using preplanned care plans that simply require editing. Survey findings support the suspicion that these types of programs, or the way they are used, tend to decrease the interactive thought processes of the team members and the individualization of the care plan when the team is not strong in the manual implementation of the care planning process.

MEDICARE DOCUMENTATION

Medicare is the principal source of healthcare insurance for persons over age 65. Persons eligible for Medicare receive Part A (Hospital and Skilled-Care Services Insurance), at no cost, but they will receive very little for long-term care. Limitations are placed on the number of days that Medicare will reimburse a skilled nursing facility (currently 100 days for a single stay). The beneficiary is covered in full for the first 20 days, then pays a coinsurance fee for days 21 to 100. The amount of this coinsurance is adjusted each year on the first day of January. This can pose a problem for facilities because most residents and family members believe they have up to 100 days of full coverage without regard to the resident's condition. When a resident exceeds the maximum benefits and is ready for discharge, eligibility for coverage ceases. Furthermore, when a resident is not improving and is not expected to improve according to his plan of care, eligibility for coverage also ends. The resident may still need skilled care; however, the resident is now identified as needing a maintenance level of care, which Medicare does not cover in a skilled nursing facility (Davis, 1993; Eliopoulos, 1992).

Preadmission requirements are also required for reimbursement for skilled care. Beneficiaries must be hospitalized in a participating hospital for medically necessary inpatient hospital care for at least 3 consecutive calendar days, not including the day of discharge. They must be in need of care after the hospital stay. Finally, they must be admitted and receive the needed care within 30 days after the day of discharge from the hospital.

The HCFA, in managing Medicare, evaluates the performance of intermediaries as well as providers. In this case, the provider is the certified skilled nursing facility. The intermediary is an agency or organization that has contracted with the Social Security Administration to process Medicare claims. The intermediary (insurance company) determines whether a claim meets the conditions for coverage, makes payment to the providers for services rendered (if the conditions have been met), and monitors the use of services.

The documentation in the clinical record must verify the necessity for provision or supervision of care by professional or technical personnel on an inpatient and daily basis in a nursing facility. If any of these conditions is not met, a nursing home stay will not be covered. Documentation must also demonstrate the validity of skilled rehabilitative care by describing a reasonable expectation of improvement or the services needed to establish a maintenance program. The amount, frequency, and duration of services must be reasonable and necessary (Eliopoulos, 1992).

Starting in July 1998, when the prospective payment system (PPS) began its 4-year phase-in, the way the MDS should be filled out will determine the reimbursement rate for Medicare residents in skilled nursing facilities. Reimbursement is based on the documentation of assessments and the services provided in a Medicare skilled unit. Documentation must communicate and substantiate a resident's health and functional status, the resident's response to treatment, the provision of services, and the quality of care. An accurately encoded MDS is the most important part of that documentation.

For Medicare residents, comprehensive assessments should be filled out more often—at the fifth, fourteenth, thirtieth, sixtieth, and ninetieth days. In addition, documentation should include any discharge, readmission, state-specific or background information sections. The facility must choose either the fifth- or fourteenth-day assessment as the admission assessment, include the RAPs, and hold the interdisciplinary care plan meeting.

PROSPECTIVE PAYMENT SYSTEM

The Balanced Budget Act of 1997, signed by President Clinton, established the PPS for nursing facilities. The PPS is the biggest change in Medicare for subacute care since its enactment in 1966. In the past, Medicare-certified nursing facilities have been paid on a cost-based system; that is, retrospectively after services have been rendered. Under the retrospective payment system, caregivers provided virtually unlimited visits, ordered therapies, and used endless amounts of supplies, all the while knowing they would be reimbursed by Medicare, regardless of resident responses and outcomes.

Under PPS, reimbursement is based on clinical documentation of assessments and the resident's response to treatments and therapy. The MDS is the tool that determines each facility's individual reimbursement rate. Assessment information on the MDS will be used to calculate and place each resident into 1 of 44 different Resource Utilization Groups, version III (RUGs III). Each RUG III category has a different reimbursement value, and each resident falls into a different category. Medicare has established only one default payment rate, which will be used if any coding errors (made by the facility) are found when the MDS is electronically submitted to the state. Therefore documentation will be critical to payment. Facilities are paid a flat daily rate based on the condition of the resident as reflected by the RUG category. Each facility must be able to produce documentation showing a comprehensive, around-the-clock, 7-days-a-week image of each resident. If not, the chances of being correctly reimbursed are diminished. Even minor variations in MDS assessments can make a huge difference in reimbursement when the MDS information is converted to RUGs codes. The difference between a resident assessed as needing "ultra-high" rehabilitation whose ADLs are coded as "moderate" and another resident assessed as needing "ultra-high" rehabilitation who is erroneously

marked as "independent" can mean thousands of dollars of lost reimbursement each month. Although this kind of error can be corrected, the lost revenue cannot be collected retroactively. Nurses and clinicians are now effectively determining reimbursement while they gather the information, make the assessment, and fill out the MDS. Undercoding can result in a monetary loss to the facility, and overcoding can throw up "red flags" to survey teams (in some cases, resulting in fines of up to $5000 per incident).

Documentation requirements are increased under PPS, and documentation must support the care planning decisions. The Initial, Annual, and Significant Change care plan decisions must reflect the RAP assessment. Quarterly notes and summaries must evaluate the resident's progress toward reaching goals and correcting problems. Each facility will need to develop time-saving techniques to avoid redundancy while still supporting MDS information and the care planning decisions and accurately reflecting the RAP assessments.

LONG-TERM CARE LIABILITY ISSUES

Between 1986 and 1996 the amount of litigation involving nursing homes increased dramatically. A research study in 1986 showed that older patients were less likely to file a malpractice suit, and their claims, if successful, were likely to result in much less money than those filed by younger plaintiffs. Nursing home litigation was the most rapidly expanding area of litigation in the United States by 1996. Nursing home plaintiffs were being awarded money at a rate that was four times higher than other types of personal injury suits (Fox, 1997).

Factors Contributing to an Increase in Lawsuits

The following factors have combined to result in the explosion of nursing home litigation:

1. The Nursing Home Reform Act of 1987 (OBRA, 1987) has had a great impact by more precisely defining the standard of care. The creation of the MDS and RAPs provided a uniform way to assess the needs of residents. Recognizing a failure to adequately assess the needs of a resident and implementing a plan to address the priority needs is now easier.
2. As the focus of health care has shifted away from hospitals and more people are receiving care in alternative settings, the number of legal cases involving long-term care is increasing (Fiesta, 1996a).
3. Tort reform on state and federal levels, which has reduced the ability of plaintiff attorneys to bring litigation in more traditional areas of law, has stimulated the investigation of injuries sustained in long-term

care facilities. In addition, some states have liberalized the laws in an effort to deter substandard care and increase the ability of nursing home residents to obtain legal counsel. Legislation in some states has resulted in the courts being allowed to award punitive damages and reimbursement to plaintiffs for legal fees (Fox, 1997).

4. Aging "baby boomers" may be more likely to bring suit when an institutionalized parent or relative is harmed in a long-term care facility. Baby boomers are less likely to place doctors and nurses on a pedestal and view them as above reproach, as did many of their parent's generation.
5. According to Fox (1997), many physicians are not interested in providing long-term care and thus may provide substandard care or avoid the facility.
6. The media is paying more attention to legal issues in long-term care (Feutz-Harter, Laughlin, 1998).

The government's attempt to improve the quality of care that is delivered in nursing homes occurred through the enactment of OBRA '87, which regulates the way that nursing homes deliver care, provide staff, train nursing assistants, monitor the quality of care, and protect the resident's rights. Facilities that do not comply with the regulations are fined and payment for Medicare and Medicaid services can be withheld. The regulations of OBRA emphasize the importance of avoiding negative outcomes. The remainder of this chapter will describe examples of negative outcomes and will be illustrated by case law. A full description of the liability issues which affect long-term care is beyond the scope of this text.

Liability Issues

In order to identify the types of cases that are litigated on behalf of long-term care residents, verdicts that were published in the national medical malpractice verdicts journal *Medical Malpractice Verdicts, Settlements and Experts* were reviewed (Iyer, 1996). The verdicts and settlements involving nursing homes from January 1993 to September 1995 were analyzed. Figure 14-10 shows the results of that analysis. Although they are not included in the figure, data from the same journal for the period from January 1997 to May 1998 was also reviewed to determine whether the trends identified in the period (1993 to 1995) were still evident in the more recent cases. The cases that involved allegations of malpractice solely by physicians were excluded from the sample.

The reader should be cautious about drawing any conclusions from the study reported above. Obviously any cases that were screened for malpractice and not filed, as well as any cases that were dropped before settlement, are not reported in jury verdict publications. (The editor of *Medical Malpractice Verdicts, Settlements and Experts* surveys many jury verdict publications, but clearly many

long-term care cases are not reported in this journal.) The sample size is small for each type of liability issue, and it is not necessarily representative of these types of cases. This study is descriptive, and no attempt has been made to draw statistical correlations between the types of cases and verdicts. When reviewing the award ranges, note that the amount of some of the settlements was kept confidential; therefore the amounts do not appear in the award range. However, observations can be drawn from both samples. The following comments relate to the sample from 1993 to 1995 unless otherwise noted:

1. Falls were the most frequently litigated issue for this population. This trend continued in the 1997 to 1998 data.
2. Most falls do not result in fractures; however, when fractures occurred, they were commonly associated with litigation. The plaintiffs won the majority of these cases in both studies (1993 to 1995 and 1997 to 1998).
3. Decubitus ulcer cases were not as successful for the plaintiff as falls cases. A roughly even split was observed in verdicts for this malpractice issue in the 1993-1995 timeframe. In the decubitus ulcer cases reported from 1997 to 1998, the plaintiffs won all of the cases. The highest verdict was $83 million (as described later in this chapter).
4. The plaintiffs have a high success rate in choking cases. Residents choked on food, tube feeding solution, and soil. Furthermore, two individuals were strangled by a chest restraint. All of these cases resulted in the death of the resident. One choking case was reported from 1997 to 1998, resulting in punitive damages (Laska, 1997h).
5. Plaintiffs also did well in cases involving infections. The range of awards for verdicts in favor of the plaintiffs was lower than that of ulcer and choking cases, which resulted in verdicts of $2.7 million and $2.4 million, respectively.
6. All cases involving residents who wandered off the premises of the facility resulted in the death of the resident. The defense won only one of these reported cases. Three "wandering" cases were presented in the 1997 to 1998 sample, all of which resulted in the death of the resident and were won by the plaintiffs.
7. Assault cases involved abuse by the nursing home staff or another resident. This category of case resulted in the highest monetary awards ($3.6 million) among the cases that were reviewed in the 1993-1995 time frame. The plaintiffs prevailed in every case involving assault or abuse.
8. Medication errors resulted in the death of the resident in three out of the four cases that were reported. The plaintiffs won in 75% of these cases.
9. In contrast, failure to prevent suicide resulted in defense verdicts in all three cases that were reported.

LONG-TERM CARE VERDICTS

TYPE OF INJURY	# of CASES	PLAINTIFF VERDICT	AWARD RANGE	DEFENSE VERDICT
FALLS	**28**	**24**	**$3,739 - $526,000**	**4**
Clinical Outcome 1. Fractures 2. Death 3. Lacerations	22 4 2			
DECUBITUS ULCERS	**9**	**5**	**$75,000 - $2.7 million**	**4**
Clinical Outcome 1. Death 2. Amputation 3. Other	6 2 1			
CHOKING	**10**	**9**	**$100,000 - $2.4 million**	**1**
Clinical Outcome 1. Death	10			
DEV. of INFECTIONS	**7**	**6**	**$145,000 - $503,734**	**1**
Clinical Outcome 1. Amputations 2. Death 3. Surgery 4. Nerve damage 5. Hospital stay	3 2 1 1 1			
WANDERING	**6**	**5**	**$38,500 - $407,259**	**1**
Clinical Outcome 1. Death	6			

Figure 14-10   Analysis of liability cases. (From Iyer P, ed: *Nursing malpractice,* Tucson, 1996, Lawyers and Judges Publishing Company.)   *Continued*

10. Cases involving weight loss, malnutrition, and obstruction of the intestines were less predictable in their success. The plaintiff and the defense had an approximately equal chance of prevailing in these types of cases.

11. The two reported burn cases were won by the plaintiff and had relatively high monetary awards. The 1997 to 1998 data also included one burn case, which was won by the plaintiff.

Sources of Liability in Long-Term Care

The next section of the chapter provides a discussion of some of the liability issues identified in Figure 14-10, such as falls, pressure ulcers, burns, wandering, abuse, neglect, and scope-of-practice issues. Cases drawn from the samples described above will be used to illustrate the malpractice issues involved in these types of resident injuries. Some of the material in this section was originally reported by Iyer (1996), but all of the cited cases were published in 1997 or 1998.

Falls

Most nursing homes have a very high percentage of confused elderly residents. A 1995 report on mental health in nursing homes outlined the depth of resident mental health problems that nursing home staffs must face (Foltz-Gray, 1995). This report states that as many as 88% of all nursing home residents exhibit mental health problems, such as dementia, depression, or Alzheimer's disease. More than one half of residents exhibit behaviors such as

TYPE OF INJURY	# of CASES	PLAINTIFF VERDICT	AWARD RANGE	DEFENSE VERDICT
ASSAULT	**6**	**6**	**$200,000 - $3.6 million**	**0**
Clinical Outcome 1. Death 2. Bruises 3. Inflammation of skin 4. Rape 5. Other	1 2 1 1 1			
MEDICATION ERRORS	**4**	**3**	**$50,000 - $850,000**	**1**
Clinical Outcome 1. Death 2. Respiratory distress	3 1			
FAILURE TO PREVENT SUICIDE	**3**	**0**	**0**	**3**
Clinical Outcome 1. Death 2. Multiple trauma	2 1			
GASTROINTESTINAL (obstruction, weight loss)	**5**	**3**	**$200,000 - $1.3 million**	**2**
Clinical Outcome 1. Death	5			
BURNS	**2**	**2**	**$613,300 - $950,000**	**0**
Clinical Outcome 1. Third-degree burns 2. Death	1 1			

Figure 14-10, cont'd   Analysis of liability cases. (From Iyer P, ed: *Nursing malpractice,* Tucson, 1996, Lawyers and Judges Publishing Company.)

wandering or leaving the facility. Alzheimer's disease affects a high percentage of residents in long-term care facilities.

One of the most dramatic changes in the standard of nursing care involves the use of physical and chemical restraints. An awareness of the hazards of restraints increased in the late 1980s, which led to an effort to reduce the routine use of restraints. Research on the hazards of restraints, arguments concerning the ethics of restraining residents, and restrictions on the use of restraints have all had a profound effect on the use of restraints. The use of restraints is now strictly controlled in long-term care, and the use of restraints in acute care is becoming increasingly restricted by the Joint Commission for the Accreditation of Healthcare Organizations (JCAHO) and state regulations as well.

Physical restraints include the use of siderails, geriatric chairs (referred to as "geri chairs"), belts, chest vests, leather restraints, and homemade devices, such as gauze bandages or sheets (Moretz, Dommel, Deluca, 1995). Chemical restraints include the use of sedation to reduce violent, disruptive, or unsafe behavior.

Concerns about liability certainly should have an influence on the use of restraints in long-term care facilities, because these cases can result in large verdicts. In the review of long-term care cases involving falls that were published from January 1997 to May 1998, the verdicts and settlements ranged from $112,000 to $1,250,000. "Long standing fears place a wedge between caregivers and more humane solutions. Will combative residents endanger workers or other residents? Will the facility be liable if injuries occur? The threat of lawsuits haunts administrators and directors of nursing who are embarking on a restraint-free path" (Foltz-Gray, 1995).

Documentation Issues and Cases

Until recently, many facilities have not had reasonable alternatives to the use of restraints to prevent injury to patients. Long-term care facilities have been more active than hospitals in developing strategies to prevent falls and lessen their reliance on restraints. An increasing variety of devices can be used in long-term care to remind residents not to climb out of bed or off of chairs, including lap buddies and wedges. Much effort has been made to educate nurses about restraints and to change attitudes about their use (Schott-Baer, Lusis, Beuregard, 1995; Thomas, Redfern, John, 1995; Bradley, Siddique, Dufton, 1995; Mason, O'Connor, Kemble, 1995).

Many facilities have implemented documentation forms that address the use of restraints. The use of restraint flow-sheets permits the caregivers to document the release of restraints, provision of toileting needs, and other information, as described in Chapter 4. Many long-term care facilities have also implemented a form that permits family members to explicitly consent to the use of restraints, or conversely to prohibit the use of restraints, including siderails. A siderail release form was the focus of a hotly contested case that recently occurred in Florida, which resulted in a verdict on behalf of the plaintiff:

> An 87-year-old resident of a nursing home fell out of bed and broke his hip. He died 13 months after the fall. His wife claimed that the defendant was negligent in failing to put the siderails up. The resident gave a videotape deposition detailing the incident before he died. Allegations were made that the defendants had altered the records to make it appear that the man had more ability than he actually did, and that he had signed a consent form to allow the siderails to be left down. The jury returned a $112,000 verdict for the plaintiff (Laska, 1998c).

What is not clear in the description of the case is which records the plaintiff alleged to have been altered (i.e., that described the resident's abilities). Note that "OBRA established significant penalties for falsification of MDS information. An individual who willfully or knowingly causes another individual to certify a material and false statement in the resident assessment document is subject to a civil monetary penalty of not more than $5000 with respect to each assessment (Federal Nursing Home Requirements, OBRA 42)" (Fox, 1997).

A recent case involving altering of the medical record was associated with death caused by strangulation on a vest restraint:

> A 31-year-old blind, mentally retarded resident of a long-term care facility was found strangled on a vest restraint that was tied to her bed. She had managed to drag her bed partially into the hallway outside of her room before she died. Staff members told police investigating the incident that they had been short of staff on the night of her death, and that someone normally would have heard her call for help.

> Evidence was also presented that her records had been altered after her death to show that she had received more staff monitoring than actually took place. The plaintiffs alleged negligence and gross negligence against the nursing home and its owner. The claims included inadequate monitoring, failure to provide adequate staffing, failure to properly train the staff in the use of restraints, and conscious indifference to the risk of improper use of restraints. The plaintiffs attempted to show that the defendant's use of the restraints violated the manufacturer's instructions for the use of the vest restraint. These instructions included a prohibition of the use of the vest for restless, agitated patients, close monitoring, and the use of siderails with the restraints. A $1 million settlement was reached (Laska, 1998a).

The issues associated with tampering with the medical record are discussed in more detail in Chapter 6.

Documentation of conversations in which the family was advised of the need for restraints can have a great impact on the defense of a nursing malpractice case, as described in the following example:

> The staff of a long-term care facility proposed the use of a Posey restraint to prevent a 78-year-old resident from falling. The plaintiffs refused to allow the use of the restraints. The woman fell repeatedly, and the plaintiffs were notified each time, but they still refused to allow the restraints. Two days before her death, the resident fell from her wheelchair, striking her head. An evaluation in the emergency department showed no indication of cerebral compromise. The resident was returned to the long-term care facility, where her condition remained normal until 2 days later, when it began to deteriorate. The staff contacted her doctor about the change in her condition. She was later found dead.

> The plaintiffs alleged that the nursing home staff was negligent for failing to prevent the fall from the wheelchair. The defendants contended that the plaintiffs refused to allow the use of restraints to prevent injuries from the fall. The plaintiffs also alleged that the staff was negligent in not monitoring her after the fall. The defendants contended that no medical symptoms were present until shortly before her death. The verdict was for the defense (Laska, 1997g).

From the description of this case, nursing documentation clearly played a crucial role in defining both the pattern of the family's refusal to allow use of restraints as well as in the evaluation of the resident's condition after the fall. In the following recent case a plaintiff unsuccessfully argued that she should have been restrained to prevent a fall:

> An 82-year-old woman was admitted to a skilled-care nursing home, where she fell and fractured her right hip. At the time of her admission her doctor had ordered that her bed rails be placed up while she was in bed. The resident had a documented history of falling before entering the facility. After her admission one bed rail was kept up and one was kept down. The resident was given Percocet (oxycodone) and Elavil (amitryptyline). She claimed that she got out of bed on her own to use the bathroom at approximately

4:00 AM because no one responded to her use of the call light. When the fracture occurred, she was on her way to the bathroom in her room. She claimed to have slipped in a puddle of water.

In the course of the trial the woman (plaintiff) alleged that the long-term care facility was negligent for the following: (1) failing to follow the doctor's order regarding the positioning of the bed rails; (2) allowing water to be present on the floor; and (3) failing to respond to the call light when she requested help. The defendants countered by contending that the plaintiff had a right to refuse restraint, and that she had specifically requested that one rail be placed up and one be placed down to enable her to sit on the edge of her bed. According to the defendants the plaintiff did not attempt to use the call light before getting out of bed despite the fact that she had been instructed to do so on at least three other occasions. The defendants denied that there was water on the floor, and asserted that the plaintiff's fall was consistent with her previous history of falling. The jury returned a verdict for the defense (Laska, 1997c).

One can assume that the long-term care staff would have documented their instructions to the resident about using the call bell for help.

Pressure Ulcers

Frail, elderly residents of nursing homes are at risk for developing pressure ulcers. Lawsuits related to skin breakdown were one of the most common allegations in the published verdicts and settlements from 1997 to 1998. The verdicts and settlements ranged from $75,000 to $83 million, and six of the nine cases won by the plaintiffs resulted in monetary awards of between $400,000 and $640,000. The importance of prevention has been given much attention in recent years, and research has focused on new technologies for preventing and healing existing pressure sores.

Documentation Issues and Cases

Having become attuned to the liability issues associated with the development of bedsores, nursing home staffs are also becoming more aware of the need to document the condition of the resident's skin when he or she arrives at the facility. These baseline data permit comparison of the resident's skin over time and provide a defense when the resident enters the facility with preexisting skin breakdown. In *State v. Whittle,* 454 S.E. 2d 688 (N.C. Ct. App 1995) a nurse was charged with one felony count of falsifying the admission record of a long-term care resident named Mr. Keller. The nurse altered the admission documentation to indicate that Mr. Keller had stage IV decubitus ulcers on his heels and feet at the time of admission when, in fact, the ulcers did not develop until after his admission to the facility. In addition, the nurse, who was the director of nursing for the long-term care facility, was charged with two misdemeanor counts of failing to establish nursing proce-

dures related to special skin care protocols for Mr. Keller's decubiti. She was also charged with failing to institute nursing procedures related to the daily documentation of the status of his ulcers. This case emphasizes the importance of complete and accurate documentation. Criminal penalties, as well as successful medical malpractice claims, can result from falsification of a patient's record (Feutz-Harter, Laughlin, 1998).

The issue of where skin breakdown developed was a factor in the following case, which resulted in the largest long-term care verdict reported between 1997 and 1998:

> The 83-year-old resident was mentally alert but unable to walk while she was being cared for at a long-term care center. She was also diabetic. While she was at the facility, she became severely dehydrated and was hospitalized. After her return to the long-term care facility, she developed pressure sores and was hospitalized again. The woman died from an infection caused by the bed sores. The plaintiff alleged negligence, gross negligence, and fraud, alleging that the dehydration was caused by a failure to provide water. The plaintiff maintained that the problems with the water were partially caused by a lack of available staff, and they pointed to medical problems at the facility (18 residents were sent to the hospital during the weeks before the decedent's death). The defendant denied any negligence and maintained that the pressure sore, which became infected, developed and became infected in the hospital. The defendant maintained that the woman's diabetes caused her systems to break down. The jury found negligence and fraud, and they awarded $13 million in compensatory damages and $70 million in punitive damages (Laska, 1998b).

Documentation of the presence of preexisting skin breakdown should follow the commonly used staging system described in Chapter 2. Appropriate treatment should be delivered and documented according to nationally accepted standards of care. In the following case a hospital and a nursing home were both named as defendants in a pressure ulcer case:

> The plaintiff, age 88, was sent to the defendant hospital to have his leg amputated. While he was in the hospital, he developed two small bedsores. He was then released to the defendant nursing home, where the bedsores were noticed but not treated. The plaintiff's condition deteriorated to the point at which it became life threatening, and he was transferred back to the hospital. After a 47-day stay in the hospital, the plaintiff died from septicemia caused by the bedsores. The verdict was against both defendants (hospital and nursing home) for $450,000 (Laska, 1997b).

Once a pressure ulcer begins to develop, nursing home nurses frequently use a flowsheet to document the size and stage of the ulcer over time. Another flowsheet is commonly used to document the implementation of the treatments designed to help the ulcer heal. Of particular importance are instructions given to the non-professional staff in the use of these treatment forms to ensure that the care they provide can be appropriately documented.

As can be seen from these cases, the development of bedsores can lead to illness, death, long periods of treatment, and liability risks.

Burns

Burns are a major source of injury to residents. They can occur in a number of ways, including spills of hot food or liquids, fires, electrical equipment (Box 14-1), outlets, and hot baths or soaks. The nurse is expected to assess the risk of burns and take precautions to reduce this hazard. Burn injuries to individuals over age 60 occur with a frequency that is out of proportion to that of all other age groups (except the very young), and elderly victims experience higher morbidity and mortality from burn injuries than any other age group. The majority of these injuries are preventable. The elderly are at particular risk for burns because of the following factors:

1. Decreased circulation, which affects the resident's perception of the temperature of things such as hot liquids
2. Sensory impairment, which diminishes the resident's awareness of heat

---

Box 14-1

Tips for Documenting After a Burn from Electrical Equipment

1. If a piece of equipment is not functioning properly, take steps to resolve the problem and document what was done.
2. If equipment fails while in use, document the entire incident. Describe interventions on behalf of the resident and notify the risk manager of the incident.
3. Inspect the resident's skin before and after any type of heating pad is applied. Carefully monitor the resident when heating pads are applied to his or her skin. Several cases in which patients were burned from prolonged use of heating pads have been documented. Do not exceed 20 minutes of application time. Take prompt action to report skin changes that could have resulted from heat. Burns from heating pads are serious clinical and risk-management problems that warrant prompt follow-up.
4. The Safe Medical Devices Act of 1990 mandates that hospitals and other facilities must report incidents in which a medical device caused or contributed to the death, serious illness, or injury of a patient. The law requires that facilities report device-related incidents resulting in death to the Food and Drug Administration (FDA) and the manufacturer (if known). Incidents resulting in serious illness or injury should be reported to the manufacturer or to the FDA (if the manufacturer is not known).

---

3. Cognitive impairment, which decreases the resident's awareness of being burned and also places the residents in high-risk situations
4. Delayed reaction time and impaired mobility, which prevent residents from getting away from the source of heat
5. Tremors of the hand and trunk

Burns involving 20% to 30% of the resident's body surface are lethal to the majority of people over the age of 60. Individuals with burns that cover more than 40% of their body surface, or those that cover 20% and are combined with smoke inhalation, have the poorest prognosis for survival. This is particularly true if the individual has preexisting cardiac or pulmonary conditions. The long-term care facility is obligated to provide care to reduce the risk of burns (Petro, 1989).

Documentation Issues and Case

In addition to careful supervision of the elderly, patient education is helpful in reducing the risk of burns. Document the patient education initiated to reduce the risk of burns following the guidelines presented in Chapter 5; for example:

1. Resident noted to have severe tremors of hands. Instructed to wait until a staff member is available to assist her in opening hot liquids and foods. Verbalized understanding.
2. Resident has decreased sensation in feet. Taught to test bath water with her wrist before getting into tub. Said she understood and would do this.
3. Explained to resident that his medication can cause sleepiness, and he should not smoke when feeling drowsy. Said he would comply.

As more facilities become smoke-free—providing residents comply with these rules—the risk of burns from smoking will eventually decrease (Box 14-2). The nurse should periodically reevaluate the resident for risk factors for burns.

Box 14-2

What to Do When the Resident Smokes

When the resident smokes, document an assessment of risk factors for burns and the interventions that were implemented. Include, as appropriate, the following interventions:

- Instruct the resident to smoke in safe, supervised areas.
- Remove smoking materials from residents who are unable or unwilling to comply with safe smoking practices.
- Instruct the family in the hazards of the resident's smoking.
- Request that the family not bring cigarettes or other smoking materials.
- Stay with the resident when he or she is smoking.

A recent case resulted in a large award to the plaintiff after burns occurred in the nursing home:

> The 75-year-old schizophrenic nursing home resident was addicted to cigarette smoking. The woman was to be supervised by an aide when she smoked, and she was not allowed to have cigarettes or matches of her own at any time. She would normally be brought into the TV room (a designated smoking area), where an aide was required to be in the room. From time to time, she was able to obtain additional cigarettes, which had resulted in various fire incidents with burns to outer clothing. Although it had been recommended that she wear a fire-retardant safety garment, she was never given one. On the day of the incident, she was brought to the TV room and placed in a chair with a belt restraint. Her aide searched her for cigarettes and matches and found none. The aide then stepped out, leaving her in the room with an elderly resident who neither smoked nor was able to walk.
>
> Fifteen minutes later, another aide found the woman engulfed in flames. She suffered second- and third-degree burns over 20% of her body on the left side. She survived for 84 days in a burn unit, remaining conscious until a few days before her death. The plaintiff alleged lack of proper supervision, failure to perform an adequate search for matches and cigarettes, and failure to observe the resident while she was smoking. The plaintiff also claimed that a safety apron should have been used. The defendant maintained that supervision was adequate, and that the cigarette had been obtained in a way that they could not control. The suit was settled for $387,500 before the closing arguments were made (Laska, 1998e).

Wandering Resulting in Injury

Wandering is a purposeful behavior that represents an attempt to fulfill a particular need in the wanderer. Wandering is initiated by a cognitively impaired and disoriented individual and is characterized by excessive ambulation, often leading to safety or nuisance-related problems (Thomas, 1995).

Wanderers generally have a higher level of cognitive impairment than non-wanderers. Short-term and long-term memory problems can result in the inability of wanderers to remember how to get back to their rooms. Wanderers are often unable to remember the correct date or where they are. From a liability perspective, wandering behavior is often associated with negative outcomes for both the resident and the staff. The negative outcomes are the result of safety issues created by the wanderer's need to leave the facility (Thomas, 1995). The dimensions of this problem were documented in a study by Gaffney (1988). Twenty-eight wanderers were observed for 15 hours. An astounding 457 attempts to leave the unit and 274 attempts to use an exit were observed. The number of attempts to leave a facility, as documented by Gaffney's study, show that the long-term care staff can never relax its vigilance over wanderers.

Documentation Issues and Cases

The long-term care facility's best defense when taking care of wandering residents is to prevent injury through the detection of potential escapes. The clinical record should reflect the strategies that are being used to control this problematic behavior. Facilities caring for Alzheimer's patients must have a system in place to detect patients who are attempting to leave the building. Should an Alzheimer's patient be successful in wandering out of a residential facility, one of the issues in the case will likely be whether the home was the appropriate setting for such a patient and whether safeguards had been instituted to prevent wandering. Consider the following case:

> In a Texas case, an 84-year-old resident of a long-term care facility suffered from Alzheimer's disease. He attempted to leave the facility on four separate occasions. On the day in question an employee of the long-term care facility left the ignition key in her car. The resident drove 25 miles away from the facility. Approximately 1 month later, his body was found in the car in a grove of trees adjacent to the road. The plaintiff alleged that the defendant was negligent for failing to provide adequate supervision and training of its residents and employees. The defendant claimed that the standard of care was not breached and that the employee who left the keys in her car was not acting within the scope of her employment when the keys were left. A $300,000 settlement was reached (Laska, 1997a).

The consistent use of strategies must be documented in the medical record. Electronic monitoring systems, which sound alarms when a resident attempts to leave, provide one solution to wandering behavior.

> A Michigan woman wandered away from her nursing home in January despite wearing a monitoring device. She was found frozen to death outside the back door the following day. The manufacturer of the monitoring device contributed $20,000 to the settlement, and the nursing home provided $180,000 (Laska, 1997e).

Whether the monitoring device was defective or simply was not heeded by the staff is unclear in this case. Once a resident is discovered to be missing, the efforts of the facility to locate the resident must be thorough and meticulously documented, as discussed elsewhere in this text.

A review of cases involving wandering shows that death can result from by being hit by a car, fractures, freezing to death in inclement weather, and other severe injuries.

> In a Illinois case a resident eloped from a long-term care facility and was found 24 hours later—laying on railroad tracks in a weak, confused, and severely dehydrated state. He developed pneumonia and died. The jury returned a verdict of $137,371 (Laska, 1997f).

Abuse and Neglect

Abuse may be financial, physical, or emotional. Few issues stir deeper emotions in the public than images of helpless elderly persons who are not receiving appropriate care or are being abused. This type of litigation is one of the more complex areas of nursing malpractice. Abuse cases may be difficult to detect and prove. The true incidence of abuse is unknown. Both the residents and the long-term care staff may deny that mistreatment is occurring. Residents who do not have family members visiting them on a routine basis are particularly vulnerable. Bruises may be covered by clothing and thus be out of the sight of even regular visitors. The cognitively impaired resident may be unable to communicate that physical abuse is occurring. In many cases the resident must rely on observant staff members who are able to detect abuse or neglect and are willing to report it, often at risk to their own jobs. The HCFA regulations require that nursing homes report the abuse to the state department of health when it is detected. The Office of Protective Services and the Office of the Ombudsman may become involved when suspected cases of abuse are uncovered. Facilities that fail to report abuse or cover it up can be cited for deficiencies and required to develop a corrective plan.

Neglect is the refusal or failure to fulfill a caretaking obligation, including abandonment; denial of food, clothing, or medical assistance; or withholding of medications or assistive devices. The failure of a facility to meet the needs of a resident is generally accepted as a form of maltreatment. Neglect may be intentional, such as when a caretaker deliberately fails to fulfill caretaking responsibilities to harm or punish a resident (e.g., not feeding a resident). Unintentional neglect results from a lack of knowledge or an inability to provide care (Fiesta, 1996b).

Documentation Issues and Cases

Provision of appropriate care according to the standards of care, coupled with thorough documentation in the medical record, are the best defense to charges of abuse and neglect, as the following case illustrates:

> An Oregon case illustrates the concept of abandonment. The 82-year-old woman was living in an elderly residential facility. When the resident's son signed up for the services, he was told that the facility monitored the attendance of residents at evening meals and would check on residents who missed the meal. The woman fell in the bathroom of her unit and was wedged between the toilet and wall. She lay there without attention for nearly 3 days, in a trapped position on her side, until she was found by her son. The plaintiffs contended that during that time she attempted to call out and was not heard. She pulled on the emergency cord, which only partially activated and was not effective. Furthermore, she missed three evening meals in the dining room. When she was discovered, 2 days' worth of morning newspapers were outside the door of her unit. The woman

suffered severe dehydration, decubitus ulcers, heart fibrillation, and incontinence as a result of the incident. She became confined to a wheelchair and required assistance because of residual weakness and dementia. Before the accident she was mentally active and able to take care of her own financial affairs. A verdict of $962,500 was returned by the jury (Laska, 1998d).

Many of the pressure ulcer cases cited earlier in the chapter could also be categorized as neglect cases. In the final case to be discussed in this section, the development of pressure ulcers, pneumonia, and hyperglycemia were all cited as evidence of neglect:

> A 77-year-old diabetic man was admitted to a nursing home to recover from pneumonia. After approximately 6 weeks, the man was found to be suffering from bedsores, pneumonia, and high blood sugar. He was admitted to a hospital, which found him dehydrated and encrusted with fecal material. The patient died about 10 days later from pneumonia, complications from bedsores, an uncontrolled blood sugar level, and dehydration. The defendant contended that the decedent had been properly monitored while he was under their care. A jury awarded $605,523. The owners of the nursing home settled out of court for a confidential amount (Laska, 1997d).

Scope of Practice Issues

In addition to the liability issues described above (i.e., falls, pressure ulcers, burns, wandering, abuse, and neglect), an additional source of liability for long-term care nurses involves stepping outside of the scope of nursing practice. A fine line often exists between medical and nursing diagnoses. Levenson (1993) noted that both nurses and physicians are involved in recognizing a change in the resident's condition, in precisely defining the problem, and in determining the cause of the problem. Nurses have a greater responsibility for determining the wishes of the resident and family related to care management. Both nurses and doctors evaluate the patient's responses to treatment.

Nurses practicing in a long-term care facility are placed in the position of making clinical judgments without a physician readily at hand. Long-term care nurses have the option of sending the patient to the emergency room of the local hospital for an evaluation, if warranted. Many long-term care nurses welcome the opportunity to exercise their nursing judgment and autonomy. This is both a source of satisfaction and liability when the nurse's clinical judgment is not used or is incorrect. Documentation of the assessment process, the information conveyed to the physician (who is usually off site), and the actions taken is essential to proving that the nurse was acting within the scope of practice.

The following case is instructive because of allegations that the nurses acted without physician's orders:

The 91-year-old Texas woman was a new resident of the defendant nursing home. She was not placed in a secure wing of the facility, and she wandered away on her second day there. The defendant charge nurse allegedly brought her back and had her restrained without doctor's orders. The nurse allegedly also took another patient's liquid Valium (diazepam) and injected it into the woman's neck with the help of another defendant nurse. The patient was restrained for 55 days without doctor's orders. The patient claimed that another resident kept untying the restraints, and because of her age and her weakness from having been restrained, she suffered repeated falls, which resulted in disabling injuries. She also claimed that the defendants never charted the first incident and failed to notify the doctor of the falls. When the incident was finally reported, the County Sheriff's Department and the Texas Department of Human Services became involved. Sanctions were imposed on the nursing home, and a settlement of $1,250,000 was reached (Laska, 1997).

Going beyond the legal limitations of the nurse practice (as it appears these Texas nurses did when they administered Valium) means the nurse is effectively practicing medicine without a license. Similar actions resulted in criminal charges against two Colorado nurses, as described in the following case:

Two long-term care nurses in Colorado stepped over the line dividing nursing and medical practice and were subject to criminal charges. In *People v. Nygren*, 696 P2d 270 (CO 1985), William Fentress was a patient at a long-term care facility. On the morning in question, William was upset, making it difficult for a housekeeper to clean his room. A nurse and a nurses aide strapped him to his bed with a restraining belt. Later that morning, the nurses aide overheard a conversation between the director of nursing and the charge nurse in which they discussed giving William a shot of Thorazine (chlorpromazine, a major tranquilizer). Later that day the aide heard them discussing the advisability of still another injection of Thorazine.

William died later that day. The resident's physician testified that he had never prescribed Thorazine for the resident while he was at the nursing home. He also stated that because Mr. Fentress was mentally retarded, he was incapable of giving informed consent to the administration of the drug. The medical evidence showed that Thorazine was in Mr. Fentress' blood after his death. The level of Thorazine was consistent with the stupor and impaired physical and mental functioning he displayed after the injections. The nurses were found guilty on criminal charges (Tammelleo, 1985).

In both of these cases the nurses went beyond the limits of nursing practice. An adequate understanding of the limits of the nursing practice act is essential for the functioning of the long-term care nurse.

SUMMARY

This chapter reviews the essentials of documentation in the long-term care setting. The computerization of the chart and electronic submission of the MDS places greater responsibility on facilities to standardize, evaluate, and improve the quality of services provided to clients and residents. Medicare- and Medicaide-funded facilities will receive reimbursement based on the nursing assessment as reflected through the RAI process, interdisciplinary team care planning, and outcomes. Documentation is crucial in capturing resident information needed for the MDS and making appropriate clinical decisions.

Gale and Steffl (1992) express the importance of accurate nursing documentation this way: "Nurses need to become aware of their potential as income-producing as well as traditional caregiving professionals. Their role now must include fiscal responsibilities and budgetary accountability. Their time and service must produce income, and they need to know how to assess and document for it. Agencies will not be reimbursed for nursing services unless nurses can identify, demonstrate, and document their worth. This includes documentation such as assessment of a patient's condition, whether it is likely to change, complications or problems with medications, treatments, and health teaching outcomes."

The increasing frequency with which nurses are being sued places greater emphasis on the delivery of quality care. Medical records are scrutinized in the event of a poor outcome or injury; therefore documentation must establish that the care was delivered according to the standards of care. This will become increasingly important as our population ages and attention is increasingly directed toward evaluating the quality of care in long-term care facilities.

REFERENCES

AHCA: *HCFA resident assessment instrument training manual and resource guide,* Washington, DC, 1990, the Association.

Bradley L, Siddique C, Dufton B: Reducing the use of physical restraints in long-term care facilities, *J Gerontol Nurs* p 21, September 1995.

Davis WE: *The introduction to health care administration,* Bossier, La, 1993, Publicare Press.

Federal Register, vol 54, February 2, 1989.

Federal Register, vol 56, February 26, 1991a.

Federal Register, vol 56, September 26, 1991b.

Federal Register, vol 57, September 23, 1992.

Federal Register, vol 62, December 23, 1997.

Fiesta J: Legal issues in long term care: part I, *Nurs Manage* 27(1):18, 1996a.

Fiesta J: Legal issues in long term care: part II, *Nurs Manage* 27(2):18, 1996b.

Feutz-Harter S, Laughlin S: Legal issues in long-term care, *J Nurs Law* 5(1):57, 1998.

Foltz-Gray D: Breaking free from restraints, *Contemp Long Term Care* 48, July 1995.

Fox S: *Primum non nocere* (first do no harm): nursing home litigation: part II, *J Legal Nurse Consult* 8(4):8, 1997.

Gaffney J: Toward a less restrictive environment, *Geriatr Nurs* (7):94, 1988.

Gale BJ, Steffl BM: The long term care dilemma: what nurses need to know about medicare, *Nurs Health Care* 1:34, 1992.

HCFA: *Long term care facilities resident assessment instrument (RAI) user's manual,* Version 2.0, Washington, DC, 1995, The Association.

Iyer P, ed: *Nursing malpractice,* Tucson, 1996, Lawyers and Judges Publishing Company.

Laska L, ed: Ninety-one-year-old Texas woman restrained in Texas nursing home without physician involvement, *Medical Malpractice Verdicts, Settlements and Experts* p 33, March 1997.

Laska L, ed: Alzheimer's patient killed in accident after taking nursing home employee's vehicle from parking lot, *Medical Malpractice Verdicts, Settlements and Experts* p 28, October 1997a.

Laska L, ed: Bedsores not treated, leading to septicemia and death, *Medical Malpractice Verdicts, Settlements and Experts* p 27, August 1997b.

Laska L, ed: Failure to properly restrain patient, *Medical Malpractice Verdicts, Settlements and Experts* p 27, December 1997c.

Laska L, ed: Michigan man dies after a six-week stay in nursing home, *Medical Malpractice Verdicts, Settlements and Experts* p 29, June 1997d.

Laska L, ed: Ninety-four year old Michigan woman wanders away from nursing home, *Medical Malpractice Verdicts, Settlements and Experts* p 27, August 1997e.

Laska L, ed: Patient elopes from nursing home, *Medical Malpractice Verdicts, Settlements and Experts* p 28, January 1997f.

Laska L, ed: Repeated falls in nursing home, *Medical Malpractice Verdicts, Settlements and Experts* p 30, June 1997g.

Laska L, ed: Seventy-nine year old Texas nursing home resident dies of respiratory arrest following repeated episodes of aspiration pneumonia, *Medical Malpractice Verdicts, Settlements and Experts* p 34, March 1997h.

Laska L, ed: Death from strangling on vest restraint, *Medical Malpractice Verdicts, Settlements and Experts* p 27, April 1998a.

Laska L, ed: Diabetic resident in nursing home not given adequate water due to staff shortage, *Medical Malpractice Verdicts, Settlements, and Experts* p 27, April 1998b.

Laska L, ed: Resident of Florida nursing home falls out of bed and breaks hip, *Medical Malpractice Verdicts, Settlements and Experts* p 30, May 1998c.

Laska L, ed: Woman in elderly residential facility lies in bathroom almost three days before found by son, despite representation that persons absent from dinner would be checked on, *Medical Malpractice Verdicts, Settlements and Experts* p 27, February 1998d.

Laska L, ed: Woman not properly supervised while in smoking area, *Medical Malpractice Verdicts, Settlements and Experts* p 27, February 1998e.

Levenson S: *Medical direction in long term care,* ed 2, Durham, NC, 1993, Carolina Academic Press.

Markides S, ed: *Aging and health perspectives on gender, race, ethnicity, and class,* Newberry Park, Calif, 1989, Sage Publications.

Mason R, O'Connor M, Kemble S: Untying the elderly: response to quality of life issues, *Geriatr Nurs* p 68, March/April 1995.

Matteson MA, McConnell ES: *Gerontological nursing concepts and practice,* Philadelphia, 1988, WB Saunders.

Moretz C, Dommel A, Deluca K: Untied: a safe alternative to restraints, *Medsurg Nurs* 4(2):128, 1995.

New Jersey Register, August 20, 1990.

Petro J et al: Burn accidents and the elderly: what is happening and how to prevent it, *Geriatrics* 44(3):26, March 1989.

Schott-Baer D, Lusis S, Beuregard K: Use of restraints: changes in nurses' attitudes, *J Gerontol Nurs* p 39, February 1995.

Tammelleo A, ed: Thorazine injected, patient dies, criminal charges, *Regan Rep Nurs Law* p 4, May 1985.

Thomas D: Wandering: a proposed definition, *J Gerontol Nurs* p 35, September 1995.

Thomas A, Redfern L, John R: Perceptions of acute care nurses in the use of restraints, *J Gerontol Nurs* p 32, June 1995.

Vlasses FR: Computerized documentation systems: blessing or curse? *Orthop Nurs* 12(1):1993.

SUGGESTED READINGS

Danzon P: *New evidence on the frequency and severity of medical malpractice claims* (Pub No R-3410 ICJ: 18-19), Santa Monica, Calif, 1996, Rand Corporation, Institute for Civil Justice.

Eggland ET: Nursing administration manual for long term care facilities, Glen Arm, Md, 1992, Health Education Network.

Fiesta J: *Legal issues for long-term care providers,* New York, 1996, Delmar.

Marek K, Rantz M, Fagin C, Krejc J: OBRA 1987: has it resulted in positive change in nursing homes? *J Gerontol Nurs* 12:32, 1996.

Sullivan G: Long-term care on trial, *Contemp Long Term Care* p 38, March 1996.

Index